WHEATER'S
PATHOLOGY

A TEXT, ATLAS AND REVIEW OF HISTOPATHOLOGY

WHEATER'S
PATHOLOGY

A TEXT, ATLAS AND REVIEW OF HISTOPATHOLOGY

SIXTH EDITION

Geraldine O'Dowd, BSc(Hons), MBChB(Hons), FRCPath

Consultant Diagnostic Pathologist
Lanarkshire NHS Board
Honorary Clinical Senior Lecturer
University of Glasgow
Glasgow, UK

Sarah Bell, BSc Med Sci(Hons), MBChB(Hons), DipFMS, FRCPath

Consultant Pathologist
Department of Pathology
Queen Elizabeth University Hospital
Glasgow, UK

Sylvia Wright, BSc(Hons), MBChB(Hons), FRCPath, DipFMS, PG Cert Mol Path

Consultant Pathologist
Department of Pathology
Queen Elizabeth University Hospital
Glasgow, UK

For additional online content visit StudentConsult.com

ELSEVIER   Edinburgh   London   New York   Oxford   Philadelphia   St Louis   Sydney   2020

First edition 1985
Second edition 1991
Third edition 1996
Fourth edition 2003
Fifth cdition 2010

Notices

ISBN: 978-0-7020-7559-9
eBook ISBN: 978-0-7020-7555-1
International ISBN: 978-0-7020-7560-5

Content Strategist: Alexandra Mortimer
Content Development Specialist: Trinity Hutton
Project Manager: Julie Taylor
Design: Miles Hitchen
Illustration Manager: Muthu Thangaraj
Marketing Manager: Michele Milano

Printed in China

Last digit is the print number: 9   8   7   6   5   4   3   2   1

ELSEVIER

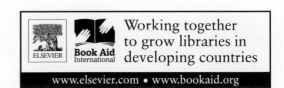

Working together to grow libraries in developing countries

www.elsevier.com • www.bookaid.org

CONTENTS

PREFACE

As we set out to write this new edition of Wheater's Pathology, our aspirations were two-fold. We wished to retain the clarity and simplicity of the existing text, supported by high quality photomicrographs, in order to provide a solid introduction for beginners in pathology and to illustrate key features of major pathological processes and diseases for slightly more advanced trainees, either in pathology or in other specialities. Alongside this, we were aware of the need to update some aspects of the text (such as classification systems and molecular diagnostic techniques), to expand other areas (such as the clinical textboxes which were added in the previous edition) and, where appropriate, to provide additional content such as macroscopic images and normal histology for comparison. It has been possible to incorporate many of these features in the printed textbook without greatly increasing its original size. However, the addition of new electronic platforms has provided us with the opportunity to expand the available educational content considerably, without the risk of producing an immense and unwieldy tome. Throughout this new edition, we have provided links to a range of online materials: normal histology images from Wheater's Functional Histology; a large number of high quality macroscopic pathology images of common pathological processes (kindly provided by Professor Robin Cooke); some additional clinical, histological and molecular data where appropriate; and also a bank of self-assessment questions to accompany each chapter.

Two new authors have joined us for the production of this edition. Our colleague of many years, Dr Barbara Young, has recently retired following her career-long involvement in the Wheater's series and Dr Willie Stewart has left the team to pursue his considerable commitments in other areas. We wish them well in their new endeavours. Our new authors, Dr Sarah Bell and Dr Sylvia Wright, have brought great energy and drive to this new production, as well as their considerable knowledge in rapidly evolving fields such as molecular pathology.

Although the general format of this new edition remains broadly similar, it has been thoroughly updated throughout. We have added a new introductory chapter covering basic histology techniques, as well as the principles of immunohistochemistry, molecular testing and digital pathology. Some chapters have been completely revised, whilst others include less comprehensive but important updates and further clinical and molecular textboxes. Throughout, we have inserted links cross-referencing additional online material, including normal histology images for comparison (from the companion text Wheater's Functional Histology, denoted 'E-Fig. X.X**H**'), gross images of common disorders (kindly used with the permission of Professor Robin Cooke, denoted 'E-Fig. X.X**G**') and some further clinical, molecular and histological online content. We hope that the revised end of chapter reviews, as well as our new bank of self-assessment questions, will be helpful revision aids.

We hope that this new edition remains a useful and concise introduction to pathology. Whilst it is aimed primarily at medical students, we recognise that it may be of use for those commencing specialist training in pathology and in a range of other specialities. It remains as short as possible but the linked material available online should facilitate additional learning for those with a developing interest in this field. The book may be read in any order and each of the chapters stands alone, although it is also a good read from beginning to end. We hope that this *Text, Atlas and Review of Pathology* will stimulate your interest and may perhaps lead some of you to a career in this field.

Glasgow 2018
Geraldine O'Dowd
Sarah Bell
Sylvia Wright

PREFACE TO THE FIRST EDITION

Histopathology is an essential component of pathology teaching in all medical and dental courses, nevertheless the scope, content and emphasis on microscopy vary considerably between different centres. Adding to this diversity are the different stages in the preclinical and/or clinical years when the subject matter is presented. This book has been designed to meet as closely as possible the requirements of these many differing courses. We believe that practical microscopy is an important part of pathology teaching, and therefore we have chosen to centre our discussion around appropriate colour photomicrographs as might be done in the lecture room or microscope laboratory. The text has been designed as a series of amplified captions explaining not only the features visible in the labelled colour plates, but also providing some background text in order to relate the subject matter to the theoretical and clinical implications of the pathological processes. Consequently this book should not be regarded as a copiously illustrated introductory textbook of pathology, but rather it is intended as a histopathology companion to any of the many excellent standard pathology textbooks; the text, though more than normally found in an atlas, is thus by no means comprehensive.

The subject matter has been divided into two sections, the first covering basic pathological processes and the second encompassing the common diseases encountered in systems pathology. In general, our material has been taken from both surgical and necropsy specimens of common clinical conditions. Uncommon conditions have been included only where they illustrate important pathological principles. The haematoxylin and eosin staining method has mainly been employed as is standard practice in pathology laboratories, but special staining methods have been occasionally used where appropriate. Rather than specifying numerical magnification factors, each micrograph has been designated as low power, medium power or high power by the abbreviations LP, MP and HP respectively as this is probably more relevant to student needs.

It is our hope that this book will be useful both as a guide in formal practical classes, as well as assisting the student in private study. Although the book is primarily aimed at preclinical and clinical medical and dental students, it would also prove useful for other groups such as veterinary science students, medical laboratory scientists specialising in histopathology, and candidates for post-graduate examinations in surgery and pathology.

Nottingham, 1985 P.R.W.
H.G.B.
A.S.
J.L.

ACKNOWLEDGEMENTS

We are greatly indebted to many individuals who have helped and supported us in the creation of this new edition of Wheater's Pathology. Our colleagues in our local laboratories have kindly allowed us access to their cases for slide photography and, in many instances, they have recommended suitable material for us to illustrate specific entities. We are immensely grateful also to the biomedical scientists and technical staff (far too many to name individually) in our laboratories (the Departments of Pathology at Queen Elizabeth University Hospital (QEUH), Glasgow, and at University Hospital Monklands, NHS Lanarkshire). Without your high quality sections, production of this illustrated work would have been impossible.

Particular thanks are due to the following for their contributions to specific figures used in the text and as online resources: Prof Robin Cooke, formerly of the University of Queensland, Australia, for his very kind permission to utilise a large number of his superb gross pathology images in the accompanying online material; Dr Frances Gallagher, Mr Allan Wilson and the laboratory staff of NHS Lanarkshire for Fig. 1.1A–H; Mr Thomas Kerr of Molecular Diagnostics in the Queen Elizabeth University Hospital, Glasgow, for Fig. 1.8A and B, and Fig. 12.25; Mr John Theunissen of Phillips Digital Pathology Solutions for Fig. 1.9; Dr Lorna Cottrell of the Department of Pathology, Crosshouse Hospital, Kilmarnock, for Fig. 15.20E and F; Dr David Millan of the Department of Pathology, QEUH, Glasgow, for Fig.17.22 and Fig. 17.30; and Dr Girish Gupta of the Department of Dermatology, NHS Lanarkshire, and Mr John Biagi and the staff of the Department of Medical Illustration, NHS Lanarkshire, for the online clinical photographs accompanying Chapter 21; Ms Gillian Thatcher and colleagues in Special Stains at QEUH, Glasgow, for assistance in the preparation of Appendix 1; and Mr Thomas Morin and staff in the Archives of Pathology Department, QEUH, Glasgow, for their immense help in retrieving suitable material from the files for many of the new photomicrographs. We would like to thank Dr Lorna Cooper for Fig. 20.13. We also extend our thanks to the many contributors who provided material for earlier editions, as mentioned previously.

It is appropriate to reiterate our appreciation for the efforts of our colleague, Dr Barbara Young, who has retired from writing the text with this edition. Her commitment and personal contribution to the Wheater's books throughout her career in pathology should not be understated and we are immensely grateful for her ongoing input and support during the planning and development stages of this sixth edition of Wheater's Pathology. Over the years, her skill as a teacher and her excellent photomicrography skills have helped shape Wheater's into a highly respected resource for those beginning their studies of microscopy. We have aimed to retain these key features in this new edition and hope that we have produced a text worthy of the Wheater's title.

Finally, we are grateful to the staff of Elsevier for their help and support in the writing of this edition.

DEDICATION

For John Paul and Francis, with all my love.
GO'D

For Graeme, Leo, Una, Isla and Struan.
SB

For my husband, Jonnie, and my children, Ottavia and Theo. I love you more!
SW

For our colleague and friend, Barbara Young, with thanks and very best wishes for the future.
GO'D, SB and SW

PART I

BASIC PATHOLOGICAL PROCESSES

ACCESS ADDITIONAL MATERIAL AT STUDENTCONSULT.COM

- Bonus normal histology images
- Macroscopic images of common pathological processes
- Self assessment questions

1 Introduction to pathology

Overview of the practice of pathology

Pathology, also referred to as histopathology, anatomical pathology or morbid anatomy, is the study of abnormal or diseased tissues and organs. This book is intended for the student approaching histopathology for the first time and aims to give a thorough but concise grounding, both in basic pathological processes and in specific diseases of the various organs and systems. Pathology is fundamental to the study, understanding and diagnosis of disease and therefore to successful treatment. We assume in this text that the student has already studied histology, the microscopic appearances of normal tissues, and has a basic understanding of the workings of the microscope (see Appendix 1 in Wheater's Functional Histology, 6th edition). Most student doctors who use this text will not become specialist pathologists, but almost all will have regular interactions with pathologists as part of their normal work and a basic understanding of pathology, even if only an ability to understand written pathology reports, is vital. For instance, what is the difference between adenocarcinoma, adenomatoid tumour and carcinoid tumour? These are three very different tumours with different behaviours requiring very different treatments and the non-pathologist receiving such a report needs to understand the difference.

As part of the diagnostic process, the pathologist uses a range of techniques. Many pathological changes can be identified by routine histological staining methods (see Appendix 1). If these do not allow specific identification of the disease then the pathologist has at their disposal a range of ancillary techniques, including *immunohistochemistry*, *electron microscopy* and various molecular tests. These allow precise diagnosis of many conditions that otherwise have similar clinical manifestations. For this reason, a *biopsy* is often carried out to obtain tissue for diagnostic purposes. This may be an incisional biopsy, i.e. removing a small sample of a lesion, or an excisional biopsy, which removes the entire lesion and may also be a curative procedure.

The pathologist's role may also include autopsies or post-mortem examinations, some of which may be forensic, i.e. investigation of suspicious or unexplained deaths. Furthermore, *molecular pathology* has an increasing role in the diagnosis of diseases, guiding targeted therapies and providing prognostic information.

The other, equally important branches of pathology, such as haematology, clinical chemistry and microbiology are not covered here.

Basic histology techniques

In this chapter we aim to give an overview of the basic techniques used in histopathology so that the reader will have a basis for understanding the subsequent chapters.

Histopathology works with tissue samples and *cytopathology* with cell samples. Both end up with the examination of biological material from a patient on a glass slide using a microscope. Before the specimen can be examined in this way a number of steps are usually needed. In the case of a histopathology specimen, after removal from a patient, the tissue undergoes the following steps:

■ *Fixation* (which may take up to 48 hours)

■ *Macroscopic* (gross) *examination* and selection of the parts to be submitted for microscopic examination (depending on the size of the specimen)

■ *Processing* – takes from 2 hours to overnight

■ *Embedding* in paraffin wax

■ *Microtomy* (cutting very thin slices) and placing sections onto a glass slide

■ *Staining* and *cover-slipping*

The finer details of how these procedures are carried out are available in technical texts and form part of the role of an essential profession allied to pathologists, known as *biomedical scientists.* The steps are briefly summarised in Fig. 1.1. Following all of these processes, the final product is a slide or set of slides ready for examination by a pathologist. The number of paraffin blocks, and therefore slides, depends on the size of the specimen. A core biopsy of a breast lesion will generate one block whereas a wide local excision or lumpectomy from the breast may generate several blocks, including blocks containing the tumour, the surgical margins, any lymph nodes removed at the time of surgery and normal breast tissue adjacent to the lesion.

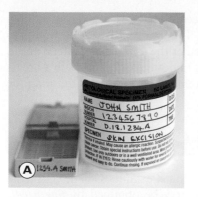

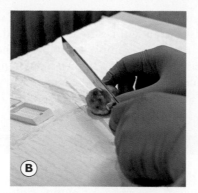

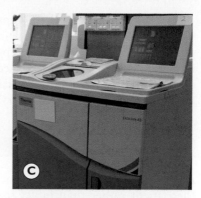

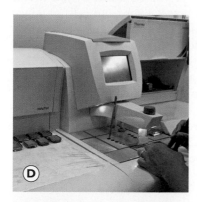

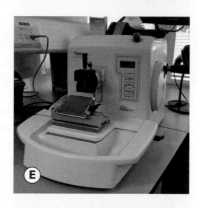

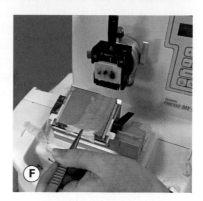

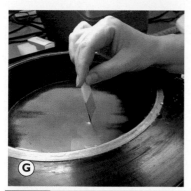

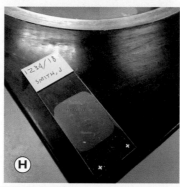

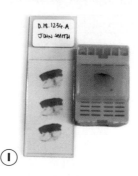

Fig. 1.1 **Processing steps. (A)** Specimen receipt and labelling; **(B)** dissection; **(C)** tissue processing machines; **(D)** block embedding; **(E)** microtome; **(F)** microtomy; **(G)** transfer of section via water bath; **(H)** unstained section on glass slide; **(I)** final products – haematoxylin and eosin (H&E) stained slide and paraffin wax block.

The production of a block and slide of high quality is essential for pathologists to do their job effectively and the technical side of pathology has its own dedicated career pathway for biomedical scientists. There are often *national quality assurance schemes* in place to ensure that all laboratories work to the same high standard. As such, many laboratories in the developed world undergo the rigorous process of *laboratory accreditation*.

The first step in producing a slide begins at the time of removal from the patient. Tissue must be *fixed*, usually by preservation in formalin, soon after removal to prevent *autolysis*, which would render the tissue uninterpretable (see Fig. 2.9). The specimen is then delivered to pathology and should be received in a container with both the container and accompanying form labelled with patient name, unique patient identifier and laboratory number (Fig. 1.1A). This allows tracking of the specimen throughout the laboratory. In Fig. 1.1B, the specimen is examined at the *dissection* bench by a pathologist (larger specimens), and postage stamp sized pieces of tissue sampled, or by a specially trained biomedical scientist (smaller specimens). Tissue is transferred to a labelled cassette.

The tissue then undergoes *processing* cycles (Fig. 1.1C) to render it firm enough to allow cutting into thin sections by a microtome. This involves dehydrating the tissue using a series of graded alcohols to remove all of the fluid. The tissue is then embedded in a mould of *paraffin wax* (Fig. 1.1D), which solidifies when cool and forms a wax block for the next stage.

A *microtome* (Fig.1.1E) is used to cut very thin (3–5 μm) sections from the wax block (Fig. 1.1F). These are floated on water to flatten out the section (Fig. 1.1G) and mounted onto a glass slide (Fig.1.1H). The slide can then be stained, usually with haematoxylin and eosin (H&E), although alternative staining protocols may be used for *special stains* or *immunohistochemistry* (see Appendix 1).

The finished product is a block with its corresponding H&E stained slide (Fig. 1.1I), which can be *quality control* checked before releasing the slides to the pathologist for reporting.

It should be remembered that at all stages of processing and reporting it is essential that patient and laboratory identifiers are checked to ensure there is no mix up of specimens.

Sometimes several of these steps are bypassed to perform a *frozen section* examination. This generally happens during an operation whilst the patient is still anaesthetised. The aim of a frozen section is to guide how the operation should proceed, for example to establish whether the tumour has spread and is inoperable or to establish the resection margins of a known malignant tumour. For example, in a breast cancer resection a diagnosis of cancer might trigger the surgeon to remove lymph nodes draining the tumour site as well as the primary lesion.

Cytopathology

Cytopathology is also a branch of pathology, but in this case the pathologist examines single cells from the patient rather than intact tissue. A specimen for cytopathology may be obtained by *fine needle aspiration (FNA)* when a needle is inserted into the lesion, such as a breast lump, and cells obtained by suction. Cells may also be obtained by scraping them from a surface *(exfoliative cytology)*, which is the technique used for cervical screening (the Pap smear). Fluids such as urine, sputum or a pleural effusion can also be obtained for cytological examination. The resulting specimen is smeared on a glass slide, fixed, stained and examined under the microscope. A major advantage of cytology examinations is that they require much less processing and preparation time than routine histopathology. However, great skill is required to interpret the appearances of individual cells without the advantage of seeing the tissue architecture. Several examples of FNA specimens are given throughout this book, for example bronchial brushings in the diagnosis of lung cancer (see Figs 12.17–12.21).

A list of different types of specimens that may be taken for diagnostic or treatment purposes is shown in Table 1.1 below.

Table 1.1 Types of specimens in histopathology and cytopathology.

Branch of pathology	Type of biopsy	Procedure	Examples
Histopathology	Core biopsy	Sample of a lesion removed by insertion of a needle to take a core of tissue (often uses a 'biopsy gun')	Core biopsy of breast mass Core biopsy of kidney in glomerulonephritis
	Incisional biopsy	Removes part of a lesion	Biopsy of skin rash
	Excision biopsy	Removes entire lesion	Benign breast lump
	Radical excision	Removes entire lesion plus additional tissues as required for cure or staging	Radical nephrectomy for malignant kidney tumour removes surrounding fat, adrenal gland and lymph nodes
Cytopathology	Aspiration cytology	Aspiration of a collection of fluid through a needle – may be part of a drainage procedure	Aspiration of pleural fluid to determine if the pleural fluid contains malignant cells
	Fine needle aspiration	Aspiration of a solid lesion using a very small diameter needle and suction	Aspiration of cells from a breast lump
	Exfoliative cytology	Removal of cells from the surface of tissue	Cervical screening

Introduction to immunohistochemistry

Immunohistochemistry (also known as immunocytochemistry, immunostaining and immunoperoxidase) is a technique for identifying antigens in tissues or cells and uses the principles of the *antigen–antibody reaction*. In brief, antibodies that react with a particular antigen are linked to an enzyme that converts a colourless substrate to a coloured product. Thus, if an antibody that is specific for cytokeratin is applied to tissue containing epithelial cells, the antibody binds to those cells but not to other cell types (i.e. fibroblasts and smooth muscle cells do not contain cytokeratin). The non-bound antibody is washed off the tissue section and the non-coloured substrate is added. Under suitable conditions, the enzyme attached to bound antibody is converted to a coloured product that highlights the epithelial cells only. A summary of the processes involved in immunostaining are given in Fig. 1.2.

Pathologists use immunohistochemistry in everyday practice in a variety of situations including:

■ to identify the site of origin of a primary tumour (e.g. TTF-1 in lung cancer)

■ as prognostic markers (e.g. p16 positivity in oropharyngeal carcinoma)

■ to predict the clinical response to specific treatments (e.g. HER 2 in breast cancer)

■ to aid in the diagnosis of certain tumours (e.g. CD117 in gastrointestinal stromal tumours)

■ to demonstrate invasion (e.g. basal cell markers in prostate cancer)

■ as a screening test for specific mutations (e.g. mismatch repair markers for Lynch syndrome).

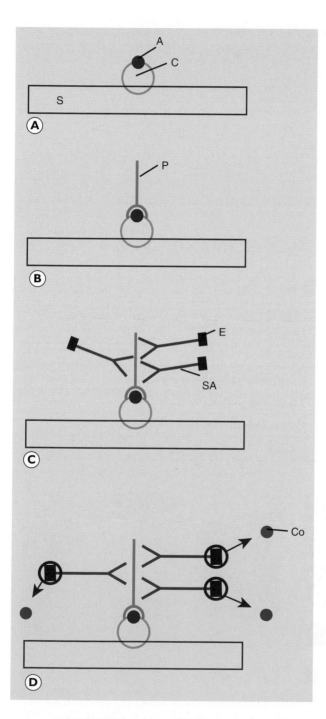

Fig. 1.2 **Basic principles of immunostaining.**
(A) Cells with antigen of interest; **(B)** primary antibody; **(C)** secondary antibody labelled with enzyme; **(D)** chromogen reaction.

Immunostains are composed of specific antibodies that should only bind to the corresponding antibody in the tissues.

In Fig. 1.2A, a slide **(S)** contains a thin section of tissue, within which there are cells **(C)** containing *antigens of interest* **(A)**. This is shown as a single cell for illustration purposes. The tissue has undergone fixation, processing and embedding prior to being mounted on the slide (Fig. 1.1). The tissue then undergoes *blocking* to stop the antibodies reacting with other non-specific antigens in the tissue, which could result in background staining. Examples include serum and commercial blocking buffers. Antigen retrieval is also carried out to *unmask* the antigens of interest that were masked by the fixation process.

There are two main methods of immunodetection. The *direct method* involves the primary antibody being conjugated to a label. The *indirect method* (illustrated) involves the primary antibody **(P)** (Fig. 1.2B) binding to a labelled secondary antibody **(SA)** (Fig. 1.2C). This requires an additional step compared with the direct method. The secondary antibody is labelled with an enzyme **(E)** *(chromogen)*, which converts a substrate to a coloured compound **(Co)** which allows visualisation of the reaction in the tissues (Fig. 1.2D). A variety of enzymes can be used for this process. The commonest is horseradish peroxidase, which results in characteristic 'brown' staining. Another example is immunofluorescence where fluorescein is conjugated to the antibody, however a fluorescence microscope is required to view this.

The final step in the process is *counterstaining* the background tissue with haematoxylin, which gives a blue hue to the cells and provides contrast to the cells stained with the antibody so that tissue morphology can be recognised.

KEY TO FIGURES
A antigen of interest **C** cell in tissue **Co** coloured compound **E** chromogen **P** primary antibody
S slide **SA** secondary antibody

Immunohistochemical interpretation

There are a vast number of antibodies used in pathology and some of these are referred to in the relevant sections of the book. To aid understanding, a summary of the common types of immunohistochemical (IHC) markers and the tissues they stain are given in Tables 1.2 and 1.3. Interpretation of immunohisto-chemical stains can be challenging. A range of factors are assessed to decide whether or not the marker is positive, including which cells are staining, which part of the cell is stained, how many cells are staining and the *intensity of staining* (weak, moderate or strong). *Patterns of staining* within the cell include nuclear, membranous, cytoplasmic, perinuclear dot or a combination. Nuclear and membranous staining patterns are illustrated in Fig. 1.3. Scoring systems exist for particular markers, such as the *Allred score* for the hormone receptors oestrogen receptor (ER) and progesterone receptor (PR) in breast cancer (see Fig. 18.12).

Table 1.2 Summary of common types of immunohistochemical markers.

Tissue type	Markers
Epithelial	CK7, CK20, CAM 5.2, EMA, AE1/3
Myoepithelial	Smooth muscle actin (SMA), S100, Calponin
Mesenchymal	SMA, Desmin (smooth muscle), Vimentin
Neuroendocrine	CD56, Synaptophysin, Chromogranin
Melanocytic	S100, Melan A, HMB45
Neural	S100, Neurofilament, GFAP
Germ cell	hCG, αFP, PLAP, OCT4
Lymphoid	Vast number of Cluster Differentiation (CD) markers, e.g. CD20 (B cell), CD3 (T cell)

Table 1.3 Organ specific immunohistochemical markers.

Marker	Organ
Thyroid transcription factor (TTF1)	Lung/ thyroid
Prostate specific antigen (PSA)	Prostate
Hepatocyte paraffin 1 (HepPar 1)	Liver (hepatocellular carcinoma)
CDX2	Gastrointestinal tract
Wilms Tumour 1 (WT1)	Ovary (serous carcinoma), mesothelium
Gross Cystic Disease Fluid Protein (GCDP 15)	Breast

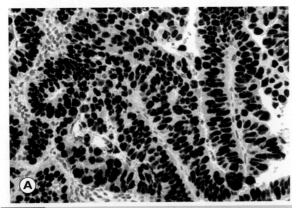 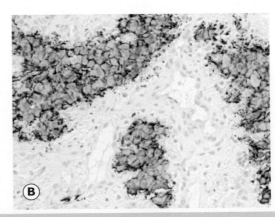

Fig. 1.3 Patterns of immunostaining. **(A)** Nuclear; **(B)** membranous.

Two common patterns of immunohistochemical staining are shown in Fig. 1.3. In Fig. 1.3A there is strong nuclear staining throughout. A nuclear pattern of staining is seen with antibodies that target the protein products of transcription factors (e.g. TTF1, CDX2), tumour suppressor genes (e.g. p53, WT1), steroid hormone receptors (e.g. ER, PR) and proliferation markers (e.g. Ki67, p16).

Cytoplasmic staining is seen in antibodies that target intermediate filaments (e.g. cytokeratins) and neuroendocrine vesicles, giving a granular appearance (e.g. chromogranin). Membranous staining (Fig. 1.3B) is a feature of markers of cell adhesion (e.g. E-cadherin) and cell surface/transmembrane receptors such as HER2 (shown here).

Electron microscopy

Since its invention in the 1930s, the *electron microscope* has provided great insights into the fine structure of cells and tissues, as well as the structure and related function of subcellular organelles such as mitochondria, the plasma membrane and the nucleus. Without electron microscopy, our knowledge of these structures would be negligible. In some cases, electron microscopy is also used for diagnostic purposes. However, many of its early applications have been replaced by immunohistochemistry, which has proven to be faster, cheaper and often more accurate. Despite this, electron microscopy remains vital for the diagnosis of many renal and skeletal muscle disorders and several examples are shown in Chapters 15 and 23 respectively.

Molecular techniques

There has been an exponential growth in knowledge and understanding of molecular biology and the genetic basis of disease in the last decade. As such, the repertoire of molecular tests utilised in pathology is expanding. These tests can be used in a variety of clinical scenarios including:

- diagnosis of cancer
- diagnosis of inherited genetic syndromes
- newborn screening
- predicting response to specific therapies
- guiding prognosis in certain cancers.

Molecular pathology is an essential component of **personalised medicine** which uses the biological features of the cancer to help decide which is the best treatment for that particular patient. Detailed discussion of the intricacies of the molecular biology of cancer are not possible here, however a summary of the main points are covered in the clinical boxes in this chapter.

Currently, the commonest tests in use are polymerase chain reaction (PCR) and in situ hybridisation (ISH/FISH) and these are summarised in Figs 1.4 and 1.5. Specific tests important to pathology practice are discussed in the relevant chapters.

MOLECULAR ORIGINS OF CANCER I
Our knowledge of the molecular origins of cancer grows at an exponential rate, such that any account of the field is destined only to be a snapshot in time of our understanding. Nevertheless, the basic principles underlying the cellular events in the development of cancers remain. In essence, all cancers arise as a consequence of non-lethal damage to DNA (i.e. the cell survives the damage). Typically, the genes damaged are in one of three classes with roles regulating the cell cycle:
- *Proto-oncogenes*, which code for proteins regulating cell growth and differentiation. Activation by either genetic damage *(mutation)* or increased expression results in the development of oncogenes.
- *Tumour suppressor genes*, which code for proteins involved in regulating the cell cycle, repairing damaged DNA or, if the DNA is damaged beyond repair, inducing programmed cell death *(apoptosis)*.
- *MicroRNAs (miRNA)*, which, unlike the other genes involved in the development of cancer, do not code for proteins but are single-stranded RNA molecules with a role in regulation of the cell cycle. Such non-lethal damage frees the cell from the normal restraints and controls on growth and maturation leading to uncontrolled, clonal expansion of the abnormal cell.

BASIC PATHOLOGICAL PROCESSES ■ INTRODUCTION TO PATHOLOGY

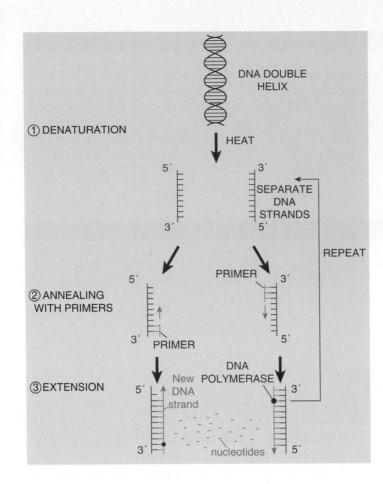

DNA DOUBLE HELIX

① DENATURATION

HEAT

SEPARATE DNA STRANDS

REPEAT

② ANNEALING WITH PRIMERS

PRIMER

PRIMER

③ EXTENSION

DNA POLYMERASE

New DNA strand

nucleotides

Fig. 1.4 **Polymerase chain reaction (PCR) steps.**

PCR involves amplification of a very small amount of DNA from cells/tissues using the enzyme **DNA polymerase**. It involves three main steps which are illustrated opposite. First, double-stranded DNA is heated and split into two separate strands **(denaturation)**. Then **primers** (short DNA sequences) are annealed to the 3' end of each strand of DNA **(annealing)** and extended along the strand by adding nucleotides with a heat-stable Taq (DNA) polymerase in a 5 prime to 3 prime direction. Once the strand is complete, the process is repeated again multiple times, which results in an exponential increase in DNA material.

In pathology laboratories, PCR can be used to establish the presence of infectious agents, e.g. human papillomavirus (HPV) within tissue samples, which is of particular importance in cases of oropharyngeal squamous cell carcinoma (see Fig. 13.2). It can also be used to identify specific genetic mutations within tumour cells or tissue samples, e.g. mutations in lung cancer (see Fig. 12.19 and corresponding clinical box 'Molecular aspects of lung cancer'). Thus it is possible to extract DNA from a tumour biopsy to permit analysis of specific markers that could indicate a specific diagnosis or prognosis for a given patient.

Another example would include the identification of *V600E BRAF* mutation in malignant melanomas, a type of skin cancer, to identify those who would benefit from BRAF inhibitor therapies.

Multiplex PCR is used to amplify multiple targets of DNA at the same time using multiple primers. An example would include detection of **microsatellite instability** (MSI) in colorectal and endometrial cancers (see clinical box 'Microsatellite instability').

MOLECULAR ORIGINS OF CANCER 2: MICROSATELLITE INSTABILITY (MSI)

There are four **mismatch repair genes** whose function is to repair DNA damage (MLH1, MSH2, MSH6, PMS2). Mutations result in inactivation of these genes and occur in two principle forms; inherited Lynch Syndrome as a result of **germline mutation** and sporadic (non-inherited) mutations usually as a result of **epigenetic** mechanisms, e.g. hypermethylation of the MLH1 gene.

Microsatellites are repetitive short sequences of DNA also known as short tandem repeats. When a mutation occurs in the tumour, these sequences of damaged DNA are not repaired and therefore accumulate. This is known as **MSI-unstable or MSI-high**. These sequences can be detected in tumour samples by **multiplex PCR**, using multiple primers at the same time to detect different sequences of DNA. There is also loss of expression of the protein product of the gene, which can be detected using immunohistochemistry.

These tests are routinely carried out in colorectal cancer specimens and endometrial cancers in many laboratories. The clinical aspects of MSI in colorectal cancer are discussed further in Ch. 13.

KEY TO FIGURES
A amplified DNA of *ERBB2* gene target

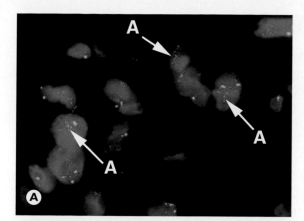

Fig. 1.5 Fluorescence in situ hybridisation.
(A) *HER2* amplification in breast cancer; **(B)** *ALK* break apart in lung cancer.

In situ hybridisation (ISH) permits the identification of a specific sequence of nucleic acid using probes designed to bind to the area of interest. ISH is used to identify Epstein–Barr virus (EBV) in some tumours such as nasopharyngeal carcinoma (see Fig. 12.3).

In *fluorescence in situ hybridisation* (FISH), the probe is bound to a fluorescent marker. If the probe binds to the target nucleic acid sequence, a signal can be detected by examining the specimen with a fluorescence microscope. FISH is used most commonly in analysis of tumours for specific mutations, e.g. in the analysis of the *ERBB2* gene *(HER2)* in certain types of breast cancer. Micrograph (Fig. 1.5A) shows fluorescence microscopy of the nuclei of breast cancer cells (stained blue). The *ERBB2* gene target normally shows a single orange and green signal, however in this case there is amplification of the gene and multiple orange signals are seen in the nuclei A, representing multiple copies (amplification) of the *ERBB2* gene and a positive test.

ALK mutation in lung cancer (Fig. 1.5B) shows similar fluorescent signals, but as a different type of probe is used, a different pattern of signals is produced. This is discussed in more detail in Fig. 12.24.

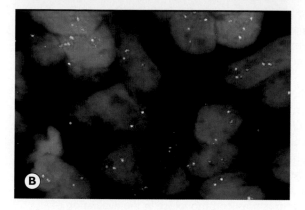

MOLECULAR ORIGINS OF CANCER 3: MORE DETAIL ON ONCOGENES

As noted above, **oncogenes** encode proteins controlling proliferation, programmed cell death **(apoptosis)** or both. Activation of these genes, with resultant abnormal production of their protein products **(oncoproteins)**, can take place in a variety of ways:

- **Point mutation**: resulting in a permanently active gene, such as in the **RAS** oncogene, which encodes a signal transduction protein. Mutations in this gene are very common, occurring in around 20% of all human cancers.

- **Translocation**: This is a common molecular abnormality in cancer cells. The result is that either the oncogene comes to lie adjacent to a gene that is constitutively expressed or relocation of the gene results in its fusion with a second gene, producing a new protein with increased activity. The former is a common event in haematological malignancies such as in **Burkitt lymphoma**, where the *C-MYC* oncogene on chromosome 8 becomes relocated adjacent to the **immunoglobulin heavy chain gene** on chromosome 14, which is constitutively expressed in mature B lymphocytes. In 95% of cases of **chronic myeloid leukaemia**, translocation results in the **ABL gene** on chromosome 9 fusing with the **BCR gene** on chromosome 22, the outcome being the **BCR-ABL** gene, also known as the **Philadelphia chromosome.** The protein product of this fused gene is constitutively active and has a role in activating proteins controlling the cell cycle.

- **Amplification**: Here, multiple copies of a gene are formed, resulting in increased production of the oncoprotein. This is of particular note in tumour progression and hence correlates with poor prognosis. One such example is the **ERBB2** (**HER2/neu**; human epidermal growth factor receptor 2) gene in breast carcinoma, where amplification of the gene correlates with poorer prognosis.

Next-generation sequencing

Next-generation sequencing (NGS) permits the amplification of large sections of DNA and RNA, including whole genomes, which can then be analysed using *bioinformatics,* a process combining computing and scientific study that puts results into clinical context. It is likely that NGS will be a routine test in molecular pathology in the coming years, providing a molecular microscope at the level of the cellular DNA and RNA within the cells.

MOLECULAR ORIGINS OF CANCER 4: THERAPY TARGETED AT ONCOGENES

Knowledge of the molecular origins of cancer, with an awareness of the genes and their protein products which drive cancerous cells, has provided researchers with targets for intervention in cancer treatment. This offers clinicians the opportunity to deliver treatment to patients based on the particular molecular signature of their specific tumour, so-called personalised or *individualised therapy*. Thus, molecular assessment of many cancers has become part of the routine pathology work-up in a growing number of cancers. Throughout this book, many examples of diagnostic molecular pathology providing insight into tumour behaviour and/or directing therapy are given. Here, we discuss the principles of these therapies using two common examples.

Those protein products which are expressed on the cell surface, in theory, provide a target for attack by appropriately designed monoclonal antibodies. This principle forms the basis of many targeted therapies in cancer. We have already mentioned the *ERBB2 (HER2/neu; human epidermal growth factor receptor 2)* gene in breast carcinoma, which, when amplified, is associated with a poorer prognosis. This protein has also provided an opportunity for development of targeted therapy through production of a monoclonal antibody to *HER2/neu* (trastuzamab; trade name *Herceptin),* which has proved successful in treatment of some patients with breast carcinoma, specifically those tumours shown to over-express the HER2/neu receptor. Thus, assessment of HER2 status is now commonplace in the evaluation of breast carcinoma.

In addition to monoclonal antibodies targeting cancer-associated proteins, a number of small molecules have been developed that can interfere with the function of oncoproteins. *Tyrosine kinases* are enzymes which phosphorylate proteins and have key roles in cell growth and differentiation (among other functions). One example where tyrosine kinase activity is increased in cancers is in relation to the *BCR-ABL* gene in chronic myeloid leukaemia (CML) where the protein product of the gene has tyrosine kinase activity. To counter this, inhibitors of tyrosine kinase have been developed and are now used in routine practice with considerable success, not only in treatment of CML, but also in other cancers where tyrosine kinase activity is implicated in the development of the tumour, such as gastrointestinal stromal tumours.

Digital pathology and image analysis

Until recently, most pathologists used traditional microscopy to analyse glass slides. With technological advances, pathologists are now able to examine virtual slides using a computer system without relying upon a traditional microscope. This is facilitated by digital scanning of glass slides. This has many advantages including the ability to share images with experts in other centres in real-time and in the interpretation of cell counts and immunocytochemistry. Many of these processes can be automated, thus improving turnaround time within the laboratory. A typical digital pathology set-up is shown in Fig. 1.6.

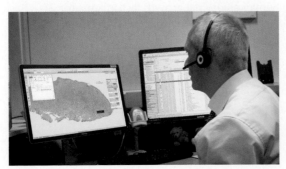

Fig. 1.6 Digital pathology workstation. (Courtesy of Mr John Theunissen, Phillips Digital Pathology Solutions.)

The microscope has been replaced by a high resolution computer screen where the pathologist is able to view digitally scanned slides. Digital pathology also allows for the application of *image analysis* techniques. These methods are more reproducible than traditional microscopy for quantitative measurements. Digital platforms are also very useful for sharing cases both locally and internationally and providing expertise to remote locations.

Personalised medicine

It is well recognised that, in the same way that each individual's appearance and personality are subtly different, their tumours also show subtle differences which can alter an individual's prognosis. As pathologists, it is our responsibility to assess accurately each tumour at the macroscopic, microscopic and molecular level and to record all of these factors within the pathology report to permit a more personalised approach to treatment.

An example would be in the treatment of lung cancer. A tumour will now be described macroscopically, its histological subtype identified with microscopy and immunohistochemistry and then, subsequently, these tumours will be tested for *EGFR* and *ALK* mutations, as well as for the presence of PD-L1 receptors on the cell surface. This allows a patient-centred treatment approach, taking into account specific biological therapies and clinical trial opportunities.

Table 1.4 Chapter review.

Introduction to pathology	Key points	Figure
Basic histology techniques	Study of tissues Variety of specimen types Processing of specimen important to create blocks and slides for pathologist review (fixation, macroscopic assessment, trimming, processing, embedding, microtomy, staining).	Table 1.1 Fig. 1.1
Cytology	Study of cells rather than tissues Includes fine needle aspirate, effusion fluid and cervical cytology	Table 1.1
Immunostaining	Identifying antigens in tissues using antigen–antibody reaction and visualising in the tissue or cell with a chromogen reaction	Fig. 1.2
Immunohistochemistry interpretation	Variety of antibodies in clinical use to help diagnose cancers, identify the primary tumour site in metastatic tumours and provide prognostic and predictive information. Many factors assessed when using IHC, such as proportion and intensity of staining.	Tables 1.2, 1.3 Fig. 1.3
Electron microscopy	Assessment of the ultrastructure of a cell including the organelles and the nucleus. Use now limited largely to renal and muscle pathology (see Ch. 15 and 23)	
Molecular techniques PCR	Amplification of DNA targets for detection, e.g. *EGFR* mutation testing in lung cancer	1.4
FISH	Detection of target using DNA probe labelled with fluorescein marker and viewed under fluorescence microscope, e.g. *ALK* mutation in lung cancer	1.5
Next-generation sequencing (NGS)	Sequencing of large sections of DNA/RNA or even whole genome	
Bioinformatics	Using applied software/statistics to analyse and interpret biological data such as those generated from NGS.	
Digital Pathology	Slides digitally scanned and assessed on a computer screen instead of microscope.	1.6

2 Cellular responses to injury

Introduction

In response to environmental changes, cells have to adapt in the face of physiological and pathological stimuli that seek to disturb their normal homeostatic milieu. This process is called *cellular adaptation* and includes mechanisms such as an increase in cell size *(hypertrophy)* or an increase in cell number *(hyperplasia)*. Other examples of cellular adaptation include *metaplasia*, which can be defined as a change in the differentiation of a cell (see Ch. 6). When there is failure of normal cellular differentiation, this can result in *dysplasia* and *neoplasia*. These concepts are covered in detail in Ch. 7.

If the change in the cellular environment is greater than the capacity of the cell to adapt, then cell injury results (Figs 2.1–2.3). This may be reversible, if the cell returns to its normal environment, or irreversible, if the environmental insult continues. Irreversible cell injury leads to cell death. Cells may die by unprogrammed means, *necrosis*, or programmed means, *apoptosis.* Not all cell death is harmful. Apoptosis is an important process by which normal cell numbers are maintained, e.g. in menstrual endometrium. *Autolysis* is a process commonly seen in post mortem tissues, by which cells breakdown by an enzymatic process of self-digestion. If the enzymes causing the cell to breakdown are derived from outside the cell, then the process is referred to as *heterolysis*.

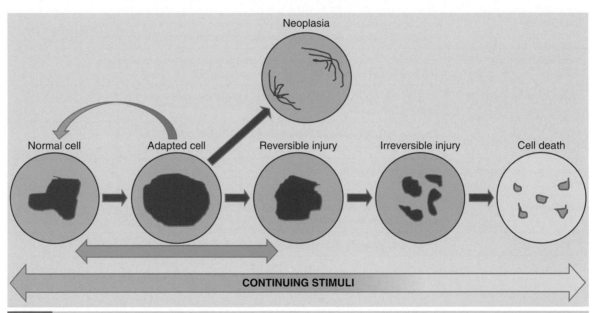

Fig. 2.1 The cellular response to injury.

Fig. 2.1 outlines the ways in which cells respond to changes in their environment. If a cell makes a successful response to an environmental change, then it will either return to normal or it may make an adaptive change. Adaptive changes are discussed in Ch. 6. This chapter will consider the morphological changes that occur when cells are exposed to pathological stimuli leading to cell damage and/or cell death.

There is a further consequence of unsuccessful adaptation to an environmental change, the development of *dysplasia* or *neoplasia*, which will be discussed in Ch. 7.

The fate of a cell exposed to harmful stimulus depends on the type, duration and magnitude of the injury and partly on how vulnerable the cell is to injury. For example, a cerebral neurone is much more vulnerable to damage following hypoxia than a fibroblast.

Host factors also contribute to the overall response: an individual who has an *immunodeficiency* disorder or poor nutrition is more likely to succumb to overwhelming infection than a well-nourished individual with a normal immune response (Fig. 2.2).

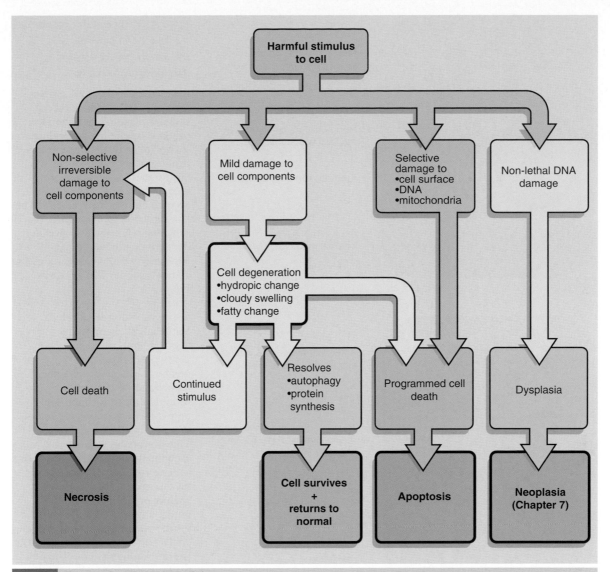

Fig. 2.2 **The response of cells to injury.**

The ultimate fate of a cell, once exposed to a harmful stimulus, depends on the type, severity and duration of the stimulus and also on the type of cell. If there is mild damage to cell components, including the energy supply, then a cell may develop morphological changes termed *cellular degeneration*. The commonest structural changes are *cloudy swelling*, *hydropic degeneration* and *fatty change* (see Figs 2.4 and 2.5). Importantly, such morphological changes are reversible if the causative harmful stimulus is removed or abates. Under such circumstances, a cell may return to normal after removal of damaged organelles through autophagy and the synthesis of new proteins. However, the outcome is not always successful and the damaged cell may still die.

If a cell develops severe, irreversible damage, usually involving many cellular components, then it is unable to respond and dies. Following cell death, a series of morphological changes take place, termed *necrosis* (see Figs 2.6 and 2.7). Necrosis may also take place if, following development of the changes of cell degeneration, the harmful stimulus does not abate.

A variety of different triggers may initiate a process of programmed cell death, known as *apoptosis* (Fig. 2.8). This is a highly organised process whereby intracellular signalling systems bring about destruction of the cell. Damage to DNA, cell surface membrane or mitochondria are potent stimuli for apoptosis. Additionally, some cells that have initially responded by showing signs of cell degeneration (sublethal cell injury) may enter programmed cell death and die through apoptosis. Apoptosis is not always pathological: it is an important mechanism in embryonic development, in regression of normal tissues such as during the normal menstrual cycle and during the maintenance and renewal of normal cells and tissues. It is still uncertain why a cell is triggered to undergo apoptosis rather than necrosis, but certain types of pathological stimuli typically initiate apoptosis, e.g. radiation damage and certain viral infections. Necrosis, on the other hand, is the usual pattern of cell death in severe hypoxia.

Although discussed later in Ch. 7, it is important to note here that some harmful stimuli to cells can cause non-lethal DNA damage that leads to mutations and development of *dysplasia* and *neoplasia*.

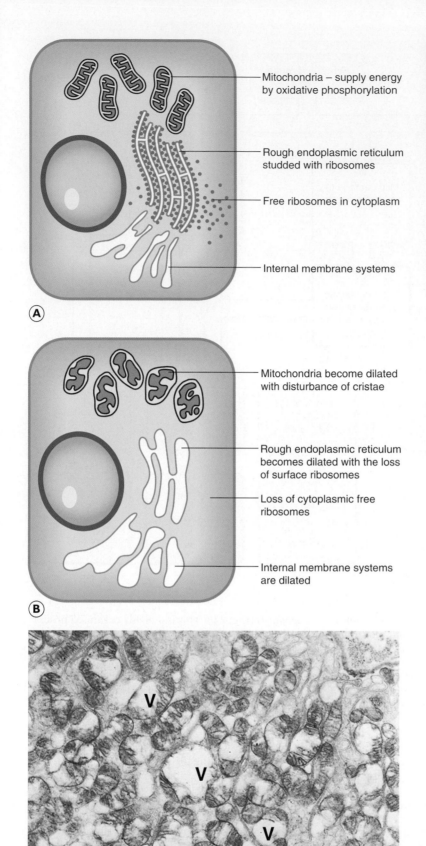

Mitochondria – supply energy by oxidative phosphorylation

Rough endoplasmic reticulum studded with ribosomes

Free ribosomes in cytoplasm

Internal membrane systems

Ⓐ

Mitochondria become dilated with disturbance of cristae

Rough endoplasmic reticulum becomes dilated with the loss of surface ribosomes

Loss of cytoplasmic free ribosomes

Internal membrane systems are dilated

Ⓑ

Ⓒ

Fig. 2.3 **Early cellular responses to injury. (A)** Normal cell; **(B)** reversible cell damage; **(C)** electron micrograph.

Reversible cell damage involves injury to one or more vital cell systems including mitochondria (leading to inability to produce energy in the form of adenosine triphosphate or ATP), cell membranes (causing loss of fluid and ion homeostasis) and accumulation of free radicals. The first ultrastructural evidence of sublethal cell damage is swelling of membrane-bound organelles, particularly endoplasmic reticulum and mitochondria as shown in Fig. 2.3B.

In Fig. 2.3C, an electron micrograph of a renal tubular epithelial cell damaged by hypoxia, most of the mitochondria are swollen. Instead of regular stacks of cristae (inner mitochondrial membrane), several of the mitochondria now contain spaces or vacuoles **(V)**, pushing the cristae apart. This is probably a result of accumulation of electrolytes and water owing to early damage to the enzymes of the membrane sodium pump. This change is potentially reversible, but further insult leads to destruction of the cristae, more severe swelling of the mitochondria and formation of electron-dense bodies. At this stage, the changes are irreversible and cell death occurs.

Another manifestation of early cell injury is loss of ribosomes from both cytosol and the surface of the rough endoplasmic reticulum.

Inner cell membrane systems, particularly the endoplasmic reticulum, become dilated and, in time, form vacuoles visible by light microscopy (see Fig. 2.4). Lethal injury is marked by progressive disintegration of other organelles, particularly lysosomes, which release hydrolytic enzymes causing autodigestion of the cell *(autolysis)* (see Fig 2.8). The cell membranes lose specialised structures such as microvilli and may form blebs that separate off from the cell.

KEY TO FIGURES
H hydropic degeneration **N** nucleus **V** vacuole

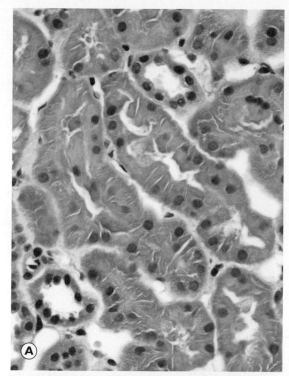

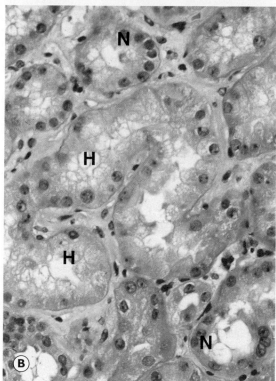

Fig. 2.4 **Hydropic degeneration. (A)** Normal renal cortex (HP); **(B)** hydropic degeneration: kidney (HP).

The earliest light microscopic evidence of cellular injury is loss of normal staining intensity of the cytoplasm, because of the swelling of membrane-bound organelles. Normal cytoplasm stained with haematoxylin and eosin is light pink with a faint tint of blue (basophilia), mainly due to the presence of ribosomal RNA. With sublethal cellular damage, ribosomes are reduced in number and the normal blue cytoplasmic tint is lost. Swelling of endoplasmic reticulum and mitochondria contributes to further cytoplasmic pallor. This is described as cloudy swelling and may be subtle and difficult to identify. With further swelling of organelles, the cell becomes waterlogged and true vacuoles appear in the cytoplasm, which now stains faintly with total loss of basophilia. At this stage, cells are said to exhibit *hydropic degeneration*. The micrograph in Fig. 2.4B shows a section of kidney (cortex) with inadequate blood flow owing to severe hypotension. The cytoplasm of the epithelial cells of the cortical tubules is pale and vacuolated and exhibits hydropic degeneration **(H)**. The nuclei **(N)** are enlarged, indicating increased protein synthesis as the cells attempt to recover and restore normal functions. Compare these tubular epithelial cells with Fig. 2.4A, a micrograph of normal renal cortex taken at similar magnification. These cells are very susceptible to hypoxia due to the very high energy demands required to produce urine. Such damage to the renal tubules may lead to acute renal failure, known as *acute tubular necrosis (ATN)*. With proper supportive measures, patients can make a full recovery.

Cloudy swelling and hydropic change reflect failure of membrane ion pumps, which allows the cell to accumulate fluid. This is due to a lack of cellular ATP as the cell diverts energy to facilitate repair mechanisms.

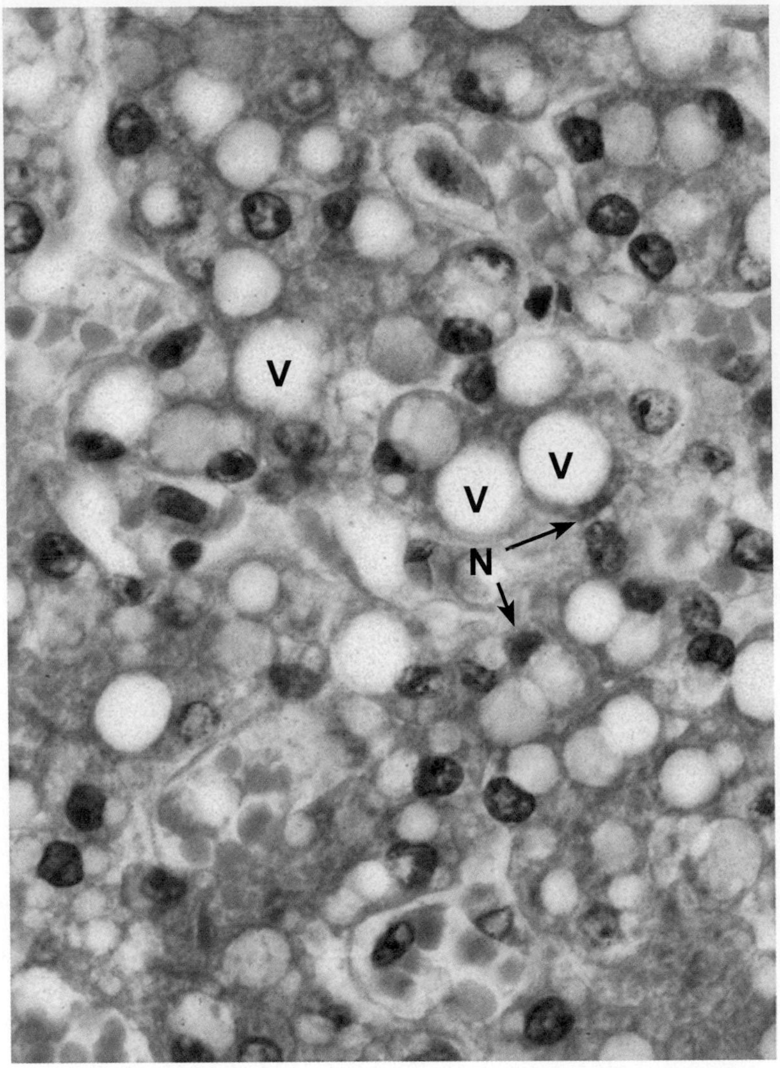

Fig. 2.5 **Fatty change: liver (HP).**

Fatty change (or *steatosis*) is another manifestation of sublethal metabolic dcrangement seen in certain cell types with high energy demand. It is most common in the liver, as in this example, but also occurs rarely in the myocardium and skeletal muscle. The common causes of fatty change in the liver are toxins (particularly alcohol and halogenated hydrocarbons such as chloroform), chronic hypoxia, diabetes mellitus and obesity. Impaired metabolism of fatty acids leads to accumulation of triglycerides (fats) that form non-membrane-bound vacuoles in cells, which may displace the nucleus from its usual location.

Fig. 2.5 is an example of liver from a patient with a history of excessive alcohol intake and shows large vacuoles (**V**) in the hepatocytes with displacement of the nucleus (**N**). In conventionally prepared tissue, organic solvents used in processing dissolve out the fat to leave empty, non-staining spaces. If necessary, frozen sections can be prepared to preserve the fat, which can then be specifically stained.

TOXIC LIVER INURY

When taken to excess as in the case of an overdose, many drugs can lead to toxic liver injury *(hepatotoxicity)*. Examples include alcohol (see Ch. 14) and carbon tetrachloride.

The drug paracetamol (acetaminophen) is a commonly used simple analgesic medication. When taken to excess *(drug overdose)*, paracetamol acts as a *hepatotoxin* causing a particular type of damage to the liver known as *centrilobular necrosis* (see Fig. 2.6A)

The hepatocyte necrosis is caused by a toxic metabolite of paracetamol (acetaminophen) called *N-acetyl-p-benzoquinone imine (NAPQI)*,which is produced specifically around the central lobular region where drug metabolism usually takes place within the liver.

Treatments for acute hepatotoxicity caused by paracetamol (acetaminophen) overdose include medical therapies such as N-acetylcysteine. In some very severe cases, a liver transplant may be performed.

KEY TO FIGURES
N nucleus **Ne** necrosis **K** karyorrhexis **Py** pyknotic nuclei **V** vacuoles

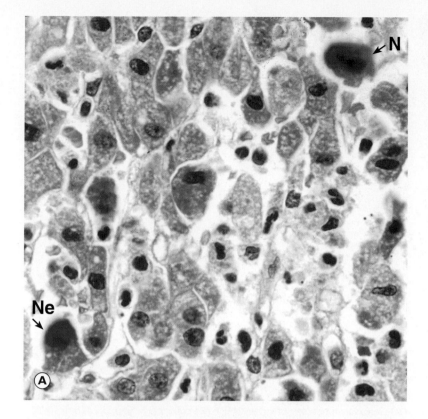

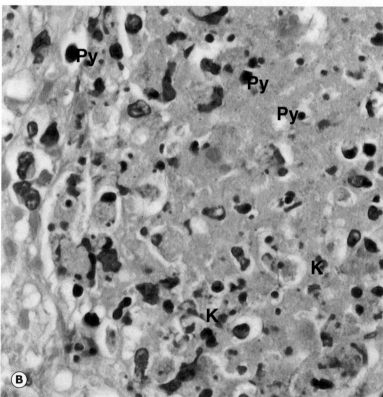

Fig. 2.6 **Cell necrosis. (A)** Liver (HP); **(B)** renal cortex (HP).

When a cell has sustained irreversible damage, a succession of histological changes occurs, which are grouped under the term *necrosis*. By definition, necrosis can only occur in a living organism.

The micrograph in Fig. 2.6A is a section of liver from a person poisoned by paracetamol (acetaminophen). Many of the hepatocytes are pale-stained and a few exhibit early cytoplasmic vacuolation, indicating hydropic degeneration. Several cells also show early histological features of necrosis **(Ne)**. The dead cells stain a bright pink (eosinophilia) and stand out from the other cells, due to degeneration of structural proteins that form a compact homogeneous mass. Compared with living cells, the nucleus of each necrotic cell is smaller, condensed and intensely stained with haematoxylin (basophilia). This nuclear condensation is termed *pyknosis* and is due to progressive chromatin clumping, possibly as a result of reduced pH resulting from terminal anaerobic metabolism.

In Fig. 2.6B, which is a micrograph of necrotic kidney, the changes of necrosis are more developed. Pyknotic nuclei **(Py)** stand out as intensely basophilic, round bodies. Note that the nuclear changes are accompanied by cytoplasmic changes. The cytoplasm has lost definition and the cell margins (plasma membranes) are indistinct. In time, the pyknotic nuclei become fragmented into several particles, which represent pieces of degenerate nuclear material, a change termed *karyorrhexis* **(K)**.

Complete breakdown of nuclear material then takes place by release of cellular hydrolytic enzymes, leading to loss of the groups that bind haematoxylin. This process is termed *karyolysis* and, when complete, leaves the dead cell as an anucleate, homogeneous, eosinophilic mass.

Many of the structural changes seen in necrosis are mediated through the action of lysosomal enzymes, liberated through breakdown of internal cell membranes.

BASIC PATHOLOGICAL PROCESSES ■ CELLULAR RESPONSES TO INJURY

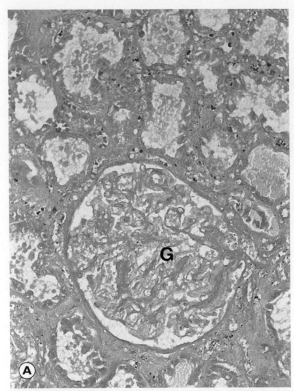
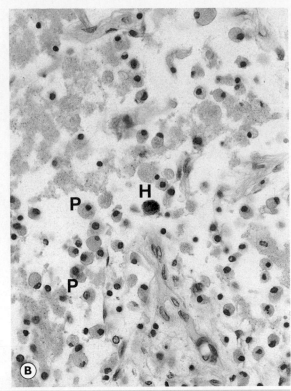

Fig. 2.7 **Patterns of tissue necrosis. (A)** Coagulative necrosis of kidney (MP); **(B)** colliquative necrosis of brain (HP).

Traditionally, three main patterns of tissue necrosis are described: *coagulative*, *colliquative* and *caseous*. Each term describes the macroscopic appearance of necrotic tissue. In coagulative necrosis, the tissue appears firm, as if cooked. In colliquative necrosis, the dead tissue appears semi-liquid, while in caseous necrosis, the dead tissue has a soft consistency, reminiscent of cream cheese. These gross patterns correlate closely with histological appearances.

In areas of coagulative necrosis, much of the cellular outline and tissue architecture can be discerned histologically even though the cells are dead. The commonest cause of this pattern of necrosis is ischaemia owing to loss of arterial oxygenated blood, such as in myocardial infarction.

In areas of caseous necrosis, cells die and form an amorphous proteinaceous mass in which no semblance of original architecture can be discerned. Caseous necrosis is typically seen in tuberculosis, several examples of which are shown in Ch. 5 (see Figs 5.3–5.6).

The term colliquative necrosis was originally used to describe the macroscopic appearance of necrosis in the brain as a result of arterial occlusion (cerebral infarction) at a stage when the necrotic area was occupied by semi-liquid material. This appearance, however, is not a specific form of necrosis, but results from dissolution of tissue after an initial coagulative phase, which is common to all tissues immediately

following cell death. The subsequent liquefaction of dead tissue reflects both tissue composition and the cause of necrosis. In the brain, the relative lack of extracellular structural proteins (reticulin and collagen) leads to rapid loss of tissue architecture as autolysis occurs, resulting in the early formation of a semi-liquid mass of dead cells. Otherwise, liquefaction of dead tissues is virtually confined to cases of necrosis associated with *pyogenic* (pus-producing) bacteria, such as in an abscess (see Fig. 3.12).

Fig. 2.7A is an example of coagulative necrosis in an area of kidney subject to infarction. Note that the architecture of a glomerulus **(G)** and surrounding tubules is still recognisable despite the dissolution of nuclear material, except for a few pyknotic and karyorrhectic remnants.

Fig. 2.7B illustrates the liquefaction phase in a cerebral infarct where no residual tissue architecture is preserved; the earlier phase of coagulative necrosis in brain can be seen in Fig. 23.2. The necrotic brain is now largely replaced by wisps of pink-staining cellular debris, with phagocytic cells **(P)** engulfing degenerate material. Some of these contain haemosiderin pigment **(H)**, which is a breakdown product of haemoglobin and is indicative of haemorrhage into the tissue.

A fourth type of necrosis, known as *fibrinoid necrosis*, is principally seen in the walls of blood vessels and is discussed in Ch. 11.

KEY TO FIGURES
A apoptotic bodies **G** glomerulus **H** haemosiderin pigment **P** phagocytic cells

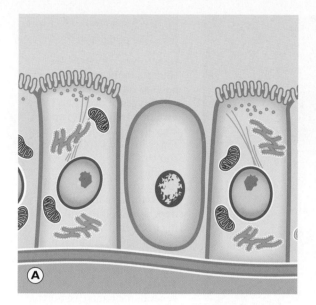

(A)

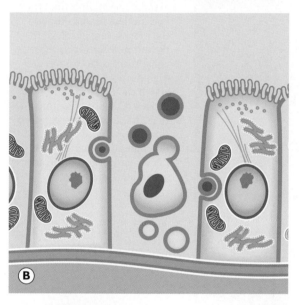

(B)

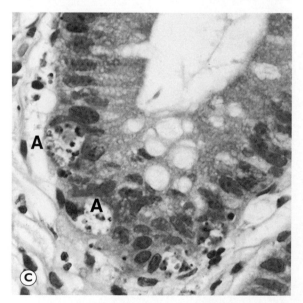

A

A

(C)

Fig. 2.8 **Apoptosis. (A)** Early stage; **(B)** later stage; **(C)** apoptosis in colonic glands (HP).

Certain stimuli to cells lead to their controlled elimination by *programmed cell death* in a process called *apoptosis*. Although apoptosis is a normal physiological process, for example in embryonic development and normal cell turnover, it is also an important mechanism for elimination of damaged or diseased cells (E-Figs 2.1 **H** and 2.2 **H**). Apoptosis may be triggered by the *intrinsic or extrinsic pathways:* for example, absence of a necessary growth factor triggers the intrinsic pathway of apoptosis, while binding of signalling molecules such as tumour necrosis factor to its receptor (one of the *death receptors*) on the cell surface, triggers the external pathway.

Increased permeability of mitochondrial outer membranes and release of cytochrome c into the cytoplasm is a common step in apoptosis whatever the trigger. Cytochrome c is able to activate the early or initiation members of the caspase cascade. Caspases, which are proteases, cleave cellular proteins and activate endonucleases that break down chromatin. Caspases are present in all cells as proenzymes and form an enzymatic cascade system analogous to the blood clotting system or the complement system. They represent the final effector mechanism of apoptosis.

When apoptosis is triggered, cells undergo a distinct set of structural changes that correspond to the biochemical changes occurring in the cell. Fig. 2.8A illustrates how the cell loses specialised surface features and attachments to other cells and structures, becoming 'rounded up'. The nucleus becomes shrunken with dense condensation of chromatin beneath the nuclear membrane.

Fig. 2.8B illustrates the rapid fragmentation of the cell into multiple small *apoptotic bodies*, each one being membrane-bound and many containing nuclear remnants. Each fragment is still a vital entity. The surface membranes express factors that facilitate phagocytosis by adjacent cells and macrophages.

Many stimuli can activate apoptosis. Cell membrane damage, damage to mitochondria, damage to DNA, viral infection and immune-mediated attack are all common triggers. The benefit of eliminating cells by apoptosis is that individual cells can be removed in a way that does not stimulate an inflammatory response.

Fig. 2.8C shows apoptosis in colonic glands in a patient who had a bone marrow transplant (graft) and is suffering from graft-versus-host disease, in which donor immune cells attack host tissues, in this case the colonic epithelial cells. These late apoptotic cells represented by multiple dot-like *apoptotic bodies* **(A)** are seen.

In tumour pathology, apoptosis is a major factor that limits the growth of a neoplasm. The production by tumour cells of factors that prevent apoptosis is an important mechanism in the development of uncontrolled growth, e.g. *follicular lymphoma*.

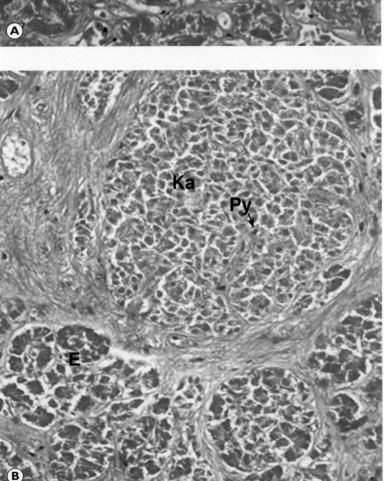

Fig. 2.9 Autolysis. (A) Kidney (HP); **(B)** pancreas (HP).

In autolysis, irreversible changes to the nucleus occur and are similar to those seen in other types of necrosis. These include pyknosis **(Py)** and karyolysis **(Ka)** as pictured in Fig. 2.9B and karyorrhexis (not shown).

When stained with haematoxylin and eosin, the autolytic cell shows intense hypereosinophilia and loss of nuclear detail.

Autolysis is commonly seen in tissue samples obtained in the investigation of death, during an *autopsy* procedure. In general, the pancreas, adrenal glands, spleen, intestinal tract and kidneys tend to show the most severe autolysis in the autopsy setting as the constituent cells contain a high proportion of enzymes which can drive the autolytic process. Autolysis is more readily seen with an increased time interval after death and in temperate climates, with higher temperatures advancing enzymatic digestion.

KEY TO FIGURES
E hypereosinophilic cytoplasm **Ka** karyolysis **Py** pyknosis.

Table 2.1 Chapter review.

Pathological process	Causes	Clinical presentation	Main histological features	Figure
Overview of cellular response to injury				2.1, 2.2
Acute reversible cell damage	Acute ischaemia Toxins	Acute failure/malfunction of organ, e.g. acute renal failure	Swelling of cell cytoplasm Vacuolation of cells	2.3, 2.4
Fatty change	Toxins, e.g. alcohol,	Initially normal Later develop organ failure to varying degrees	Clear vacuole within cells containing excess lipid May expand to completely fill cytoplasm	2.5, 14.2, 14.5A
Overview of necrosis				2.6
Necrosis – coagulative	Ischaemia	Organ malfunction, e.g. myocardial infarction	Maintenance of tissue architecture, loss of cell nuclei, cytoplasm becomes eosinophilic, eventually develops fibrous scar	2.7A
Necrosis – colliquative	Ischaemia – only affects brain	Organ malfunction, e.g. cerebral infarction (stroke)	Damaged area replaced by cyst filled with fluid, surrounding brain has increased glial cells (gliosis)	2.7B
Necrosis – caseous	Mycobacterial infection (tuberculosis)	Low grade fever, malaise, organ malfunction – can affect any organ, very variable clinical presentation	Classic epithelioid granulomas with central featureless necrotic material, surrounded by a zone of lymphocytes; later there is fibrosis and scarring	5.3, 5.4, 5.5, 5.6, 5.7
Necrosis – fibrinoid	Damage to blood vessel walls due to accelerated hypertension or immune mechanisms	Vessel malfunction – blockage due to thrombosis and/or haemorrhage due to rupture	Deposition of plasma proteins within the vessel wall- appears as an eosinophilic deposit, may be associated with inflammation and/or thrombus	11.2, 11.7
Apoptosis (programmed cell death)	May be physiological or pathological	Destruction of virus-infected cells, graft versus host disease, elimination of old/worn-out cells	Drop-out of individual cells often surrounded by lymphocytes, apoptotic bodies	2.8
Autolysis	Usually seen in the post mortem setting	Due to enzymatic digestion of tissues.	Intense hypereosinophilia and loss of nuclear definition	2.9

3 Acute inflammation, healing and repair

Introduction

Inflammation is an almost universal response to tissue damage by a wide range of harmful stimuli, including mechanical trauma, tissue necrosis and infection. The purpose of inflammation is to destroy (or contain) the damaging agent, initiate repair processes and return the damaged tissue to useful function. Inflammation is somewhat arbitrarily divided into *acute* and *chronic inflammation*, but, in reality, the two often form a continuum. Many causes of tissue damage provoke an acute inflammatory response but some types of insult may bring about a typical chronic inflammatory reaction from the outset (e.g. viral infections, foreign body reactions and fungal infections). Acute inflammation may *resolve* or *heal by scarring* but may also progress to chronic inflammation and it is common for a mixed acute and chronic response to co-exist. This chapter describes acute inflammation and its sequelae, while chronic inflammation is discussed in Ch. 4. Many examples of acute and chronic inflammation are illustrated throughout this book.

There are three major and interrelated components of the acute inflammatory response

■ **Vascular dilatation**

– Relaxation of vascular smooth muscle leads to engorgement of tissue with blood *(hyperaemia)*

■ **Endothelial activation**

– Increased endothelial permeability allows plasma proteins to pass into tissues

– Expression of adhesion molecules on the endothelial surface mediates neutrophil adherence

– Production of factors that cause vascular dilatation

■ **Neutrophil activation and migration**

– Expression of adhesion molecules causes neutrophils to adhere to endothelium

– Chemotactic factors drive emigration from vessels into surrounding tissues

– Increased capacity for bacterial killing

These are outlined in Fig. 3.1.

| Fig. 3.1 | **Outline of acute inflammation.** *(Illustration opposite)* |

Acute inflammation may develop over minutes or hours, depending on the type and severity of the tissue damage, and generally lasts hours to days. Vascular dilatation, increased vascular permeability and neutrophil activation and migration are interdependent processes and all three are required for the full response. Immediately after the tissue damage has occurred there may be a brief phase of constriction of arterioles, but this is followed within seconds by arteriolar and capillary dilatation, increasing blood flow to the area. This is mediated by histamine and nitric oxide, released by tissue mast cells (E-Fig. 3.1**H**) and endothelial cells (E-Fig. 3.2**H**) respectively. At much the same time, gaps form between endothelial cells of the post-capillary venules, allowing protein-rich plasma to leak into the tissue. The dilated capillaries and venules become engorged with red cells and blood flow slows and then stops. The slowing of blood flow brings neutrophils (E-Figs. 3.3**H** and 3.4**H**) into contact with the endothelial cells, which have been activated to increase expression of *adhesion molecules* on their surface membranes, including selectins and integrin receptors. As the neutrophils contact with the endothelium, adhesion molecules on the neutrophil cell membrane bind to their complementary molecules on the endothelial cells and become stuck. Activation of neutrophils plays a role here, in that activated neutrophils are more likely to stick. The neutrophils pass through the basement membrane of the endothelium and

move along a concentration gradient of *chemotactic factors*. When they arrive at the site of injury, the activated neutrophils phagocytose necrotic tissue debris and any pathogenic organisms. The activation of the neutrophils makes them more efficient at phagocytosis and bacterial killing.

Opsonisation of bacteria by complement and immunoglobulins renders them more readily phagocytosed.

Meanwhile, in the tissues, the plasma-derived proteins undergo various changes. The *complement cascade* is initiated (via the alternative pathway) forming components, such as C5a and C3a, with a wide range of activities. *Immunoglobulins* bind to any causative organisms, immobilising them and forming immune complexes that further activate complement (via the classical pathway). *Fibrinogen* is cleaved to form monomers, which then polymerise to form a network of *fibrin* that impedes the movement of any pathogenic organisms present and also provides a framework for the movement of neutrophils. The increased fluid in the tissue causes an increased flow of lymph to carry immune complexes and antigenic material to the lymph nodes, where a specific immune response is initiated over the next few days.

This entire process is orchestrated by a plethora of chemical mediators derived from injured tissues, bacteria, plasma proteins and leukocytes. The most important of these mediators are indicated at their sites of action. Note that some mediators have multiple actions.

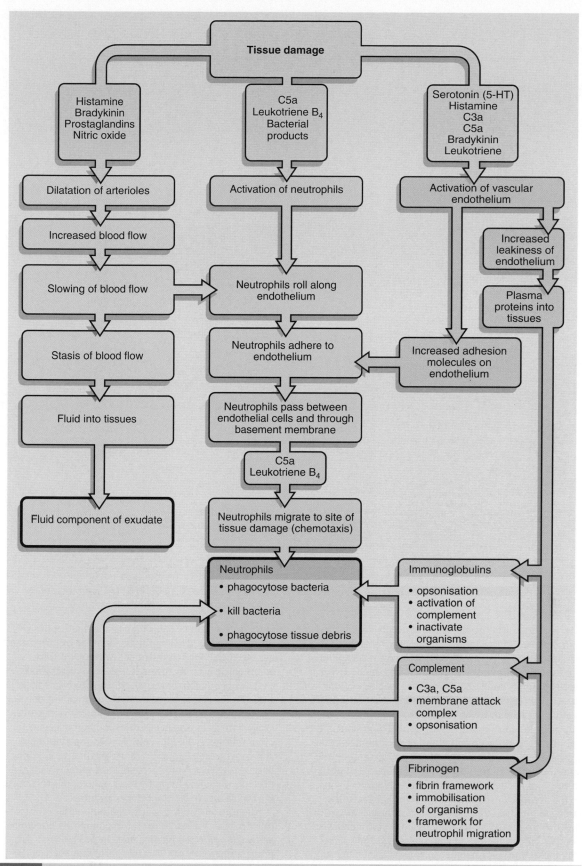

Fig. 3.1 **Outline of acute inflammation.** *(Caption opposite)*

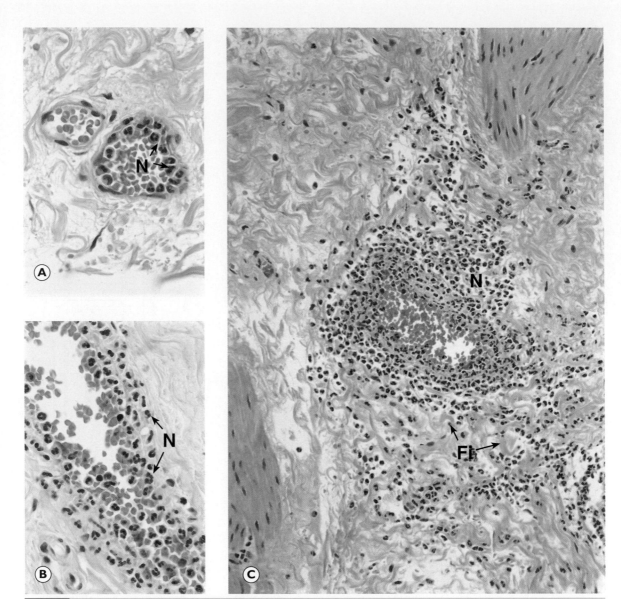

Fig. 3.2 **Formation of the acute inflammatory exudate. (A)** Early vascular changes (HP); **(B)** migration of neutrophils (HP); **(C)** early formation of exudate (LP).

Fig. 3.2 illustrates the sequence of events during the initial phases of the acute inflammatory response described in Fig. 3.1. In Fig. 3.2A, two small capillaries are shown. Both vessels are dilated and, in the larger, neutrophils **(N)** line up around the periphery of the vessel, a process termed *pavementing*. Neutrophils are easily identified in tissue sections by their lobulated nuclei and inconspicuous cytoplasm. These neutrophils are adherent to the endothelium, a process facilitated by increased expression of adhesion molecules on the endothelium and on the neutrophils. The surrounding fibrous connective tissue contains clear spaces owing to the accumulation of fluid *(oedema)* between the collagen bundles. Plasma proteins, although not visible, are also found free within the tissue. These include components of the blood coagulation cascade, acute phase reactants, complement proteins and circulating immunoglobulins.

The neutrophils pass through the vessel wall by extending a pseudopodium between adjacent endothelial cells. The neutrophils then penetrate the endothelial basement membrane and move into the perivascular connective tissue as shown in Fig. 3.2B.

Once in the extravascular tissues, the neutrophils **(N)** are attracted to the site of tissue damage by chemotactic agents, such as the complement component *C5a*, and migrate actively towards higher concentrations of these agents *(chemotaxis)*; this is shown in Fig. 3.2C. At the site of tissue damage, neutrophils play an important role in destruction of micro-organisms. Phagocytosis of organisms is promoted by a coating of immunoglobulin and complement *(opsonisation)* and activated neutrophils are more effective at killing pathogens. These three components, namely water, proteins including fibrin **(Fi)** and neutrophils **(N)**, form the typical *acute inflammatory exudate*.

Chemical mediators, although not visible, control this process. Vasodilatation is mediated by *histamine*, *prostaglandins* and *nitric oxide*. Increased vascular permeability is controlled by substances such as the vasoactive amines, serotonin (5-hydroxytryptamine (5-HT)) and histamine, complement components *C5a* and *C3a*, *leukotrienes C$_4$, D$_4$* and *E$_4$* and *platelet activating factor (PAF)*. Leukocyte activation and chemotaxis are influenced by *C5a*, *leukotriene B$_4$*, various *chemokines* and bacterial products.

KEY TO FIGURES
A alveolus **C** alveolar capillary **F** interlobar fissure **Fi** fibrin **M** alveolar macrophage **N** neutrophils

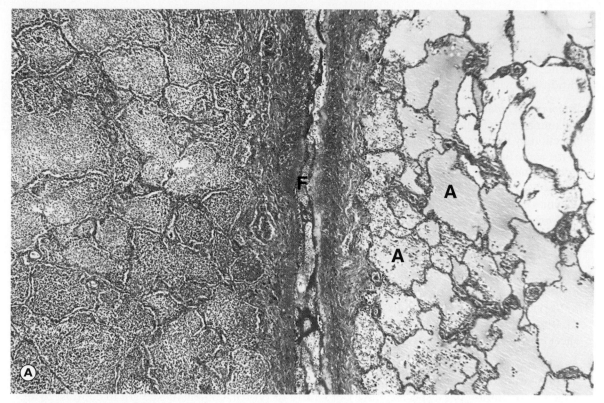

Fig. 3.3 **Established acute inflammation: lobar pneumonia. (A)** LP; **(B)** MP.

Fig. 3.3 is an example of an established acute inflammatory reaction in the lung parenchyma, namely lobar pneumonia. This pattern of pneumonia is most commonly caused by the pneumococcus *(Streptococcus pneumoniae)*. In lobar pneumonia, which is becoming less common, a whole lobe becomes solidified due to a massive outpouring of fluid, fibrin and neutrophils into the alveolar spaces. By far the most common type of pneumonia is bronchopneumonia (see Fig. 12.7) where infection spreads from the bronchi into adjacent lung tissue.

In Fig. 3.3A, a portion of lung is shown with an interlobar fissure **(F)** running vertically. The lung tissue on the left shows obliteration of alveolar spaces by purple-staining masses of inflammatory cells (mainly neutrophils) with associated fibrin; this is termed ***consolidation***. Alveolar walls can still be discerned. The dense inflammatory exudate is sharply limited by the interlobar fissure. The lung on the right of the fissure shows the earliest changes of acute inflammation, with faint pink-staining serous exudate in alveoli **(A)** and early neutrophil migration giving rise to a few scattered cells within the alveolar spaces.

At higher magnification in Fig. 3.3B, alveolar wall capillaries **(C)** are seen engorged with blood.

The alveolar spaces are obliterated by an acute inflammatory exudate rich in neutrophils and lesser amounts of wispy pink-stained fibrin. Occasional large, rounded mononuclear cells, macrophages **(M)**, can also be seen, but these are few in the acute phase of the disease.

If untreated, there are various possible outcomes to lobar pneumonia: death may occur (as in this patient), there may be complete resolution (see Fig. 3.7) or, very rarely, the exudate may become organised with consequent permanent fibrosis of the lung tissue, or lung abscess or empyema may develop.

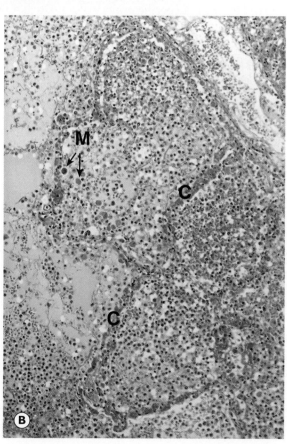

Morphological patterns of acute inflammation

While the basic process of acute inflammation is the same in all tissues, there are frequently qualitative differences in the inflammatory response seen under different circumstances. Terms describing these variations are widely used in clinical practice and are summarised below:

■ **Suppurative inflammation (purulent inflammation)** refers to acute inflammation in which the acute inflammatory exudate is rich in neutrophils. Suppurative inflammation is most commonly seen due to infection by bacteria where the mixture of neutrophils (viable and dead), necrotic tissue, and tissue fluid in the acute inflammatory exudate form a semi-liquid material referred to as *pus*, hence the term *purulent inflammation* (see Fig. 3.4). Within tissues, a circumscribed collection of semi-liquid pus is termed an *abscess* (see Fig. 3.12). The destruction of tissue may be due as much to release of neutrophil lysosomal enzymes as to tissue destruction by bacteria. Bacteria that produce purulent inflammation are described as *pyogenic bacteria.* They initiate massive neutrophilic infiltration with subsequent destruction of infected tissues. Pyogenic bacteria include staphylococci, some streptococci *(Streptococcus pyogenes, S. pneumoniae), Escherichia coli* and the neisseriae *(Neisseria meningitidis, N. gonorrhoeae).*

■ **Fibrinous inflammation** refers to a pattern of acute inflammation where the acute inflammatory exudate has a high plasma protein content (see Fig. 3.4). Fibrinogen, derived from plasma, is converted to fibrin, which is deposited in tissues. This pattern is particularly associated with membrane-lined cavities such as the pleura, pericardium and peritoneum, where the fibrin strands form a mat-like sheet causing adhesion between adjacent surfaces.

■ **Serous inflammation** describes a pattern of acute inflammation where the main tissue response is an accumulation of fluid with a low plasma protein and cell content. This is often called a *transudate*, which by definition has a specific gravity of <1.012 or protein content of <25 g/L in contrast to an *exudate,* with a specific gravity of >1.020 and protein content of >25 g/L. This pattern of response is most commonly seen in the skin in response to a burn.

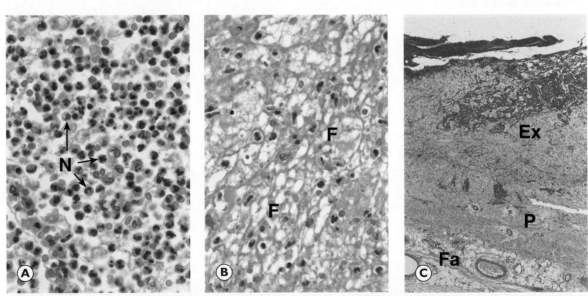

Fig. 3.4 **Acute inflammatory exudate. (A)** Neutrophilic exudate (HP); **(B)** highly fibrinous exudate (HP); **(C)** fibrinous inflammation: acute pericarditis (LP).

The micrographs in Fig. 3.4 contrast purulent and fibrinous inflammation. Fig. 3.4A shows a purulent acute inflammatory exudate in which neutrophils **(N)** are the main component (i.e. pus). This is the typical pattern of acute inflammation when the damaging stimulus is a pyogenic bacterial infection. After migration into the tissues, neutrophils phagocytose and kill the causative organisms. At the site of inflammation, the activated neutrophils generate a **respiratory burst** to produce the hydrogen peroxide and other reactive oxygen species used to kill bacteria; the neutrophils then die by apoptosis. Mature neutrophils only survive for 3 days but their numbers are maintained in acute inflammation by new arrivals from the circulation. The systemic response to acute inflammation is release of neutrophils from bone marrow into the blood, resulting in a **neutrophil leukocytosis.** Apoptotic neutrophils can be recognised by condensation *(pyknosis)* and fragmentation *(karyorrhexis)* of their nuclei and,

eventually, cytoplasmic disintegration; the neutrophil debris is usually phagocytosed by macrophages. Good examples of purulent inflammation include lobar pneumonia (see Fig. 3.3), bronchopneumonia (see Fig. 12.7) and acute appendicitis (see Fig. 13.17) and many other examples are found throughout this text.

An acute inflammatory exudate on a serosal surface usually contains plentiful fibrin. Fig. 3.4B shows an acute inflammatory exudate consisting of fibrin **(F)** with very few neutrophils *(fibrinous exudate)*, sometimes described as 'bread and butter pericarditis'. Macroscopically, a shaggy layer of fibrin coats the formerly smooth surface as in acute pericarditis (Fig. 3.4C). In this low-magnification micrograph, the exudate **(Ex)** is well established on the pericardial aspect of the pericardium **(P)**. No myocardium is seen in this micrograph, but epicardial fat **(Fa)** is readily identifiable. Acute pericarditis most commonly occurs after death of underlying cardiac muscle *(myocardial infarction)*.

Clinical features and nomenclature of acute inflammatory processes

The vascular and exudative phenomena of acute inflammation are responsible for the clinical features and were described by Celsus in the first century AD. The *cardinal signs of Celsus* are:

- **redness** (rubor) caused by hyperaemia

- **swelling** (tumor) caused by fluid exudation and hyperaemia

- **heat** (calor) caused by hyperaemia

- **pain** (dolor) resulting from release of bradykinin and PGE_2.

   Virchow later added:

- **loss of function** (functio laesa) caused by the combined effects of the above.

   Clinically, patients who have significant acute inflammation feel unwell and have a fever. This is mediated by cytokines released into the blood *(interleukins 1 and 6 (IL-1 and IL-6* respectively), *tumour necrosis factor (TNF)* and prostaglandins), acting on the hypothalamus. Laboratory investigations commonly reveal a raised neutrophil count in the blood (neutrophil leukocytosis).

   The nomenclature used to describe inflammation in different tissues employs the tissue name (or its Greek or Latin equivalent) and the suffix '-itis'. For example, inflammation of the appendix is referred to as *appendicitis*, inflammation of the Fallopian tube is termed *salpingitis* and inflammation of the pericardium is termed *pericarditis*. Notable exceptions to this rule include *pleurisy*, for inflammation of the pleura and acute *cellulitis* for inflammation of subcutaneous tissues. Many examples of acute inflammatory diseases are presented in the systematic pathology chapters, which form the second half of this book. Common examples are outlined in Table 3.1.

Table 3.1 **Nomenclature and aetiology of common types of inflammation.**

Tissue	Acute inflammation	Typical causes
Meninges	Meningitis	Bacterial and viral infections
Brain	Encephalitis	Viral infections
Lung	Pneumonia	Bacterial infections
Pleura	Pleurisy	Bacterial and viral infections
Pericardium	Pericarditis	Bacterial and viral infections, myocardial infarction
Oesophagus	Oesophagitis	Gastric acid reflux, fungal infection (*Candida albicans*)
Stomach	Gastritis	*Helicobacter pylori* infection, reflux/chemical gastritis
Colon	Colitis	Bacterial infections, inflammatory bowel disease
Rectum	Proctitis	Infections, ulcerative colitis
Appendix	Appendicitis	Faecal obstruction
Liver	Hepatitis	Alcohol abuse, viral infections
Gallbladder	Cholecystitis	Bacterial infections, chemical irritation
Pancreas	Pancreatitis	Obstructed pancreatic duct, alcoholism, shock
Urinary bladder	Cystitis	Bacterial infections
Bone	Osteomyelitis	Bacterial infections
Subcutaneous tissues	Cellulitis	Bacterial infections
Joints	Arthritis	Infections, autoimmune diseases
Arteries	Arteritis	Immune complex deposition
Kidney	Pyelonephritis	Bacterial infections
Peritoneum	Peritonitis	Spread from intra-abdominal inflammation, e.g. appendicitis, salpingitis Ruptured viscus, e.g. perforated peptic ulcer

KEY TO FIGURE
Ex exudate   **F** fibrin   **Fa** pericardial fat   **N** neutrophils   **P** pericardium

Outcomes of acute inflammation

The process of acute inflammation is designed to neutralise injurious agents and to restore the tissue to useful function. There are four main outcomes of acute inflammation (if the patient survives): *resolution*, *healing by fibrosis*, *abscess formation* and *progression to chronic inflammation*. Three factors determine which of these outcomes occurs:

■ the severity of tissue damage

■ the capacity of stem cells within the damaged tissue to divide and replace the specialised cells required, a process termed *regeneration*

■ the type of agent that has caused the tissue damage.

Resolution involves complete restitution of normal tissue architecture and function. This can only occur if the connective framework of the tissue is intact and the tissue involved has the capacity to replace any specialised cells that have been lost (regeneration). Neutrophils and damaged/dead tissue are removed by phagocytosis by macrophages (E-Fig. 3.5**H**), which leave the tissue via the lymphatics. Regeneration of tissues plays an important part in resolution, for example re-growth of alveolar lining cells following pneumonia: this regrowth is dependent on the intrinsic ability of resident stem cells to divide and differentiate into mature tissue cells. Examples of resolution are recovery from sunburn (acute inflammatory response in the skin as a result of ultraviolet radiation exposure) and the restitution of normal lung structure and function following lobar pneumonia (see Figs 3.3 and 3.7).

Healing by fibrosis (scar formation) occurs when there is substantial damage to the connective tissue framework and/or the tissue lacks the ability to regenerate specialised cells. In these instances, dead tissues and acute inflammatory exudate are first removed from the damaged area by macrophages (see Fig. 3.6), and the defect becomes filled by ingrowth of a specialised vascular connective tissue called *granulation tissue* (see Fig. 3.8). This is called *organisation*. The granulation tissue gradually produces collagen to form a *fibrous (collagenous) scar*, constituting the process of *repair* (see Figs 3.8 and 3.9). Despite the loss of some specialised cells and some architectural distortion caused by the fibrous scar, structural integrity is re-established. Any impairment of function is dependent on the extent of loss of specialised cells. Modified forms of fibrous repair occur in bone after a fracture when new bone is created (see Fig. 3.11), and in brain with the formation of an astrocytic scar (see Fig. 23.2).

Abscess formation takes place when the acute inflammatory reaction fails to destroy/remove the cause of tissue damage and continues, usually with a component of chronic inflammation. This is most common in the case of infection by pyogenic bacteria. As the acute inflammation progresses, there is liquefaction of the tissue to form *pus.* At the periphery of this acute abscess, a chronic inflammatory component surrounds the area and fibrous tissue is laid down, walling off the suppuration (see Fig. 3.12).

Chronic inflammation may result following acute inflammation when an injurious agent persists over a prolonged period, causing concomitant tissue destruction, inflammation, organisation and repair. Some injurious agents elicit a chronic inflammatory type of response from the outset. Chronic inflammation is discussed fully in Ch. 4.

INFLAMMATION OUT OF CONTROL

Inflammation can do harm as well as good. In most people, inflammation is activated appropriately in response to some kind of adverse stimulus and terminated promptly when the infective organisms have been eliminated and tissue damage repaired. In some individuals, control of the inflammatory process is lost; this is called *autoimmune disease*.

One of the major stimuli of acute inflammation is a type of adaptive immune response where *specific* antibodies recruit components of the acute inflammatory response as effector mechanisms, thereby directing the non-specific components of the acute inflammatory system at *specific* targets (E-Fig. 3.6).

Normally, the immune system is programmed to ignore antigenic stimuli within the individual's own body, a process known as *self-tolerance*. When this self-tolerance is lost for one or more antigens, *autoimmune disease* results. These may be organ-specific antigens as in the organ-specific autoimmune disease *Hashimoto's thyroiditis* (see Fig. 20.3) or, at the other end of the spectrum, the antigens triggering the response may be widespread in many tissues, as in *systemic lupus erythematosus (SLE)*, where the body reacts to double-stranded DNA as well as many other cellular antigens, causing systemic disease.

In many autoimmune disorders, inflammation and pain may cause major morbidity. Also, the misdirection of the immune response causes local tissue damage such as pain and swelling in the joints in rheumatoid arthritis (see Fig. 22.11) or renal failure due to renal damage in SLE. Many anti-inflammatory drugs are available but side effects are common and can be potentially serious. Recently, immunomodulating therapies have been used to treat some inflammatory conditions, e.g. anti-TNF antibodies in rheumatoid arthritis and inflammatory bowel disease. These therapies can have side effects, including an increased propensity to some infective organisms such as *Mycobacterium tuberculosis*, highlighting the complex immunomodulating role of biological therapies.

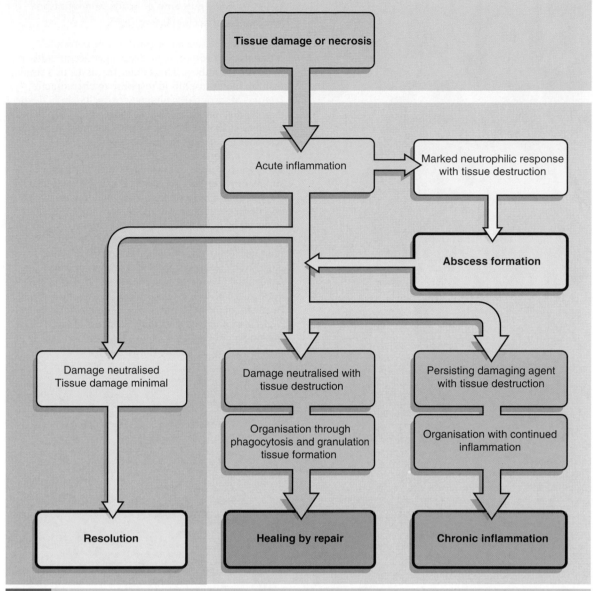

Fig. 3.5 **Outcomes of acute inflammation.**

The flow chart in Fig. 3.5 summarises the main outcomes following acute inflammation. If the tissue damage is minimal, as in mild acute inflammation then resolution is possible, but complete resolution is uncommon. Acute inflammation usually leads to tissue damage.

If the inflammation then resolves, the inflamed area heals with formation of a fibrous scar. If the inflammation persists and there is ongoing tissue damage, chronic inflammation ensues (see Ch. 4).

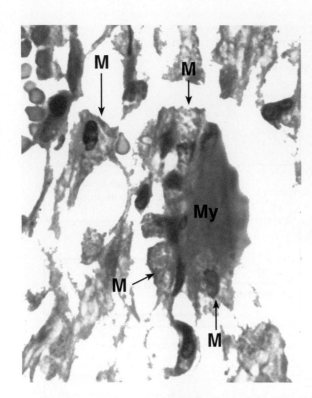

Fig. 3.6 **Early outcome of acute inflammation: macrophage accumulation (HP).**

As early as the second or third day of the acute inflammatory response, macrophages accumulate in increasing numbers. These enter the tissue in a similar fashion to neutrophils in response to chemotactic factors. Macrophages phagocytose cell debris, dead neutrophils and fibrin. At the same time, lymphocytes begin to enter the damaged area, reflecting an immune response to any introduced antigens.

Fig. 3.6 shows an area of cardiac muscle that has undergone necrosis following blockage of its arterial supply *(myocardial infarction)*. The acute inflammatory response has almost run its course, and the neutrophils and fibrin predominant in the earlier stages have been removed by macrophages. All that remains is a soft, loose tissue containing a few necrotic myocardial remnants **(My)**, one of which is shown here being engulfed by macrophages **(M)**. The macrophages can be identified under these circumstances by the foamy appearance of their cytoplasm, which also often contains brownish pigment granules. These brown granules are iron-containing pigments *(haemosiderin)* derived from haemoglobin. Further details of the events following myocardial infarction are shown in Fig. 10.2.

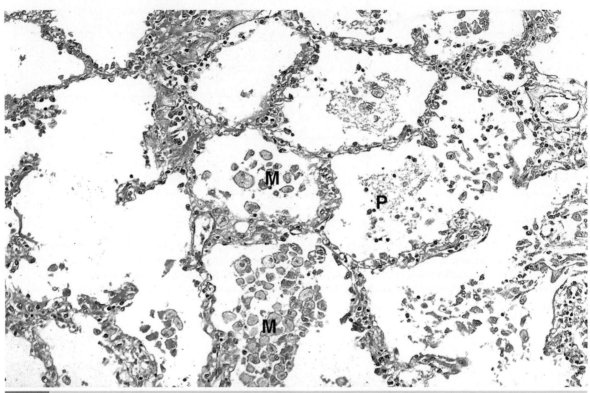

Fig. 3.7 **Resolution of acute inflammation: lobar pneumonia (MP).**

Occasionally, a damaging stimulus might excite a strong acute inflammatory response with minimal tissue damage. In such circumstances, resolution of the exudate might occur without any need for organisation and repair, thereby leaving no residual tissue scarring.

This phenomenon occurs in lobar pneumonia (Fig. 3.7), in which the acute inflammatory response is due to infection by a bacterium, commonly the pneumococcus (see Fig. 3.3). The alveoli of one or more lobes of the lung are filled with acute inflammatory exudate and the loss of respiratory function may be so great as to cause fatal *hypoxia*. In the pre-antibiotic era, this was a common cause of death in previously fit young people.

Bacteria are engulfed by neutrophils and fibrin strands are broken down by *fibrinolysins* derived from plasma and neutrophil lysosomes. Macrophages **(M)** are recruited and phagocytose apoptotic neutrophils, extravasated red cells and other cell debris. Fluid and degraded proteinaceous material **(P)**, together with the macrophages, are then resorbed into the circulation via alveolar wall vessels and interstitial lymphatics or may be coughed up as brown-coloured sputum. Alveolar spaces are thus cleared of exudate and can participate in gas exchange. Regeneration of alveolar lining cells completes the return to normal structure and function.

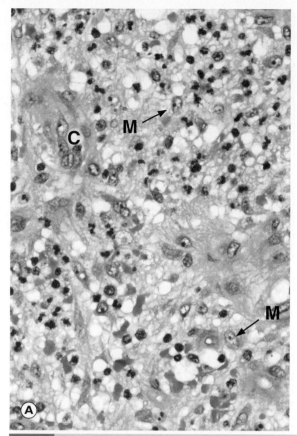

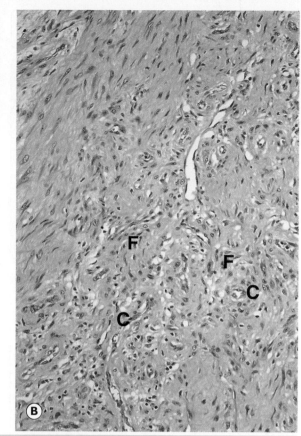

Fig. 3.8 **Granulation tissue.** **(A)** Vascular granulation tissue (HP); **(B)** fibrous granulation tissue (MP).

Where there is significant damage to the connective tissue framework, the first phase of the healing process is the formation of **granulation tissue**, a mixture of proliferating capillaries, fibroblasts and inflammatory cells. Formation of a network of new capillaries **(C)** **(angiogenesis)** occurs by a combination of budding from vessels at the periphery of the damaged area and from endothelial precursor cells. This is stimulated by growth factors such as **vascular endothelial growth factor (VEGF)**. In this early form, called **vascular granulation tissue** (Fig. 3.8A), the spaces between the capillaries are occupied by macrophages, lymphocytes, proliferating fibroblasts and loose oedematous extracellular matrix. The capillaries are thin-walled and relatively leaky, leading to extravasation of erythrocytes and fluid into the tissue. Students often confuse granulation tissue with **granulomas** (see Ch. 4) but the two are quite different.

Over time, most of the vessels regress, collagen is laid down, and the inflammatory cells return to the circulation. The effect of this progression is seen in Fig. 3.8B, where numerous plump activated

fibroblasts **(F)** can be seen with a few residual lymphocytes and relatively inconspicuous capillaries **(C)**. This is called **fibrous granulation tissue** in recognition of the presence of mature collagenous fibrous tissue. Collagen, laid down by the fibroblasts, becomes remodelled in an orderly pattern (upper left area of micrograph) and the fibrous granulation tissue takes on the characteristics of an early **fibrous scar** (see Fig. 3.10).

Granulation tissue is also involved in healing of wounds, whatever the cause and site of the tissue defect. In the case of a simple skin incision, where the wound edges are in close apposition and the actual defect is minimal, healing occurs quickly with a small amount of granulation tissue and is termed **healing by primary intention**. In other situations, the tissue defect will be large and filled with blood clot and a variable amount of tissue debris. In this case, described as **healing by secondary intention**, organisation and filling of the defect by granulation tissue take considerably longer (Fig. 3.9).

DELAYED WOUND HEALING
Many factors can delay or stop healing. A common factor is continuing inflammation where the initial stimulus to inflammation persists: a good example of this would be an infected wound or persistent peptic ulceration due to *Helicobacter pylori* infection (see Ch. 13). The presence of dead tissue or a foreign body in a wound can delay healing, as well as host factors such as poor nutrition, poor circulation, pre-existing diabetes mellitus or medications such as steroids.

KEY TO FIGURES
C capillary   **F** fibroblasts   **M** macrophage   **My** myocardial remnant   **P** proteinaceous debris

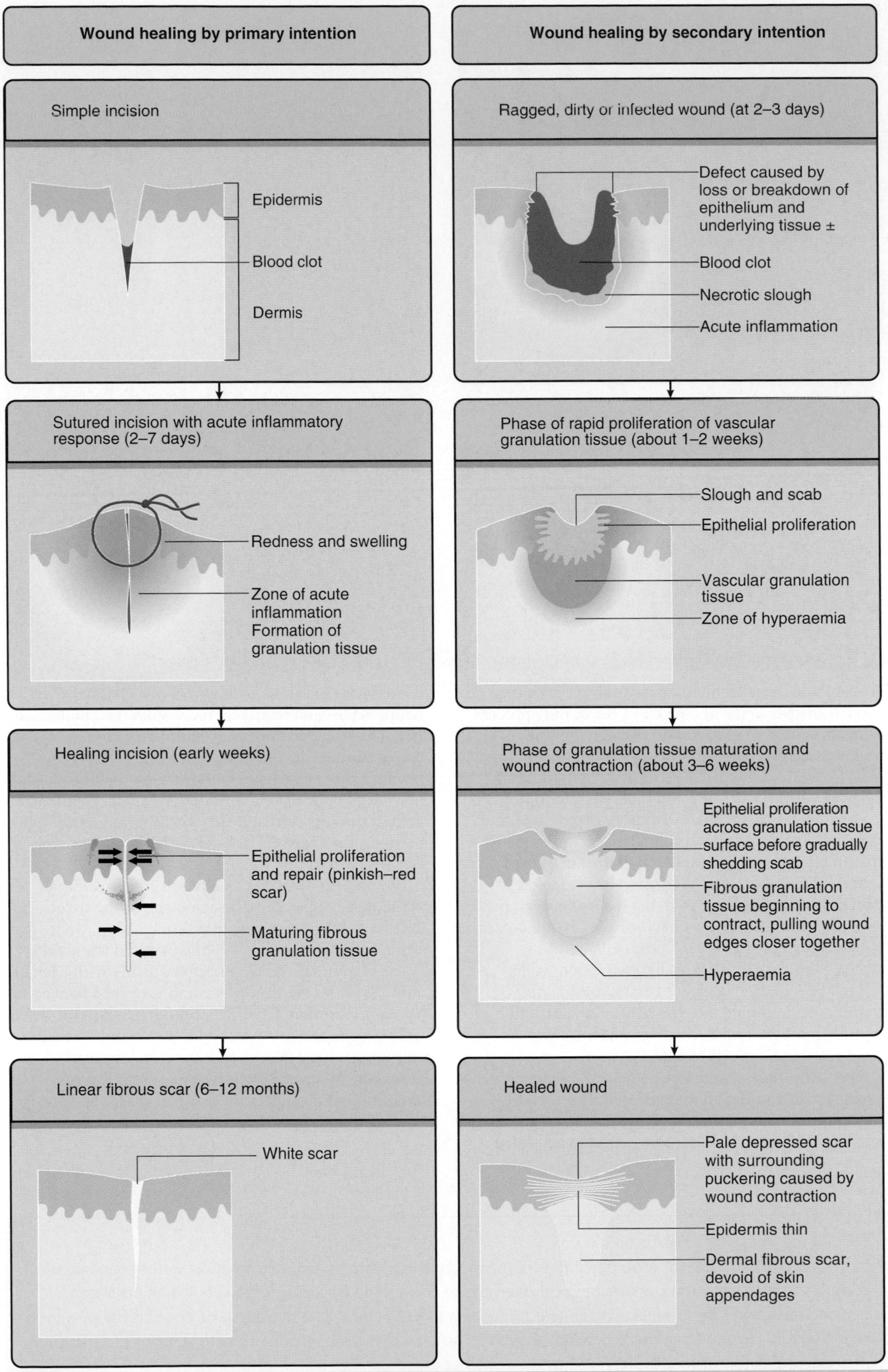

Wound healing by primary intention

Simple incision

Epidermis

Blood clot

Dermis

Sutured incision with acute inflammatory response (2–7 days)

Redness and swelling

Zone of acute inflammation
Formation of granulation tissue

Healing incision (early weeks)

Epithelial proliferation and repair (pinkish–red scar)

Maturing fibrous granulation tissue

Linear fibrous scar (6–12 months)

White scar

Wound healing by secondary intention

Ragged, dirty or infected wound (at 2–3 days)

Defect caused by loss or breakdown of epithelium and underlying tissue ±

Blood clot

Necrotic slough

Acute inflammation

Phase of rapid proliferation of vascular granulation tissue (about 1–2 weeks)

Slough and scab

Epithelial proliferation

Vascular granulation tissue

Zone of hyperaemia

Phase of granulation tissue maturation and wound contraction (about 3–6 weeks)

Epithelial proliferation across granulation tissue surface before gradually shedding scab

Fibrous granulation tissue beginning to contract, pulling wound edges closer together

Hyperaemia

Healed wound

Pale depressed scar with surrounding puckering caused by wound contraction

Epidermis thin

Dermal fibrous scar, devoid of skin appendages

Fig. 3.9 **The processes involved in wound healing.** The left column shows the process of wound healing by primary intention. This process would occur in incised, somewhat shallow wounds. The right column shows healing by secondary intention, a process that usually occurs in ragged, deeper wounds or wounds that are infected.

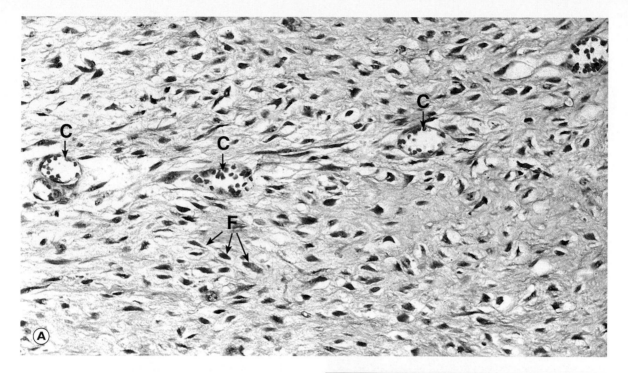

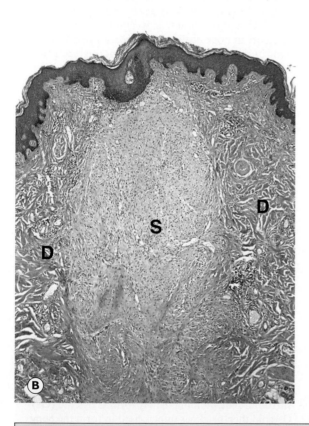

Fig. 3.10 **Fibrous scar.** **(A)** Fibrous scar tissue (HP);
(B) skin scar (LP).

The deposition of collagen within fibrous granulation tissue occurs over a period of many weeks. Collagen is remodelled in an appropriate orientation to withstand the tensile stresses placed on the area of repair. With time, the previously plump and metabolically active fibroblasts regress and become relatively inconspicuous, as shown in Fig. 3.10A, a micrograph of a typical area of early fibrous scar. Note the condensed nuclei of inactive fibroblasts **(F)**. Some capillaries **(C)** persist, accounting for the red appearance of recent scars.

The micrograph in Fig. 3.10B illustrates, at low magnification, a recent area of scarring in the skin after healing of a simple incision for biopsy of a skin tumour. Immature collagenous tissue forms a pale scar **(S)**, which interrupts the normal pink collagen of the dermis **(D)** on either side. There are no skin appendages in a skin scar. During the ensuing months and years, the cellularity of the scar diminishes, there is progressive loss of capillary vessels and the scar contracts so that after many years, a skin scar may be virtually undetectable with the naked eye. Note that healing of skin of mucous membrane involves epithelialisation of the surface by proliferation of epithelium at the edges of the defect (i.e. epithelial regeneration).

KELOID

Keloid is the name given to excessive formation of scar tissue. Some individuals have a tendency to form excessive amounts of collagen. When this occurs but does not extend beyond the bounds of the pre-existing wound, it is called a ***hypertrophic scar***. However, when is extends beyond the pre-existing scar, it is called ***keloid*** and can give rise to a very unsightly appearance. Unfortunately, attempts to remove the excessive scar tissue surgically can give rise to even more keloid formation and a poor cosmetic outcome.

KEY TO FIGURES
C capillaries   **D** dermis   **F** fibroblasts   **S** scar

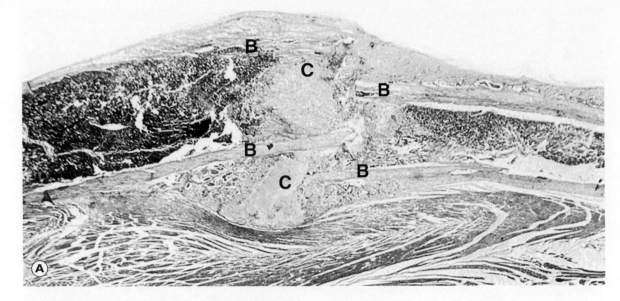

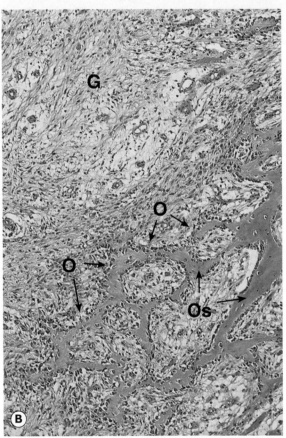

Fig. 3.11 **Specialised healing in bone. (A)** LP; **(B)** HP.

In most tissues, fibrous scar forms a functionally adequate, albeit unspecialised, replacement for damaged tissues. In bone, the replacement of damaged tissue by fibrous scar is inadequate for restoration of function (e.g. weight bearing) and therefore in bone healing the processes that form bone during embryonic development are reactivated. This leads to new bone formation, a process of *regeneration* rather than *repair*. As in other forms of wound healing, the process is carefully controlled and orchestrated by an array of mediators, including platelet-derived growth factor (PDGF), transforming growth factor β (TGFβ), fibroblast growth factors (FGF) and bone morphogenetic proteins (BMPs).

Immediately following fracture, there is bleeding in and around the fracture site resulting in a mass of coagulated blood, a *haematoma*. An initial acute inflammatory response is rapidly followed by organisation of the haematoma with formation of granulation tissue as described in Fig. 3.8. In the case of bone fracture, this granulation tissue is termed *provisional* or *soft tissue callus* **(C)** and forms around the broken ends of the bone **(B)**, loosely uniting them; this is seen at low magnification in Fig. 3.11A. Mesenchymal stem cells found in the cambium layer of the periosteum are activated and divide and differentiate into *chondrocytes* and *osteoblasts* to produce cartilaginous matrix and osteoid, the organic matrix of bone, respectively. This is seen in Fig. 3.11B where typical granulation tissue **(G)** at the top of the field gives way to osteoblasts **(O)**, which surround pink-staining, newly formed osteoid **(Os)**. Osteoid then becomes mineralised to form the *bony callus* between the two fractured ends. This initial bone is haphazardly arranged (known as *woven bone*) and, over the next few months, undergoes extensive remodelling by osteoclasts and osteoblasts to form lamellar bone with trabecular architecture, best suited to resist local stresses. The end result is normal bony architecture and function.

KEY TO FIGURES
B bone **C** provisional callus **Ca** capillaries **F** fibrin **G** granulation tissue **N** neutrophils
O osteoblasts **Os** osteoid

NON-UNION OF FRACTURES

While most fractures heal completely and well with modern management, in some individuals, there is delay in complete healing of a fracture; in others there may be cessation of the healing process without restitution of functional bone, known as **non-union**. A wide range of factors may contribute to delayed or failed healing, the most important of which are poor immobilisation, poor blood supply, poor nutrition (lack of protein, vitamin C, etc.), the presence of infection and foreign bodies or fragments of necrotic bone in the fracture. Old age, drugs such as steroids and non-steroidal anti-inflammatory drugs (NSAIDs), diabetes mellitus, burns and irradiation may also delay or stop healing.

TYPES OF FRACTURE

Fractures are described as **complete** or **incomplete** depending on whether the entire thickness of the bone is fractured. In **closed** fractures the overlying skin is intact, while **compound** fractures include disruption of the overlying skin. A **comminuted** fracture has multiple separate bone fragments. **Pathological fractures** occur in bone with pre-existing disease, such as osteoporosis or metastatic tumour. **Greenstick fracture** is an incomplete fracture where there is initial bending with partial fracture of the side under tension: it typically occurs in children.

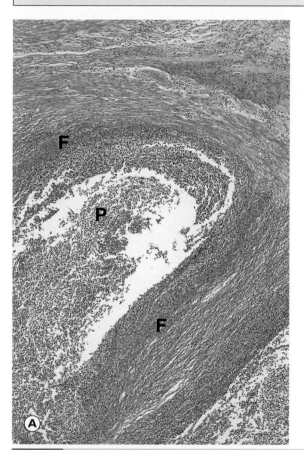

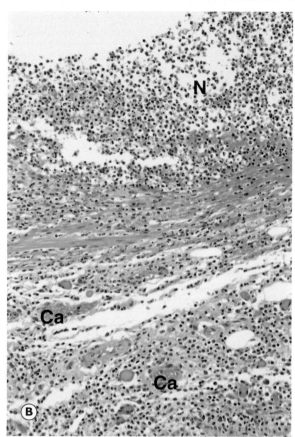

Fig. 3.12 **Abscess formation. (A)** LP; **(B)** HP.

An abscess is a localised collection of pus, which usually develops following extensive tissue damage by one of the pyogenic bacteria, such as *Staphylococcus aureus*. Such organisms excite an inflammatory exudate in which neutrophils predominate. In these circumstances, large numbers of neutrophils die, releasing their lysosomal enzymes and undergoing autolysis; the resulting viscous fluid, **pus**, contains dead and dying neutrophils, necrotic tissue debris and the fluid component of the acute inflammatory exudate with a little fibrin. Pyogenic bacteria often remain viable within the abscess cavity and may cause enlargement of the lesion, which is described as an **acute abscess**. At an early stage, expansion of the lesion is limited by the processes of organisation and repair at the margins of the abscess. Thus, the abscess may become walled off, isolating the bacteria-containing pus and preventing further spread; an

abscess encapsulated by granulation and fibrous tissue is termed a **chronic abscess**. On the other hand, if the bacteria are highly virulent and present in large numbers, such attempts at organisation and repair may be overwhelmed and expansion of the abscess ensues with destruction of surrounding tissue. The coexistence of active tissue damage and attempts at repair are typical of **chronic inflammation** (see Ch. 4).

Fig. 3.12A shows an abscess in the wall of the colon. The centre consists of a collection of pus **(P)**. At its margin is a pink-staining zone of fibrin **(F)**. As yet, there is little evidence of organisation at the margins of the abscess; this therefore represents an acute abscess. Fig. 3.12B shows the wall and lumen of a chronic abscess at high power, illustrating the neutrophils **(N)** and tissue debris in the cavity of the abscess and the capillaries **(Ca)** in the inflamed granulation tissue of the wall.

Table 3.2 Chapter review.

Concept	Definition/main features	Figure
Three major components of the acute inflammatory response	1. Oedema due to increased fluid in tissue 2. Dilated vessels 3. Infiltration by inflammatory cells: mainly neutrophils in the early stages and macrophages later	3.1, 3.2, 3.3, 3.4
Five cardinal signs of acute inflammation	1. Redness 2. Heat 3. Pain 4. Swelling 5. Loss of function	
Mediators of acute inflammation	1. Vasodilatation: histamine, prostaglandins, nitric oxide 2. Increased vascular permeability: serotonin (5-HT), histamine, C5a, C3a and leukotrienes 3. Leukocyte activation and chemotaxis: C5a, leukotriene B4, various chemokines and bacterial products	3.1, 3.2
Outcomes of acute inflammation	1. Complete resolution 2. Healing by fibrosis (scar) 3. Abscess formation 4. Progression to chronic inflammation 5. Loss of self-tolerance leading to autoimmune disease	3.5, 3.6, 3.7, 3.8, 3.12 and clinical box (Inflammation out of control).
Wound healing	■ May be by primary or secondary intention ■ Results in fibrous scar formation ■ Process differs in specialised tissues such as bone	3.9, 3.10, 3.11

4 Chronic inflammation

Introduction

In developed countries, where the major pyogenic infections have been brought more or less under control, chronic inflammatory conditions result in a huge burden of morbidity and mortality. In less industrialised countries, certain infections, such as tuberculosis, typically cause a chronic inflammatory response and are responsible for a large amount of disease. By definition chronic inflammation lasts longer than acute inflammation. Different stimuli may cause variations in the morphological appearances but, overall, in the chronic inflammatory infiltrate lymphocytes, macrophages and plasma cells predominate, in contrast to acute inflammation where the major cell type is the neutrophil. The hallmark features of chronic inflammation are ongoing tissue damage, a chronic inflammatory infiltrate and fibrosis. Chronic inflammation may be subdivided as follows:

- **Non-specific chronic inflammation**: arises following non-resolution of acute inflammation, e.g. chronic peptic ulcer, chronic abscess

- **Specific (primary) chronic inflammation**: arises *de novo* in response to certain types of injurious agents, e.g. rheumatoid arthritis, idiopathic pulmonary fibrosis

- **Granulomatous inflammation**: is a subset of specific chronic inflammation characterised by the presence of granulomas, e.g. sarcoidosis, tuberculosis (see Ch. 5).

Non-specific chronic inflammation

Chronic inflammation may arise following an episode of acute inflammation (see Ch. 3) where the acute inflammatory response has not been adequate to neutralise or destroy the noxious stimulus. In this situation, tissue damage, acute inflammation, granulation tissue, tissue repair and chronic inflammation co-exist. There may be active tissue damage in one area with ongoing acute inflammation, while in adjacent areas fibrosis and a chronic inflammatory infiltrate are seen. The chronic inflammatory infiltrate is dominated by tissue macrophages, lymphocytes and plasma cells (Fig. 4.1), in contrast to the marked preponderance of neutrophils in the acute inflammatory response. This type of chronic inflammation represents a dynamic balance between tissue destruction and repair. The course of the disease might include repeated acute phases when tissue damage is predominant and intervening chronic phases when chronic inflammation smoulders along with ongoing tissue repair. The outcome of non-specific chronic inflammation depends on whether local and systemic factors favour the injurious agent or the process of healing (Table 4.1). Chronic inflammation usually heals by fibrosis.

Table 4.1 Factors that affect healing.

Factors that impair resolution and healing	Factors that aid resolution and healing
Poor nutrition	Administration of appropriate antibiotics
Immunosuppression	Surgical removal of foreign material
Persisting tissue damage and/or infection	Surgical removal of dead tissue
Retained foreign material	General attempts to improve nutrition
Sequestered dead tissue	Drugs that specifically modify the inflammatory response
Poor blood supply	
Deficiency of intrinsic anti-inflammatory factors	
Diabetes mellitus and other chronic illnesses	
Certain medications, such as corticosteroids	
Older age	

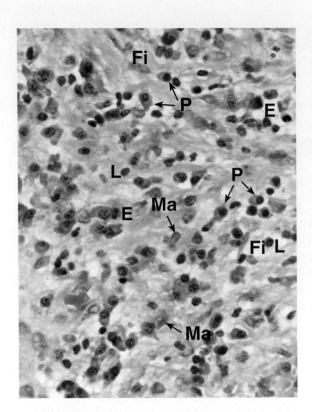

Fig. 4.1 Cells in chronic inflammation (HP).

In chronic inflammation, the major infiltrating cells types are **macrophages**, **lymphocytes** and **plasma cells** (sometimes collectively called **mononuclear cells**) as well as **eosinophils**, **mast cells** and some **neutrophils**. These cells may be derived from resident tissue populations and/or migrate into the tissue from the circulating blood. As well as killing and disposing of infective organisms, inflammatory cells secrete a wide variety of soluble factors that regulate the inflammatory and healing processes.

In Fig. 4.1, plasma cells **(P)** are identified by their amphophilic (purple) cytoplasm and eccentric 'clock face' nuclei. Plasma cells are differentiated B lymphocytes that are committed to antibody production. Lymphocytes **(L)** are seen as dark, rounded nuclei with a thin, almost invisible, rim of basophilic cytoplasm. These are the effector cells of the specific immune response and include both helper and cytotoxic T cells as well as B cells. Macrophages **(Ma)** are recognised by their oval or kidney-bean-shaped nuclei and pale cytoplasm. Eosinophils **(E)** have bilobed nuclei and brightly eosinophilic granules in their cytoplasm. When stimulated, eosinophils release their granule contents, including major basic protein, a substance that is effective in killing parasites. Some neutrophils and many active fibroblasts **(Fi)** are also commonly found in chronic inflammation.

Fibroblasts secrete the components of the extracellular matrix including collagen. When the damaging stimulus has been removed and repair is completed, often after weeks or months, these cells progressively disappear from the tissue.

Fig. 4.2 Chronic peptic ulcer. (A) Entire ulcer (LP); **(B)** surface layers of ulcer (MP); **(C)** deep layers of ulcer (MP). *(Illustrations opposite)*

A common example, which illustrates the principles of non-specific chronic inflammation, is the localised chronic ulceration of the stomach or duodenum, most often in individuals infected by ***Helicobacter pylori***; such lesions are collectively referred to as chronic peptic ulcers. By definition, an ***ulcer*** extends through the full thickness of the mucosa; an ***erosion*** is a lesion involving only the superficial mucosa.

Ulceration is caused by an imbalance between damaging factors (gastric acid and peptic enzymes) and protective factors (gastric mucus secretion, local secretion of alkali).

H. pylori does not invade the tissues but inhabits the protective mucus layer that covers the surface of the mucosa (see Fig. 13.9). It has a unique ability to survive the acid environment of the stomach because of a bacterial enzyme, ***urease***. This allows it to produce ammonia by splitting urea, raising pH in the immediate vicinity of the organism. It typically colonises the antrum and, by producing a localised alkaline environment here, *H. pylori* interferes with normal physiological control of gastric acid secretion. The falsely high antral pH stimulates secretion of ***gastrin*** by the antral G cells, which acts upon the oxyntic cells in the corpus to increase acid production still further. This excess acid production overwhelms normal mucosal defence mechanisms, leading to the formation of an acute ulcer. If the process proceeds unchecked, the ulcer can burrow through the full thickness of the stomach or duodenal wall, leading to perforation and escape of gut contents into the peritoneal cavity (see Fig. 13.10).

Often, the destructive process is arrested by an acute inflammatory response. Tissue repair then begins with the formation of granulation tissue; if conditions are favourable, repair may be effective, leaving a fibrous scar. If tissue destruction continues, the concurrent organisation and repair result in chronic inflammation. A chronic peptic ulcer reflects this dynamic balance between tissue destruction and repair. A section through a chronic ulcer is shown in Fig. 4.2A (see E-Fig. 4.1**H**). The ulcerated surface is covered in a slough **(Sl)**, composed of a pink-staining layer of necrotic debris combined with the fibrin and neutrophils of an acute inflammatory exudate. Beneath the slough is a zone of vascular granulation tissue **(V)**; these features are seen at a higher magnification in Fig. 4.2B. The next layer is a zone of fibrous granulation tissue **(F)**, seen in detail in Fig. 4.2 C. Deeper still in the ulcer base, is a fibrous scar **(Sc)**. In this deep ulcer, the muscular wall **(M)** is completely replaced by the ulcer crater, granulation tissue and scar. If a large blood vessel is present in the ulcer base, erosion into the vessel leads to bleeding into the stomach, giving rise to ***haematemesis*** (vomiting blood) or ***melaena*** (black, tar-like faeces composed of altered blood).

The outcome of chronic peptic ulceration depends on whether conditions favour ongoing tissue damage or repair. If healing is favoured, fibrous tissue gradually repairs the ulcer crater and mucosa regenerates from the ulcer margins to cover the epithelial defect and protect the fibrous tissue from further damage. A healed peptic ulcer thus consists of an area of fibrous scarring replacing all or part of the thickness of the stomach wall. Internally, the regenerated mucosa is usually puckered because of contraction of the underlying scarred wall (E-Fig. 4.2**G**).

KEY TO FIGURES
E eosinophil   **F** fibrous granulation tissue   **Fi** fibroblast   **L** lymphocyte   **M** muscular wall
Ma macrophage   **P** plasma cells   **Sc** scar   **Sl** necrotic slough   **V** vascular granulation tissue

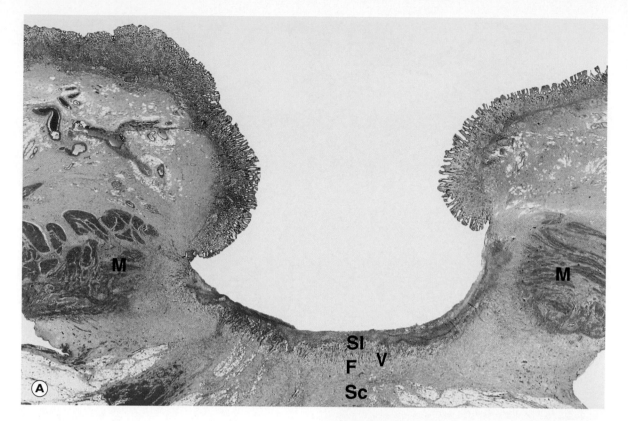

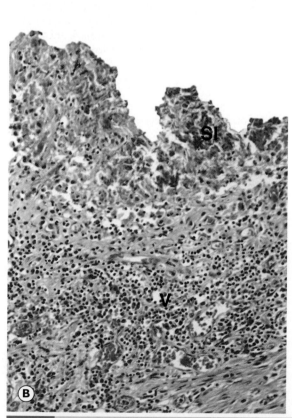

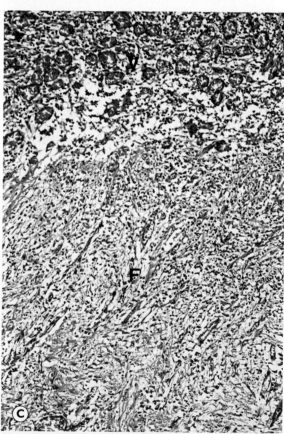

Fig. 4.2 **Chronic peptic ulcer.** (*Caption opposite*)

CLINICAL MANAGEMENT OF PEPTIC ULCER DISEASE

Understanding of the role of *H. pylori* has revolutionised management of peptic ulceration. In the past, peptic ulcers were treated by surgical procedures, which aimed to reduce acid production, such as partial gastrectomy (to remove the antral source of gastrin) or vagotomy and pyloroplasty (removing the vagal-driven pathway of acid secretion but requiring release of the pylorus since the vagus also controls gastric emptying). Such operations were associated with considerable morbidity. Conventional medical management of peptic ulcer disease employed a range of drugs, from simple alkalis to neutralise excess acid, through various drugs, which interfere with normal physiological control of acid secretion (e.g. adrenergic antagonists and histamine (H2) receptor blockers) to the more recent use of *proton pump inhibitors (PPIs)*, which effectively block the final common pathway of acid production. Although acid-blocking drugs were usually effective, treatment had to continue for the rest of the patient's life. Now, treatment usually requires only a short course of eradication therapy, using a combination of two antibiotics with a proton-pump inhibitor *(triple therapy)*.

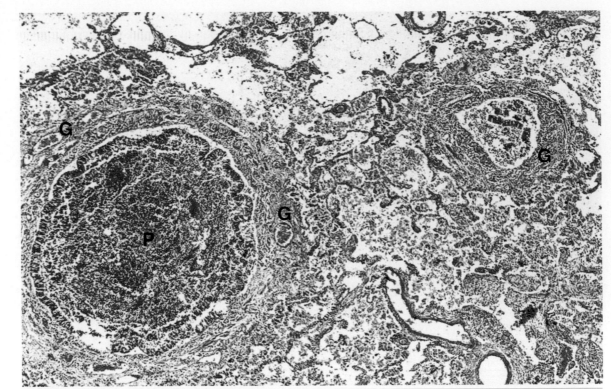

Fig. 4.3 Bronchiectasis (LP).

Bronchiectasis is a chronic inflammation of the bronchi associated with destruction of the wall and permanent dilatation (E-Fig. 4.3 **G**). In most cases, repeated episodes of infection and obstruction lead to progressive destruction of the normal elastic and muscular components of the airway wall. Obstruction may be due to foreign bodies in bronchi, tumour, structural abnormalities or stasis of secretions, perhaps related to ciliary malfunction or cystic fibrosis. The elastic and muscular components of the bronchial wall are replaced by granulation tissue and later by fibrous tissue. This process weakens the wall,

leading to dilatation of the airway, which in turn predisposes to stagnation of secretions and further episodes of bacterial infection, creating a vicious cycle.

In this micrograph, two abnormal bronchi are seen (E-Fig. 4.4 **H**), each with the lumen filled with pus (**P**). The wall of each affected bronchus is formed of fibrovascular granulation tissue (**G**), in which there is a heavy infiltrate of dark-staining cells, just visible at this magnification; these cells are a mixture of plasma cells and lymphocytes. Bronchiectasis exemplifies the concept of co-existing tissue damage and attempts at repair, which are the hallmarks of chronic inflammation.

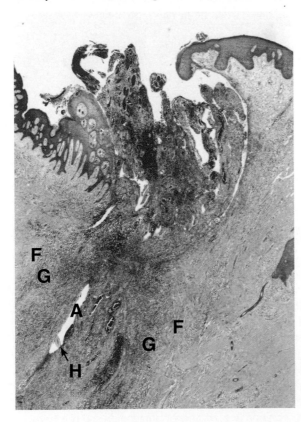

Fig. 4.4 Pilonidal sinus (LP).

A common example of a chronic abscess is the pilonidal sinus (Fig. 4.4). In this condition, a chronic subcutaneous abscess forms, most commonly seen in the sacrococcygeal area. Hair shafts (**H**), derived from locally destroyed follicles and shed body hair, are present in the abscess and act as a focus for chronic inflammation. Successful healing and repair are hindered by the persistence of the hairs, which are resistant to phagocytosis. Secondary infection may further complicate the process. As part of the attempt at healing, surface epithelium proliferates and comes to line the tract leading down into the abscess cavity (not seen in this micrograph); such a tract is known as a *sinus*.

In this micrograph, note the subcutaneous abscess cavity (**A**), the wall of which is formed by granulation tissue (**G**), heavily infiltrated by lymphocytes and plasma cells. There is surrounding fibrosis (**F**) in the dermis as a result of previous attempts at fibrous repair.

A pilonidal sinus, like any other chronic inflammatory lesion, will only heal if the source of persistent irritation is removed; surgical excision or laying open the complex of sinuses and abscess cavities is usually the only satisfactory method in this situation.

Specific (primary) chronic inflammation

This type of chronic inflammation arises by different mechanisms from non-specific chronic inflammation. Primary chronic inflammation may be either *granulomatous* or *non-granulomatous*. A key feature in chronic inflammation is the activation of macrophages, which orchestrate the chronic inflammatory response. Macrophages may become activated by either immune or non-immune mechanisms. Activated macrophages not only become more efficient at phagocytosis and killing of organisms, but also secrete a wide range of factors that control the behaviour of other inflammatory cells (e.g. chemotactic factors, lymphokines) and which induce fibrosis (e.g. fibrogenic cytokines, growth factors). The types of agent that can invoke primary chronic inflammation include:

■ Immunological

- Low-toxicity organisms such as *Treponema* sp., the causative organism of syphilis and yaws

- Infective organisms that grow within cells, e.g. viruses, *Mycobacteria*

- Hypersensitivity reactions such as hypersensitivity pneumonitis

- Autoimmune conditions such as systemic lupus erythematosus

- Infections by fungi, protozoa and parasites.

■ Non-immunological

- Foreign body reactions

- Inert noxious materials such as silica, talc, asbestos or beryllium.

Primary chronic inflammation of the immune type may be either granulomatous or non-granulomatous. A good example of the non-granulomatous immune type is hepatitis B virus infection (HBV) (see Fig. 14.3). Virus-infected cells in the liver incite a cell-mediated immune response, producing cytotoxic T lymphocytes, which kill virus-infected hepatocytes. Some individuals mount an effective immune response and clear the infection, whilst in others there is ongoing infiltration of the liver by lymphocytes over months or years, a condition known as *chronic active hepatitis*. In these people, there is continuing destruction of hepatocytes and fibrosis of the liver, which may eventually cause cirrhosis. As in many examples of chronic inflammation, the tissue damage is due to the inflammatory response rather than the virus itself. In non-immune type primary chronic inflammation, the mechanisms are less clear. However, certain materials such as silica can directly activate macrophages to release mediators that induce an inflammatory reaction and fibrosis.

Granulomatous inflammation

The defining feature of granulomatous inflammation is the presence of activated *epithelioid macrophages* and *multinucleate giant cells* derived from macrophages. Epithelioid macrophages are so named because they bear some resemblance histologically to epithelial (squamous) cells. These cells may form well-circumscribed *granulomas* (clusters), which are generally surrounded by lymphocytes, macrophages, fibroblasts and varying degrees of fibrosis. Granulomatous primary chronic inflammation may arise by either immune or non-immune mechanisms. The immune type, known as the *delayed hypersensitivity response*, is epitomised by tuberculosis (see Ch. 5). T lymphocytes responding to mycobacterial antigens are activated and divide and mature to produce helper T cells. The helper T cells in turn secrete lymphokines (e.g. interferon (IFN)-γ) that induce the transformation of macrophages into activated epithelioid macrophages and giant cells.

Non-immune granulomatous inflammation is exemplified by the foreign body reaction, for example in response to suture material after a surgical procedure, or when a rose thorn becomes embedded in the skin. Fig. 4.9 is an example of such a reaction and shows plant material (from faeces) embedded in the wall of the bowel in a patient with diverticular disease. In some granulomatous conditions such as Crohn's disease and sarcoidosis, the mechanism is unclear: infective causes have been postulated but never proven.

The term granuloma needs some clarification. In general, granuloma means a cluster of epithelioid macrophages as opposed to granulation tissue as defined in Ch. 3. However, in the past, 'granuloma' was applied to both a granuloma and granulation tissue and a few examples remain in current terminology where the old usage persists. Examples include an *apical granuloma* referring to a mass of granulation tissue at the root of a tooth and a *pyogenic granuloma* (lobular capillary haemangioma), which is a mass of granulation tissue in a healing wound.

KEY TO FIGURES
A abscess cavity **F** fibrosis **G** granulation tissue **H** hair shaft **P** pus

Some granulomas develop necrosis in their central area. The classical form is caseous necrosis, which is almost always found in tuberculosis (see Ch. 5). Caseous necrosis appears creamy macroscopically (caseous means 'like cream cheese'). By light microscopy, caseous necrosis is featureless and eosinophilic, containing few cells. Some other granulomatous conditions, such as atypical mycobacterial infection, also develop central necrosis but the necrosis is suppurative with plentiful neutrophils, often called *suppurating* or *necrotising granulomas*. Some common types of granulomatous inflammation are characterised by their lack of necrosis; examples of this type are Crohn's disease and sarcoidosis.

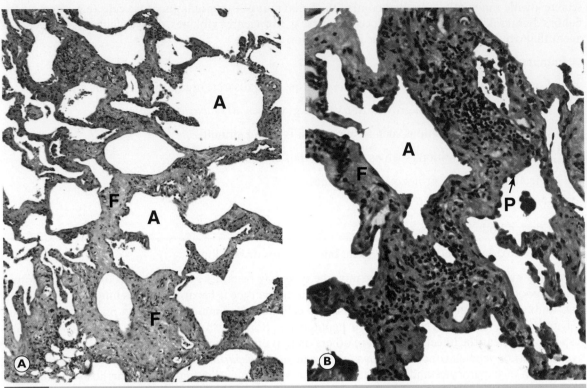

Idiopathic pulmonary fibrosis (or *cryptogenic fibrosing alveolitis*) is a good example of a chronic inflammatory condition that in its earliest phases has a chronic inflammatory infiltrate. At this early stage, it may be called *interstitial pneumonitis* (or *usual interstitial pneumonia*), where an unknown damaging agent repeatedly triggers the inflammation of the alveolar walls (E-Fig. 4.5 **H**) leading to extensive fibrosis as part of the healing process. Idiopathic pulmonary fibrosis is one of a group of disorders known as interstitial pneumonias.

The later stages of this process are well illustrated in these micrographs where the alveolar walls are thickened because of the deposition of dense fibrous tissue **(F)**. The thickened alveolar walls are distorted and less permeable to gases. In the final stages, there may be great distortion of alveoli, giving rise to greatly enlarged alveolar spaces **(A)**, known as *honeycomb lung* (see

Fig. 12.13, E-Fig. 4.6 **G**). In addition, there is damage to the alveolar lining cells and these are replaced by hyperplastic or regenerating type II pneumocytes. In Fig. 4.5A, the inflammatory infiltrate of lymphocytes and plasma cells is readily seen, as well as type 2 pneumocyte hyperplasia **(P)**, shown in Fig. 4.5B.

The usual presentation of idiopathic pulmonary fibrosis is of insidious onset of breathlessness associated with finger clubbing. However, a histologically identical picture may arise as an end stage of *diffuse alveolar damage* owing to oxygen toxicity in premature infants, i.e. *hyaline membrane disease* (see Fig. 12.12) and acute viral pneumonitis. The condition may also follow a range of other conditions such as hypersensitivity pneumonitis, drug toxicity, miliary tuberculosis, connective tissue disorders and sarcoidosis. Some of these disorders are associated with early granulomatous inflammation and this may still be apparent at the end stage.

CHRONIC FIBROSIS

Chronic fibrosis, whatever the cause, can be a cause of great morbidity and sometimes mortality. Fibrosis and scar formation are normal parts of tissue healing after significant damage. However, in some individuals, in association with certain insults, there is a tendency to develop excess fibrosis such that the fibrous tissue impairs organ function. Idiopathic pulmonary fibrosis as described above is one example; others include keloid scars and intra-abdominal adhesions that may arise and persist after abdominal surgery.

The underlying immune basis of a group of unusual fibrosing disorders (including retroperitoneal fibrosis, Riedel's thyroiditis, chronic sclerosing sialadenitis and autoimmune pancreatitis) has recently been recognised. These are now described using the term *IgG4 related disease.* All of these disorders are linked by the tendency to form tumour-like lesions with numerous lymphocytes and plasma cells, many of them IgG4 positive plasma cells, prominent *storiform* fibrosis (with the cells arranged in a cartwheel/woven pattern) and obliterative phlebitis (inflammation obliterating small veins). Some patients also have a raised serum IgG4 level.

Other instances of excessive fibrosis result from known causes (e.g. infections such as tuberculosis (see Ch. 5) and fibrosis of a transplanted kidney in chronic rejection.

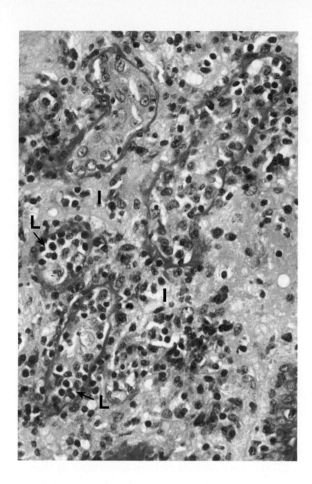

Fig. 4.6 Transplant rejection: kidney (LP).

Organ transplantation introduces non-self antigens into the recipient. Specifically, the HLA antigens (human leukocyte antigens) of the donor are rarely identical to those of the recipient, except in the case of transplantation of organs between identical twins. The HLA antigens of the donor excite both *antibody-* and *cell-mediated immune responses* in the recipient in an attempt to rid the body of the foreign material by killing donor cells. This is, of course, a gross simplification of the many and complex faces of transplant rejection, which are dealt with in more detail in Ch. 15. Fig. 4.6 illustrates a cell-mediated immune response to a transplanted kidney. There is an infiltrate of lymphocytes, most of which are T cells, in the interstitium (**I**) of the kidney. The tubules are atrophic and widely separated. Lymphocytes (**L**) can be seen within the tubular basement membrane between the tubular epithelial cells *(tubulitis)*. These lymphocytes are attacking the tubular epithelial cells, causing tubular damage and eventual loss of tubules. Loss of any part of the nephron leads to loss of the entire nephron so that the transplanted kidney is unable to function. As in many cases of chronic inflammation, tissue damage is caused primarily by the inflammatory infiltrate. The transplanted kidney makes no attack on the recipient and, if left alone by the immune system, does nothing but good. Various combinations of immunosuppressant drugs are used to suppress the cell-mediated immune response to the transplanted kidney to allow it to function, thus freeing the recipient from a life of dialysis.

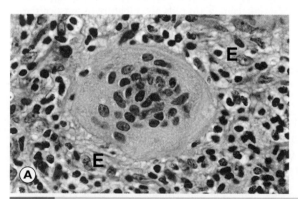

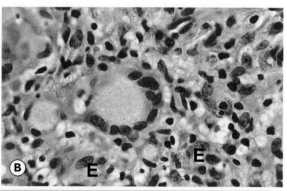

Fig. 4.7 Giant cells. **(A)** Foreign body giant cell (HP); **(B)** Langhans' giant cell (HP).

As described in the introduction, multinucleate giant cells are formed by the fusion of epithelioid macrophages and are a highly characteristic, though not universal, feature of chronic granulomatous inflammation. These micrographs illustrate typical appearances of giant cells. Fig. 4.7A is a good example of a *foreign body-type giant cell*, which is characterised by a central group of nuclei similar to those seen in adjacent epithelioid macrophages (**E**). These cells may be found in association with implanted foreign material, for example a remnant of a surgical suture or a rose thorn in the skin (see Fig. 4.9). These cells are usually found in association with epithelioid macrophages, although they may not form the discrete granulomas seen in other types of granulomatous inflammation.

The second important form of giant cell is the *Langhans' giant cell*, said to be characteristic of tuberculosis. As shown in Fig. 4.7B, the multiple nuclei of Langhans' giant cells are arranged in a horseshoe formation around the periphery. Again, epithelioid macrophages (**E**) are seen in the surrounding tissues.

Both epithelioid macrophages and giant cells are specialised secretory cells, rather than phagocytic cells. The plentiful eosinophilic cytoplasm seen in both cell types is indicative of abundant rough endoplasmic reticulum, as opposed to the pale foamy cytoplasm of phagocytic macrophages. Although Langhans' giant cells and foreign body cells are said to be more or less specific for different types of granulomatous inflammation, in practice this is not so.

KEY TO FIGURES
A enlarged alveolar space   **E** epithelioid macrophage   **F** fibrous tissue   **I** interstitium   **L** lymphocytes
P type 2 pneumocyte hyperplasia

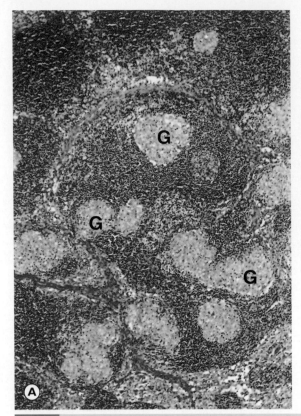

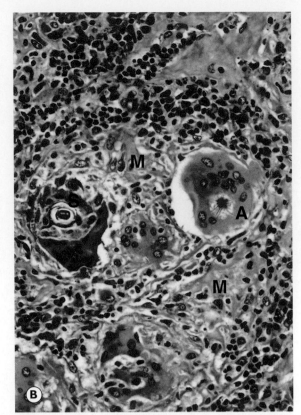

Fig. 4.8 **Sarcoidosis. (A)** Sarcoidosis in a lymph node (MP); **(B)** sarcoid granulomas (HP).

Sarcoidosis is a chronic granulomatous disease of unknown aetiology, characterised by the formation of multiple discrete granulomas in many tissues. In marked distinction to classic tuberculous granulomas (see Ch. 5), those of sarcoidosis do not typically undergo central caseous necrosis, although small foci of necrosis may be seen in large granulomas.

Sarcoidosis may occur in any organ or tissue, notably the spleen, liver, skin and lymph nodes, but frequently also involves the lungs, which may be peppered with numerous granulomas. In most cases of pulmonary sarcoidosis, the hilar lymph nodes are also grossly enlarged by masses of granulomas; such massive nodes are a useful diagnostic feature when visible on chest imaging.

Fig. 4.8A illustrates part of a typical lymph node (E-Fig. 4.7**H**). Note the scattered non-caseating granulomas **(G)**. Since there is no central mass of caseation, the sarcoid granuloma differs from the tuberculous granuloma by having a much broader zone of epithelioid macrophages. As in tuberculosis, sarcoid granulomas are surrounded by a zone of lymphocytes, although this feature is much less

obvious in sarcoid lesions. In tissues other than lymph nodes, the granulomas are described as being 'naked', i.e. lacking a rim of lymphocytes and fibroblasts.

Fig. 4.8B shows a typical sarcoid granuloma at high magnification. Note the epithelioid macrophages **(M)**. Multinucleate giant cells are a feature of most of the granulomas. The cytoplasm of sarcoid giant cells may contain inclusion bodies of two types: eosinophilic star-shaped *asteroid bodies* **(A)** or small, laminated calcified concretions called *Schaumann bodies* **(S)**. In practice, these inclusion bodies are rare. Although characteristic of sarcoid giant cells, such inclusion bodies are not pathognomonic of sarcoidosis (i.e. not exclusive to sarcoidosis) and are occasionally found in other chronic inflammatory granulomas.

Sarcoidosis has many possible clinical presentations, including no clinical symptoms; in persistent cases, the granulomas undergo progressive fibrosis, although some giant cells still remain. In the lungs, this may culminate in pulmonary fibrosis and honeycomb lung (see Fig. 4.5) and may lead to chronic respiratory failure.

KEY TO FIGURES
A asteroid body   **F** foreign body giant cells   **G** non-caseating granuloma   **L** lipogranuloma
M epithelioid macrophages   **P** plant material   **S** Schaumann body

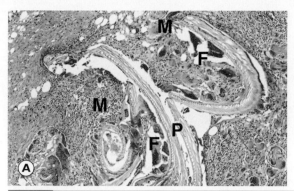

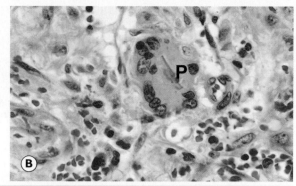

Fig. 4.9 **Foreign body reaction. (A)** Foreign body granuloma (LP); **(B)** giant cell with inclusion (HP).

The presence of certain non-soluble foreign materials in tissues may excite a chronic granulomatous inflammatory response, with or without discrete granuloma formation. Common examples of such *foreign body reactions* are those produced by suture material, wood or other vegetable matter, metal or glass splinters, and inorganic materials such as silica and beryllium, inhaled deep into the lungs during industrial dust exposure. Inhaled materials are of particular clinical importance because of their tendency to produce progressive pulmonary fibrosis, similar to that which may occur in idiopathic pulmonary fibrosis. Many of these foreign bodies are refractile when viewed with polarised light and can thus be identified within the granulomas or giant cells.

At low magnification, Fig. 4.9A shows plant material **P**, derived from faeces, that has become embedded in the wall of the colon in a patient with *diverticulitis*. Diverticular disease is a condition where the mucosa of the bowel herniates through the muscular wall, forming a pouch or diverticulum in which faecal material may become impacted, leading to inflammation and sometimes perforation (see Ch. 13). The pale, incompletely digested plant material is surrounded by aggregates of foreign body giant cells **(F)** and epithelioid macrophages **(M)** as well as other inflammatory cells. At high power in Fig. 4.9B, a fragment of plant material **(P)** can easily be seen within the cytoplasm of a Langhans' type giant cell.

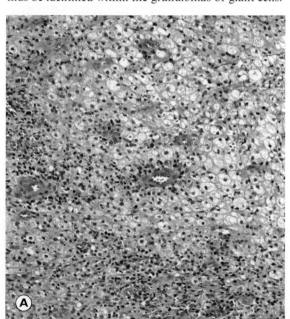

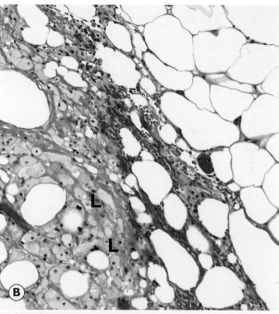

Fig. 4.10 **Xanthogranulomatous inflammation and lipogranuloma. (A)** Xanthogranulomatous cholecystitis (MP); **(B)** lipogranuloma in fat necrosis (HP).

Xanthogranulomatous inflammation is a rare condition most often seen in the kidney or the gallbladder (E-Fig. 4.8 **H**). Although rare, these are important lesions as they may form a mass that can be mistaken for a malignant tumour. Fig. 4.10A shows xanthogranulomatous inflammation in the gallbladder at medium power. The lesion consists of sheets of macrophages whose cytoplasm is loaded with droplets of lipid, thus giving it a foamy appearance. The lipid in the macrophage gives the lesion an orange-yellow appearance macroscopically. Interspersed among the foamy macrophages are lymphocytes, plasma cells, eosinophils and, sometimes, a few neutrophils. Older lesions are often very fibrotic and the

gallbladder may become shrunken and thick walled. Xanthogranulomatous pyelonephritis tends to occur in patients with *Proteus* urinary tract infection and has similar histological appearances (E-Fig. 4.9 **G**).

Another much more common appearance is the accumulation of lipid-laden macrophages in areas where fat is released from adipocytes, often in areas of fat necrosis. Fig. 4.10B shows such an area where necrotic fat cells are easily identified by their lack of nuclei. Interspersed among the fat cells are sheets of foamy macrophages, often with very few other inflammatory cells. Occasional lipogranulomas **(L)** may be seen, consisting of a droplet of lipid surrounded by foamy macrophages.

Table 4.2 Chapter review.

Type of chronic inflammation	Histological features	Some examples	Figure
Non-specific: follows on from unresolved acute inflammation	Mixed inflammatory response with lymphocytes, plasma cells, eosinophils, neutrophils. Characterised by mixture of acute inflammation, chronic inflammation and attempts at healing (granulation tissue, fibrosis)	Chronic peptic ulcer Bronchiectasis (E-Fig. 4.3 **G**) Pilonidal sinus Ulcerative colitis	4.2 4.3 4.4 13.18
Specific chronic inflammation (non-granulomatous)	The inflammatory infiltrate consists predominantly of lymphocytes, plasma cells and macrophages. Sometimes there are variable numbers of eosinophils and mast cells	Viral infections Idiopathic pulmonary fibrosis (E-Fig. 4.6 **G**) Cellular rejection of transplanted kidney Lichen planus	5.12–5.14 4.5 4.6 21.7
Specific chronic inflammation (granulomatous)	This type of inflammation is characterised by the formation of granulomas: aggregates of epithelioid macrophages, with or without giant cells	Sarcoidosis Foreign body giant cell reaction Tuberculosis Leprosy Crohn's disease	4.8 4.9 5.3–5.7 5.9 13.16

KEY TO FIGURES
L lipogranulomas

5 Infections of histological importance

Introduction

A number of infections may be diagnosed from the characteristic appearances seen in biopsy specimens. In some cases, the diagnosis may first be suspected when a biopsy is examined by light microscopy. In other cases, the clinician suspects an infective agent and seeks confirmation by biopsy as well as by other means. Although histological appearances are often characteristic, it is usually necessary to confirm the presence of the infective agent by other techniques such as microbiological cultures or serology. In addition, the pathologist may employ a wide variety of techniques such as electron microscopy, immunohistochemical staining with specific monoclonal antibodies and a range of special stains to confirm the diagnosis.

Many infections that are otherwise difficult to diagnose arise in immunosuppressed patients, for example patients with HIV/AIDS and organ transplant recipients and, as the number of such patients increases, so the role of histopathology in diagnosis of infection expands. This chapter aims to give an overview of infections that are important in routine diagnostic pathological practice, to illustrate the appearances of these organisms in the tissues and to consider the patterns of tissue damage they cause. As prion disease specifically affects the central nervous system, this is discussed in Ch. 23.

Bacterial infections

Most bacteria cause disease by exciting an acute exudative inflammatory response *(pyogenic bacteria)*. This inflammatory exudate is responsible for many of the clinical features of the disease (e.g. lobar pneumonia, see Fig. 3.3; bronchopneumonia, see Fig. 12.7). The pattern of tissue damage is similar irrespective of the pyogenic bacteria causing it and the organism can only be identified by microbiological methods. More complex mechanisms are involved in the tissue damage caused by infection with bacteria such as *Helicobacter pylori*, which cause inflammation by interfering with the normal physiological regulation of gastric acid secretion (see Figs 4.2 and 13.9). Other bacteria cause disease by producing toxins, which induce necrosis of cells and tissues (e.g. *Clostridium difficile* toxins destroy the surface epithelium of the colon (E-Fig. 5.1**G**) (Fig. 5.1), and some bacteria initiate a type IV hypersensitivity reaction (e.g. *Mycobacteria* and some *Treponema* organisms) and so produce characteristic changes.

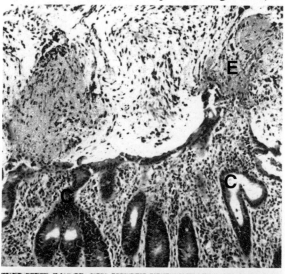

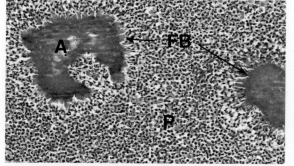

Fig. 5.1 Pseudomembranous colitis.

In pseudomembranous colitis, there is focal necrosis of the surface epithelium of the colon. This necrotic epithelium is replaced by an area of membrane, which is composed of a predominantly fibrinous acute inflammatory exudate. Typically, it occurs in older people following treatment with certain antibiotics. The antibiotic destroys the natural bacterial flora, allowing uncontrolled multiplication of *Clostridium difficile*. This bacterium produces a toxin, which causes extensive colonic epithelial necrosis and may be fatal.

The pattern of superficial mucosal necrosis is characteristic. There are multiple focal lesions of necrosis with tufts of exudate (**E**), likened to an erupting volcano. The deep components of the mucosa remain largely intact, but the superficial parts of the colonic crypts (**C**) appear acutely inflamed and atrophic (E-Fig. 5.2**H**)

Fig. 5.2 *Actinomyces* organisms.

These bacteria are filamentous bacteria, which grow in characteristic fungal-like colonies, appearing grossly as yellow *sulphur granules* and causing chronic abscesses and *fistulation.* Typical sites of infection include oral cavity, lung, GI tract and female genital tract (linked to use of intrauterine contraceptive devices). Fig. 5.2 shows the *Actinomyces* (**A**) lie within a pool of pus (**P**) and appear encrusted by eosinophilic material (the *Splendori–Hoeppli phenomenon*). The filamentous shape of the bacteria (**FB**) can be seen at the edges of these colonies.

KEY TO FIGURES

A *Actinomyces*   **C** colonic crypts   **E** inflammatory exudate   **FB** filamentous bacteria   **P** pus

Mycobacterial infections

Infections caused by various *Mycobacteria* can frequently be diagnosed histologically because of the tissue reaction to their presence. The organisms are difficult and slow to grow in microbiological culture and therefore biopsy often plays an important role in early diagnosis. *Mycobacterium tuberculosis* causes **tuberculosis**, a disease that is increasing in incidence because of the emergence of drug-resistant strains. *Mycobacterium leprae* is the cause of **leprosy** (Fig. 5.9). There are other pathogenic *Mycobacteria* (called atypical *Mycobacteria*) that cause a range of disorders.

Important points to note about the histology of mycobacterial infections are:

- Most show a **granulomatous** pattern of chronic inflammation (see Ch. 4) due to a delayed type hypersensitivity reaction.
- **Caseous necrosis** (Fig. 5.3) is particularly associated with *M. tuberculosis* infection.
- Suppurating granulomas (with neutrophils in the central necrotic area of the granuloma) may occur in infections by atypical *Mycobacteria* (Fig. 5.8). These organisms are also referred to as **Mycobacteria other than tuberculosis (MOTT)** or **non-tuberculous Mycobacteria (NTM).**
- The causative organism can sometimes be identified in histological sections by the use of special stains (Ziehl–Neelsen, Wade–Fite) as shown in Appendix 1.

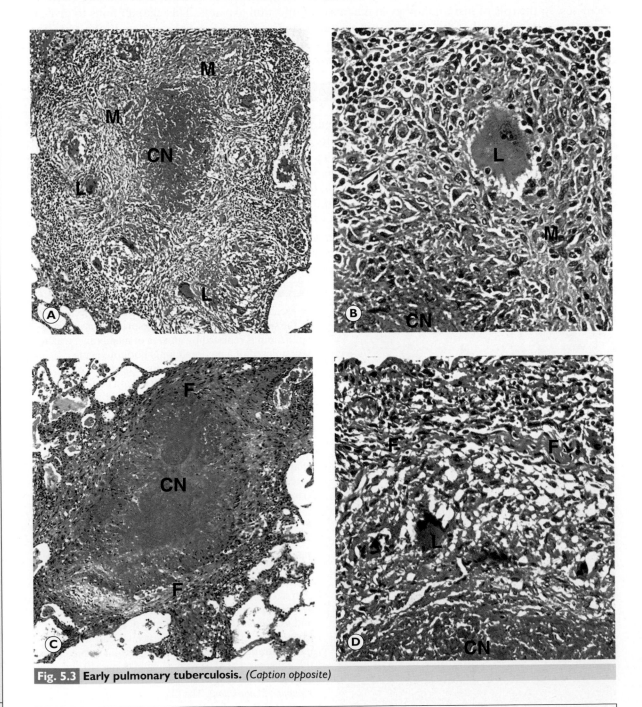

Fig. 5.3 **Early pulmonary tuberculosis.** *(Caption opposite)*

KEY TO FIGURES
CN caseous necrosis **F** fibroblasts **L** Langhans' giant cell **M** epithelioid macrophages **W** fibrous wall

Fig. 5.3 **Early pulmonary tuberculosis. (A)** Early tubercle (MP); **(B)** early tubercle (HP); **(C)** later tubercle (MP); **(D)** later tubercle (HP). *(Illustrations opposite)*

The characteristic histological lesion in tuberculosis is the granuloma, which in this case is known as a *tubercle*.

When mycobacteria gain access to the lungs by inhalation, they tend to localise in the periphery of the lung where they excite a transient neutrophil response. The organisms survive neutrophil enzyme activity, probably because of their thick and resistant glycolipid cell wall. They are then ingested by macrophages where they may initially continue to divide within macrophage cytoplasm. The macrophages present mycobacterial antigen to T lymphocytes, which become activated and initiate a cell-mediated (type IV hypersensitivity) response. The sensitised lymphocytes produce various soluble factors *(cytokines)*, which attract and activate the macrophages, enhancing their ability to secrete substances that kill mycobacteria. Such activated macrophages become large and develop granular, eosinophilic cytoplasm. As a result of their supposed resemblance to epithelial cells, they are known as *epithelioid macrophages* (see Ch. 4). These cells form a major component of all granulomas, including tubercles.

Fig. 5.3A shows an entire tubercle at an early stage, and Fig. 5.3B illustrates a sector of the same tubercle at higher magnification. At the centre of the tubercle is an area of caseous necrosis **(CN)** containing mycobacteria. These can only be demonstrated by specific staining methods for acid-fast bacilli (Fig. 5.10). The caseous area is surrounded by a zone of epithelioid macrophages **(M)** with abundant eosinophilic cytoplasm. Some of the macrophages fuse to produce multinucleate giant cells called *Langhans' giant cells* **(L)**; a typical Langhans' giant cell is shown in more detail in Fig. 4.8. Peripheral to the macrophages, there is a rim of lymphocytes.

Progressive, central, caseous necrosis results in enlargement of the tubercle and the zone of peripheral macrophages and lymphocytes becomes relatively thinner. These changes can be observed by comparing Fig. 5.3A with Fig. 5.3C, which shows a more advanced tubercle. With further development, spindle-shaped fibroblasts **(F)** appear in the peripheral lymphocytic zone of the tubercle, where they are stimulated by factors produced by epithelioid macrophages to lay down collagen in the extracellular tissue; this process is evident in Fig. 5.3C and at higher magnification in Fig. 5.3D.

At this stage, further changes in the tubercle can occur in one of two ways. If the organisms are virulent and present in large numbers, particularly if the body's resistance is low (as, for example, in a debilitated or immunosuppressed patient), then the tubercle rapidly enlarges owing to increasing caseous necrosis. The macrophage–lymphocyte–fibroblast defensive reaction is overwhelmed, failing to confine the infection. This can result in tuberculous bronchopneumonia (Fig. 5.6). On the other hand, if the balance of resistance and attack is reversed, the macrophage–lymphocyte–fibroblast barrier resists enlargement of the tubercle and proliferation of fibroblasts produces a firm shell confining the infection. Production of collagen by these fibroblasts further strengthens this capsule, imprisoning the necrotic tissue and its contained mycobacteria and isolating the organisms from other susceptible tissue (Fig. 5.4). Calcium salts may become deposited in the collagenous shell and necrotic centre. In the lung, carbon is also taken up by the macrophages of the granuloma.

In primary tuberculous infection, the initial tubercle in the lung is known as a *Ghon focus* and is usually situated in the subpleural area in the mid-zone of the lung. This lesion rarely attains a large size and undergoes the process of fibrosis described above. Before the lung lesion is walled off, however, mycobacteria pass via lymphatics to regional lymph nodes in the lung hilum, where tubercles develop in a manner identical to the Ghon focus in the lung (E-Fig. 5.3**G**). The outcome of the infection depends on what happens to this tuberculous infection of the hilar lymph nodes. Possible outcomes are discussed in Figs 5.4 to 5.7.

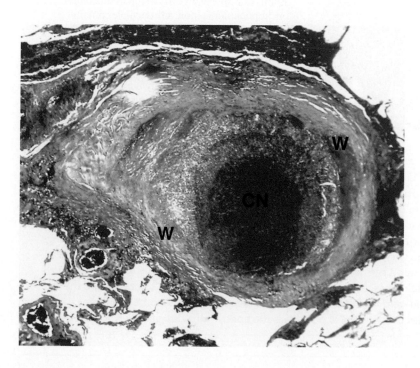

Fig. 5.4 **Fibrocaseous tuberculous nodule (LP).**

In most cases of primary tuberculosis, the Ghon focus heals by fibrosis leaving a small fibrous nodule, which is often calcified.

Some individuals are unable to contain the initial infection and develop *post-primary tuberculosis*. Others contain the initial infection but later, because of relatively suppressed immunity, further active infection occurs due to reactivation. In either case, a variety of lesions may result, including a localised lesion at the apex of the lung known as an *Assmann focus*. This may progress to spread the infection further or may be contained by chemotherapy, giving rise to a *fibrocaseous nodule*. A thick fibrous wall **(W)** completely encircles a mass of caseous necrotic material **(CN)**. In this case, there is little calcification.

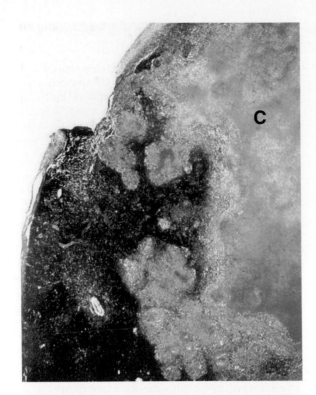

Fig. 5.5 Tuberculous lymph node (LP).

With the formation of a Ghon focus in a child's lung, tubercle bacilli pass via lung lymphatics to regional lymph nodes where they initiate caseous necrosis and tubercle formation similar to that in the lung. The combination of a Ghon focus in the lung and tuberculous regional (peribronchial) lymph nodes is called a *primary complex* or *Ghon complex*. The outcome of infection depends on the fate of the lymph node lesion. If defences are strong, healing of the tubercles occurs by fibrosis, leaving only small fibrocalcific nodules in the lung periphery and regional lymph nodes. If defence mechanisms are inadequate, the lymph node tubercle enlarges due to extensive caseous necrosis, tending to overwhelm the surrounding macrophage–lymphocyte–fibroblast reaction. The lymph node enlarges until its capsule is breached then ruptures, discharging many tubercle bacilli into the surrounding tissues. The enlarging node may ulcerate into nearby bronchi, causing tuberculous bronchopneumonia (Fig. 5.6), or into blood vessels (Fig. 5.7), leading to extensive systemic spread of the organisms. Here, the tubercle has greatly enlarged so that the lymph node has almost been destroyed by caseous necrosis (C) and the zone of cellular reaction around it is very thin.

Necrosis has almost reached the lymph node capsule and rupture is imminent.

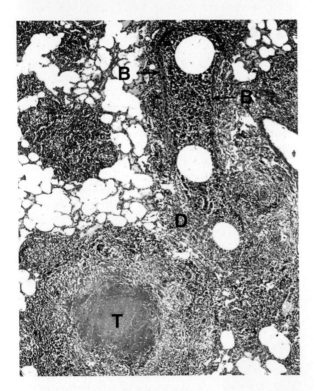

Fig. 5.6 Tuberculous bronchopneumonia (MP).

When the wall of a bronchus is eroded by an enlarging tuberculous node or an apical Assmann focus, tubercle bacilli pass into the bronchial lumen from which they may be spread in various ways. If coughed up in sputum, the infection may be transmitted to other susceptible persons by droplet infection, sometimes infecting the patient's larynx *(tuberculous laryngitis)* on the way. Infected sputum may be swallowed and subsequently produce **tuberculous oesophagitis** or **ileitis.** Infected sputum may also gravitate to lower areas of the same or opposite lung where, by destruction of a bronchiolar wall, the organism may invade peribronchial lung tissue to form further caseating tubercles. This is called **tuberculous bronchopneumonia**.

In this example of an early lesion in tuberculous bronchopneumonia, note a bronchiole containing infected material. The walls of the bronchiole are indicated by the arrows marked (B). A segment of the bronchiolar wall has been destroyed (D), permitting access of bacilli which have initiated a caseating tubercle (T) in the nearby lung parenchyma. Large numbers of such lesions may form, merging with one another to produce a wide area of rapidly enlarging caseation, usually in the lower lobes of the lungs. This is the pathogenesis of the once dreaded *'galloping consumption'*.

SOME OTHER ASPECTS OF TUBERCULOSIS

In all cases of suspected tuberculosis, material should be submitted for culture. Culture of *M. tuberculosis* is difficult and time-consuming and may take 6 weeks or more. When the organisms have been cultured successfully, this allows assessment of antimicrobial resistance and sensitivity. It is often necessary to begin treatment empirically whilst awaiting microbiological confirmation and so initial histological findings supportive of this diagnosis can be very valuable. Histological identification of the organisms using special staining techniques is dependent upon the nature of the mycobacterial cell wall. This lipid-rich coating allows the organisms to retain certain dyes, even upon heating with acid and alcohol solutions, and therefore mycobacteria are often called **acid and alcohol fast bacilli** (see Fig. 5.10). Another name for *M. tuberculosis* which is sometimes used in clinical practice is the eponymous designation **Koch's bacillus.**

KEY TO FIGURES

B bronchiole **Bo** bony trabeculae **C** caseous necrosis **D** destroyed wall **G** granuloma
L Langhans' giant cell **T** tubercle

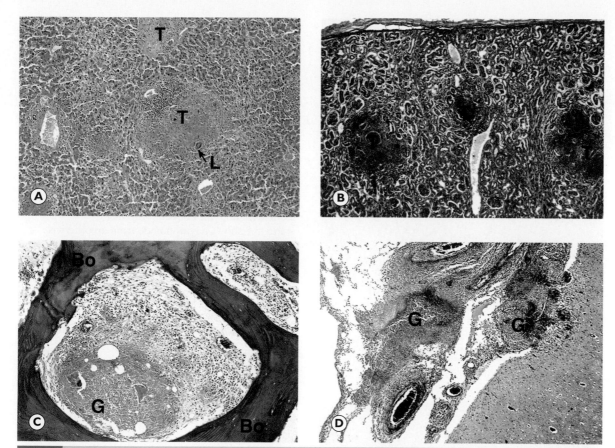

Fig. 5.7 **Disseminated tuberculosis. (A)** Liver (MP); **(B)** kidney (MP); **(C)** bone (MP); **(D)** tuberculous meningitis (MP).

If a ruptured tuberculous lymph node (or a rapidly enlarging focus of post-primary tuberculosis) erodes a blood vessel wall, masses of mycobacteria are discharged into the circulation and lodge in the microvasculature. When the eroded vessel is a branch of the pulmonary artery, the organisms pass to other areas of the lung, but when a pulmonary venous tributary is involved, they are spread in the systemic circulation to many organs, notably the liver, kidney and spleen. In this way, vast numbers of new tubercles may be produced throughout the body. Such multiple lesions rarely attain any great size because this occurrence usually produces rapid clinical deterioration and death. Because the gross appearance of individual lesions resembles millet seeds, this condition is known as *miliary tuberculosis*.

Fig. 5.7A shows several miliary tubercles **(T)** in the liver (E-Fig. 5.4**H**). One of the tubercles exhibits Langhans' giant cells **(L)** and the larger tubercle shows early central caseous necrosis.

It seems that a relatively small number of organisms can be disseminated by the bloodstream to various organs without causing overt disease, only to become reactivated at a later date when the host's immune status is impaired. These organisms remain viable but quiescent and active tuberculosis may then reappear in tissues remote from the original lesion many years later. This phenomenon is known as *metastatic* or *isolated organ tuberculosis* and most commonly involves the kidneys, adrenals, meninges, bone, Fallopian tubes, endometrium and epididymis.

Fig. 5.7B illustrates renal involvement (E-Fig. 5.5**H**) with the formation of small tubercles **(T)** in the renal cortex. Continuation of this process results in destruction of much of the renal cortex and medulla,

with eventual rupture of large confluent tubercles into the pelvicalyceal system, which becomes distended with caseous material. This condition is known as *tuberculous pyonephrosis*. In more advanced cases, infection spreads to involve the ureter and bladder. Renal tuberculosis is frequently bilateral and may result in renal failure.

Bone tuberculosis *(tuberculous osteomyelitis)* most frequently affects the long bones, associated joints and the vertebrae *(Pott's disease)*. In long bones, infection may produce a localised, painful swelling, which may drain to the skin to form a chronic sinus. Joint involvement *(tuberculous arthritis)* is most common in children and often affects the hips or joints associated with the vertebrae *(tuberculous spondylitis)* as part of Pott's disease of the spine. As in other tissues, Fig. 5.7C shows the characteristic caseating granulomas **(G),** which cause progressive destruction of the bony trabeculae **(Bo)**. The infection tends to spread extensively in the cancellous medullary bone, leading to necrosis of surrounding cortical bone (E-Fig. 5.6**H**).

Tuberculous meningitis is an uncommon but frequently fatal complication of tuberculosis. Most often, it affects the meninges around the base of the brain and the spinal cord. As shown in Fig. 5.7D, tuberculous granulomas **(G)**, with characteristic central areas of caseation, develop in the leptomeninges and adjacent brain tissue (E-Fig. 5.7**H**) where they may damage cranial and spinal nerves. The presence of numerous lymphocytes in CSF obtained from lumbar puncture is useful in distinguishing tuberculous meningitis from purulent (bacterial) meningitis. In the latter, neutrophils are the major cell type present.

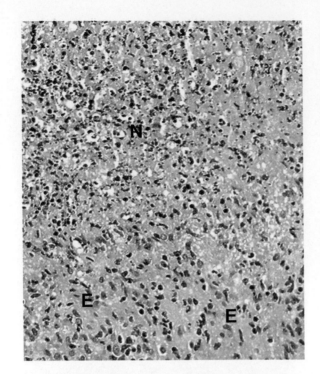

Fig. 5.8 Atypical mycobacterial infection involving lymph node (MP).

Infection with non-tuberculous mycobacteria (also known as atypical mycobacteria or mycobacteria other than tuberculosis, MOTT) is not uncommon in the cervical lymph nodes of young children. Another group at risk from these organisms are patients with AIDS who, because of severe immunosuppression, commonly develop widespread infections involving the liver, lymph nodes and spleen. In these patients, there is usually a deficient immune response and the histological appearance may simply be of aggregates of epithelioid cells or even foamy macrophages in the tissue with no lymphocytic component.

Fig. 5.8 shows a lymph node from an otherwise healthy child with MOTT infection. The lymphoid tissue is replaced with a granulomatous inflammatory response, consisting of confluent sheets of epithelioid macrophages (**E**). In contrast to *M. tuberculosis*, the granulomas in MOTT infection show suppurative necrosis with aggregates of neutrophils (**N**), rather than caseous necrosis. As in this example, giant cells may be sparse.

Fig. 5.9 Leprosy. (A) Dermal infiltration (LP); (B) nerve involvement (HP).

Leprosy is a disease caused by infection with *M. leprae*. The tissue reaction to the bacillus depends on the immune response of the infected person. In the ***tuberculoid*** form of the disease, there is an active cell-mediated immune response and granulomas are formed that are similar to those seen in tuberculosis, but without evidence of caseation. In the ***lepromatous*** form, there is no effective cell-mediated immune response and tissues are infiltrated with macrophages colonised by large numbers of bacteria. Intermediate forms of leprosy exist with both tuberculoid and lepromatous features.

Clinically, people with the lepromatous form of the disease have nodular dermal and subcutaneous deposits of macrophages filled with bacteria and lipid. The disease affects the face, ears, arms, knees and buttocks, as the leprosy bacilli require cooler areas of the body for proliferation. In contrast, the tuberculoid form of the disease gives rise to macular or plaque-like skin lesions and, in addition, causes extensive inflammatory destruction of peripheral nerves. This typically gives rise to anaesthesia (loss of sensation) in the limbs, which then become prone to damage through repeated non-perceived injury.

Fig. 5.9A is a micrograph of the skin (E-Fig. 5.8**H**) of a person with tuberculoid leprosy. Histiocytic granulomas (**G**) with a heavy surrounding lymphocytic infiltrate are present at all layers throughout the dermis, but particularly in relation to small nerves. This is illustrated at higher magnification in Fig. 5.9B. Here, a small dermal nerve (**DN**) is shown surrounded by a cuff of lymphocytes. There is an associated granuloma (**G**).

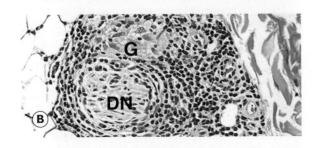

KEY TO FIGURES
C carbon pigment   **DN** dermal nerve   **E** epithelioid macrophages   **G** granuloma   **N** neutrophils

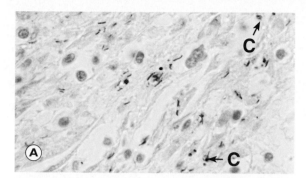

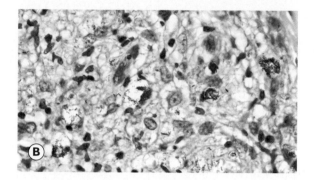

Fig. 5.10 **Special staining for mycobacteria.**
(A) Ziehl–Neelsen stain in tuberculosis (HP);
(B) Wade–Fite stain in lepromatous leprosy (HP).

M. tuberculosis and atypical mycobacteria are not visible on routine H&E stains. To demonstrate the presence of mycobacteria in tissue, the Ziehl–Neelsen (ZN) staining method is employed. The stain is taken up by the cell walls of the mycobacteria and remains despite treatment with acid and alcohol. This is the origin of the term *acid and alcohol fast bacilli*, which is used in describing mycobacteria. In a very high-power micrograph (Fig. 5.10A), scattered magenta-coloured, rod-shaped organisms can be seen in the lung of an immunocompromised patient. Some carbon pigment **(C)** can be identified within alveolar macrophages. In an immunocompetent individual, these organisms may be very sparse and difficult to find, but even a single organism in the appropriate background of a caseating granuloma is diagnostic. In immunosuppressed individuals (as shown here) and also in MOTT infection, the organisms are often much more numerous.

The micrograph of lepromatous leprosy (Fig. 5.10B) shows the Wade–Fite stain, which is a modified version of the ZN stain. Again, it stains the organisms red. The similarity in appearance between *M. tuberculosis* and *M. leprae* can be readily appreciated.

Spirochaete infections

The major form of spirochaete infection worldwide is **syphilis**, due to *Treponema pallidum*. **Yaws** and **pinta** are further important treponemal infections, but these are rare except in specific tropical regions. Although now relatively uncommon, late-stage syphilis is still regarded as one of the classical examples of specific chronic inflammation. The infecting organism, the spiral-shaped spirochaete *T. pallidum*, resists usual tissue defences and excites a progression of fascinating pathological and clinical phenomena, which represent typical chronic inflammatory responses with superimposed hypersensitivity reactions mounted by the immune system. The condition usually proceeds through three stages over a long period.

In brief, the organism usually gains access to the body by penetrating the genital mucosa where it produces a single, small primary lesion known as a **chancre**. The chancre is a raised, reddened nodule caused by an intense local accumulation of plasma cells and lymphocytes in the subepithelial connective tissue. The chancre may ulcerate at this stage, but it is often painless and may easily pass unnoticed. By the time the chancre has developed, the organism has multiplied extensively and has been disseminated to regional lymph nodes and thence into the bloodstream, causing a generalised bacteraemia. The chancre and concomitant bacteraemia *(primary syphilis)* are followed some weeks or months later by a transient **secondary stage**. This is characterised by a widespread, variable skin rash, often with moist, warty, genital lesions and ulceration of the oral mucosa. These various mucosal lesions are histologically similar to the primary chancre and are full of treponemal organisms. The disease is now at its most contagious, yet the patient usually feels well and the only other evidence of a generalised infection is a widespread lymphadenopathy and positive serological findings.

In most untreated cases, the infection is effectively resolved by body defences and, in many of these patients, even serological evidence of previous infection disappears. Unfortunately, a proportion of untreated cases proceed from the secondary stage to develop **tertiary syphilis**, after a variable interval from one to many years. The lesions of tertiary syphilis may be either focal or diffuse and it is the focal lesion of tertiary syphilis, known as the **gumma**, which exhibits many of the features of a granulomatous inflammation. Tertiary lesions may occur in almost any organ or tissue and the clinical consequences vary enormously. The diffuse form of tertiary syphilis most notably involves the cardiovascular system, particularly the ascending aorta and, less commonly, the central nervous system; the well-known **tabes dorsalis** and **general paresis of the insane (GPI)** are two of the manifestations of neurosyphilis. In the focal form of tertiary syphilis, gummas may develop in the liver, bone, testes and other sites. The clinical outcome depends upon the nature and extent of local tissue destruction.

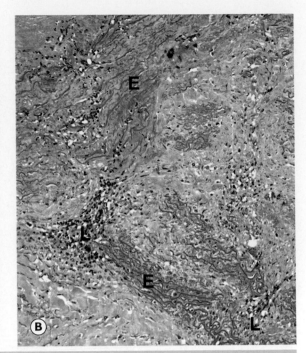

Fig. 5.11 **Syphilis. (A)** Syphilitic gumma of the liver (LP); **(B)** syphilitic aortitis (MP).

Fig. 5.11A illustrates the classic appearance of a gumma with central, homogeneous, coagulative necrosis (**N**) surrounded by a zone of epithelioid macrophages, lymphocytes, plasma cells and plump fibroblasts. Fibrous healing of liver gummas may produce a pattern of coarse, deep scars dividing the liver surface into numerous irregular lobules. This condition is known as *hepar lobatum*.

Fig. 5.11B illustrates *syphilitic aortitis*, the most common form of diffuse tertiary syphilitic lesion. The characteristic feature of syphilis is a low-grade, chronic vasculitis of small vessels with thickening of the wall, particularly the endothelium, and a perivascular cuff of

lymphocytes and plasma cells (*endarteritis obliterans*). In the aorta, the vasculitis affects the vasa vasorum of the tunica adventitia and their smaller branches that extend into the tunica media. The blue-stained areas in the tunica media represent lymphocytic cuffing (**L**) around numerous small vessels. The smooth muscle and elastic fibres of the media degenerate, probably because of ischaemia, and the aortic wall is replaced by collagen. Residual elastin (**E**) is stained deep pink. The loss of elasticity and contractility in the aortic wall allows progressive stretching with the formation of an *aneurysm* (see Chs 8 and 11), usually affecting the ascending aorta or aortic arch.

Viral infections

Viruses cause disease in three main ways:

- By causing death of the cell they infect, either by a direct effect or by modifying the genome such that the host cell is recognised as foreign and is destroyed by the host immune system.
- By causing excessive proliferation of the infected cell line, which may result in the development of malignant tumours. *Human papillomavirus* (HPV) is particularly important in this respect.
- By integrating themselves in the cell nucleus where they produce latent infection.

Although viral culture and the demonstration of rising titres of antibodies against the virus remain the mainstays of diagnosis, some viral infections can be diagnosed by characteristic histological appearances. Individual viruses are too small to be seen by light microscopy, but when congregating together in enormous numbers within the host cell, they are visible as *viral inclusion bodies* and may be either intranuclear, intracytoplasmic or both. Inclusion bodies provide a histological clue to the causative virus and this can be confirmed by electron microscopy and immunohistochemistry.

One viral infection of particular importance is the *human immunodeficiency virus* (HIV), which is the cause of the *acquired immune deficiency syndrome* (AIDS). As well as producing certain characteristic histological changes, particularly affecting lymph nodes, HIV compromises the host immune system and so a range of other unusual infections may result. HIV-1 is a lymphotropic virus that gains access to cells by way of the CD4 surface protein, normally found on T helper cells as well as on most monocytes and other macrophages. Infection with HIV-1 is associated with several clinical and pathological syndromes. Some patients develop fever, weight loss, diarrhoea and generalised lymph node enlargement *(lymphadenopathy)* in which there is generalised follicular hyperplasia. In patients with the full-blown immunodeficiency state of AIDS, lymph nodes show loss of follicles, lymphocyte depletion, vascular proliferation and fibrosis.

KEY TO FIGURES
E elastin **I** inclusion body **L** lymphocytes around vessels **N** necrosis **S** syncytial cells **V** vesicle

The two main consequences of the immunodeficiency state seen in AIDS are:
- Predisposition to opportunistic infections, particularly
  - *Pneumocystis* pneumonia (Fig. 5.17)
  - Cytomegalovirus infection (Fig. 5.13)
  - Mycobacterial infections, tuberculosis (Figs 5.3–5.7) as well as atypical *Mycobacteria* (Fig. 5.8)
  - Mucocutaneous and other fungal infections (Fig. 5.15) including *Cryptococcus* (Fig. 5.18)
  - Toxoplasmosis
- Predisposition to certain tumours, particularly
  - Kaposi's sarcoma (Fig. 11.11)
  - Non-Hodgkin's lymphoma, especially diffuse large B-cell lymphoma (see Ch. 16).

CLINICAL FEATURES OF HERPES VIRUS INFECTION

Herpes simplex virus types 1 and 2 (HSV-1 and HSV-2) cause the common skin eruptions known as ***cold sores*** and genital herpes, whilst the chicken pox virus (Herpes zoster) is responsible for ***shingles***. In immunocompetent individuals, Herpes viruses may remain latent in nerve cells with intermittent episodes of reactivation when the virus replicates within and destroys either epidermal cells or the epithelial cells of mucous membranes. Clinically, this gives rise to the typical appearance of groups of vesicles on an erythematous background. Most lesions heal spontaneously although the latent viral DNA remains in the nerve cells and can emerge in subsequent clinical episodes. In immunosuppressed patients, such as those with AIDS or those on immunosuppressive treatment, herpetic infection may result in widespread skin or visceral infections, rather than the self-limiting rash seen in the immunocompetent.

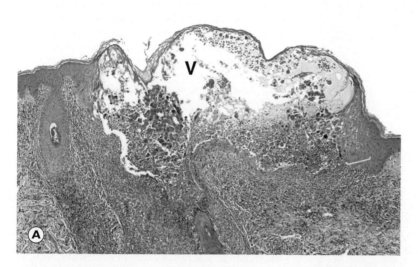

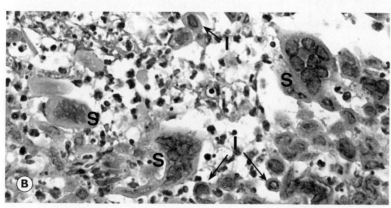

Fig. 5.12 Herpes virus infection. (A) Skin (LP); **(B)** oesophagus (HP).

Fig. 5.12A shows a skin biopsy from a patient with HSV-2 infection. At low power, there is ***vesiculation* (V)** due to hydropic degeneration and necrosis of epithelial cells (E-Fig. 5.8**H**).

Fig. 5.12B shows a high power image of an oesophageal biopsy from a patient undergoing chemotherapy for gastric carcinoma. There is severe inflammation of the squamous mucosa and numerous intranuclear eosinophilic ***inclusion bodies* (I)** can be seen within the nuclei, pushing the hyperchromatic host chromatin to the periphery. These consist of masses of virus particles. Another characteristic feature is fusion of epithelial cells to form multinucleate ***syncytia* (S)**. These nuclei contain inclusions and typically mould together within the cells.

If there is active infection, neonates can become infected during passage through the birth canal and may succumb to a severe, generalised infection of the lymph nodes, spleen, lungs, liver, adrenals and central nervous system.

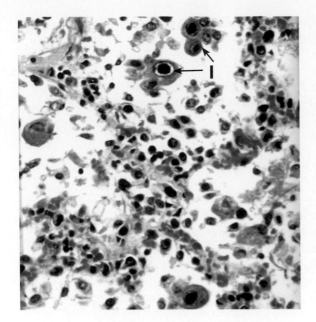

Fig. 5.13 Cytomegalovirus infection (HP).

Cytomegalovirus (CMV), another of the Herpes virus group, causes a mild, non-specific infection in immunocompetent individuals. Most adults will have been exposed to this virus by late middle age and will have specific serum antibodies. CMV infects white blood cells and may remain latent in leukocytes for many years. If the individual then becomes immunosuppressed for any reason, widespread systemic infection may result. Common sites of infection include the lungs, brain, retina, gastrointestinal tract and kidney.

CMV pneumonitis is shown in Fig. 5.13. The characteristic feature is markedly enlarged cells with large, dark-staining, intranuclear inclusion bodies (**I**). These are surrounded by a clear halo. Cytoplasmic inclusions may be seen but are not illustrated in this micrograph. There is sometimes focal necrosis, but there is usually minimal, if any, inflammation. Cytomegalic inclusions are usually seen in epithelial cells, endothelial cells and in macrophages and, as is the case in other Herpes virus infections, these inclusions may be sparse.

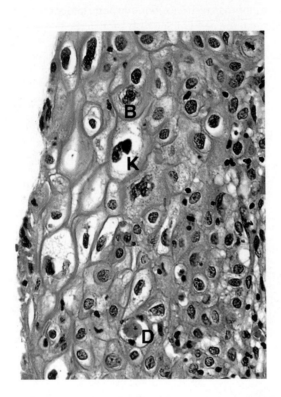

Fig. 5.14 Human papillomavirus (HP).

Human papillomavirus (HPV) is the causative agent of the common viral skin warts and genital warts. High risk types of the virus are closely associated with cervical intraepithelial neoplasia (CIN) and with invasive squamous cell carcinoma of the cervix, vagina, vulva, anogenital region and other sites such as oropharynx (see clinical box 'Human papillomavirus (HPV) and cancer' in Ch. 17).

HPV infects squamous epithelial cells and causes characteristic morphological changes in the cervical squamous epithelium, as shown in Fig. 5.14 (E-Fig. 5.9**H**). The epithelium is usually thickened (acanthotic) or may have the papillary appearance of an exophytic wart *(condyloma acuminatum)*. Infection of cells in the upper layers of the epithelium produces enlargement of the nuclei, which are hyperchromatic and have a folded appearance. A prominent cytoplasmic halo is also seen. These cells are called *koilocytes* (**K**). In addition, the epithelium contains binucleate cells (**B**) and *dyskeratotic cells* (**D**) (i.e. individual cell keratinisation).

Such changes are usually seen in association with low-grade CIN, as in this specimen from a woman with CIN I. In high-grade CIN, these changes are usually less apparent, being overshadowed by more advanced dysplastic changes. HPV infection can be demonstrated by molecular techniques in almost all high-grade CIN lesions (see also Figs 17.6 and 17.7.).

Fungal infections

Fungal infections range from minor localised skin infections to life-threatening systemic diseases in immunosuppressed patients. The inflammatory reaction in fungal infections may have one of three patterns. The classical appearance is of a granulomatous inflammation, which may exhibit central suppurative necrosis. A second pattern is of acute inflammation with an infiltrate consisting primarily of neutrophils. This pattern is seen in *Candida* infection of the oesophagus. The third is a very minimal inflammatory response, as in superficial infections of the skin by dermatophytic fungi.

Fungi are not usually obvious on routine H&E staining, but the thick cell walls are highlighted by special stains such as periodic–acid Schiff (PAS) or silver stains. Some fungi are easily recognised histologically because of the characteristic shape and structure of the hyphae and the pattern of budding of the yeast forms. Despite this, culture techniques are preferable for definitive identification of fungal species. An important diagnostic point is that the presence of fungal yeast forms, such as *Candida* at a mucosal surface or on the skin, does not necessarily indicate active infection, as these agents are common commensals. Evidence of active invasion must be demonstrated and, in most cases, there is an appropriate inflammatory response.

CLINICAL ASPECTS OF FUNGAL INFECTION

Many superficial forms of fungal infection are very indolent and slow growing and, as a result, treatment with anti-fungal drugs may need to extend over a prolonged period. It may be important to identify the precise type of fungus that is causing infection in order to ensure that the organism is sensitive to the form of treatment chosen. As fungi tend to have different growth requirements from bacteria, the microbiology laboratory must be informed if fungal infection is suspected so that appropriate cultures can be undertaken.

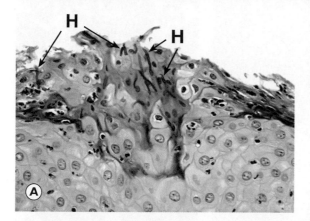

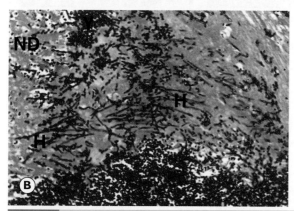

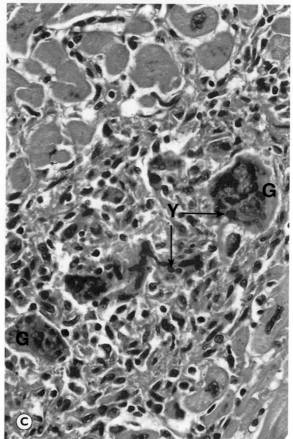

Fig. 5.15 **Candidiasis. (A)** Oral candidiasis (PAS) (HP); **(B)** oesophageal candidiasis (PAS) (HP); **(C)** myocardial candidiasis (PAS) (HP).

Candida albicans is a ubiquitous commensal fungus on the epithelial surfaces of the skin, mouth and genital tract. It exists in both a hyphal/mycelial form and as rounded yeasts. Although usually commensal, it can become pathogenic, usually producing reddening and soreness of the affected epithelium, often with a whitish surface membrane comprising excess keratin production and fungal hyphae.

The common sites for this are the mouth (oral candidiasis or thrush) and the vulvo-vaginal region (candidal vulvo-vaginitis). Both may be precipitated by debilitation or as a complication of systemic antibiotic therapy destroying the normal bacterial flora and allowing overgrowth of the fungus.

More severe infections can occur in patients who are immunosuppressed. Surface epithelial infections are more extensive and symptomatic, with large numbers of organisms in both hyphal and yeast forms (see Fig. 5.15B). Organisms may also gain access to the bloodstream and in immunosuppressed patients

may produce disseminated candidiasis, with organisms in many organs.

Fig. 5.15A shows candidal infection, mainly in hyphal forms **(H)**, on the surface of the buccal epithelium from a case of oral thrush in a patient taking antibiotics.

Fig. 5.15B shows abundant candidal infection, both in hyphal **(H)** and yeast **(Y)** forms, in the oesophagus of an elderly man debilitated by terminal cancer. There is also abundant necrotic debris **(ND)** forming a thick surface membrane. The infection had started as severe oropharyngeal thrush, but had spread down his oesophagus.

Fig. 5.15C shows *Candida* yeast forms **(Y)** in giant cells **(G)** in the myocardium (E-Fig. 5.10**H**), forming a small granuloma. Often, bloodstream spread of *Candida* produces small abscesses filled with neutrophils (pus), but this patient was severely immunosuppressed and was unable to mount an acute inflammatory reaction.

KEY TO FIGURES
B binucleate cell   **D** dyskeratotic cell   **G** giant cell   **H** hyphae   **I** inclusion body   **K** koilocyte
ND necrotic debris   **Y** yeast forms

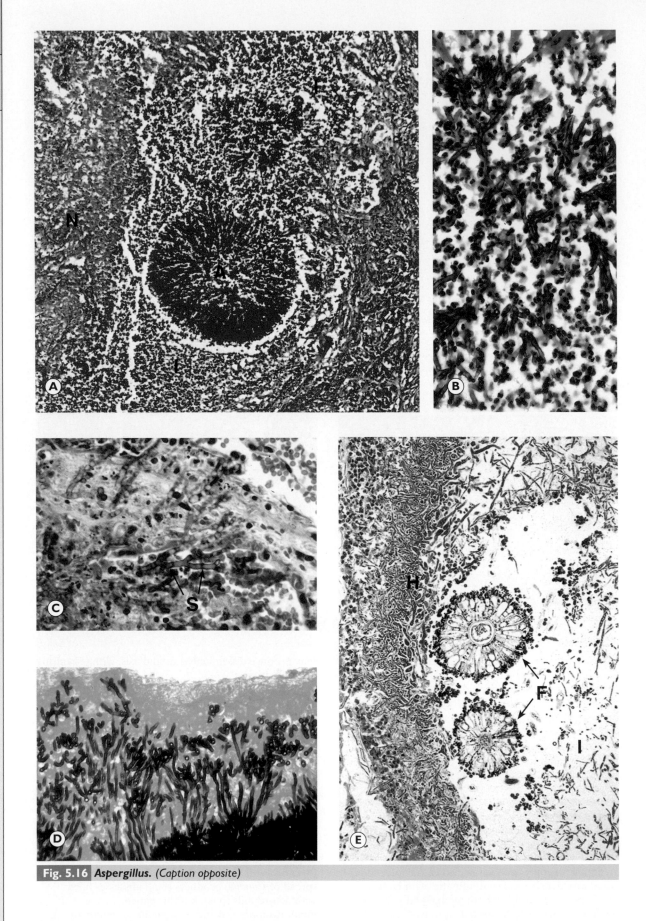

Fig. 5.16 *Aspergillus.* (Caption opposite)

KEY TO FIGURES
A *Aspergillus* hyphae   **E** exudate   **F** fruiting bodies   **H** hyphae   **I** inflammatory cells   **L** lymphocytes
N necrotic tissue   **S** septa

Fig. 5.16 *Aspergillus.* **(A)** MP; **(B)** HP; **(C)** HP; **(D)** silver stain (HP); **(E)** *Aspergillus niger* (MP). *(Illustrations opposite)*

Aspergillus is a ubiquitous fungus that may cause an allergic pulmonary response in otherwise healthy individuals. This is known colloquially as brewer's lung and belongs to the group of diseases known by the term ***extrinsic allergic alveolitis***. In this case, the *Aspergillus* does not colonise or invade the lung.

Asthmatic individuals may have their bronchial tree colonised by *Aspergillus* without invasion. They are then likely to suffer from an exacerbation of their asthma as a result of ***allergic bronchopulmonary aspergillosis***. This is a hypersensitivity response to *Aspergillus* antigens to which they are constantly exposed.

Aspergillus may also colonise pre-existing abscess cavities, classically old tuberculous cavities, where it may form a fungus ball *(aspergilloma)*. Invasive *Aspergillus* infections occur in individuals who are immunosuppressed.

Fig. 5.16A shows a medium-power view of invasive *Aspergillus* infection in the lung. A mass of *Aspergillus* hyphae **(A)** is surrounded by an inflammatory infiltrate **(I)** consisting mainly of neutrophils. Adjacent to this, there is a zone of necrotic lung tissue **(N)**. The high power micrograph (Fig. 5.16B) shows the mass of *Aspergillus* hyphae. These characteristically branch at an acute angle as is shown in Fig. 5.16C. The hyphae are also **septate,** i.e. the hyphae have divisions or septa **(S)** that divide them into segments. The typical appearance of *Aspergillus* on a silver stain is shown in Fig. 5.16D, which shows the fungal hyphae clearly.

Fig. 5.16E shows a mass of hyphae of *Aspergillus niger* **(H)** and inflammatory cells **(I)** from the external ear canal of a patient with chronic otitis externa. In the centre of the field there are two characteristic ***fruiting bodies* (F)** or ***conidia***. These are similar to the fruiting bodies of other *Aspergillus* species except that they are pigmented. The brownish-black pigment is visible around the periphery of the fruiting body and gives rise to the name *Aspergillus niger*. This is a common cause of chronic otitis externa, an infection of the outer ear, mainly the auditory canal.

OTHER FUNGAL INFECTIONS – ZYGOMYCOSIS

Zygomycosis (also termed **mucormycosis**) is a form of opportunistic fungal infection caused by one of a range of environmental fungi of the class **Zygomycetes**. These organisms pose no threat to immunocompetent individuals but can cause very serious and often life-threatening infections in those who are immunocompromised, particularly in patients with diabetes in whom the organisms may infect the nose and paranasal sinuses, invading from this site to involve the orbits and cerebrum *(rhinocerebral mucormycosis)*. In cases of mucormycosis, the hyphae are broad and irregular, branching at near right angles (in contrast to the acute angles seen in *Aspergillus* infection). Also, the hyphae typically appear open and non-septate in routine preparations. Often, the fungi invade into artery walls and may then give rise to thrombosis and tissue necrosis.

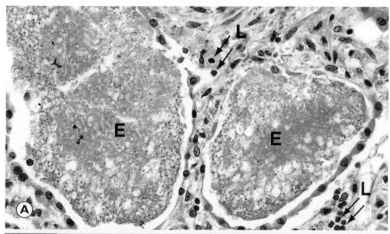
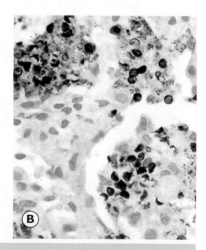

Fig. 5.17 *Pneumocystis* in the lung. **(A)** H&E (MP); **(B)** silver stain (HP).

The organism *Pneumocystis jirovecii* (formerly known as *Pneumocystis carinii*) was previously classified as a protozoan, but more recently it has become clear that it is a member of the fungal family. It is a ubiquitous organism and can be demonstrated in the lungs of most normal individuals where it causes no disease. *Pneumocystis* has, however, been brought into the spotlight by AIDS, although it may infect patients with immunosuppression from other causes. In patients with AIDS, *Pneumocystis* causes a diffuse patchy pneumonia, which may be the presenting feature of full-blown AIDS and is often fatal. Diagnosis may be difficult and transbronchial lung biopsy is often required. With routine H&E staining, as in Fig. 5.17A, the organisms may not be apparent **(E-Fig. 5.11H)**.

The alveoli are often filled by a foamy, acellular exudate **(E)** with an interstitial infiltrate of lymphocytes **(L)** in the alveolar wall. The inflammatory infiltrate may be minimal or more severe, showing features of diffuse alveolar damage (see Fig. 12.12) with hyaline membranes, capillary dilatation and exudation of red cells. Demonstration of the organisms requires a silver stain as shown in Fig. 5.17B. The organisms are cup-shaped and measure 4–6 μm.

Giemsa and toluidine blue stains may also be used. The above stains may also be carried out on sputum samples and bronchial washings. Patients with AIDS frequently have concurrent infections with other organisms such as cytomegalovirus (Fig. 5.13).

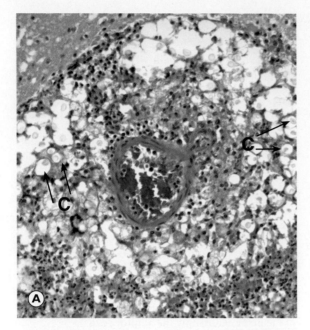

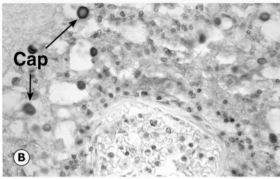

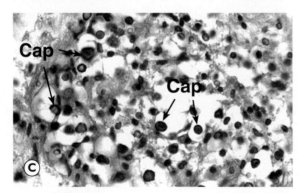

Fig. 5.18 *Cryptococcus.* **(A)** Brain H&E (MP); **(B)** alcian blue stain (HP); **(C)** mucicarmine stain (HP).

Cryptococcus neoformans is another yeast that causes serious infections in many tissues, mainly in immunosuppressed individuals such as patients with AIDS, haematological malignancy and transplant recipients. Occasionally, however, it may cause meningitis, meningoencephalitis or lung infection in an otherwise well individual.

Fig. 5.18A shows the typical appearance of *Cryptococcus* in the brain. The organisms are seen forming a cyst in a Virchow–Robin perivascular space. These lesions are known as 'soap bubble' lesions. The cryptococci **(C)** have a thick surrounding capsule that appears as a clear space. This capsule is an important virulence factor as it inhibits phagocytosis of the organisms and reduces normal leukocyte migration. Typically, there is a minimal inflammatory response, which may be due to the immunosuppressed state of the patient. However, in chronic infections in non-immunosuppressed individuals, the organisms may incite a granulomatous response.

Techniques employed in demonstrating cryptococci are highly dependent upon the thick capsule of the organisms. One simple method uses India ink to create a negative image, showing the organism with a clear capsular halo against a dark background.

Figs 5.18B and C show other special staining techniques that are useful in highlighting cryptococci. The organism's thick polysaccharide capsule **(Cap)** can be stained using Alcian blue as illustrated in Fig. 5.18B. Here, the nuclei of surrounding cells are counter-stained red. Fig. 5.18C shows brain tissue stained using the mucicarmine method. The cryptococci organisms are surrounded by a thick, magenta-coloured capsule **(Cap)**.

In the lung, *Cryptococcus* may cause a diffuse infection or it may form a solitary mass lesion in previously healthy individuals. Focal lesions such as this may lead to suspicion of other pathologies, such as bronchial carcinoma. In this case, the lesion is actually a large granuloma with a jelly-like centre, formed by a mass of organisms surrounded by a thick layer of macrophages, lymphocytes and giant cells.

Protozoa and helminths

Of the wide range of ***protozoa*** that are of pathological importance, only a few are usually diagnosed histologically. Many of these organisms are major causes of morbidity and mortality in particular geographic regions in the developing world. Increasingly, such infections may be seen elsewhere as a result of more widespread travel and migration. Protozoa are unicellular organisms that may reproduce asexually or sexually. Many have a complex life cycle involving one or more animal hosts. ***Giardia lamblia*** is a common protozoan infecting the small intestine in communities worldwide (Fig. 5.19). ***Trichomonas vaginalis*** is another protozoan parasite that is a common cause of female genital tract infection (Fig. 5.20). This organism is frequently encountered in cervical cytology screening. ***Malaria*** and ***amoebiasis*** are also described in this chapter (Figs 5.21 and 5.22). A wide variety of ***helminths*** infect humans, many primarily infecting the gut, although they may pass through other anatomical sites en route. Some helminths, such as the nematodes ***Enterobius vermicularis*** and ***Toxocara canis***, are found worldwide, while others, such as ***Wuchereria bancrofti***, have a more limited tropical distribution. ***Enterobiasis*** is fairly commonly seen in routine practice (Fig. 5.24) and ***Schistosomiasis*** is of particular histological importance (Fig. 5.23). These infections are illustrated.

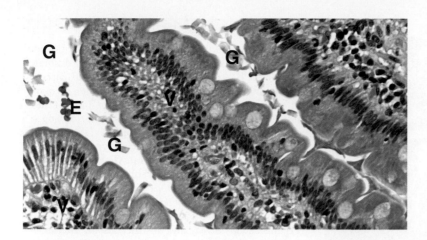

Fig. 5.19 Giardiasis (HP).

Giardia lamblia is a common protozoan parasite that causes diarrhoea. The organism is spread via contaminated water and is more common in institutionalised and immunocompromised patients. Diagnosis is commonly made by biopsy of the small intestine (Fig. 5.19). The *Giardia* organisms (**G**) are seen on the surface of the villi (**V**). A few erythrocytes (**E**) are also seen. The mucosa may appear normal or may be inflamed, sometimes resembling coeliac disease (see Fig. 13.15).

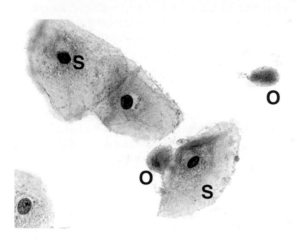

Fig. 5.20 *Trichomonas vaginalis* (Papanicolaou stain) (HP).

This flagellated protozoan parasite commonly infects the female genital tract, presenting with itching and a frothy greenish vaginal discharge. The organism is motile and can be demonstrated in wet preparations but is most commonly noted at the time of examination of a routine cervical smear test (Pap test). In Fig. 5.20, the organisms (**O**) are pear-shaped or ovoid and are somewhat smaller than the surrounding squamous epithelial cells (**S**). The organisms stain a smudgy grey-green colour. Indistinct nuclei and red cytoplasmic granules may be seen. Flagellae are not usually identifiable on routine preparations. The surrounding epithelial cells may show reactive changes and scattered neutrophil polymorphs may be present.

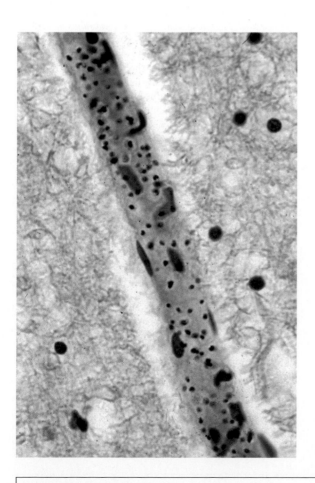

Fig. 5.21 Cerebral malaria (HP).

Malaria, which is caused by four species of the protozoan *Plasmodium*, is common in the tropics and subtropics and is a major cause of mortality. After entering the blood via the proboscis of a mosquito, the merozoites enter erythrocytes. Further cycles of division occur within the erythrocytes, which rupture, allowing further cycles of infection. The sexual phase of the life cycle occurs within the mosquito. *Plasmodium falciparum* is the most virulent form of malaria, with cerebral involvement being a major cause of death. The cerebral tissue is characteristically congested, as shown in Fig. 5.21, where a dilated small blood vessel is packed with erythrocytes within which the malarial parasites can be seen as dark brown dots. Falciparum malaria has the property of causing erythrocytes to adhere to endothelium, thus obstructing blood flow. The congested vessels often rupture to cause 'ring haemorrhages' (not shown here). Without specific treatment, cerebral malaria is almost always fatal and the increasing incidence of drug resistance makes it difficult to treat. Malarial parasites can be seen within erythrocytes in any other tissues and the diagnosis is usually made by examination of a blood smear. The different species can be identified by their characteristic appearance. The other species that cause malaria, namely *P. vivax, P. ovale* and *P. malariae*, cause a much milder illness that may be recurrent. *P. falciparum* may cause severe anaemia, pulmonary oedema, renal failure, shock, hypoglycaemia and cerebral disease.

KEY TO FIGURES
C Cryptococci **Cap** capsule **E** erythrocytes **G** *Giardia* **O** *Trichomonas* organism
S squamous cell **V** villus

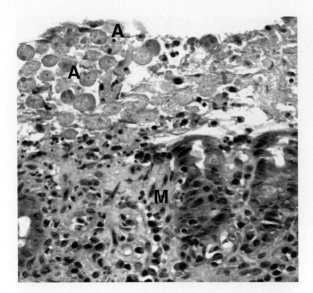

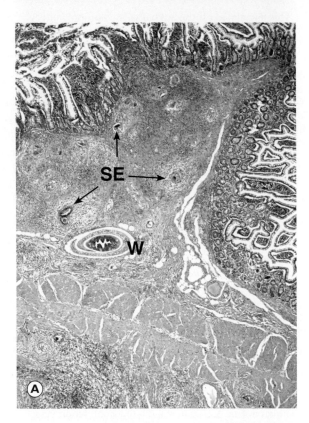

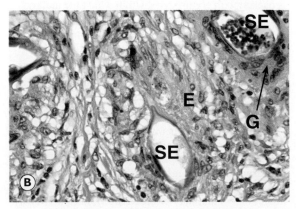

Fig. 5.22 Amoebiasis (HP).

Infections with *Entamoeba histolytica* occur worldwide. The organism is restricted to humans and it is estimated that about 10% of the world's population may carry the organism in the colon. The most common form of infection is **amoebic dysentery**, where the *Entamoebae* invade the mucosa of the colon and rectum, causing painful, bloody diarrhoea. Pathologically, the mucosa is extensively undermined, producing typical flask-shaped ulcers, which may perforate (E-Fig. 5.2**H**). Fig. 5.22 shows organisms (**A**) adherent to colonic mucosa (**M**). The *Entamoebae* are slightly larger than a macrophage and characteristically phagocytose erythrocytes (visible within the organisms). The organisms may invade and obstruct colonic arteries, causing superimposed ischaemic necrosis. The organism may spread to the liver, causing an **amoebic abscess**, and thence to the lung or pleural, peritoneal or pericardial cavities. Venereal infections of the cervix and penis also occasionally occur.

Fig. 5.23 Schistosomiasis. (A) MP; (B) HP.

Schistosomiasis is a systemic parasitic infection caused by the organism *Schistosoma*, a genus of **trematode worms (flukes)**. Three species are of pathological importance. Their life cycle includes water snails (the intermediate host), with humans (the definitive host) becoming infected by bathing or working in water containing the larvae or **cercaria** released from snails. The cercaria penetrate the skin, in the process converting to **schistosomules**, and then migrate via the venous system to the pulmonary vessels where they mature for 4 weeks before entering the systemic circulation. From here, they migrate to the hepatic branches of the portal vein (*Schistosoma mansoni* and *Schistosoma japonicum*) or the pelvic veins (*Schistosoma haematobium*) where they mature and may persist for several years or even more. In their chosen location, the adult worms mate with the females, producing up to 3000 eggs per day. Some eggs leave the body in urine or faeces and, on reaching still or gently flowing fresh water, hatch into a ciliated form called **miracidia** and thus reach their intermediate snail hosts. Other eggs lodge in the tissues (*S. mansoni* and *S. japonicum* in the small and large intestine and thence to the liver; *S. haematobium* in the bladder and rectum), exciting a florid granulomatous reaction progressing to extensive fibrosis. In the liver, there is severe fibrosis of the portal tracts where the eggs lodge. Schistosomiasis is the major cause of portal hypertension worldwide. *S. haematobium* causes a similar reaction in the bladder, with a number of manifestations including papillomas, ulcers and bladder contractures. Chronic inflammation predisposes to dysplasia and malignancy. Eggs may also be found at many other sites such as the lungs and CNS.

Fig. 5.23A shows a low-power view of schistosome eggs (**SE**) in the small intestine. Unusually, part of the adult worm (**W**) is seen. Fig. 5.23B shows two schistosome eggs (**SE**) at high power. The groups of eggs are surrounded by epithelioid cells (**E**), giant cells (**G**) and eosinophils. The eggs of each species can be identified by their size and the position of the spine, which in this case is terminally located and therefore likely to come from *S. haematobium*.

KEY TO FIGURES

A amoebae **AP** alar projection **C** cuticle **E** epithelioid cells **G** giant cell **L** longitudinal section through worm **M** mucosa **SE** schistosome eggs **W** transverse section adult worm

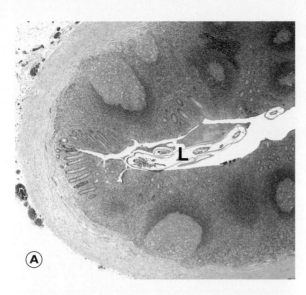

(A)

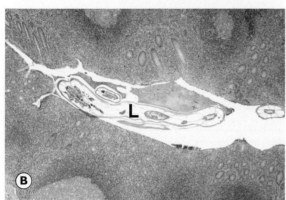

(B)

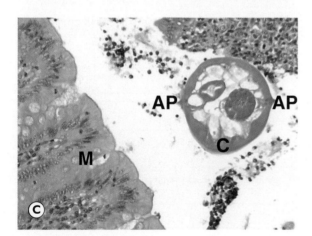

(C)

Fig. 5.24 *Enterobius vermicularis* **in appendix. (A)** LP; **(B)** MP; **(C)** HP.

Enterobius vermicularis is also known as pinworm or threadworm. The organism is spread by the faecal-oral route and is commonly present within the lumen of the bowel, particularly in children. The organisms do not invade the tissues. The female worm lays eggs in the peri-anal area and symptoms, if any, tend to be of perineal irritation. The adult worms inhabit the ileocaecal area and are most commonly identified in the appendix.

Fig. 5.24A shows the tip of the appendix, sectioned longitudinally (E-Fig. 5.12**H**). Adult worms are visible within the lumen, one shown in longitudinal section **(L)**. Note the normal reactive lymphoid tissue within the wall of the appendix. Typically, there is no tissue reaction associated with the presence of the parasites and the normal appendiceal mucosa with its associated lymphoid tissue can been seen at higher magnification in Fig. 5.24B.

Fig. 5.24C shows a transverse section through an adult worm, lying within the lumen of the appendix. Again, note that there is no invasion of the mucosa **(M)**. The thick cuticle **(C)** of the worm has a typical alar projection **(AP)** on each side and the oesophagus and other internal structures of the worm can also be seen.

Table 5.1	Chapter review.	
Disorder	**Main features**	**Figure**
Bacterial infections		
Clostridium difficile E-Fig.5.1**G**	Pseudomembranous colitis with focal epithelial necrosis due to toxin. 'Volcano' pattern with inflammatory exudate	5.1
Actinomyces	Filamentous bacteria forming 'sulphur granule' colonies with encrusted proteinaceous material	5.2
Mycobacterium tuberculosis E-Fig. 5.3**G**	Granulomatous inflammation with caseation and Langhans' giant cells Ghon complex. May progress to miliary disease if immunosuppressed	5.3–5.7, 5.10A
Atypical mycobacteria (MOTT, NTM)	Often in immunocompromised patients. Suppurative granulomas	5.8
Mycobacterium leprae	Pattern depends upon immune status (tuberculoid/lepromatous). Granulomatous inflammation of skin and dermal nerves	5.9, 5.10B
Treponema pallidum	Primary, secondary and tertiary syphilis. Chancre, gumma, endarteritis obliterans	5.11
Viral infections		
Herpes simplex virus	Types 1 & 2. Oral and genital herpes. Disseminated in immunosuppressed. Vesiculation with syncytial giant cells and intranuclear inclusions	5.12
Varicella zoster virus	Cause of chickenpox and shingles. Morphology similar to HSV	Like 5.12
Cytomegalovirus	Non-specific symptoms normally. Disseminated in immunosuppressed. Very large cells with intranuclear and intracytoplasmic inclusions	5.13
Human papilloma-virus	Many types, causes common wart. Oncogenic forms cause cervical cancer Koilocytosis, binucleation, dyskeratosis and dysplasia (CIN)	5.14, 17.6, 17.7
Fungal infections		
Candida	Common, often affects mucous membranes. Typically neutrophil response. Yeast forms and branching pseudohyphae	5.15
Aspergillus	Mostly lung disease. Allergic, colonising and invasive forms Narrowing septate hyphae with branching at acute angles	5.16
Zygomyces	Mucormycosis. Typically sinonasal disease in diabetic patients. Invades vessels. Broad and non-septate hyphae with right-angle branching	
Pneumocystis	Environmental fungus, pathogenic in immunocompromised, e.g. AIDS. Foamy exudate in alveoli, cup-shaped organisms on silver stains	5.17
Cryptococcus	Mostly in immunocompromised patients. Can cause lung disease in normal people. Yeasts with thick outer capsule	5.18
Protozoa and helminths		
Giardia lamblia	Cause of infective diarrhoea. Protozoan parasite infecting small intestine. Small sickle-shaped organisms on mucosal surface	5.19
Trichomonas vaginalis	Common cause of vaginal discharge and irritation, often seen in cervical smear tests. Pear-shaped protozoan parasites with flagellae	5.20
Plasmodium sp.	Cause of malaria. Intracellular parasites with complex life cycle, spread by mosquito. Pigmented organisms in erythrocytes, vascular complications	5.21
Entamoeba histolytica	Very common cause of dysentery worldwide. Invades colorectal mucosa. Flask-shaped ulcers and organisms larger than macrophages, PAS positive	5.22
Schistosoma sp.	Important worldwide. Complex lifecycle involving snail. Eggs lodge in various tissues and cause granulomatous inflammation	5.23
Enterobius vermicularis	Threadworm or pinworm. Common, colonises ileocolic area. Worms do not invade. Eggs cause perianal irritation. Often seen in appendix	5.24

6 Disorders of growth

Introduction

Cells exist in, and must adapt to, an environment that is continually changing, reflecting not only physiological processes but also external influences such as drugs or toxins. As briefly discussed in Ch. 2, if the stimulus is overwhelming, the cells undergo degeneration or cell death. However, many less noxious stimuli cause cells to adapt by altering their pattern of growth. This may occur in three main ways:

- alteration in the size of cells

  - *hypertrophy*: increase in size of existing cells

  - *atrophy*: decrease in size of existing cells

- increase in the number of cells *(hyperplasia)*

- change in the differentiation of cells *(metaplasia)*.

In an organ composed of different types of cell, only one of the cell types may be affected, leading to a marked change in tissue appearance and function.

In all tissues, there is a population of undifferentiated cells *(stem cells)* that differ from mature cells throughout the body in three ways:

- they are capable of dividing and renewing themselves (self-renewal)

- they are unspecialised

- they can give rise to specialised cell types.

Extrinsic to the cell, factors such as blood supply, innervation, hormonal stimulation, physical stress or biochemical alterations will determine the normal pattern of cell growth in an organ or tissue. Depending on the intrinsic characteristics of a particular cell type, a change in environment may result in a change in the growth pattern. Such responses are now recognised as being under the control of various growth factors that act upon specific cell surface receptors. Alterations in the concentrations of growth factors or the expression of growth factor receptors will result in altered cell growth.

CELL AND GENE THERAPY

Stem cells are undifferentiated cells with the capacity for self-renewal and differentiation into other specialised types of cells. Harnessing the regenerative/reparative characteristics of stem cells in treating disease is the subject of a large field of clinical research.

Stem cell therapy involves transferring intact, whole cells into a patient either from their own body *(autologous)* or from another person/donor *(allogeneic)*. Gene therapy involves transfer of DNA or RNA into a patient via a vector such as a virus or carrier cell. Gene and stem cell therapies are often used in combination to target diseases by altering the genetic structure of the cell before transfer into the patient.

The most common clinical application of stem cell therapy is bone marrow transplantation for the treatment of a variety of haematological diseases including forms of leukaemia, lymphoma and myeloma. However, the therapeutic repertoire of stem cell therapy is expanding to include treatment of diseases such as Parkinson's disease, myocardial infarction and other types of cancer.

In bone marrow transplantation, the bone marrow must first be cleared of cells through a process known as *myeloablation* using a combination of both chemotherapy and radiotherapy. This process removes any remaining, diseased marrow and reduces the likelihood of transplant rejection. As above, stem cells can be sourced from the patient's own marrow or blood *(autologous transplant)* or from a donor *(allogeneic transplant)*. The harvested haematopoietic stem cells can then be introduced to the patient through an intravenous infusion. Allogeneic transplants use stem cells collected from a donor with a tissue type that closely matches that of the recipient, often a family member. This reduces the risk of transplant rejection, known as *graft versus host disease*, where donor immune cells mount a response to the recipient's tissues, particularly the skin, gastrointestinal tract and liver.

Increased cell mass

Organs may respond to environmental stimulation by an increase in functional cell mass through hyperplasia and/or hypertrophy (Fig. 6.1). Hyperplasia occurs where cells are capable of dividing to generate an increased number of cells. In contrast, hypertrophy is typified by increase in cell size without an increase in cell number (Fig. 6.2). An important feature of these forms of increased cell mass is that, following removal of the environmental stimulus, the altered pattern of growth ceases and the tissue may revert to its former state. Hypertrophy and hyperplasia can, in many circumstances, be regarded as normal physiological adaptations, as exemplified by exercise-induced skeletal muscle hypertrophy and the hyperplasia and hypertrophy of the myometrium during pregnancy.

Many pathological stimuli invoke the responses of hypertrophy and hyperplasia and it appears these responses occur in many cases by the same mechanism that induces the normal physiological response (Fig. 6.3). Thus, in the first part of the menstrual cycle, the endometrium proliferates with elongation of glands and increased numbers of epithelial cells. When an excessive concentration of oestrogen acts on the endometrium, such as during the menopause or owing to injudicious hormone replacement therapy, similar but more pronounced changes occur, leading to crowding of endometrial glands. Removing the stimulus to this excess growth can result in a regression. This contrasts with the abnormal, uncontrolled proliferation of cells associated with the development of cancers, referred to as *neoplasia* (see Ch. 7) where growth is independent of any external stimuli. Therefore, hyperplastic tissue is not of itself neoplastic but may carry with it an increased risk of neoplastic change. Thus, hyperplastic endometrium is more likely than normal endometrium to progress to cancer. This risk is increased further when the hyperplasia is combined with cytologic atypia (termed *atypical hyperplasia*) (E-Fig. 6.1**G**).

For poorly understood reasons, the process of hyperplasia may not be uniform throughout an organ or tissue and, in these instances, nodules of excessive cell growth arise in between areas of unaltered cell growth. This phenomenon, known as *nodular hyperplasia*, is seen in the thyroid gland (see Fig. 20.5), the adrenal gland (see Fig. 20.9) and the prostate gland (see Fig. 19.8).

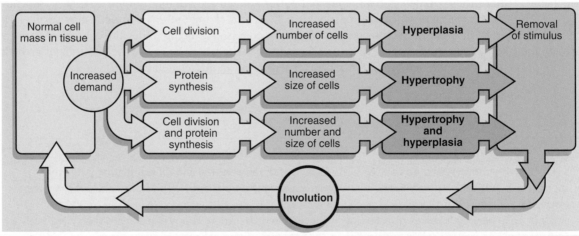

Fig. 6.1 **Increased functional cell mass.**

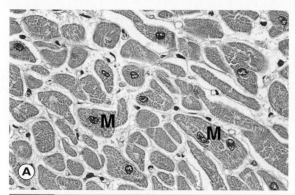

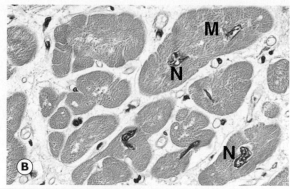

Fig. 6.2 **Hypertrophy. (A)** Normal myocardium (MP); **(B)** hypertrophic myocardium (MP).

Pure hypertrophy, without co-existing hyperplasia, is virtually only seen in muscle, where the stimulus is an increased demand for work. An example is adult myocardium, the cells of which are incapable of division and are therefore unable to undergo hyperplasia. As such, myocardium becomes hypertrophic when it is subjected to an increased haemodynamic load over a period of time, such as in systemic hypertension or valvular stenosis.

Fig. 6.2A shows normal myocardium **(M)** (E-Fig. 6.2**H**) while Fig. 6.2B, which is at the same

magnification, shows enlargement of myocardial cells **(M)** and their nuclei **(N)**. This enlargement is due to increased synthesis of proteins and filaments, permitting an increased workload; thus the size and weight of the heart are increased (E-Fig. 6.3**G**).

Other examples of muscular hypertrophy include bowel wall smooth muscle in chronic obstruction of the bowel by tumour, bladder detrusor muscle in chronic obstruction due to prostatic hyperplasia and in regularly exercised skeletal muscles.

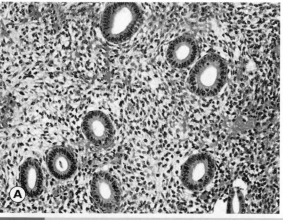

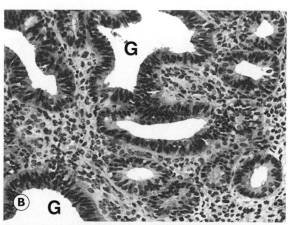

Fig. 6.3 **Hyperplasia. (A)** Normal proliferative phase endometrium (HP); **(B)** hyperplasia of endometrium (HP).

Endometrial hyperplasia occurs when there is abnormal oestrogenic stimulation. Fig. 6.3A shows normal proliferative phase endometrium responding to normal ovarian oestrogenic stimulation (E-Fig. 6.4**H**). In contrast, in Fig. 6.3B, the endometrial glands are markedly hyperplastic and continued increase in the number of cells in each gland has resulted in some glands **(G)** showing cystic dilatation. In addition, there is irregularity and crowding of the glands as well as crowding of the epithelial cells lining the glands. This example is from

a woman on hormone replacement therapy where the effects of oestrogen were not counterbalanced by progestogens, resulting in persisting growth of the endometrium. Similar changes may also be seen in the endometrium of women with oestrogen secreting ovarian tumours. Thus, hyperplasia results from exaggeration of a normal physiologic mechanism.

In such examples, removal of the abnormal oestrogenic stimulation restores the normal pattern of endometrial growth.

KEY TO FIGURES
G gland **M** myocardial cell **N** nucleus

Reduction in functional cell mass

When the functional cell mass in a tissue is reduced, the tissue is said to have undergone **atrophy**. The mechanisms of atrophy may involve reduction in cell volume and/or in cell number, both leading to a reduction in functional capacity. Macroscopically, the appearance of the tissue depends on whether the functional cells lost are replaced by other tissue. Commonly, when atrophy occurs, the lost cells are replaced by either adipose or fibrous tissue, often maintaining the overall size of the organ. When adipose or fibrous replacement does not occur, the overall size of the organ is reduced. Examples are the testis in the elderly (Fig. 6.4) and the adrenal gland when suppressed by exogenous steroid administration (see Fig. 20.9). Atrophy may occur as a physiological event (termed **involution**), such as in embryologic development or the normal involution of the thymus during adolescence.

A variety of causes of atrophy is recognised, in general conditions opposite to those causing hypertrophy or hyperplasia. Thus, disuse of skeletal muscle will result in a loss of cell mass **(disuse atrophy)**. Removal of endocrine stimulation causes atrophy in target organs. Reduction in blood supply to a tissue may result in loss of functional cells **(ischaemic atrophy)**, a situation commonly encountered in the kidney.

Atrophy must be distinguished from **hypoplasia,** a condition where there is incomplete growth of an organ, and **agenesis**, where there is complete failure of growth of an organ during embryological development.

In many atrophic tissues a granular, brown pigment **(lipofuscin)**, which is composed of degenerate lipid material in lysosomal granules, may accumulate within the shrunken cells. It is most readily identified in atrophic myocardial fibres of the hearts of elderly people, giving rise to the term **brown atrophy**.

Hyaline is a term used to describe replacement of tissue by an amorphous pink-staining material similar to basement membrane matrix. It is a common end result of atrophy or cell damage, being frequently accompanied by fibrosis.

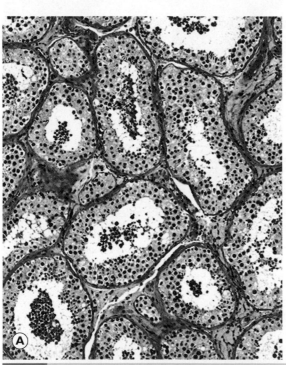
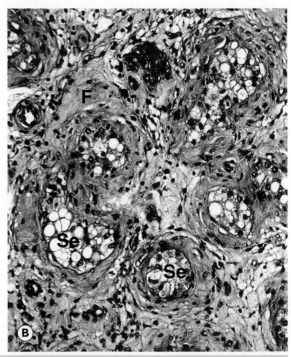

Fig. 6.4 **Atrophy. (A)** Normal testis (HP); **(B)** atrophic testis (HP).

Atrophy of a tissue occurs by shrinkage of cells, with reduction of cytoplasmic components such as organelles and enzyme proteins, and also by loss of cells by apoptosis.

Fig. 6.4B illustrates atrophy of the testis in a 94-year-old man. Compared with the normal testis in Fig. 6.4A (E-Fig. 6.5**H**), the seminiferous tubules

of the atrophic testis show almost no spermatogenic activity; however, the Sertoli cells **(Se)** are still easily identified. The basement membranes of the tubules are thickened and pink stained **(hyalinised)**. The interstitial tissue shows an increased deposition of fibrous tissue **(F)**.

Change in cell differentiation

Under certain circumstances, cells may undergo a change in differentiation to another, mature, differentiated cell type *(metaplasia)*. This is thought to be an adaptive response that produces cells better equipped to withstand an environmental change (usually pathological). For example, in the bronchi the specialised columnar respiratory epithelium may be replaced by squamous epithelium under the influence of chronic irritation by cigarette smoke *(squamous metaplasia)*. Similarly, in response to environmental changes during the reproductive cycle, the normal columnar endocervical epithelium is replaced by a stratified squamous epithelium (Fig. 6.5A).

In the lower oesophagus, the normal stratified squamous epithelium may, in response to acid reflux from the stomach, be replaced by gastric *(gastric metaplasia)* or small intestinal *(intestinal metaplasia)* mucosa (Fig. 6.5B). In common with metaplasia at other sites, the basic alteration appears to occur in the stem cells of the tissue such that, rather than differentiating into a squamous cell, they mature instead into a mucus-producing columnar cell that is better able to protect itself from an acid environment. When the stimulus is removed, the stem cells may revert to producing differentiated cells of the original type.

Metaplasia most commonly occurs in epithelial tissues but may also be seen in mesodermal tissues; for example, areas of fibrous tissue exposed to chronic trauma may form bone *(osseous metaplasia)*. Metaplasia may co-exist with hyperplasia and, more importantly, *dysplasia* (see Ch. 7).

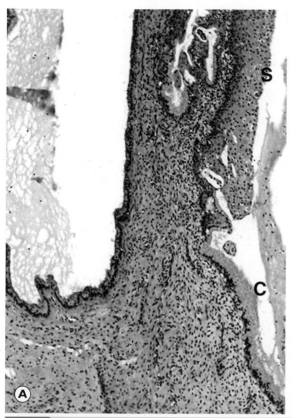 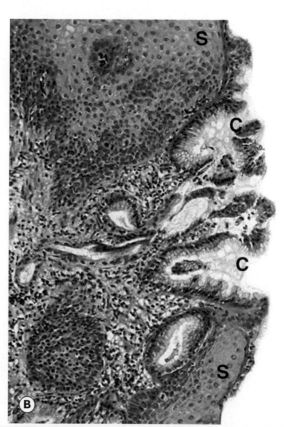

Fig. 6.5 **Metaplasia.** **(A)** Squamous metaplasia of cervix (MP); **(B)** gastric metaplasia of lower oesophagus (MP).

Squamous metaplasia of the cervix is so common it may almost be regarded as physiologically normal. During a woman's reproductive life, the shape of the cervix changes cyclically, exposing the endocervical columnar epithelium to the environment of the vagina. This *ectropion*, often incorrectly referred to as an *erosion*, is apparent macroscopically as an area of velvety pink epithelium at the external os.

In response to this change of environment, the endocervical epithelium is replaced by stratified squamous epithelium as shown in Fig. 6.5A. At the top, the surface is covered by mature stratified squamous epithelium **(S),** which overlies endocervical glands lined by the normal mucus-secreting columnar epithelium **(C),** which is also present at the surface at the bottom. In time, the metaplastic squamous epithelium may extend into the glands. Inflammation of the cervix accelerates this process.

In Fig. 6.5B, the reverse change is occurring in the lower oesophagus where normal native squamous epithelium **(S)** at the top and bottom is being replaced by gastric-type columnar epithelium **(C),** which is able to produce mucus to protect the epithelium from acid reflux. This is known as *Barrett's oesophagus*.

KEY TO FIGURES
C columnar epithelium **F** fibrous tissue **S** squamous epithelium **Se** Sertoli cells

Table 6.1 Chapter review.

	Main features	Examples	Figure
Hypertrophy	Increase in size of existing cells	Myocardium in hypertension	6.2
		Skeletal muscle with exercise	
Hyperplasia	Increase in number of cells	Endometrium under oestrogenic stimulation	6.3
Atrophy	Reduction in cell size and/or number	Ischaemic atrophy of kidney	
		'Brown atrophy' of myocardium	
		Testicular atrophy	6.4
Metaplasia	Change of differentiation in a cell	Squamous metaplasia of cervix	6.5A
		Gastric/intestinal metaplasia of lower oesophagus	6.5B

7 Dysplasia and neoplasia

Cellular atypia and dysplasia

In the previous chapter, we considered cellular adaptations to a variety of stimuli resulting in alterations in their pattern of growth, whilst still achieving full differentiation/maturation. Occasionally, cells have an increased rate of division such that they do not have time to reach complete maturation (with full development of cytoplasmic specialisation) before another cycle of cell division supervenes. This leads to a population of cells that are structurally abnormal, having a high nuclear to cytoplasmic ratio with large nuclei containing abundant, dark-staining chromatin and prominent, occasionally multiple, nucleoli. These nuclear changes are associated with evidence of incomplete maturation of the cytoplasm, which may be lacking in the specialised structures normally seen in that cell type, such as mucin vacuoles or surface cilia. This is called *failure of differentiation* and the cells are said to show *atypia*.

   Cellular atypia may be a consequence of rapid multiplication of cells as a response to cell destruction due to a persistent damaging stimulus. In this case, atypia is a result of the high turnover of cells attempting to regenerate damaged epithelium. When the damaging stimulus is removed, these abnormalities should revert to normal with full differentiation of the cells returning. However, sometimes the atypia is persistent and is not simply the result of regeneration. In these cases, the population of atypical cells may eventually be the focus from which invasive cancer develops. This type of persistent cellular atypia is called *dysplasia* (Fig. 7.1). The problem for the pathologist is in distinguishing between cellular atypia, representing a reactive, regenerative response to tissue damage, and dysplasia, which is indicative of early pre-cancer. There is no simple answer.

   Dysplasia often arises in metaplastic tissues and it is likely that the stimuli that cause dysplasia are also responsible for metaplastic change. Thus metaplastic epithelium in the cervix and Barrett's oesophagus is at risk of dysplasia and subsequent neoplasia. In dysplastic cells, molecular biological techniques have demonstrated some of the genetic abnormalities found in invasive neoplasms. Because of the sinister association of dysplasia with the subsequent development of neoplasia, treatment of dysplastic conditions is undertaken to minimise the risk of subsequent development of a malignancy. Recognition of dysplastic changes by cytological examination of cervical smears forms the basis of screening for cancer of the cervix (see clinical box 'Screening and pathology' and Fig. 17.6).

SCREENING AND PATHOLOGY
Screening is an important part of disease prevention and involves assessing a subset of the population for a disease or condition using a relatively non-invasive test. This allows early detection and treatment and therefore improves survival rates. It is important to remember that screening tests only identify those at high risk of having the disease/condition and a further diagnostic test, usually in the form of a biopsy, is required for confirmation and/or treatment. Most developed countries now offer several different screening programmes, examples of which are given below. Pathologists can be involved in assessing the screening test sample itself or the diagnostic test sample (e.g. a core biopsy), which follows a positive screening result.

Disease/condition	Screening test	Diagnostic test
Cervical cancer	Cervical smear: cytology	Biopsy or large loop excision of transformation zone (LLETZ)
Breast cancer	Mammography	Fine needle aspirate (FNA) or core biopsy
Colorectal cancer	Faecal occult blood (FOB) test +/- colonoscopy	Removal of polyp/ biopsy of lesion
Prostate cancer	Prostate specific antigen (PSA) blood test and digital rectal examination	Trans-rectal ultrasound (TRUS) and core biopsy

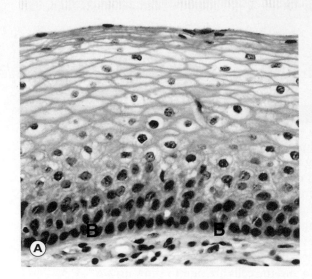

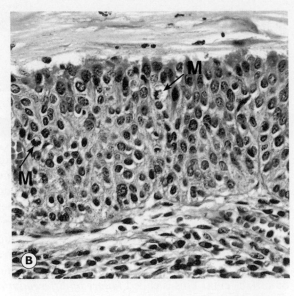

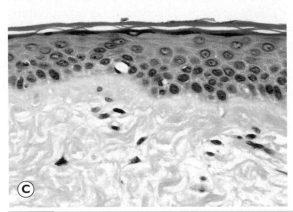

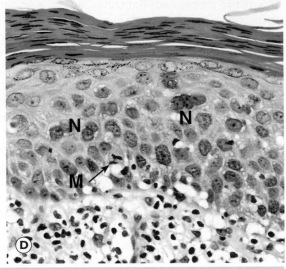

Fig. 7.1 **Dysplasia. (A)** Normal cervix (HP); **(B)** dysplasia in the cervix (HP); **(C)** normal skin (HP); **(D)** dysplastic skin (HP).

Dysplasia is a morphological feature characterised by increased cellular proliferation with incomplete maturation of cells. It occurs most commonly at the uterine cervix and in the skin.

Fig. 7.1A illustrates normal stratified squamous epithelium from the cervix (E-Fig. 7.1**H**). Cellular proliferation is confined to the basal layer **(B)** where the cells are small, uniform and darkly stained. As the cells mature towards the surface, their cytoplasm expands and becomes more eosinophilic. Near the surface, the cells become progressively flattened. The ratio of nucleus to cytoplasm diminishes as the cells pass from the basal to surface layers.

In contrast, Fig. 7.1B shows dysplastic cervical epithelium where there is disruption of the normal orderly maturation sequence. Cells in all layers now exhibit larger than normal nuclei, some with prominent nucleoli. Mitotic figures **(M)** may be seen well above the basal layer. The nuclei of the cells

are more variable in shape and size than normal *(pleomorphism)* and the nuclear to cytoplasmic ratio is greater than normal. It is the presence of such surface cells with large nuclei that alerts the cytologist to underlying dysplasia in a cervical smear (see Fig. 17.6).

Figs 7.1C and D demonstrate similar features in normal (E-Fig. 7.2**H**) and dysplastic skin, respectively. Note how the normal cellular stratification is disrupted in the dysplastic specimen by cells with large, darkly staining nuclei and multinucleated cells **(N)** extending into the middle strata. In addition, a disturbed pattern of maturation is reflected in the development of a thick layer of keratin, which contains purple-stained nuclear remnants *(parakeratosis)*. It is this keratin layer that becomes clinically evident as thickening and scaling of the skin. Mitotic figures **(M)** are also apparent above the basal layers.

Both of these conditions have a greatly increased tendency to develop into invasive carcinoma.

KEY TO FIGURES
B basal layer   **M** mitotic figure   **N** multinucleated cells

In a neoplasm, cellular proliferation and growth occur in the absence of any continuing external stimulus. Therefore, the term *neoplasia* (from the Greek for new growth) describes a state of autonomous cell division and the abnormal mass of cells that results is termed a *neoplasm.* The state of neoplastic growth contrasts with *hyperplasia*, discussed in Ch. 6, where, although there is abnormal proliferation of cells, this ceases with removal of the causative stimulus.

As well as abnormal cell proliferation, neoplasia is characterised by abnormal maturation of cells. A feature of normal tissue growth is the maturation of constituent cells into a form adapted to a specific function. Such adaptation may involve the acquisition of specialised structures such as mucin vacuoles, neurosecretory granules, microvilli or cilia. This process of structural and functional maturation is called *differentiation*. A fully mature cell of any particular cell line is said to be *highly differentiated*, whereas its primitive precursor cells are described as being *undifferentiated*. In any given tissue, the normal cells have a characteristic state of differentiation. In contrast, neoplastic cells exhibit variable states of differentiation and commonly fail to achieve a highly differentiated state. Neoplasms are divided clinically into two main groups (Table 7.1):

■ *benign neoplasms* grow slowly and remain localised to the site of origin

■ *malignant neoplasms* grow rapidly and may spread widely.

There is a broad correlation between histological appearances and biological behaviour, allowing prediction of the likely prognosis. In general, the cells of benign neoplasms are well differentiated. In the case of malignant neoplasms, there is a variable degree of differentiation. At one end of the spectrum, the constituent cells may closely resemble the tissue of origin, in which case the tumour is described as being a *well differentiated malignancy*. Alternatively, the constituent cells may bear little resemblance to the tissue of origin, in which case the neoplasm is described as being *poorly differentiated*. At the extreme end of the spectrum, neoplasms that exhibit no evidence of differentiation are termed *anaplastic* and, in many cases, it may not be possible to identify the cell of origin on morphological grounds alone. Generally, the degree of differentiation of a neoplasm is related to its behaviour. A poorly differentiated neoplasm tends to be more invasive and more aggressive than a well differentiated neoplasm.

CARCINOGENESIS

Transformation from normally functioning and growing cells to cancer, called *carcinogenesis*, is regarded as a complex multistep process involving acquisition of genetic mutations, failure of normal DNA repair mechanisms and reduced apoptosis, along with developing the capacity for invasion and metastasis.

As discussed in Chapter 1, the consequences of a mutation in a single oncogene invariably would be overcome by otherwise normally functioning tumour suppressor genes. This concept is summarised by the *Knudson hypothesis*, which states that multiple mutations, or 'hits', are required for cancer to develop. In the typical example of familial cancer syndromes, the first hit is in inheriting the abnormal DNA which is balanced by normally functioning genes until the second hit, where these too are damaged and cancer develops.

In addition to a growing list of inherited cancer syndromes, a considerable number of environmental agents associated with the development of cancer are now recognised, including chemical agents, ionising radiation and infections such as viruses. These are known as *carcinogens* and examples of these are given below.

Inherited cancer syndromes		Chemical agents		Infections	
Gene	Association	Agent	Association	Agent	Association
NF1, NF2	Neurofibromatosis types 1 and 2	Asbestos	Mesothelioma, lung cancer, GI tract cancers	HPV	Cervical carcinoma
APC	Familial adenomatous polyposis, colon cancer	Nitrosamines	Gastric carcinoma	EBV	Burkitt, Hodgkin lymphomas
BRCA1/ BRCA2	Breast and ovarian cancers	Benzene	Leukaemia, Hodgkin lymphoma	Hep B/C	Hepatocellular carcinoma
RB	Retinoblastoma	Nickel	Lung cancer	HHV8	Kaposi's sarcoma
P53	Li-Fraumeni syndrome	Azo dyes	Bladder cancer	*H. pylori*	Gastric carcinoma MALT lymphoma

Carcinoma in situ

The term *carcinoma in situ* is used when an epithelial tissue shows the cytological and histological features of carcinoma (architectural and cytological abnormalities such as cell crowding, pleomorphism, increased and abnormal mitotic activity, which may involve the full thickness of the epithelium), but there is no evidence that the basement membrane bounding the abnormal epithelial tissue has been breached and there is no encroachment of atypical cells into the underlying stroma. The process whereby tumour cells breach the basement membrane and extend into the surrounding tissues is described as *invasion*. Thus, with carcinoma in situ the epithelial cells show the cytological, but not the behavioural, characteristics of malignancy. However, many forms of carcinoma in situ will become invasive if left untreated.

Certain benign epithelial tumours may progress to form an invasive malignant tumour by development and selective persistence of mutations in key oncogenes. A sequence from benign neoplasm through increasing severity of dysplasia to carcinoma in situ and on to invasive carcinoma is well recognised in certain sites.

Carcinoma in situ is synonymous with severe/high grade dysplasia. However, terminology varies depending on the anatomical location. For example, the term carcinoma in situ is used in the skin (see Fig. 21.14) and bladder (see Fig. 15.21). At other sites such as the cervix, carcinoma in situ is called CIN3 (cervical intraepithelial neoplasia; see Fig. 17.7), in the vulva, VIN3 (vulval intraepithelial neoplasia) and in colonic adenomatous polyps, 'high grade dysplasia' (see Fig. 13.21). It also occurs in solid glandular organs, most notably the breast (ductal and lobular carcinoma in situ; see Figs. 18.9 and 18.11).

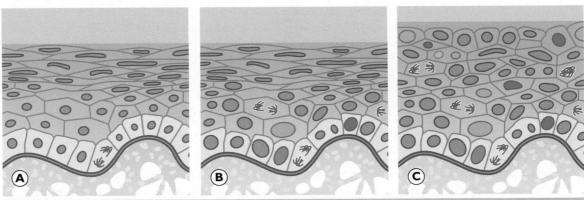

Fig. 7.2 **Carcinoma in situ. (A)** Normal; **(B)** dysplasia; **(C)** carcinoma in situ.

Fig. 7.2A shows the regular architecture of a normal stratified squamous epithelium. The layered epithelium is formed by mitotic replication of the basal layer, producing layers of regular cells, which differentiate and flatten as they approach the surface (stratification). The cells are regular in shape and size, as are the nuclei, and mitotic activity is confined to the basal layer.

Fig. 7.2B shows an epithelium in which there is dysplasia in the lower layers. The cells and their nuclei are irregular in shape and size and the nuclei occupy more of the cell. Mitoses are present in layers other than the basal layer. The cells still differentiate and eventually mature near the surface.

Fig. 7.2C shows fully developed carcinoma in situ. The dysplastic epithelial cells now occupy the full thickness of the epithelium and stratification and differentiation are largely lost. Mitoses can be present in any of the layers, even in surface cells. Although all the cells in this epithelium show cytological characteristics of malignancy (cellular and nuclear pleomorphism, high nuclear to cytoplasmic ratio, nuclear hyperchromasia and increased abnormal mitotic activity), the epithelial cells as yet show no tendency to invade across the basement membrane into the stroma.

In certain anatomical locations, the dysplastic changes shown in Figs 7.2B and C are acknowledged by applying a numerical value, with 1 regarded as low grade and 2 or 3 regarded as high grade. Therefore, in the squamous epithelium of the uterine cervix, the changes in Fig. 7.2C would be called CIN 3 (cervical intra-epithelial neoplasia 3), whereas those in Fig. 7.2B would be called CIN 2. A similar scheme exists in the nomenclature of dysplastic/in situ neoplastic changes in the vulva (VIN) and vagina (VAIN).

General characteristics of neoplasms

As mentioned before, the property whereby a malignant tumour can grow into the surrounding tissue is termed invasion. A further property of malignant neoplasms is distant spread of neoplastic cells away from the main neoplasm (the *primary tumour*) to form subpopulations of neoplastic cells that are not in continuity with the primary tumour. Distant spread of tumour from a primary site is termed *metastasis*. The *secondary tumours* that result from this distant spread are termed *metastases*.

In general terms, a benign tumour will behave in a relatively innocuous manner and a malignant tumour will have deleterious effects, often leading to death. There are, however, exceptions to these generalisations and factors other than the biological growth pattern of a tumour may be important in influencing the outcome. Of these, the most notable is the location of the tumour. For example, a benign tumour of the brain stem may lead to rapid death, whereas a malignant tumour of the skin may progress slowly over many years.

In addition to local effects, malignant tumours can cause a variety of systemic symptoms such as weight loss *(cachexia)*, loss of appetite, fever and general malaise. In most cases, the pathophysiology is poorly understood, but includes effects of secreted cytokines such as *tumour necrosis factor*. Some tumours, benign and malignant, retain the function of their organ of origin. If this happens to be an endocrine function, then the tumour may exert harmful effects by secretion of excess hormone. Other tumours secrete hormones not usually secreted by that tissue, for example the secretion of parathyroid hormone by lung carcinomas. This is known as *ectopic hormone secretion* and the clinical manifestations are described as *paraneoplastic syndromes* (see clinical box 'Paraneoplastic syndromes').

Table 7.1 Summary of features of neoplasms.

	Benign	Malignant
Behaviour	Expansile growth only; grows locally	Expansile and invasive growth; may metastasise
	Often encapsulated	Not encapsulated
Histology	Resembles cell of origin (well differentiated)	May show failure of cellular differentiation
	Few mitoses	Many mitoses, some of which are abnormal forms
	Normal or slight increase in ratio of nucleus to cytoplasm	High nuclear to cytoplasmic ratio
	Cells are uniform throughout the tumour	Cells vary in shape and size (cellular pleomorphism) and/or nuclei vary in shape and size (nuclear pleomorphism)

PARANEOPLASTIC SYNDROMES

In addition to direct, local invasion and metastatic spread, cancers may give rise to distant symptoms and/or signs through two main mechanisms:

- An immune response to the malignancy producing antibodies to tumour cells, which cross-react with normal cells. In many cases, the antibodies may target normal neurones producing well characterised, complex neurological presentations.

- Release of cytokines/hormones by malignant cells, such as ectopic adrenocorticotrophic hormone (ACTH; see Ch. 20), which may be released by a variety of cancers, including pulmonary carcinomas.

The associated clinical syndromes may precede, follow or present at the same time as the primary malignancy.

Histological assessment of neoplasms

Histological assessment of a tumour provides a useful guide to its behaviour, i.e. whether the tumour is benign or malignant, and provides a rational basis for treatment. Histological assessment should establish the following features:

■ **The type of tumour.** This is based on the presumed tissue of origin and/or differentiation of the tumour.

■ **The degree of differentiation** (Fig. 7.10). This is known as *grading* and takes into account some or all of the following features:

  – the similarity of the tumour to the supposed tissue of origin both architecturally and cytologically *(differentiation)*

  – the degree of variability of cellular shape and size *(pleomorphism)*

  – the proportion of mitotic figures (dividing cells).

■ **The extent of spread of tumour** *(staging)* is partly assessed histologically, particularly:

  – size of the primary tumour

  – histological assessment of local, vascular, lymphatic and perineural invasion

  – the presence of metastatic tumour deposits, for example in lymph nodes and bones.

■ **The presence or absence of other prognostic factors.** For instance, the presence of oestrogen receptors in breast carcinoma cells confers an improved prognosis. The expression of certain oncogenes is increasingly being related to prognosis in some tumours.

Tumour nomenclature and classification

The classification and nomenclature of neoplasms have developed from gross morphological, histological and behavioural observation. Ideally, the name given to a tumour should convey information about the cell of origin and the likely behaviour (either benign or malignant). While this is the case for the majority of tumours of epithelial and connective tissues, there are many tumours that are given eponymous or semi-descriptive names out of either poor understanding of pathogenesis or long-established tradition. Some tumours have several different names that are synonymous, but derive from different classifications.

Tumours of epithelial origin

■ Benign neoplasms of surface epithelia, for example skin, are termed *papillomas.* This term is preceded by the cell of origin, for example squamous papilloma of skin or larynx.

■ Benign neoplasms of both solid and surface glandular epithelia are termed *adenomas.* This is prefixed by the tissue of origin, for example thyroid adenoma, salivary gland adenoma. Frequently, a benign tumour of surface glandular epithelium (almost always in the large bowel) assumes a papillary growth pattern, termed a *villous adenoma.*

■ A malignant tumour of any epithelial origin is termed a *carcinoma.* Tumours of glandular epithelium (including that lining the gut) are termed *adenocarcinomas.* Tumours of other epithelia are preceded by the cell type of origin, for example *squamous cell carcinoma* and *transitional cell carcinoma.* To classify a carcinoma further, the tissue of origin is added, for example adenocarcinoma of prostate, adenocarcinoma of breast and squamous cell carcinoma of larynx.

The nomenclature of epithelial tumours is summarised in Table 7.2.

Table 7.2 Nomenclature of epithelial tumours.

Tissue of origin	Benign	Malignant
Surface epithelium	Papilloma/adenoma	Carcinoma
Examples:		
Squamous	Squamous cell papilloma	Squamous cell carcinoma
Glandular (columnar)	Adenoma (villous or tubular)	Adenocarcinoma
Transitional	Transitional cell papilloma	Transitional cell carcinoma
Solid glandular epithelium	Adenoma	Adenocarcinoma
Examples:		
Thyroid	Thyroid adenoma	Thyroid adenocarcinoma
Kidney	Renal adenoma	Renal cell carcinoma
Liver	Hepatic adenoma	Hepatocellular carcinoma

Tumours of connective tissue origin

In connective tissues, there is a simpler and more descriptive classification of neoplasms. First, the tissue of origin is designated, with the addition of the suffix *-oma* for a benign tumour or *-sarcoma* for a malignant tumour. As an example, a benign tumour of adipose tissue is termed a lipoma, whilst a malignant tumour of the same origin is termed a liposarcoma. A summary of other connective tissue tumours is shown in Table 7.3.

Table 7.3 Nomenclature of connective tissue tumours.

Tissue of origin	Benign	Malignant
Fibrous tissue	Fibroma	Fibrosarcoma
Bone	Osteoma	Osteosarcoma
Cartilage	Chondroma	Chondrosarcoma
Adipose tissue	Lipoma	Liposarcoma
Smooth muscle	Leiomyoma	Leiomyosarcoma
Skeletal muscle	Rhabdomyoma	Rhabdomyosarcoma
Blood vessel	Haemangioma	Haemangiosarcoma

Nomenclature of other tumours

There are other neoplasms that do not fit into either the epithelial or the connective tissue category described above and these are grouped according to their tissue of origin. The main categories are as follows:

■ **Melanoma:** tumours of melanocytes (Fig. 7.8 and Ch. 21)

■ **Lymphomas:** tumours of solid lymphoid tissue (Fig. 7.7 and Ch. 16)

■ **Leukaemias:** tumours derived from haematopoietic elements that circulate in the blood and only rarely form tumour masses (see Ch. 16)

■ **Gliomas:** tumours derived from the non-neural support tissues of the brain (see Ch. 23)

■ **Germ cell tumours:** tumours derived from germ cells in the gonads (Fig. 7.9, Ch. 17 and Ch. 19)

■ **Neuroendocrine tumours**: tumours derived from cells of the neuroendocrine system. Examples include phaeochromocytoma (see Fig. 20.11), carcinoid tumour (see Fig. 12.22) and medullary carcinoma (see Fig. 20.7).

Finally, there is a group of tumour-like lesions known as **hamartomas** that represent non-neoplastic overgrowths of tissues indigenous to the site of their occurrence. These are thought to be developmental abnormalities. A common example is the 'port-wine stain' of the skin composed of blood vessels and known as a **haemangioma.** An example of a haemangioma in the liver is shown in Fig. 11.8.

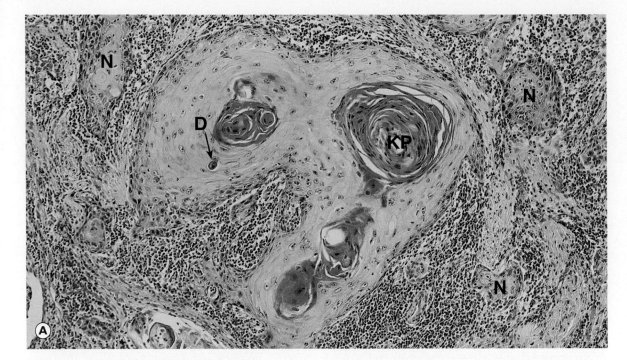

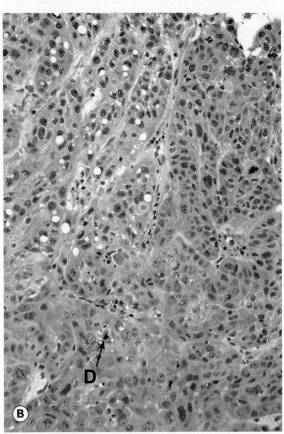

Fig. 7.3 **Squamous cell carcinoma. (A)** Well differentiated (HP); **(B)** poorly differentiated (HP).

Squamous cell carcinomas may arise in any site of native stratified squamous epithelium (E-Fig. 7.3**H**), for example skin, oesophagus or tongue. They may also arise in stratified squamous epithelium that has formed by the process of metaplasia, for example in the bronchus or urinary bladder.

The degree of differentiation varies widely. Well differentiated tumours, as seen in Fig. 7.3A, have cytological features similar to the prickle cell layer of normal stratified squamous epithelium. The cells are large and slightly fusiform in shape and the nuclei exhibit a moderate degree of pleomorphism. Mitotic figures are infrequent. The cells are commonly arranged in broad sheets and large nests **(N)**. At very high magnification, intercellular bridges (typical of normal prickle cells) may be visible. The most characteristic feature of well differentiated squamous carcinomas is the formation of keratin, which may be seen within individual cells (known as *dyskeratosis* **(D)**), but which more often forms lamellated, pink-stained masses known as *keratin pearls* **(KP)**.

In contrast, poorly differentiated squamous carcinomas, as in Fig. 7.3B, lose most of their resemblance to normal prickle cells and have a high nuclear to cytoplasmic ratio. Keratin pearl formation is not seen, although individual dyskeratotic cells **(D)** may be present. In the most anaplastic squamous carcinomas, the only evidence of the cell of origin may be intercellular bridges, which are only visible at high magnification after a careful search, or the detection of certain types of cytokeratin by immunohistochemistry.

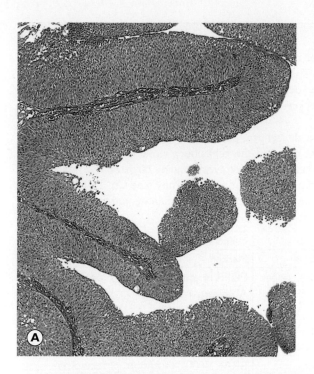

Fig. 7.4 **Transitional cell (urothelial) carcinoma.**
(A) Low grade/grade 1 (LP); **(B)** high grade/grade 3
(HP).

These tumours arise almost exclusively from native
transitional epithelium in the urinary tract (E-Fig. 7.4 **H.**).

Low grade lesions usually adopt a papillary growth
pattern (see Fig. 15.22) and the cytological features
may be almost indistinguishable from those of normal
transitional epithelium. Fig. 7.4A shows a typical
papillary tumour resembling normal urothelium,
but with slight nuclear pleomorphism and minimal
evidence of mitotic activity.

As transitional cell carcinomas become less differentiated, the growth pattern becomes more solid and
nuclear pleomorphism becomes more marked. In
anaplastic tumours, it may not be possible to determine
the tissue of origin except by knowing that the tumour
has arisen in the urinary tract. Fig. 7.4B shows a high
grade solid tumour from the bladder wall. Note the
nests of highly pleomorphic tumour cells **(T)** invading
between bundles of smooth muscle **(M).**

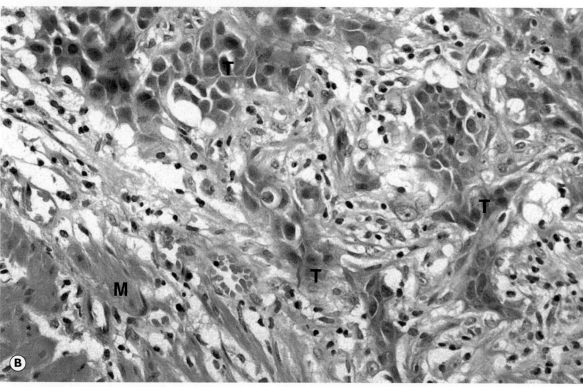

KEY TO FIGURES
D dyskeratotic cell   **KP** keratin pearl   **M** smooth muscle   **N** cell nest   **T** tumour cells

TUMOUR MARKERS

Tumour markers are substances produced by cancer cells, usually in large quantities and can be detected by biochemical assays of the blood or urine. These markers are also produced by normal cells usually at much lower levels and also by benign conditions, therefore the markers are not particularly sensitive or specific. Tumour markers can be used in screening for cancers, monitoring response to therapy and detecting recurrent disease.

There are a variety of types of tumour markers in clinical use, including hormones and specific proteins; examples of which are shown below. More recently, there has been a marked increase in molecular tests for specific genetic signatures in certain cancers to help with guiding targeted therapy and in predicting response to treatments such as chemotherapy and immunotherapy (see Ch. 1). Furthermore, there is currently a large field of research involving the detection of circulating tumour DNA in the blood as a possible method of early cancer detection.

Hormones		Proteins		Molecular	
Marker	Tumour(s)	Marker	Tumour(s)	Marker	Tumour(s)
hCG	Choriocarcinoma, germ cell tumours	PSA	Prostate cancer	EGFR mutation and ALK gene rearrangement	Non–small cell lung cancer
Calcitonin	Medullary thyroid carcinoma	Ig	Multiple myeloma	HER2 amplification	Breast cancer, gastric cancer
αFP	Hepatocellular carcinoma, germ cell tumours	CA 125	Ovarian carcinoma	BRAF V600E mutation	Melanoma
Gastrin	Gastrinoma	CA 19.9	Pancreatic cancer, cholangiocarcinoma	KRAS mutation	Colorectal cancer
ER/PR	Breast cancer	Chromogranin A	Neuroendocrine tumours	PD-L1 expression	Non–small cell lung cancer

---

Fig. 7.5 **Colonic adenocarcinoma. (A)** Well differentiated (MP); **(B)** poorly differentiated (HP); **(C)** signet ring (HP); **(D)** mucinous (MP). *(Illustrations opposite)*

Carcinomas that derive from surface glandular epithelium, such as colon (E-Fig. 7.5 **H**) and stomach Fig. 7.6 **H**), tend to exhibit a glandular pattern of growth and are known as *adenocarcinomas.* The same is true of carcinomas arising in solid glandular tissues, such as kidney, breast and prostate, and of tumours of the liver (which in embryological terms develops as an outgrowth of primitive gut epithelium).

Fig. 7.5A illustrates a typical well differentiated colonic adenocarcinoma. Although it is a carcinoma, it still exhibits a glandular pattern **(G)** reminiscent of normal colon. The cell nuclei are, however, hyperchromatic, with a high nuclear to cytoplasmic ratio and numerous mitoses **(M)** are seen. Unlike the normal colon, the glandular pattern is irregular and there is little evidence of mucin secretion.

Poorly differentiated adenocarcinomas, as shown in Fig. 7.5B, display a minimal tendency to form a glandular pattern and the cells are extremely pleomorphic. The only evidence of glandular origin is

the presence of occasional cells with secretory vacuoles **(V)** containing mucin.

Two other patterns of adenocarcinoma, seen much more commonly in other tissues than in colon, are *signet ring cell* and *mucinous* forms. In signet ring cell carcinoma, as shown in Fig. 7.5C, the tendency to produce mucin-filled cytoplasmic vacuoles is greatly exaggerated such that the majority of cells have their nuclei **(N)** pushed to one side by a mucin-filled vacuole **(V)**. This pattern is much more common in the stomach (see Fig. 13.12) than in the colon, although focal areas of this pattern may be seen in adenocarcinomas from a wide variety of tissues. In contrast, in a mucinous carcinoma, as shown in Fig. 7.5D, excessive secretion of mucin **(Mu)** results in so-called mucin lakes in which small nests of tumour cells **(T)** are found. This pattern of adenocarcinoma is not uncommon in the colon and is also well recognised in the breast (see Fig. 18.10).

KEY TO FIGURES

G glandular pattern   **M** mitotic figure   **Mu** mucin   **N** nucleus   **T** nest of tumour cells   **V** mucin vacuole

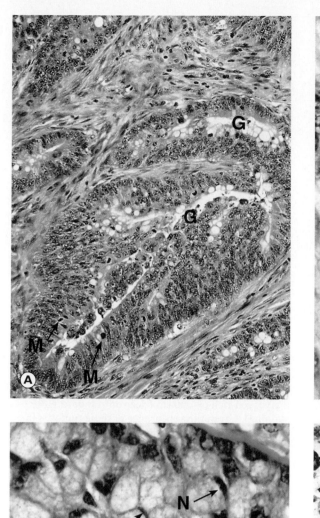

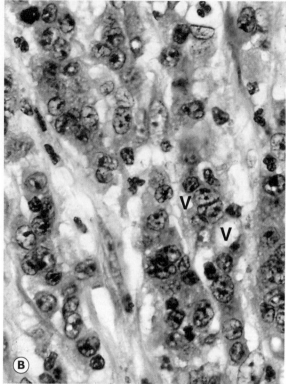

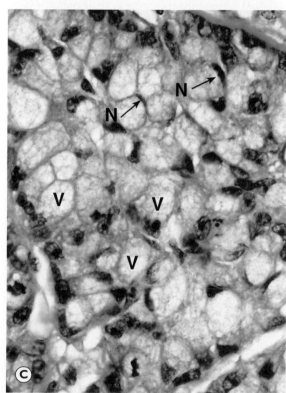

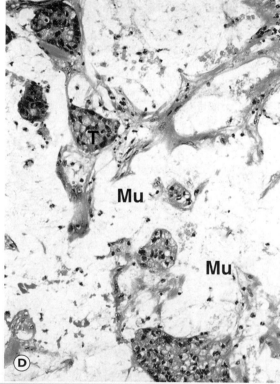

Fig. 7.5 **Colonic adenocarcinomas.** (*Caption opposite*)

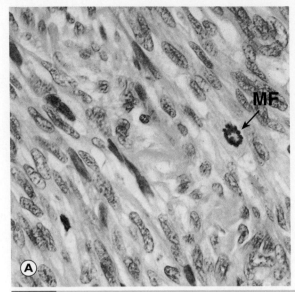

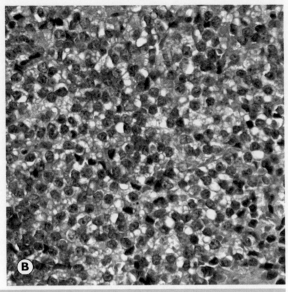

Fig. 7.6 **Sarcomas. (A)** Leiomyosarcoma (HP); **(B)** Ewing's sarcoma (HP).

Sarcomas are malignant tumours derived from connective tissues, including adipose tissue, bone, cartilage and smooth muscle. Many sarcomas resemble the tissue of origin either cytologically, structurally or by producing characteristic extracellular materials such as collagen and ground substance. For example, liposarcomas have intracellular lipid vacuoles and chondrosarcomas produce cartilaginous ground substance.

Fig. 7.6A shows an example of a uterine *leiomyosarcoma*, a sarcoma derived from smooth muscle. The tumour cells are spindle-shaped and resemble normal smooth muscle cells. However, they have large pleomorphic nuclei with evident mitoses including an abnormal, ring-form mitotic figure **(MF)**.

Fig. 7.6B shows a typical *Ewing's sarcoma*. This malignant tumour typically arises in the medullary cavity of long or flat bones in children, though the cell of origin is unknown. As shown here, the tumours consist of sheets of small round cells with a glycogen-rich cytoplasm (clear on standard H&E staining). Given the appearance of these tumours in H&E, they are often described, with other primitive, poorly differentiated tumours, **as** *small round blue cell tumours*. Ewing's tumours are aggressive and may metastasise early. Treatment with combinations of surgery, chemotherapy and radiotherapy can improve the outcome.

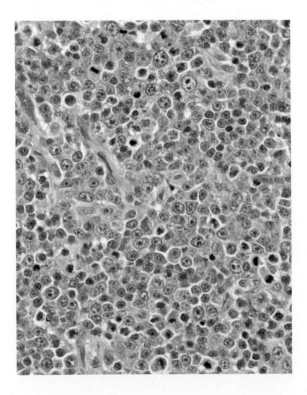

Fig. 7.7 Lymphoma (HP).

Lymphomas are solid tumours derived from cells of the lymphoid system. The majority arise in lymphoid organs such as lymph nodes, spleen and bone marrow, but may spread to other tissues, particularly the skin, liver and CNS. Primary lymphomas may also arise at extranodal sites, often in tissues where a longstanding chronic inflammatory or autoimmune response is present such as the small intestine in coeliac disease or the thyroid in Hashimoto's thyroiditis.

Histologically, lymphomas consist of sheets of lymphoid cells arranged either diffusely or in a follicular pattern. Lymphomas are discussed in detail in Ch. 16.

Fig. 7.7 illustrates a diffuse large B cell lymphoma **(DLBCL),** characterised by sheets of large atypical lymphoid cells. DLBCL is the commonest type of high grade lymphoma (see Fig. 16.9).

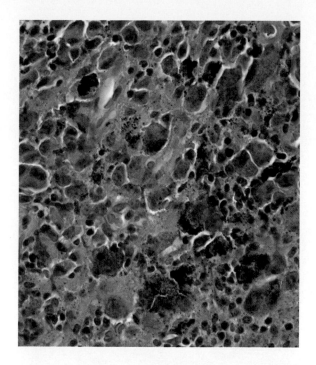

Fig. 7.8 Melanoma (HP).

Melanomas are malignant tumours of melanocytes, most often arising in sun-exposed skin, though examples arising in sites not traditionally associated with sun exposure do occur, such as bowel and dura. Clinically, melanomas appear as irregular, variably pigmented, raised or flat lesions that may be prone to bleeding.

In the example shown here, the tumour cells are large, irregularly shaped and have abundant cytoplasmic melanin pigment. Unfortunately, this 'typical' appearance may not always be apparent, particularly in metastatic tumour, for example in a lymph node specimen where the primary may be unknown. For this reason, melanomas are often regarded as the classic 'mimic metastases', in that they can assume the morphological features of almost any other malignancy. Under such circumstances a careful and thorough search for melanin pigment, combined with the judicious use of immunohistochemistry stains, can be helpful in achieving a diagnosis.

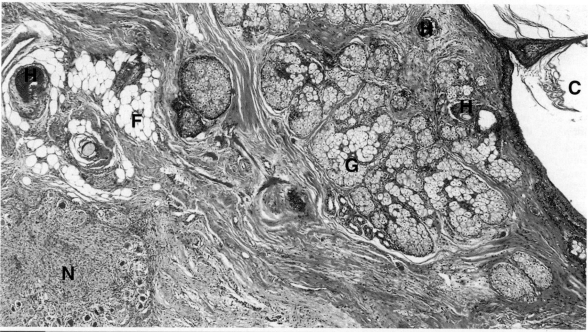

Fig. 7.9 Teratoma (MP).

Teratomas are tumours derived from germ cells and most commonly arise in the testis or ovary. The tumours contain neoplastic tissues derived from all of the three germ cell layers, i.e. endoderm, mesoderm and ectoderm (including neuroectoderm), and thus can contain tissues as diverse as skin, teeth, thyroid, brain and muscle. The tumours range from benign to highly malignant.

A benign teratoma of the ovary is shown in this micrograph. Epidermis-type epithelium, including hair follicles (H) and sebaceous glands (G), has formed a cystic space (C). Connective tissue elements including fat (F) are also seen. Neural tissue (N) is present in the form of well differentiated clusters of ganglion cells. Teratomas arising in the ovary are usually benign, whereas those in the testis are usually malignant and contain more primitive, immature tissue such as primitive mesenchyme (see Ch. 19).

KEY TO FIGURES
C cystic space   **F** fat   **G** sebaceous glands   **H** hair follicles   **MF** abnormal mitotic figure   **N** neural tissue

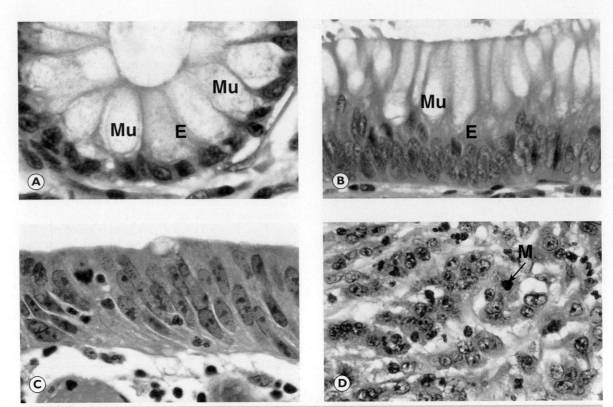

Fig. 7.10 **Degrees of tumour differentiation: colon. (A)** Normal mucosa (HP); **(B)** benign neoplasm (HP); **(C)** well differentiated malignant neoplasm (HP); **(D)** poorly differentiated neoplasm (HP).

The series of micrographs in Fig. 7.10 demonstrates the variable degree of differentiation that may be seen in tumours arising from the same cell of origin.

Note the similarity between normal colonic mucosa in Fig. 7.10A and a benign neoplasm *(tubular adenoma)* in Fig. 7.10B. In both cases, the epithelial cells **(E)** are tall, columnar and regular in form. The main points of difference are that the cells of the benign neoplasm contain less mucin **(Mu)** and their nuclei are larger and more crowded.

The cells of the well differentiated malignant neoplasm shown in Fig. 7.10C are also tall and columnar, but the nuclei are more irregular in shape and arrangement with no mucin secretion, most of each cell being occupied by the nucleus. The nuclei are crowded and are no longer arranged along the basal parts of the cells. The nucleoli are also large and irregular in size and shape. In contrast, in the poorly differentiated colonic neoplasm in Fig. 7.10D, the cells bear little resemblance to the tissue of origin and are arranged haphazardly. The cells show a great variability in size and nuclear shape, mitoses **(M)** are seen and there is little evidence of mucin secretion.

Modes of spread of malignant neoplasms

There are four main modes of tumour spread:

■ **Local invasion.** Invasive tumours tend to spread into surrounding tissues by the most direct route. Examples include carcinoma of the breast invading overlying skin or deeply into underlying muscle and carcinoma of the cervix invading rectum or bladder.

■ **Lymphatic spread.** Tumours may spread via lymphatic vessels draining the site of the primary tumour. Neoplastic cells are conducted to local lymph nodes where they may form secondary tumours, e.g. breast cancer spreading to lymph nodes in the axilla or carcinoma of the tongue spreading to lymph nodes in the neck.

■ **Vascular spread.** Tumours can spread via the veins draining the primary site. Gut tumours tend to spread via the portal vein to the liver where secondary tumours are very common. In the systemic circulation, neoplastic cells may be trapped in the lung to form pulmonary metastases (Fig. 7.16).

■ **Transcoelomic spread.** Certain tumours can spread directly across coelomic spaces, for example across the peritoneal or pleural cavities. Carcinoma of the ovary may spread transcoelomically to produce large numbers of metastatic deposits on the peritoneal surfaces.

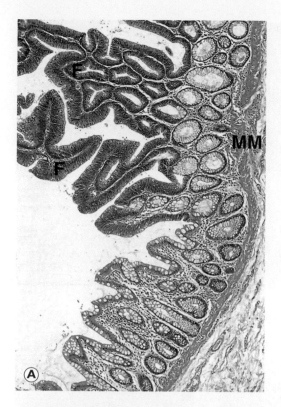

Benign neoplasms of surface epithelia usually grow in the form of warty, papillary or nodular outgrowths and show no tendency to infiltrate downward into the submucosa. Fig. 7.11A shows one form of benign colonic neoplasm. This *villous adenoma* has grown into the lumen in the form of papillary fronds (**F**) with a stromal core covered by moderately dysplastic epithelial cells. The underlying muscularis mucosae (**MM**) is intact and there is no downward tumour spread.

Malignant neoplasms not only form a mass in the lumen, but also spread across the epithelial basement membrane into subepithelial tissues. In Fig. 7.11B of a colonic *adenocarcinoma*, the tumour cells (**T**) have grown in complex, abnormal gland formations (**G**) within the mucosa. Malignant glands are also seen invading into the submucosa (**SM**), having breached the muscularis mucosae (**MM**), and have spread beneath the adjacent normal mucosa (**Muc**). Even at low power, it is obvious that the malignant cells are disorganised, crowded together and less differentiated than are the cells of the benign adenoma. Note the nuclear hyperchromasia of both benign and malignant lesions in comparison to the normal.

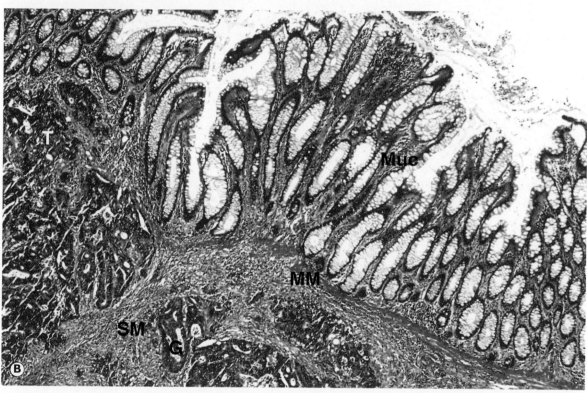

KEY TO FIGURES
E epithelial cells **F** papillary fronds **M** mitotic figure **MM** muscularis mucosae **Mu** mucin **Muc** normal mucosa **SM** submucosa **T** tumour

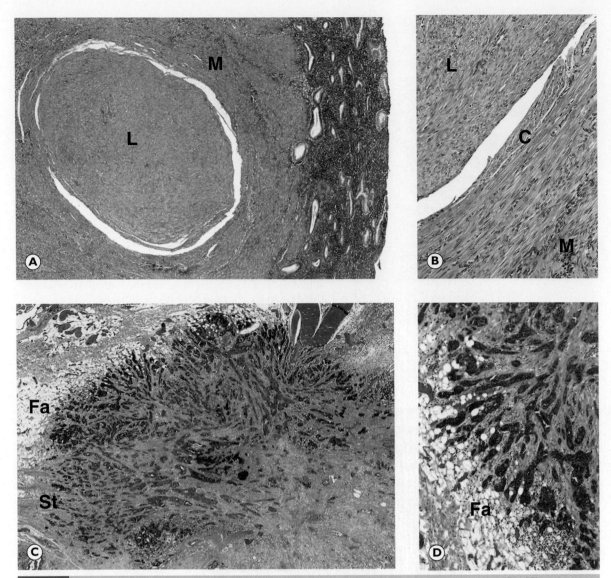

Fig. 7.12 **Local invasion. (A)** Benign neoplasm of myometrium (LP); **(B)** margin of lesion in (A) (MP); **(C)** malignant neoplasm of breast (LP); **(D)** margin of lesion in **(C)** (MP).

The micrographs in Fig. 7.12 compare the local growth patterns of benign and malignant neoplasms within solid organs. Fig. 7.12A shows a benign neoplasm of the uterine smooth muscle, a *leiomyoma* (L), surrounded by normal myometrium (M). The tumour margin is shown at higher magnification in Fig. 7.12B. Note that the neoplasm is well circumscribed and shows no evidence of local invasion. This neoplasm has expanded symmetrically and compressed the supporting stroma of the myometrium to form a *pseudocapsule* (C).

Fig. 7.12C illustrates a breast carcinoma. Note the neoplasm has an irregular outline with tongues of neoplastic cells invading the fatty tissue (Fa) and collagenous stroma (St) of the breast. There is no tendency to form a capsule. The ill-defined tumour margin is illustrated in Fig. 7.12D in which hyperchromatic malignant cells can be seen infiltrating the surrounding adipose tissue.

KEY TO FIGURES
C pseudocapsule   **Fa** fatty tissue   **L** leiomyoma   **Ly** lymphatic   **M** myometrium   **MS** medullary sinuses   **S** sinus   **St** stroma   **T** tumour cells

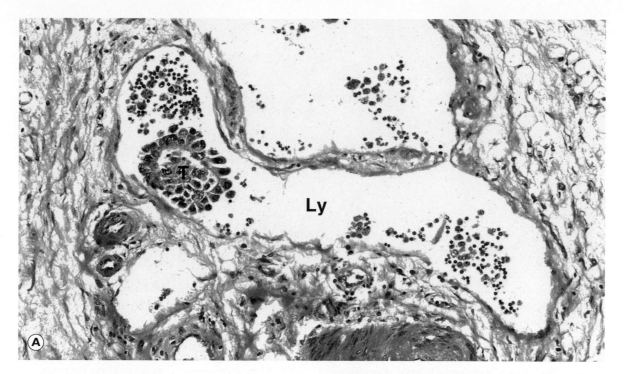

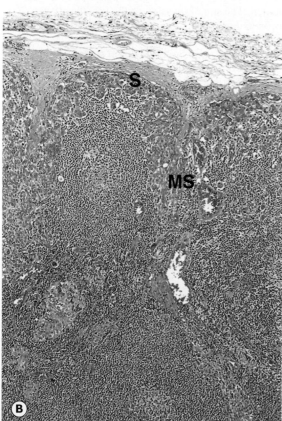

Fig. 7.13 **Lymphatic spread. (A)** Tumour in lymphatic vessel (HP); **(B)** metastasis in a lymph node (MP).

Malignant tumours may invade through the walls of lymphatics and spread either by growth of solid cores along the lumina or by fragments breaking off the intralymphatic tumour mass to form emboli, which pass to regional lymph nodes.

Fig. 7.13A illustrates a large, valved lymphatic **(Ly)** containing an embolic clump of malignant tumour cells **(T)** en route to a lymph node. Tumour spread via lymphatics to regional lymph nodes is a very common mode of spread for carcinomas.

Fig. 7.13B shows a lymph node draining a primary breast carcinoma. Tumour cells, which arrive via afferent lymphatics, lodge and proliferate in the subcapsular sinus **(S)**. From here, the malignant cells may then infiltrate down the medullary sinuses **(MS)** and go on to form solid masses in the parenchyma of the node (not illustrated here).

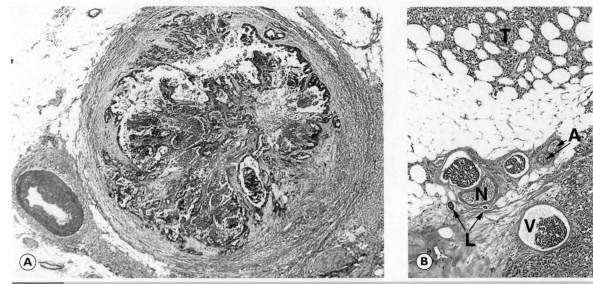

Fig. 7.14 **Haematogenous spread of malignant neoplasms. (A)** Malignant colonic neoplasm (MP); **(B)** malignant breast neoplasm (MP).

The thin-walled vessels of the venous system provide a ready means of spread for many types of malignant tumour. In contrast, invasion of arterial vessels is rare and tends to result in haemorrhage or infarction, rather than tumour spread. Malignant cells may grow along veins in solid cores from which fragments may break off to form tumour emboli, which tend to lodge in the first capillary bed encountered. The lungs and liver are frequent sites of metastatic deposition. From here, tumour cells may pass through the heart to the arterial system and spread throughout the body. Hence, brain and bone marrow are other common sites for metastatic deposits.

Fig. 7.14A shows a large serosal vein from a colon in which there was an extensive malignant neoplasm. A solid mass of tumour is growing along the vessel lumen. The site of invasion of the vessel wall was proximal to this section and, therefore, cannot be seen.

Venous invasion by carcinoma of the breast is seen in Fig. 7.14B. Solid masses of tumour cells **(T)** infiltrate the fatty tissue of the breast. Tumour emboli are seen within three small venules **(V)** and also two small lymphatics **(L)**, adjacent to a nerve **(N)**. The arterioles **(A)** close by are not affected. Vascular and lymphatic invasion by tumour is an important factor in the prognosis of many types of tumour.

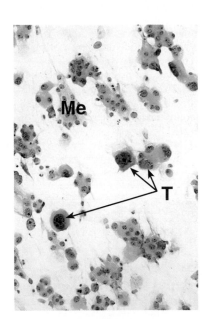

Fig. 7.15 **Transcoelomic spread of malignant neoplasms (HP).**

Malignant tumours may spread into coelomic spaces by direct extension from adjacent organs. Tumour emboli may then break free from the tumour to float in the small amount of fluid normally present in these spaces and spread to other areas of the mesothelial surface. Thus, breast and lung tumours commonly involve the pleural space. Ovarian and gastric tumours are usually responsible for peritoneal involvement.

In response to tumour growth in these serous spaces, there is commonly an inflammatory response in the lining with accumulation of protein-rich fluid and inflammatory cells, proliferation of mesothelial cells and often haemorrhage to form a *malignant pleural effusion* or *malignant ascites.*

This example is a smear of ascitic fluid from a patient with metastatic breast carcinoma. The tumour had spread through the pleural space and reached the peritoneum, probably via the diaphragm. Aspiration of the fluid serves to relieve symptoms and to confirm the diagnosis cytologically *(diagnostic paracentesis)*. Tumour cells **(T)** are present as single cells and small aggregates. They are pleomorphic with large, hyperchromatic nuclei and prominent nucleoli. Reactive mesothelial cells **(Me)** are also present and, in contrast to the tumour cells, are smaller with bland nuclear features. In this example, inflammatory cells are sparse.

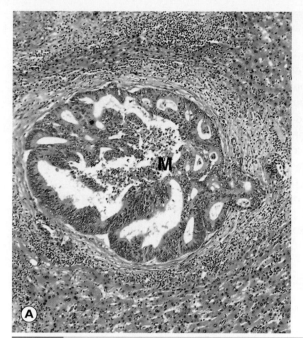
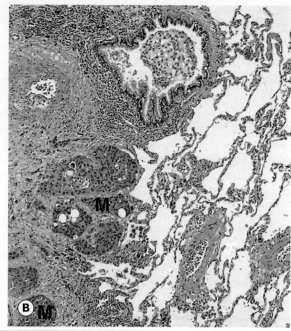

Fig. 7.16 **Metastatic tumour deposits in solid organs. (A)** Liver (MP); **(B)** lung (LP).

As noted above, metastatic deposits of tumour are frequently encountered in liver, lung, bone marrow and brain as a result of haematogenous spread. Other tissues are less common sites for deposition of metastatic tumour (e.g. heart and skeletal muscle).

However, metastases can occur in any tissue or organ. Certain types of tumour have characteristic patterns of spread. For example, malignant tumours of the prostate gland have a propensity to spread to bone. It is thought that the malignant cells and the target organ must express mutually compatible receptors and cell-surface adhesion molecules, which facilitate cellular anchorage and subsequent growth.

Figs 7.16A and B show examples of hepatic (E-Fig. 7.7 **G**) and pulmonary Fig. 7.8 **G**) blood-borne

metastases (**M**), respectively. Hepatic metastases often arise from organs drained by the portal system; the lesion in Fig. 7.16A is from a moderately differentiated adenocarcinoma of the colon. Lung metastases, on the other hand, arise from tumour emboli from the systemic venous circulation, and Fig. 7.16B is an example of secondary spread from a primary breast carcinoma. Note that both tumours have induced a stromal reaction in the form of fibrous connective tissue containing blood vessels and inflammatory cells. Without this ability to induce the formation of a vascular supply (***angiogenesis***), the growth of metastases would not be possible.

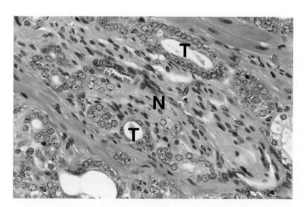

Fig. 7.17 **Perineural spread (HP).**

Spread along the course of nerve bundles is a common feature of some tumours, such as adenocarcinoma of the prostate, but may also be seen in other tumour types. Fig. 7.17 shows perineural invasion by a well differentiated prostatic adenocarcinoma. Tumour cells (**T**) in a glandular conformation are seen infiltrating around and between bundles of nerve fibres (**N**).

KEY TO FIGURES
A arterioles   **L** lymphatics   **M** metastasis   **Me** mesothelial cells   **N** nerve fibres   **T** tumour cells
V venule

BASIC PATHOLOGICAL PROCESSES ■ DYSPLASIA AND NEOPLASIA

Staging of malignant tumours

The extent of local, regional and distant tumour spread is an important determinant of tumour management and prognosis. Several systems have been devised for defining these characteristics in a standardised fashion; this is known as *staging* of a tumour. This is different from *grading,* described earlier in the chapter, which involves pathological assessment of the degree of differentiation of the tumour.

The **TNM system** is the most widely used method and involves scoring the extent of local *T*umour spread, regional lymph *N*ode involvement and the presence of distant *M*etastases. Despite advances in diagnostic techniques, the stage of a tumour is still a very good indicator of likely prognosis. Tumour stage assessment is also important in planning therapy. Tumours at an advanced stage (extensive spread) may require aggressive treatment, while early-stage tumours (localised) can be treatable by more conservative measures such as surgical excision alone. Staging is usually performed by a combination of histopathology, radiology and clinical assessments.

By way of example, the TNM (8th Edition) for colonic cancer staging is illustrated in Table 7.4.

Table 7.4 **TNM 8 staging of colonic cancer.**

T0	No evidence of primary tumour	N0	No nodes involved	M0	No distant metastases
T1	Tumour invades submucosa	N1	Spread to 1 to 3 regional nodes: N1a: 1 node N1b: 2–3 nodes N1c: no nodes positive but discontinuous tumour deposits in mesentery, sub-serosa or non-peritonealised tissues	M1	Distant metastases M1a: 1 organ without peritoneal metastasis M1b: 2+ organs without peritoneal metastasis M1c: metastasis to peritoneum
T2	Tumour invades muscularis propria	N2	Spread to 4 or more regional nodes N2a: 4–6 nodes N2b: 7+ nodes		
T3	Tumour invades subserosa				
T4	a: Tumour invades visceral peritoneum OR b: Tumour invades other organs/ structures				

From the *AJCC Cancer Staging Manual,* 8th edition.

SENTINEL LYMPH NODE BIOPSY

One common route of the spread of cancer cells is via the lymphatic system to local (regional) lymph nodes (Fig. 7.13). Cancer typically spreads in a predictable fashion to local nodes before involving more distant nodes.

Lymph node clearance *(lymphadenectomy)* of all the regional nodes in the vicinity of a tumour can result in significant morbidity for the patient due to lymphoedema (accumulation of excess tissue fluid due to disruption of normal draining after surgery). *Sentinel node* procedures aim to reduce this morbidity by identifying those patients with pathological evidence of lymph node spread and offering only these patients completion lymphadenectomy. Sentinel node biopsy can also be used to stage patients with advanced disease.

The sentinel node is the first node (or nodes) draining a tumour. In a sentinel node biopsy, radioactive tracer material is injected near to the tumour along with blue dye. A *lymphoscintigram* can be carried out pre-operatively to identify the exact location of a sentinel node on imaging. Intra-operatively, the sentinel node is identified as it should stain blue and is radioactive using a gamma probe. The node is often described as 'hot and blue' and is removed and sent to pathology for assessment. The node is often examined at multiple histological levels with additional tests such as immunohistochemistry performed to look for small groups or single tumour cells. Post-operative assessment using paraffin sections is more accurate than intra-operative frozen section in the identification of metastatic tumour cells. If metastatic tumour is present in the node, it is regarded as 'positive' and the patient will undergo a completion lymphadenectomy. Current research in this field involves rapid assessment of nodes intra-operatively by molecular techniques so that the patient only requires one operation.

Sentinel lymph node surgery is now commonplace for the surgical management of breast cancer and malignant melanoma.

Table 7.5 Chapter review.

	Definition/main features	Examples	Figure
Dysplasia	Increased cell proliferation with failure of maturation	Uterine cervix	7.1
		Skin	7.1
Carcinoma in situ	Features of carcinoma in an epithelium, but no invasion		7.2
		Uterine cervix	7.7
		Skin	21.14
		Breast	18.9
Epithelial tumours	Benign tumours either *papillomas* or *adenomas*		7.11
	Malignant tumours termed *carcinomas*		
		Squamous cell carcinoma	7.3
		Transitional cell carcinoma	7.4
		Colonic adenocarcinoma	7.5
Connective tissue tumours	Benign tumours named after tissue of origin with suffix *-oma*		7.12A
	Malignant tumours named after tissue of origin with suffix *-sarcoma*		7.6
		Leiomyosarcoma	7.6
Lymphoma	Solid tumours derived from cells of lymphoreticular system	Diffuse large B cell lymphoma	7.7
Melanoma	Tumour derived from melanocytes		7.8
Teratoma	Tumour derived from germ cells		7.9
Invasion	Spread of tumour to surrounding tissues	Breast carcinoma	7.12C
		Colonic adenocarcinoma	7.11B
		Perineural invasion	7.17
Metastasis	Distant spread of tumour by one of several mechanisms	Lymphatic spread	7.13
		Haematogenous	7.14
		Transcoelomic	7.15

8 Atherosclerosis

The wall of an artery has three layers, the intima, media and adventitia, which are separated from each other by thin elastic fibres known as the *elastic laminae* (E-Fig. 8.1**H**). The intima, the innermost layer, is composed of fibroelastic tissue and is lined by a thin layer of endothelial cells along its luminal aspect. The media contains bundles of smooth muscle and is separated from the intima by the internal elastic lamina (Fig. 8.2A). The adventitia is composed of collagen and is separated from the media by the external elastic lamina. In larger arteries, the adventitia also contains the vasa vasorum, the blood vessels which supply blood and nutrients to the arterial wall. This combination of smooth muscle, elastin and collagen permits alteration in vascular tone.

With age, the relative proportions of these components alter, resulting in a loss of elasticity and thickening of the vessel of wall due to an increase in collagen deposition and smooth muscle hypertrophy within the intimal layer. This process, commonly referred to as *arteriosclerosis* (derived from the Greek *arteria*, meaning artery, and *skleros* meaning hardening) is often used as a general descriptive term for such diseases. Arteriosclerosis can often be identified in patients with hypertension and can be seen in the arterioles within the kidney in these patients (see Figs. 11.1 and 11.2). It is illustrated in Fig. 8.1.

Fig. 8.1 **Arteriosclerosis (LP).**

Intimal thickening of arteries and arterioles is extremely common with increasing age. This may form part of the spectrum of atherosclerotic disease or may simply represent a physiological adaptation, which occurs with age.

Fig. 8.1 shows a small artery. Note the intima (**In**) is normal to the right of the image (*arrow*). The left side of the artery exhibits eccentric intimal proliferation (**IP**). The thickened intima, clearly defined by the internal elastic lamina (**IEL**), can be seen to consist of multiple cell layers and involves approximately half the circumference of the vessel. The media (**M**) and adventitia (**A**) are unremarkable.

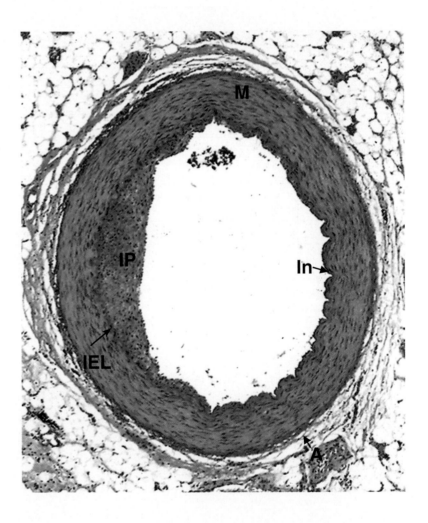

KEY TO FIGURES
A adventitia   **IEL** internal elastic lamina   **In** intima   **IP** intimal proliferation   **M** media

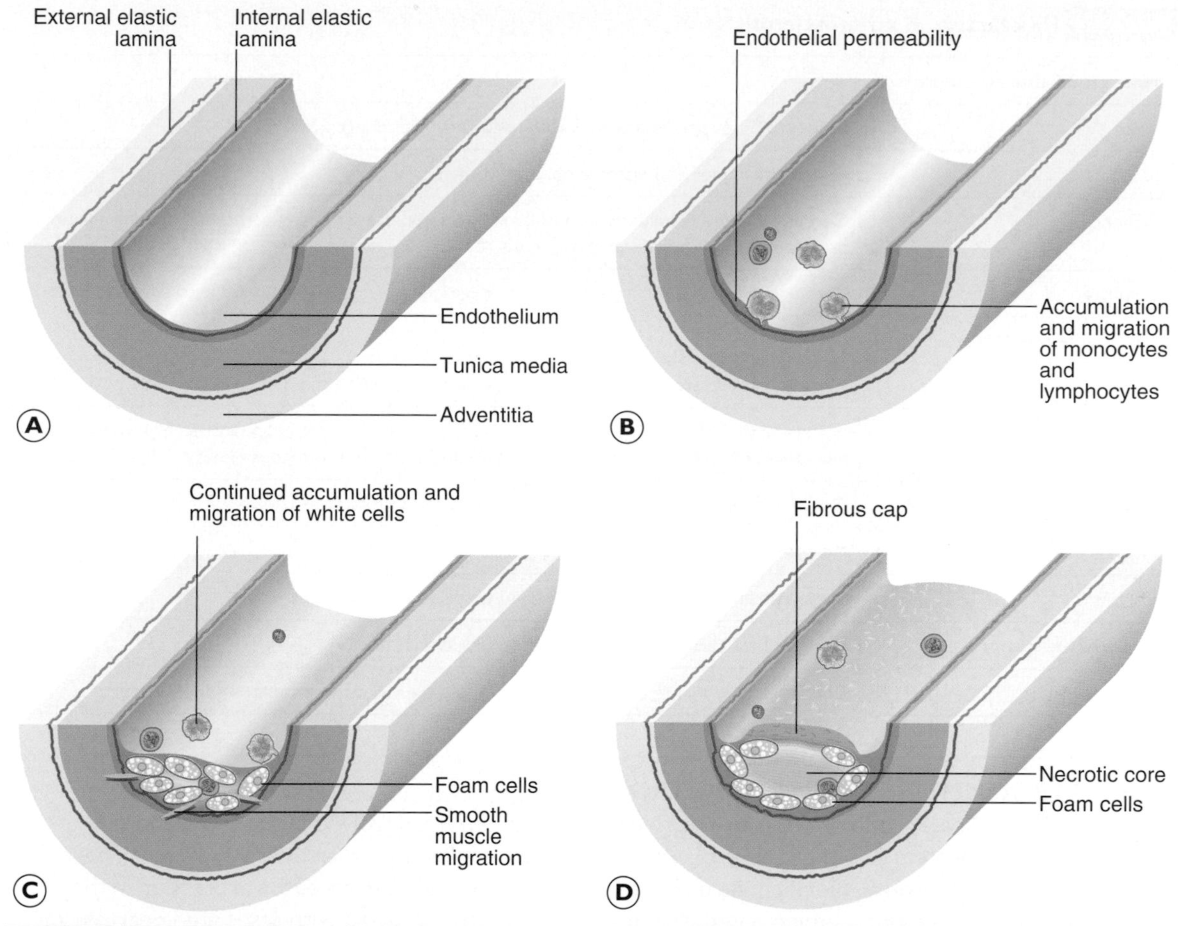

Fig. 8.2 Stages in atheroma formation.

Fig. 8.2A shows a normal *elastic artery* with a distinct internal elastic lamina. The artery is lined internally by a smooth, flat endothelium lying on a delicate, fibroelastic, loose connective tissue, which contains occasional multifunctional myointimal cells (tunica intima). Beneath the intima is a strong internal elastic lamina followed by a layer of smooth muscle containing some elastic fibres (tunica media). On the outer surface is the loose tunica adventitia.

Endothelial dysfunction (Fig. 8.2B). At certain locations in the arterial system, such as vessel branch points, turbulent flow and shear stress are associated with expression of cell adhesion factors by the endothelium, which result in the accumulation and migration of monocytes and T lymphocytes. In parallel, the endothelium may become permeable to lipoproteins.

Fatty streak (Fig. 8.2C). Continued endothelial dysfunction, with associated permeability to lipoproteins and monocyte and T-lymphocyte migration, produces an intimal collection of

lipid- laden macrophages (foam cells) and inflammatory cells. This is followed by migration of smooth muscle from the media producing the fatty streak lesion, the earliest visible stage of atherosclerosis.

Advanced/complicated atheroma (Fig. 8.2D). Further progression of the early atheromatous fatty streak sees the formation of a fibrous cap between the vessel lumen and the accumulating constituents of the mature plaque, including lipid-laden macrophages, free lipid, inflammatory cells and debris. This fibrous cap forms from modified smooth muscle cells. Over time, the plaque continues to evolve, re-model and, frequently, undergoes calcification. Complications may arise from these advanced plaques through rupture (thereby exposing the highly thrombotic plaque contents), thrombosis associated with rupture, aneurysmal dilatation of the vessel or haemorrhage into the plaque, in turn leading to rupture. Thrombosis and plaque rupture usually lead to myocardial infarction in the heart and stroke in the brain.

Atheroma (from the Greek word for porridge or gruel) affects the intima and media of large and medium-sized arteries and is the commonest type of arteriosclerosis, referred to as *atherosclerosis* (E-Figs. 8.2**G** and 8.3**G**). It is a chronic inflammatory process affecting susceptible individuals. It is a very common condition in developed societies and contributes to a large proportion of deaths. A variety of *modifiable* risk factors (those we can influence/control) and *non-modifiable* risk factors (those we have no control over) are important in the causation of this disease; these are summarised in Table 8.1.

BASIC PATHOLOGICAL PROCESSES ■ ATHEROSCLEROSIS

Table 8.1 Risk factors in atherosclerosis.

Non-modifiable risk factors	
Age	Incidence of severe disease rises with each decade after age 55
Sex	Higher risk in men and postmenopausal women
Genetic	Certain inherited conditions such as familial hyperlipidaemia and hyperhomocysteinaemia can predispose to premature atherosclerosis.
Ethnicity	People with South Asian ancestry are at increased risk, probably in part due to inherited factors
Modifiable risk factors	
Hypertension	Most important risk factor for stroke and one of most important for cardiac disease
Hyperlipidaemia	High total cholesterol, high triglycerides, high levels of low-density lipoprotein or low levels of high density lipoprotein cholesterol increase the risk of atheromatous disease
Tobacco use	Risk increased if started smoking when young, heavy smoker or female
Physical inactivity	Increases risk by up to 50%
Obesity	Major risk for cardiovascular disease and predisposes to diabetes
Diabetes mellitus	Doubles the likelihood for developing cardiovascular disease
Psychosocial	Chronic stress, anxiety and depression increase the risk of atheromatous disease

---

DRUG TREATMENTS FOR ATHEROSCLEROSIS

Statins: These are a group of drugs that act by inhibiting an enzyme involved in the production of low-density lipoprotein (LDL) cholesterol, which transports cholesterol to arteries where it can be incorporated as atheroma. Blocking the enzyme results in increased LDL receptor expression in the liver and, as a consequence, an increased clearance of LDL from the blood with associated decrease in blood cholesterol levels. There is some evidence to suggest that statins also reduce cardiovascular risk by other mechanisms.

   Aspirin/clopidogrel: These drugs both act to inhibit platelet aggregation and reduce the risk of thrombosis.

   Anti-hypertensives: Close control of blood pressure is important in patients with increased cardio-vascular risk. High blood pressure can be controlled by anti-hypertensive medications.

   Diabetic control: Poorly controlled diabetes mellitus is a risk factor for progressive atherosclerosis. Diabetic patients may take medications such as gliclazide, metformin or insulin injections to adequately control diabetes mellitus. This can be monitored using an HbA1c test to reveal what percentage of haemoglobin is bound to excess sugars within the blood (**glycosylated**).

Fig. 8.3 Atheromatous plaque development. **(A)** Early atheromatous plaque (LP); **(B)** foam cells and lipid (HP); **(C)** fibrofatty plaque (LP); **(D)** fibrous plaque (LP). (*Illustrations opposite*)

The stages in development of a mature, fibrous atheromatous plaque are illustrated in these four images. Fig. 8.3A shows a pale-staining area of thickening of the intima **(In)** composed of aggregated myointimal cells containing lipid and some intimal fibrous tissue. Macroscopically, these lesions appear as slightly raised, flat areas termed *atheromatous plaques*. Note that the medial layer of the vessel **(M)** is uniform and appears normal at this stage. Early atheroma is a disease confined to the intima.

   Fig. 8.3B reveals detail of the intimal thickening at higher power. Foam cells **(FC)** filled with lipid appear as large, pale-staining cells with vacuolated cytoplasm. These cells may be derived from either myointimal cells or macrophages. As the lesion progresses, some of the foam cells break down and liberate free lipid into the intima, which appears as non-staining, angular clefts **(C)** *(cholesterol clefts)*.

   Early intimal atheromatous lesions enlarge by further accumulation of lipid both in foam cells and free within extracellular intimal tissue. This is associated with a more marked fibrotic response in the intima, leading to increased thickening of the lesion to produce a *fibrofatty plaque* (P) as shown in Fig. 8.3C. Note the areas of non-staining lipid **(L)** surrounded by pink-staining fibrous tissue **(F)** making up the thickened intima. A zone of denser, more intensely stained fibrous tissue, sometimes termed a *fibrous cap* **(Cap)**, runs between the endothelial surface and the underlying fibrofatty aggregate.

   With progression of the lesion, the fibrous cap thickens and the intimal lesion becomes larger and more raised. Fig. 8.3D shows such a plaque **(P)**, which is mostly composed of fibrous tissue. Note that in both Figs. 8.3C and 8.3D there is early thinning of the tunica media **(M)** beneath the plaque compared with the adjacent normal vessel wall. This is the result of loss of supporting elastic tissue, atrophy of smooth muscle cells and progressive medial fibrosis. With time, the medial fibrous tissue stretches owing to loss of elastic recoil in the vessel wall and the vessel dilates. This dilatation is the basis of the formation of an atheromatous aneurysm.

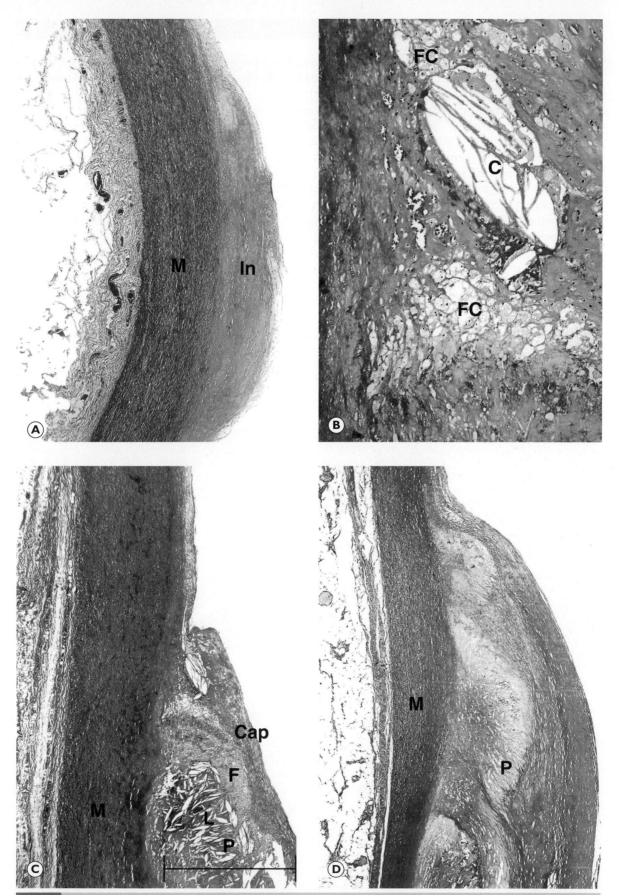

Fig. 8.3 Atheromatous plaque development. (*Caption opposite*)

KEY TO FIGURES
C cholesterol clefts **Cap** fibrous cap **F** fibrous tissue **FC** foam cells **In** intima **L** lipid
M media **P** fibrofatty plaque

Consequences of atheroma

All arterial vessels may be affected by atherosclerosis. The most commonly affected vessels are the coronary arteries (resulting in angina or myocardial infarction), the aorta (contributing to the formation of aneurysms) and the cerebral arteries (resulting in stroke).

The most important pathological and clinical sequelae of atherosclerosis are as follows:

- **Occlusion:** Narrowing of the arterial lumen produces partial or complete obstruction to blood flow; this may result in ischaemia and *infarction* of the tissue supplied by the atheromatous vessel (see Ch. 10).
- **Thrombosis:** When there is shear stress within the lumen of a blood vessel due to turbulent blood flow, endothelial disruption or ulceration can result. This can act as a nidus for the formation of a *thrombus*, an aggregate of platelets and fibrin within the lumen of a vessel wall (see Ch.9). Thrombus can obstruct the vessel wall leading to infarction of the tissue supplied (see Ch.10). In some cases, the thrombus can detach and travel with circulating blood, along the blood vessel *(embolism).* This can result in the obstruction of blood vessel lumen distal to the embolus (see Ch. 9).
- **Aneurysm:** Loss of smooth muscle and elastin from the media of an artery causes weakening of the vessel wall, predisposing to a localised area of dilatation. This is referred to as an *aneurysm* (E-Fig. 8.4**G**). As an aneurysm increases in diameter, the wall thins and the risk of rupture increases (according to the law of Laplace). Rupture of the aneurysm can lead to fatal haemorrhage, most commonly seen in the abdominal aorta (so-called ruptured abdominal aortic aneurysm). Aneurysms may also lead thrombus formation (see Ch. 9) due to blood stasis and endothelial disruption within the aneurysmal cavity.

The main complications are shown in Figs. 8.4 to 8.7.

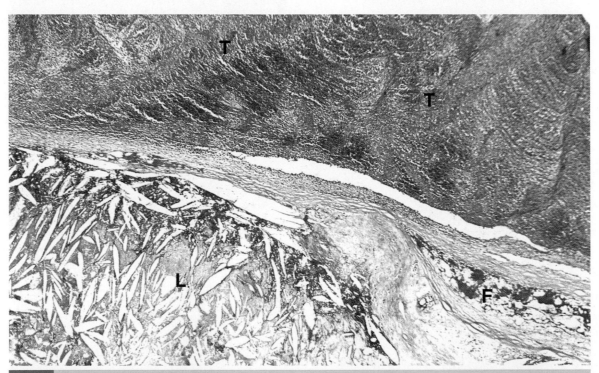

Fig. 8.4 **Complicated atheroma (MP).**

As an atheromatous plaque enlarges, it may become very thick relative to the normal thickness of the vessel wall, and, in addition to lipid, foam cells and fibrous tissue, calcium may be deposited in the lesion. With thickening and fibrosis the lesion may undergo rupture or surface ulceration. This is then described as a *complicated atheromatous plaque*. The normal smooth endothelial lining is gone and the highly thrombogenic plaque contents are exposed directly to the blood

flow. The coagulation sequence is thus activated and thrombus is formed on the vessel wall at the site of ulcerated atheroma (see Ch. 9).

Fig. 8.4 shows the top of an atheromatous plaque with foam cells (**F**) and free lipid (**L**). The surface has ulcerated and is encrusted with thrombus (**T**) composed of fibrin, platelets and entrapped blood cells. In a small vessel, for example a coronary artery, such a thrombus can occlude the lumen.

KEY TO FIGURES
A atheroma   **F** foam cells   **L** lipid   **Lu** lumen   **M** tunica media   **T** thrombus

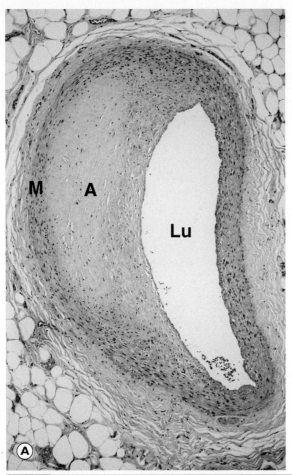 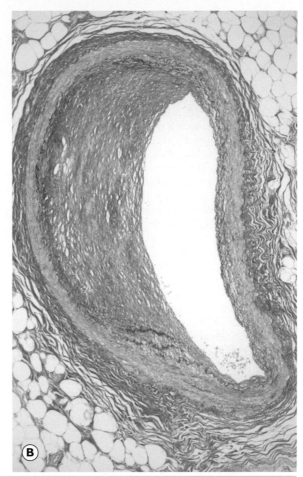

Fig. 8.5 **Arterial narrowing by atheroma (LP). (A)** H&E; **(B)** EVG.

As shown in Fig. 8.5A, the formation of a plaque of atheroma **(A)** in the intima of a small or medium-sized artery, such as this branch of a coronary artery, can greatly reduce the size of the lumen **(Lu)**. The consequent reduction in blood flow leads to ischaemia of the tissues supplied. Note that the media **(M)** underlying the atheroma is thinned. Such partly occlusive atheroma is frequent in the coronary arteries of cigarette-smoking males, particularly in the region of the bifurcation of the left coronary artery. Fig. 8.5B is stained by a special method to demonstrate elastin and illustrates the disruption of the internal elastic lamina.

A common symptom of this arterial narrowing is known as **angina pectoris**, a gripping pain in the chest particularly experienced on exertion and settling with rest. This pain is a manifestation of ischaemia.

Patients with longstanding angina often have small regions of myocardium that have been replaced by fibrous scar tissue (replacement fibrosis). This is termed **ischaemic heart disease**.

Similar luminal narrowing by atheroma occurs in many other arteries. In the leg arteries, such changes can produce severe calf pain on walking **(intermittent claudication)** and may eventually lead to the development of gangrene of the lower leg. In the cerebral arterial system (the arteries of the circle of Willis), which supplies the cerebral hemispheres, severe atheroma can produce transient ischaemia known as a **transient ischaemic attack** (or TIA). Clinically, this presents as loss of sensation or movement within the face and/or limbs that resolves within twenty-four hours of onset.

ANGIOGRAPHY AND STENTS

Where a vessel is narrowed by atheroma, typically a coronary artery, it is possible to visualise the narrowed segment by a process known as **angiography**.

During angiography, a catheter is passed along the systemic arterial system from a peripheral vessel (such as the femoral artery) to the diseased coronary artery. Once at the site of narrowing, the vessel can be visualised using contrast dye injections. If there is significant narrowing, then a stent can be deployed. This acts as a scaffold to keep the narrowed artery open. Some stents can contain medication, which is supplied directly to the site of arterial disease; these are known as a **drug eluting stents**. Research is currently focused upon stent structure and composition in order to improve their function and longevity.

BASIC PATHOLOGICAL PROCESSES ■ ATHEROSCLEROSIS

Fig. 8.6 Haemorrhage into atheromatous plaque (LP).

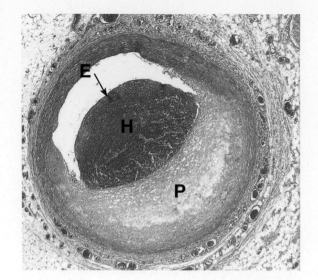

There are two possible mechanisms for the development of haemorrhage in an atheromatous plaque. First, the rigid fibrotic plaque may split under the constant trauma of pulsatile movements and allow blood from the vessel lumen to greatly expand the plaque lesion; such a process is termed *plaque fissuring*. Alternatively, small capillary vessels that develop in established plaques may rupture and lead to haemorrhage. Whatever the mechanism, because of the confined space in which such apparently trivial haemorrhage occurs, the consequences can be disproportionately devastating. In Fig. 8.6, a small haemorrhage (**H**) has occurred in the superficial area of a fibrofatty atheromatous plaque (**P**). The accumulated blood has tracked beneath the non-ulcerated endothelium (**E**), causing it to bulge markedly into the artery. This has led to even greater narrowing of a lumen already reduced to about half its normal size by the pre-existing atheromatous plaque. Such an abrupt reduction in arterial flow leads to acute ischaemia in the supplied tissues.

In this patient, the lesion was situated in the anterior descending branch of the left coronary artery and resulted in acute ischaemia of a substantial area of the anterior wall of the left ventricle and the anterior half of the interventricular septum (E-Fig. 8.5**G**). Necrosis of heart muscle ensued, a process known as *myocardial infarction*, resulting in this patient's death (see Fig. 10.2).

CORONARY ARTERY BYPASS GRAFT SURGERY (CABG)

Where atheroma in a coronary vessel is such that symptoms from the reduced flow through the stenotic segment cannot be controlled by medication and/or a stent procedure, it is possible to perform surgery to bypass the blocked segment of vessel. This is achieved by utilising a nearby vessel (e.g. internal thoracic artery) or inserting a length of vessel from elsewhere in the body (e.g. a vein from the leg) between the aorta and the diseased vessel beyond the point of stenosis. This length of vessel is sometimes referred to as the *graft*. Hence, the procedure is commonly referred to as a *coronary artery bypass graft* or, more often, by its acronym as a *CABG* (pronounced 'cabbage').

Whilst angioplasty and stenting may be favoured for disease in a single coronary vessel, bypass surgery is preferred where more than one vessel is diseased. Hence, the number of vessels bypassed may be referred to when discussing the procedure (e.g. *double bypass, triple bypass*).

Together, the procedures of angioplasty, stenting and bypass surgery are referred to as *re-vascularisation* procedures. Although these procedures have transformed outcomes in patients with coronary artery atheromatous disease, it should be borne in mind that while they may overcome the diseased arterial segment, they do not prevent further atheroma from developing. As such, following re-vascularisation, it is advised that patients do all they can to tackle the modifiable risk factors that may have contributed to the development of their atheromatous disease.

KEY TO FIGURES
C clot **E** endothelium **H** haemorrhage **P** plaque **T** thrombus

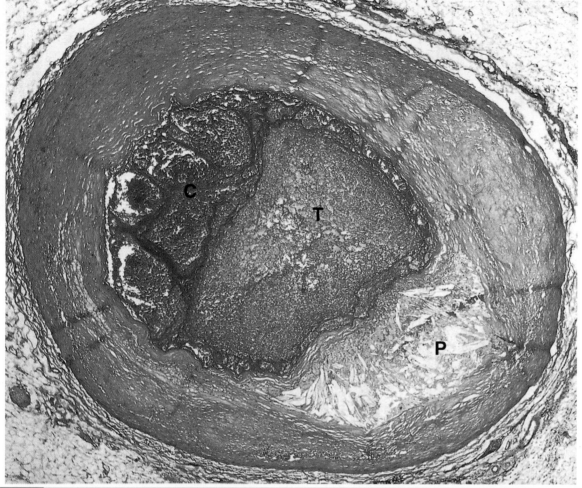

Fig. 8.7 Thrombus formation on atheroma (LP).

The most important complication of atheroma in small and medium-sized arteries is the development of a *thrombus* on the surface of an atheromatous plaque. The process of thrombus formation is discussed in detail in Ch. 9. Thrombus, which consists of a mass of platelets and insoluble fibrin, tends, in the arterial system, to form on any intimal surface that is denuded to expose the underlying tissues. Endothelial ulceration over an atheromatous plaque is the commonest cause of thrombosis in the arterial system, although plaque fissuring, as discussed in Fig. 8.6, can also initiate thrombosis.

This micrograph (Fig. 8.7) of a coronary artery shows an ulcerated atheromatous plaque (**P**), which has already significantly constricted the arterial lumen. A thrombus (**T**) has then developed on the ulcerated surface, largely obliterating the remaining lumen. The thrombus is deep pink in colour and is composed of fibrin and platelets with entrapped red blood cells.

The residual lumen is occupied by bright red post-mortem blood clot (**C**), composed entirely of tightly packed red blood cells. The naked eye distinction between genuine ante-mortem thrombus and post-mortem clot is important. Thrombus is pinkish red, granular and firm, whereas clot is predominantly dark red, shiny and jelly-like.

When thrombus formation occurs on an atheromatous lesion in a large-diameter artery, such as the aorta or carotid arteries, the thrombus may be small and cause little significant obstruction to blood flow at the site. Fragments of thrombus may, however, become detached and pass into the peripheral circulation to block a smaller vessel and cause ischaemia or infarction in its area of distribution. This phenomenon is known as *thromboembolism* and is more fully described in Ch. 9.

BASIC PATHOLOGICAL PROCESSES ■ ATHEROSCLEROSIS

Table 8.2 Chapter review.

Disorder	Definition	Main features	Figure
Arteriosclerosis	General term for loss of elasticity and hardening of vessel walls	Can occur with aging Often associated with hypertension Changes often seen in kidneys	8.1
Atherosclerosis	Commonest type of arteriosclerosis	Endothelial dysfunction leads to accumulation of macrophages, lymphocytes and lipoproteins within the intima, forming a fatty streak Progression results from smooth muscle proliferation and collagen deposition forming an atheromatous plaque There are a number of risk factors	8.2, 8.3 Table 8.1
Complications of atherosclerosis	Progression of atherosclerosis can result in clinical manifestations	Severe atheromatous plaque can result in occlusion, thrombosis or aneurysm	8.4, 8.5, 8.6, 8.7

9 Thrombosis and embolism

Thrombosis

The vascular system normally contains fluid blood. However, it is often necessary for blood to coagulate to prevent bleeding following injury to a vessel wall. To control this process of *haemostasis*, there are interacting systems that either promote or inhibit the process of blood coagulation. These systems are normally well regulated. Under certain pathological circumstances these dynamics may be disrupted, leading either to *haemorrhage* or *thrombosis*. Thrombosis is a dynamic process in which a *thrombus,* composed of a solid, tangled mass of fibrin, platelets, erythrocytes and other blood constituent cells, forms within the lumen of a blood vessel in response to disruption of the normal blood flow. Thrombosis can be differentiated from coagulation in so far as coagulation occurs within static blood, often at the site of an injury. Thrombosis is a dynamic process and can occur more frequently in certain diseased states.

Thrombosis may occur in any part of the circulation, but most commonly occur in large veins (E-Fig. 9.1 **G**), large arteries, in the heart chambers (E-Fig. 9.2 **G**) and on heart valves (Figs 11.16 and 11.17). Three major factors, alone or in combination, predispose to thrombosis. These are often referred to as *Virchow's triad*:

■ **Damage to the endothelium** is the main cause of arterial and intracardiac thrombosis: This damage may be either through physical endothelial disruption or as a consequence of endothelial cell dysfunction. Hence hypertension, turbulent blood flow and bacterial endotoxins may contribute to endothelial dysfunction and thrombus formation.

■ **Disordered blood flow.** Relative stasis is important in initiating thrombus in slow-flowing blood such as in veins. Turbulent blood flow predisposes to thrombus formation in arterial vessels and the heart through disruption of endothelial function and the creation of eddy currents in the blood with focal stasis.

■ **Abnormal haemostatic properties of the blood (hypercoagulability).** Hypercoagulable states may be either inherited or acquired. Of the inherited disorders, abnormalities in the factor V and prothrombin genes are commonest and may present with recurrent venous thrombosis. There are numerous acquired hypercoagulable states, such as those associated with changes in blood viscosity, for example in dehydration, major illness, disseminated carcinoma or in the post-operative state.

A thrombus has a defined architecture and consistency, which reflects the manner and stages of its formation and the nature of blood flow in the vicinity. For example, thrombus formed in an artery is usually dense and composed mainly of aggregated platelets and fibrin (Fig. 9.2).

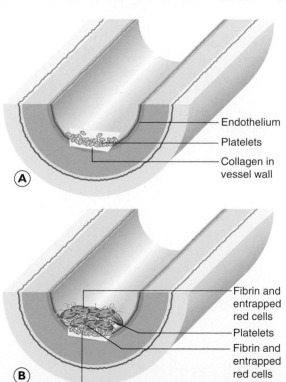

(A) Endothelium / Platelets / Collagen in vessel wall

(B) Fibrin and entrapped red cells / Platelets / Fibrin and entrapped red cells / Platelets

Fig. 9.1 Early thrombogenesis.

Following endothelial injury (Fig. 9.1A), platelets adhere to exposed subendothelial collagen (mediated by von Willebrand factor) and become activated, liberating ADP and thromboxane A2, which mediate further platelet aggregation.

Platelets undergo degranulation and their products, together with released tissue factors, activate the coagulation cascade (Fig. 9.1B). This results in generation of thrombin, which converts soluble fibrinogen to insoluble fibrin. Red cells become passively entrapped in the resultant fibrin–platelet mesh, the number depending on the circumstances of thrombus formation. In arteries, there are few red cells and more platelets and fibrin; in veins, where blood flow is slower, there are generally many more red cells.

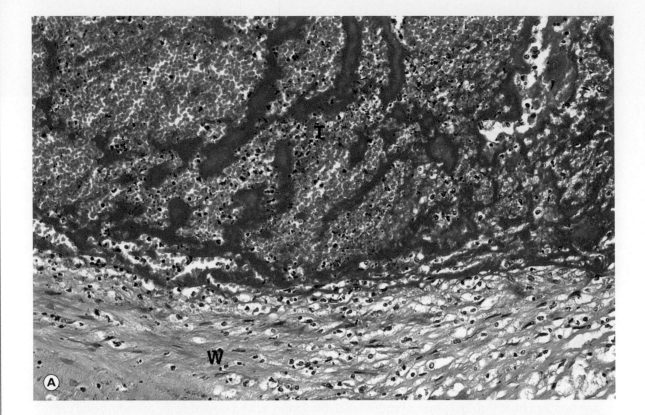

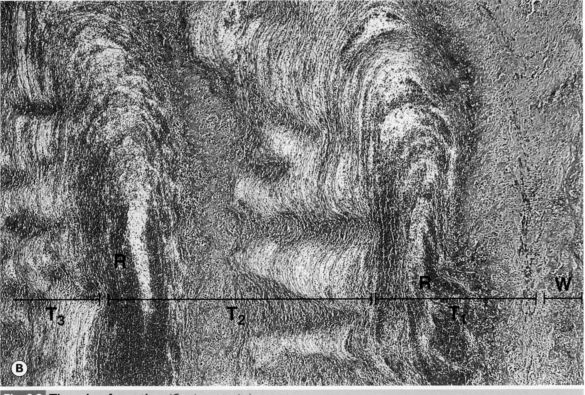

Fig. 9.2 **Thrombus formation.** (*Caption opposite*)

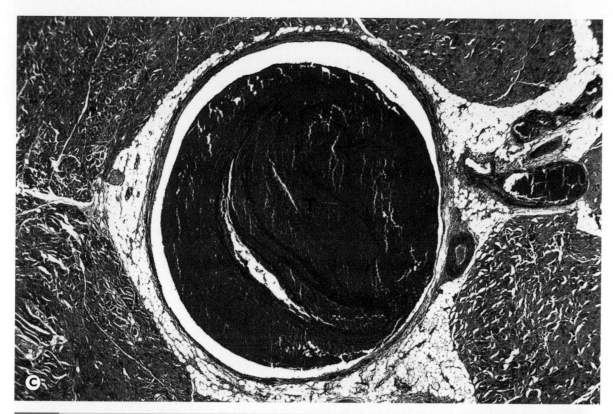

Fig. 9.2 **Thrombus formation. (A)** Early thrombus (HP); **(B)** enlargement of thrombus (MP); **(C)** thrombosis in a vein (LP). *(Illustrations (A) and (B) opposite)*

Damage to the endothelium exposes collagen fibrils within the intima, to which platelets adhere and then aggregate at the site of damage. Tissue damage and collagen exposure also activate the extrinsic and intrinsic blood clotting systems respectively, the latter system also depending on release of platelet factor 3 from aggregated platelets. The result is activation of prothrombin to thrombin, which in turn catalyses the conversion of soluble plasma fibrinogen into insoluble fibrin. Thus, the flimsy platelet aggregates become bound together into a solid, resilient mass, the thrombus.

Fig. 9.2A illustrates an arterial wall **(W)** which is damaged by atheroma. The endothelium has become ulcerated with the formation of thrombus **(T)** at the site of injury. This thrombus consists of platelet aggregates within a meshwork of eosinophilic fibrin. Entrapped erythrocytes and leukocytes are present but are not themselves involved in the specific haemostatic processes.

Small areas of thrombus formed on vessel walls may be dissolved completely by fibrinolytic mechanisms. However, under appropriate conditions, the thrombus continues to enlarge. Fig. 9.2B illustrates this process. The abnormal vessel wall **(W)** has become coated by a thin layer of fibrin and platelet thrombus **(T$_1$)**, with entrapped red cells **(R)**. This has formed the basis for the deposition of another layer of fibrin–platelet thrombus **(T$_2$)**, again with entrapped red cells. A third layer **(T$_3$)** can be seen forming at the left of the picture. Thus, thrombi enlarge by the successive deposition of a number of layers, a feature that is apparent to the naked eye in the laminated cut surface seen in an established thrombus *(lines of Zahn)*.

In the arterial system, damage to the intimal layer is the most common predisposing factor in thrombus formation but, in the venous system, the most crucial factor is the rate of blood flow; reduced flow rates increase susceptibility to thrombus formation. Vasculitis or inflammation of the vessel wall also causes thrombosis (see Ch. 11).

Fig. 9.2C shows a venous thrombus **(T)** completely occluding the lumen of a vein found in the muscle of the calf. This is known as *deep venous thrombosis (DVT)* and may be encountered in post-operative patients confined to bed.

KEY TO FIGURES
R red cells **T** thrombus **W** arterial wall

Fate of vascular thrombi

Once thrombus is formed there are several possible outcomes:

■ **Propagation:** The thrombus itself is thrombogenic and may attract more platelets and fibrin to the site, resulting in it enlarging and growing along the vessel, ultimately leading to vessel occlusion and/or embolisation if left untreated.

■ **Embolisation:** In addition to the triad of factors contributing to thrombus generation, Virchow coined the term embolus for *'fragments from the end of a softening thrombus that are carried along by the current of the blood and driven into remote vessels'*. This term is now applied not only to fragments of thrombus *(thromboemboli)*, but to any material forming in, or entering, the bloodstream and passing with the circulation to lodge in a more distal vessel.

Emboli are most commonly caused by detachment of all or part of a thrombus from its site of formation. Venous thromboembolism is of clinical importance as, for example, following deep venous thrombosis in the leg, the thrombus may propagate as far as the common iliac vein or even the inferior vena cava. Part of such a huge thrombus may readily become detached and pass via the right side of the heart to lodge in the pulmonary arterial tree as a *pulmonary embolus*, which is often fatal (Fig. 9.4) and (E-Fig. 9.3 **G**).

Systemic arterial thromboemboli most commonly arise from the heart or major arteries. In such cases, the thrombus often covers only part of the luminal wall as a plaque-like structure and is known as *mural thrombus*. Such thrombi may form on the ventricular endocardium following myocardial infarction (Fig. 9.3). Emboli arising in the arterial system impact in peripheral arterial vessels where the most dramatic outcome is necrosis of the tissue supplied *(infarction)*; this is described in detail in Ch. 10.

Whilst thrombotic emboli are the most common, emboli may also arise from other sources. These include atheromatous debris, tumour cells, bacterial vegetation from infected heart valves, fat and bone marrow after bone fracture (Fig. 9.5), air entering the circulation and, rarely, amniotic fluid in cases of complicated pregnancy. Embolisation can also have a therapeutic role (see Fig. 9.6).

■ **Resolution:** This involves the normal physiological phenomenon of fibrinolysis as well as autolytic disintegration of the cellular elements of the thrombus. The end result is complete dissolution with restoration of blood flow. This process may be enhanced by the therapeutic administration of thrombolytic drugs, a principle of the acute management of stroke (see clinical box 'Clinical management of thrombosis and embolism').

■ **Organisation:** Ingrowth of granulation tissue from the vessel wall and subsequent fibrous repair occur when fibrinolysis is ineffective in removing the thrombus. By an extraordinary mechanism, the organised thrombus may undergo recanalisation, a process whereby new vascular channels are formed to re-establish a patent lumen. The processes of organisation and recanalisation are illustrated in Fig. 9.7.

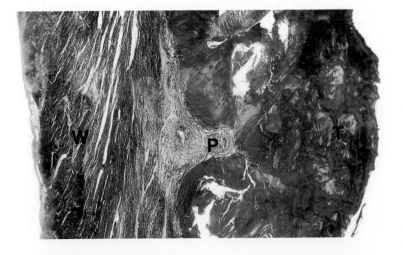

Fig. 9.3 Left ventricular mural thrombus (LP).

Thrombus within the heart chambers most commonly forms upon endocardium damaged by myocardial infarction (see Fig.10.2). Fig. 9.3 illustrates infarcted ventricular wall **(W)** with mural thrombus **(T)** laid down on the luminal surface; the thrombus surrounds a papillary muscle **(P)**.

The left ventricle is the most common site of mural thrombosis after myocardial infarction.

KEY TO FIGURES
E embolus   **P** papillary muscle   **T** thrombus   **W** ventricular wall

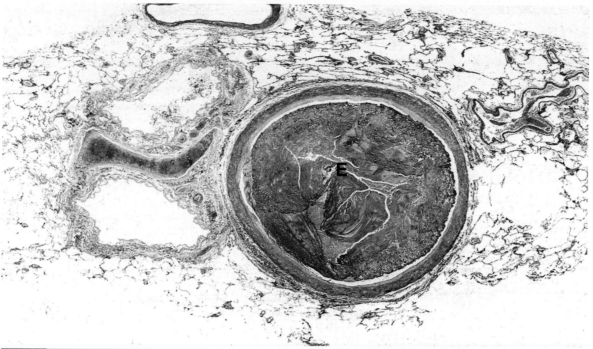

Fig. 9.4 Thromboembolism: pulmonary embolus (LP).

When fragments of thrombus become detached from their site of formation, they travel in the circulation (venous or arterial, according to site of origin) as thromboemboli. On reaching vessels of small enough calibre to prevent further passage, the thromboemboli impact, producing sudden vascular occlusion.

Depending on the size of the thromboembolus, the tissue or organ involved and the extent of alternative vascular supply, the result may be either inadequate blood flow for normal sustenance of the tissue (ischaemia) or frank tissue necrosis (infarction); these phenomena are described in Ch. 10. Fig. 9.4 illustrates lung tissue in which the pulmonary artery branch is occluded by an embolus (**E**) originating from thrombus in the deep veins of the leg.

This condition, known as *pulmonary embolism*, is an important cause of sudden death, especially in debilitated or immobilised patients who are predisposed to deep venous thrombosis.

CLINICAL MANAGEMENT OF THROMBOSIS AND EMBOLISM

To supplement the natural process of fibrinolysis and hasten dissolution of thrombus in clinical situations where early restoration of blood flow *(reperfusion)* to an organ may be indicated, a variety of pharmacological agents have been developed that aid breakdown *(lysis)* of the thrombus. Hence this treatment is known as *thrombolysis* and the drugs used are termed *thrombolytics*. These drugs act to increase the conversion of naturally occurring plasminogen to plasmin, which has powerful fibrinolytic properties. An example is recombinant tissue plasminogen activator (rt-PA).

Administration of these agents has transformed the acute management of stroke. The aim is to achieve reperfusion of the vascular bed as quickly as possible, to minimise the volume of tissue infarcted.

Embolectomy can help to treat ischaemic limbs and can prevent the need for amputation. In this process, either a surgeon or an interventional radiologist can use a catheter to remove an embolus from an artery within a limb, restoring blood flow to the ischaemic area.

Some patients take anticoagulant drugs such as *warfarin,* a coumarin-based medication, particularly if they have an irregular heart rhythm called *atrial fibrillation.* This has been shown to decrease the frequency of strokes caused by embolism of atrial thrombi into the cerebral arterial tree.

BASIC PATHOLOGICAL PROCESSES ■ THROMBOSIS AND EMBOLISM

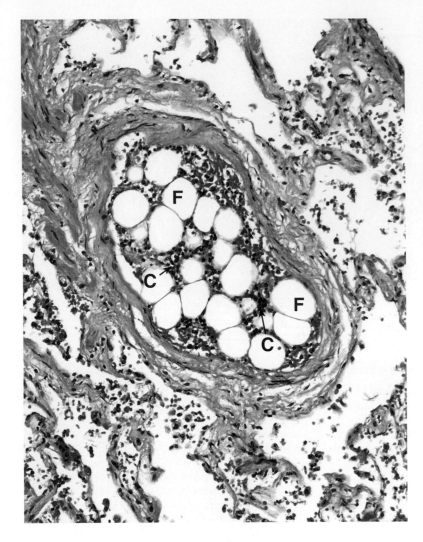

Fig. 9.5 Bone marrow embolus (MP).

As noted above, other than thrombus, there are a number of other objects that may embolise. These include atheroma, tumour, fat and bone marrow. Whatever the source, the consequence is obstruction of distal vessels with resultant partial or complete occlusion.

In Fig. 9.5, a fragment of bone marrow has embolised to the pulmonary vasculature and become lodged in a pulmonary artery branch. The lumen of the vessel contains both fat cells of bone marrow (**F**) and the cellular haematopoietic elements (**C**).

Bone marrow/fat embolism is a common complication of trauma, in particular following fracture of a long bone such as the femur. It can also occasionally occur as a complication of orthopaedic surgery. In the majority of cases, it passes without symptoms. Where symptoms occur, they most often arise in the days following injury with breathlessness, tachycardia, delirium and a petechial rash; this last observation is a useful sign in supporting the diagnosis clinically. In a small proportion of cases (approximately 10%), fat embolisation is fatal.

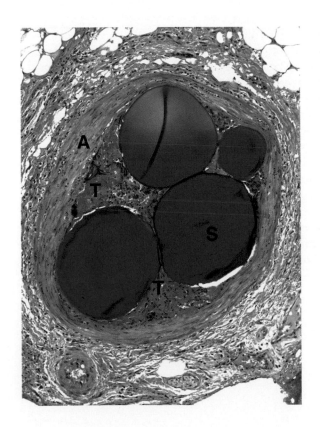

Fig. 9.6 Therapeutic embolisation (MP).

Under certain circumstances, embolisation may be used as a therapeutic manoeuvre whereby embolic agents, of which there is a variety available, are introduced to the target vasculature through a catheter sited via a peripheral vessel. Indications for this include: to control abnormal bleeding (e.g. complicating fibroids), to occlude vessels supplying a richly vascular tumour prior to chemotherapy or surgery, or to treat a vascular malformation.

In Fig. 9.6, taken from a surgical resection specimen several days after embolisation therapy, embolisation spheres (**S**) are seen almost filling the lumen of a medium-sized artery, the wall of which is clearly visible (**A**). As a result of this, thrombus (**T**) has formed around the spheres. The combination of the spheres and associated thrombus has occluded the vessel. This aids surgery by minimising the risk of intraoperative haemorrhage from a highly vascular tumour.

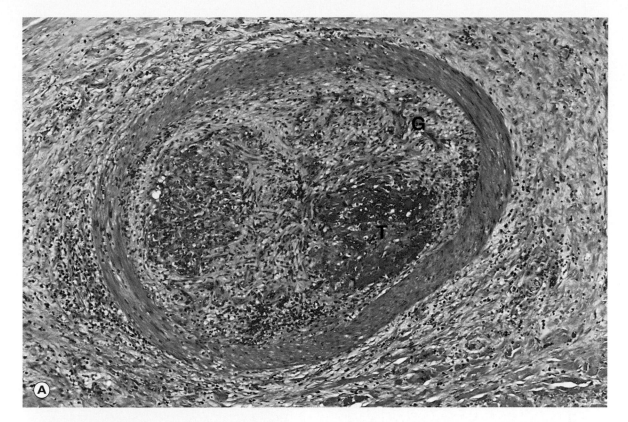

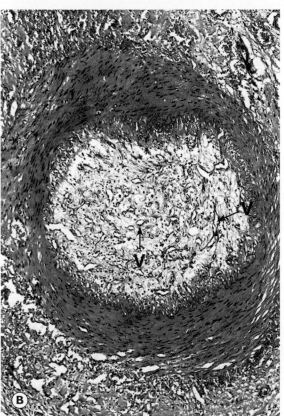

Fig. 9.7 **Fate of thrombi. (A)** Organisation (MP);
(B) recanalisation (MP).

Following occlusion of a vessel by thrombus, there is
an initial inflammatory response in the vessel wall.

Within a few days, the thrombus becomes *organised*
by ingrowth of granulation tissue from the intima of
the vessel wall. Fig. 9.7A shows a vein occluded by
thrombus (**T**). At various points, granulation tissue
(**G**) extends from the vessel wall into the thrombus.
This eventually results in replacement of the thrombus
by fibrovascular granulation tissue. In some cases,
larger vessels develop within the fibrovascular
granulation tissue of the organising thrombus and
may permit passage of blood through the damaged,
previously occluded area. This occurs most commonly
in arteries and is termed *recanalisation*.

Fig. 9.7B illustrates this process in an artery that
has been occluded by thrombus and is at a later stage
of organisation than in Fig. 9.7A. Note that the
granulation tissue in the lumen contains numerous
small blood vessels (**V**). These vessels may conduct
blood across the thrombosed area and some will
enlarge with time, acquiring smooth muscle walls.

BASIC PATHOLOGICAL PROCESSES ■ **THROMBOSIS AND EMBOLISM**

KEY TO FIGURES
A artery   **C** bone marrow cells   **F** fat   **G** granulation tissue   **S** embolisation sphere   **T** thrombus
V blood vessels

Table 9.1 Chapter review.

Feature	Definition	Figure
Thrombus	Aggregate of platelets, fibrin and blood cells formed in vessel lumen by the process of thrombosis	9.1 9.2 9.3
Virchow's triad	Factors predisposing to thrombus formation namely damaged endothelium, abnormal blood flow and hypercoagulability	
Fate of thrombi	Propagation: enlargement with growth along vessel or occlusion of vessel Embolisation: see below Resolution: dissolution of the thrombus by fibrinolysis Organisation: where fibrinolysis is unsuccessful, granulation tissue may form with subsequent fibrous repair and recanalisation	9.4 9.7
Embolus	Fragment of thrombus or other material (e.g. bone marrow, air) passing with the circulation to lodge in a distal vessel	9.5 9.6

10 Infarction

Introduction

When there is sustained occlusion of arterial blood supply or venous drainage, a type of necrosis can occur called *infarction*. Common clinical examples of infarction are myocardial infarction (affecting the heart) and cerebral infarction or stroke (affecting the brain). In these situations, the myocardial or cerebral vessels are affected by atherosclerosis, thrombosis or embolism. If the blood supply is temporarily altered, then this can lead to ischaemia of the tissues; sustained ischaemia leads to infarction.

Types of infarction

In most situations, infarction arises as a consequence of thrombotic or embolic events in the arterial system, though occlusion of venous drainage may also result in infarction.

■ **Arterial infarction** is usually due to complete blockage of an artery by thrombosis or embolism. Arterial thrombosis is generally a complication of pre-existing atheroma (see Ch. 8). Embolisation in the arterial system is most commonly from the heart, either from mural thrombus (see Fig. 9.3) or thrombus occurring on heart valves (*vegetations*; see Figs 11.16 and 11.17) or from thrombosis and/or atheroma of arteries. Examples of infarcts from the kidney and myocardium are shown in Figs 10.1 and 10.2, respectively, and from the cerebellum in Fig. 23.2.

■ **Venous infarction** most commonly arises as a consequence of mechanical compression of blood vessels, particularly in organs that receive their blood supply via a vascular pedicle. Such organs may become infarcted if the pedicle becomes twisted, for example torsion of the testis (see Fig. 19.1), or constricted by becoming entrapped in a narrow space, for example bowel infarction caused by hernial strangulation (Fig. 10.5). In such cases, venous obstruction occurs as extrinsic pressure compresses the thin-walled, low-pressure veins without initially compromising the arteries. As a consequence, tissues become massively suffused with red cells and prolonged venous obstruction eventually causes the tissue to become ischaemic owing to stasis of blood. The resulting cessation in tissue perfusion results in infarction. Venous infarction may also occur in the brain as a complication of dural sinus thrombosis.

Macroscopic appearance of infarcts

When infarction is due to simple cessation of arterial supply, the shape of the infarct reflects the arterial territory involved. In most organs (e.g. kidney, spleen or brain), the infarct appears wedge-shaped in section, with the broad part of the wedge at the periphery (E-Fig. 10.1**G**). In contrast, infarcts in the heart are not wedge-shaped, but are classified as subendocardial or transmural depending on the underlying cause (E-Figs 10.2 and 10.3**G**). Transmural infarctions, i.e. those involving the full thickness of the ventricle, are caused by an obstruction of one of the coronary artery territories. As the coronary arteries are *end arteries*, blockage of a major coronary artery branch causes necrosis of the segment of heart muscle supplied by that branch. Subendocardial infarctions can be seen in cases of global poor perfusion, such as in cases of systemic shock. As their name suggests, they do not affect the thickness of the muscle wall and are confined to the innermost aspect of the heart muscle, as this region receives its blood supply from the lumen of the ventricle.

Like most forms of tissue damage, infarction excites an acute inflammatory response followed by replacement of necrotic tissue by granulation tissue, which then undergoes fibrous repair and scarring (see Ch. 3). The appearance of infarcts histologically and to the naked eye thus depends on how far this sequence has progressed. One important exception to this process is the brain, which does not normally show the usual processes of granulation tissue formation and fibrous repair. Cerebral infarcts undergo central liquefaction known as colliquative necrosis (see Ch. 2) with reactive gliosis at the margins of the lesion (see Ch. 23). Old cerebral infarcts are usually marked by a cystic area surrounded by a zone of gliosis; brain infarction is illustrated in Figs 2.7B and 23.2.

Organs in which there are extensive capillary, sinusoidal or arteriovenous anastomoses often have infarcts that are dark red in their early stages because of congestion with blood and haemorrhage (from the Latin, *infarcire*, meaning to stuff). Important examples are the lung (Fig. 10.4) and spleen.

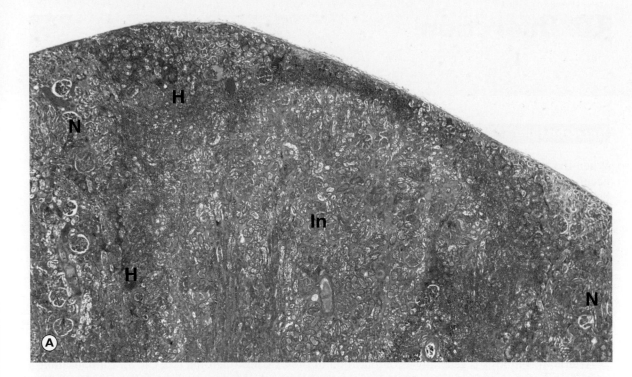

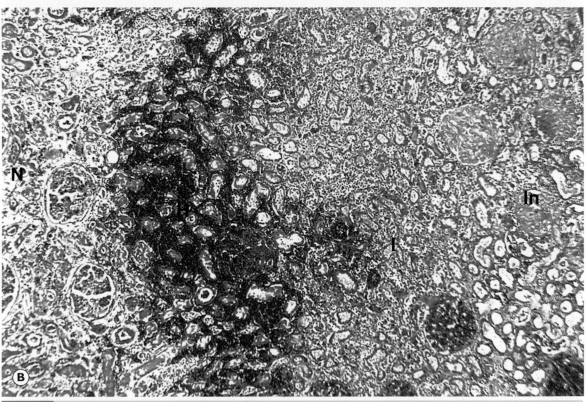

Fig. 10.1 **Renal infarction.** (*Caption opposite*)

KEY TO FIGURES
H hyperaemic zone   **I** acute inflammation   **In** infarcted region   **N** normal   **S** scar

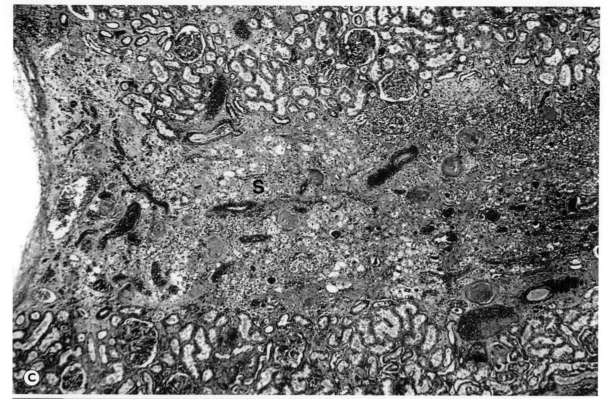

Fig. 10.1 **Renal infarction. (A)** Early infarct (LP); **(B)** margin of infarct (MP); **(C)** old renal infarct (MP). (*Illustrations (A) and (B) opposite*)

The kidneys are favoured sites for infarction, often asymptomatic, as a result of the large blood flow to the kidneys and their limited collateral circulation *(end arteries)*. The majority of renal infarcts result from emboli originating from thrombus in the left ventricle (e.g. mural thrombus after myocardial infarction) or the left atrial appendage (e.g. in atrial fibrillation).

In the very early stages (i.e. within 12 hours of infarction), gross examination shows the infarcted area to be ill defined and dark. Soon, the lesion becomes paler until it becomes a clearly defined, wedge-shaped, readily identifiable region with the base towards the cortical surface and the apex extending towards the medulla. Such established infarcts may be recognised within 24 hours of onset.

Fig. 10.1A shows the histological appearance of a typical early renal infarct. The recently infarcted necrotic area **(In)** stains less intensely than the normal cortex **(N)**, but the general architecture of the infarct remains intact with still discernible 'ghosts' of glomeruli and renal tubules. The infarcted area has become demarcated from normal cortex by a narrow hyperaemic zone **(H)** representing the earliest vascular stages of a typical acute inflammatory response. Between this hyperaemic zone and the necrotic tissue

is a purple-staining band containing the neutrophils of an early cellular acute inflammatory exudate.

Fig. 10.1B shows, at higher magnification, the edge of the infarct in Fig. 10.1A. Note that the normal cortical tissue **(N)**, with its well-defined glomeruli and tubules, gives way to a zone of hyperaemia **(H)**. Next to this is a purplish band of acute inflammation **(I)** at the margin of the infarcted area **(In)** where marked necrotic changes are evident in both glomeruli and tubules (see Fig. 2.7). The acute inflammatory zone exhibits typically dilated and congested capillaries and an influx of small, dark-staining neutrophil polymorphs.

The necrotic tissue is progressively removed by neutrophils and macrophages and replaced by granulation tissue, which eventually undergoes fibrous repair to form a small fibrous scar. This is shown in Fig. 10.1C, which illustrates the end result of a renal infarct occurring 2 months previously; the infarct was of a comparable size to that shown in Fig. 10.1A. All that now remains is a small, narrow, pink-staining, wedge-shaped scar **(S)** with its broad aspect at the capsular surface. Note that the capsular surface at the site of the scar is depressed as a result of contraction of the collagen fibres within the scar (a process known as *cicatrisation*).

TYPES OF MYOCARDIAL INFARCTIONS

Acute myocardial infarctions can be subdivided by the pattern of ECG changes noted at initial presentation, as ST elevation myocardial infarction (STEMI) and non-ST elevation myocardial infarction (NSTEMI). STEMIs tend to occur secondary to acute coronary artery thrombosis and are usually treated by a minimally invasive surgical procedure to remove the thrombus (*percutaneous coronary intervention* or *PCI*) generally followed by medical therapy. NSTEMIs may be caused by a less severe blockage of a coronary artery and, in general, can be treated with up-front medical therapy and subsequent coronary intervention.

There are other ways to describe myocardial infarctions, notably type 1 myocardial infarction and type 2 myocardial infarction. Type 1 myocardial infarction can be diagnosed when clinical features of myocardial infarction – chest pain, arm/neck pain, sweating, nausea – are present, together with a rise in *troponin,* a blood test finding indicative of myocyte damage, and ECG changes. A type 2 myocardial infarction may not present with the typical clinical features of myocardial infarction and is better termed secondary ischaemic cardiac injury.

Ischaemic heart disease is a major cause of death in all industrialised countries. Atherosclerosis of coronary arteries accounts for the vast majority of cases, hence the alternative term *coronary artery disease (CAD)*. Three main clinical syndromes are recognised:

■ *Stable angina pectoris* (from the Latin for 'choking pain' of the 'chest'). Angina describes a complex of symptoms arising from paroxysmal, often recurring and brief episodes of reversible myocardial ischaemia. Symptoms arise as a consequence of increased load on the heart (e.g. during exercise) in the face of coronary artery stenosis through atheroma. Thus, there is insufficient perfusion of the myocardium as coronary artery blood flow is limited by atheroma. Stable angina may progress to acute myocardial infarction with increasing atheromatous occlusion and/or thrombosis.

■ *Acute myocardial infarction* (heart attack). Two main pathological forms are recognised:

– *Transmural infarction.* This involves the full thickness of a segment of the ventricular wall and is associated with complete blockage of a main coronary artery by thrombosis, often superimposed on an area of atherosclerotic narrowing (see Ch. 8). Complications of an acute transmural infarction include death, cardiac dysrhythmia, ventricular aneurysm, acute valve dysfunction and pericarditis.

– *Subendocardial myocardial infarction.* In this case, myocardial necrosis is limited to cells in the inner third of the ventricular wall. The pathogenesis of infarction is limitation of flow to the end arteries supplying the inner part of the ventricular wall, rather than complete occlusion of the main arterial trunks.

■ *Sudden cardiac death* (immediately fatal myocardial infarction or dysrhythmia due to acute ischaemia resulting in death).

The histological changes following infarction are illustrated in Figs 10.2 and 10.3.

Fig. 10.2 Myocardial infarction. (A) 24-hour infarct (HP); **(B)** 3-day infarct (HP); **(C)** 10-day infarct (HP); **(D)** 14-day infarct (HP). (*Illustrations opposite*)

The most common clinical example of infarction is that of the myocardium following occlusion of a coronary artery. Using routine staining methods, the earliest histological features of infarction may be visible approximately 4 hours after infarction and are established at about 12 to 24 hours, as illustrated in Fig. 10.2A. The infarcted cardiac muscle fibres **(In)** exhibit patchy loss or blurring of cross-striations and tend to become more intensely stained by eosin than normal myocardial fibres **(M)**. At this stage there may also be a degree of early capillary engorgement, interstitial oedema and a mild neutrophil infiltrate representing the earliest stages of the acute inflammatory response.

By about 2 or 3 days, as shown in Fig. 10.2B, the infarcted fibres are intensely eosinophilic and most have lost their nuclei. There is marked infiltration by neutrophils **(N)** into the oedematous interstitium. This acute inflammatory process evolves during the succeeding days, during which time the necrotic myocardium undergoes autolysis and fragmentation. By about the 10th day, as illustrated in Fig. 10.2C, most of the necrotic muscle has disappeared due to the combined phagocytic activity of neutrophils and macrophages. The infarcted area is now largely occupied by residual macrophages, some lymphocytes

and plasma cells in a loose oedematous mesh in which a few capillaries and fibroblasts herald the early signs of granulation tissue formation.

By about the 14th day, the infarct is almost wholly replaced by fibrovascular granulation tissue **(G)**, as illustrated in Fig. 10.2D, and the necrotic myocardium has been almost completely removed by the phagocytic activity of macrophages and neutrophils.

Over succeeding weeks, the fibrovascular granulation tissue becomes progressively more fibrous and less vascular, leading to the formation of a highly collagenous and relatively acellular scar by about the end of the second month following infarction. An example of a myocardial scar is shown in Fig. 10.3.

The infarcted myocardium offers the least resistance to pressure around days 5 to 10, at which time the patient is most vulnerable to myocardial rupture. This not uncommon complication is almost invariably fatal, the ruptured ventricle wall spilling blood into the pericardial cavity (*haemopericardium*). If the interventricular septum is involved in the infarct, there may be rupture of the septum with the sudden appearance of a systolic murmur. Similarly, rupture of an infarcted papillary muscle may lead to mitral valve incompetence with the appearance of a characteristic systolic murmur.

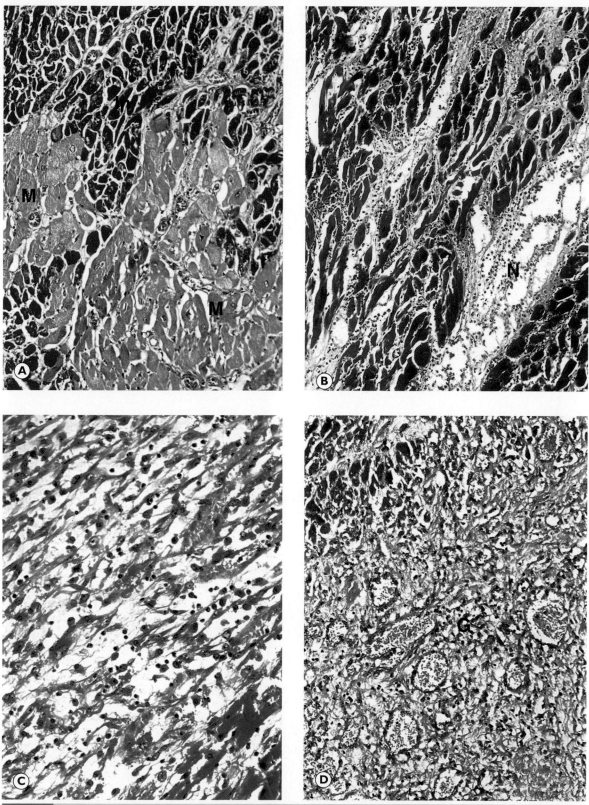

Fig. 10.2 **Myocardial infarction.** (*Caption opposite*)

KEY TO FIGURE
G granulation tissue   **In** infarcted fibres   **M** normal fibres   **N** neutrophils

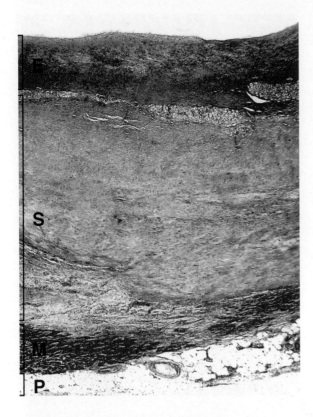

Fig. 10.3 Old myocardial infarct: full-thickness scar (LP).

Fig. 10.3 shows the appearance of a myocardial scar several months after infarction. The site of infarction is marked by densely collagenous, pale pink-staining scar (**S**), contrasting with the more eosinophilic, surviving myocardium (**M**). Continuing contraction (cicatrisation) of the fibrous scar over succeeding months leads to thinning of the infarcted area. If the scar is inadequate to withstand ventricular pressures, a ventricular aneurysm may develop by ballooning of the wall (most likely after a full-thickness infarct). With or without aneurysm formation, stasis in the region of the non-contractile scar predisposes to formation of a mural thrombus.

If the original infarct involves the endocardium (**E**), visceral pericardium (**P**) or both, as in some full-thickness infarcts, these normally delicate layers become markedly thickened as a result of their involvement in the inflammatory process and subsequent organisation and repair.

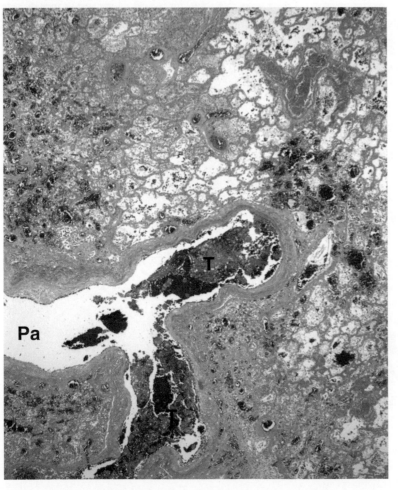

Fig. 10.4 Pulmonary infarct (LP).

Pulmonary infarcts often result from emboli (E-Fig. 10.4**G**) arising from fragments of thrombus within the deep veins of the legs. In their initial stages, pulmonary infarcts are firm, dark-red, wedge-shaped areas at the lung periphery. Their firmness and colour derive from the fact that the alveolar spaces are filled with erythrocytes, partly owing to leakage from damaged capillary walls and partly to blood carried by the unobstructed bronchial arterial circulation. The pleura often becomes involved in the resulting acute inflammatory response leading to the characteristic sharp pleuritic pain and a pleural friction rub. Larger emboli that obstruct the main pulmonary arteries can result in sudden death through acute right heart failure.

Fig. 10.4 illustrates a branch of a pulmonary artery (**Pa**) containing fragments of fibrin thrombus (**T**). Surrounding this vessel there is haemorrhage into air spaces, the walls of which are pale and without nuclei, in keeping with recent infarction.

KEY TO FIGURES
E endocardium   **M** surviving myocardium   **P** pericardium   **Pa** pulmonary artery branch   **S** scar
T thrombus

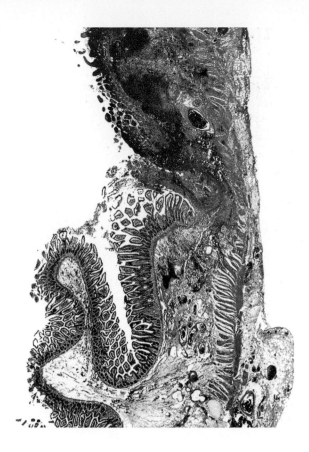

Fig. 10.5 Venous infarction of bowel following volvulus (LP).

Bowel infarction may occur either as a result of arterial occlusion (e.g. mesenteric thrombosis or embolism) or, more commonly, as a result of venous obstruction. Venous obstruction may occur through *torsion* (twisting) of a free loop of bowel around its vascular pedicle *(volvulus)*, entrapment in a tight hernial orifice (e.g. *incarcerated indirect inguinal hernia*) or obstruction by fibrous *peritoneal adhesions* (e.g. following previous surgery).

Venous obstruction initially causes the bowel to become intensely congested with blood, giving it a plum-coloured appearance on gross examination. As the dammed-back blood prevents arterial inflow, the bowel becomes progressively ischaemic. Frank necrosis follows unless the venous obstruction is relieved.

In this micrograph of a small bowel volvulus (Fig. 10.5), the necrotic bowel at the top of the picture stains bright red because of massive suffusion with blood; the outline of the necrotic mucosal villi is still apparent. Note the sharp demarcation between normal and necrotic bowel, and the marked engorgement of all vessels.

Table 10.1 Chapter review.

Disorder	Definition/example	Features	Figure
Arterial infarction	Renal infarction	Common and often asymptomatic. Typically wedge-shaped, base towards capsular surface In initial stages demarcated from surrounding, non-infarcted tissue by hyperaemic zone. Heals leaving fibrous scar.	10.1
	Myocardial infarction	Earliest histological changes detected within 4 hours; established by 12 to 24 hours.	10.2 10.3
	Pulmonary infarction	Initial stage, firm, dark red, wedge-shaped. Sharp pleuritic pain plus pleural rub. Can result in sudden death.	10.4
	Cerebral infarction	Earliest changes within hours of infarction; established at 6 to 12 hours.	2.7 23.2
Venous infarction	Torsion of testis	Twisting of spermatic cord leads to compression of thin-walled veins and subsequent infarction.	19.1
	Small bowel volvulus	Initially intensely congested with blood. Bowel becomes progressively ischaemic. Necrosis unless venous obstruction relieved.	10.5

PART 2

BASIC SYSTEMS PATHOLOGY

ACCESS ADDITIONAL MATERIAL AT STUDENTCONSULT.COM

- Bonus normal histology images
- Macroscopic images of common pathological processes
- Self assessment questions

11 Cardiovascular system

The cardiovascular system includes the heart, blood vessels and circulating blood and is often referred to as the circulatory system. In this chapter, we will focus upon diseases affecting the blood vessels (the arteries and veins) and the heart.

Diseases of the arterial system

The most common pathological abnormality of the arterial tree is thickening and hardening of the walls, known as atherosclerosis (see Ch. 8). Among the risk factors for atherosclerosis are hypertension and diabetes mellitus. In both cases, specific vascular changes may be recognised, often superimposed on the changes of atherosclerosis. Some of the important arterial wall changes associated with hypertension are illustrated in this chapter in Figs 11.1 and 11.2 and in relation to the kidney in Fig. 15.13.

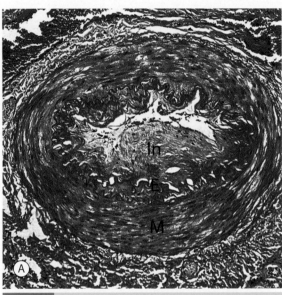
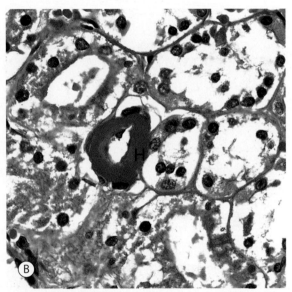

Fig. 11.1 **Essential hypertension: kidney. (A)** Medium-sized artery (MP); **(B)** renal arteriole (HP).

Hypertension, whether idiopathic (primary) or secondary, is frequently associated with changes in peripheral arterial vessels. In larger arteries this can manifest as arterial dissection (Fig. 11.3), which is a life-threatening medical emergency.

More commonly, when the onset of increase in blood pressure is moderate and gradual (*essential* or *benign hypertension*), smaller muscular arteries undergo progressive thickening of their walls. Three features are characteristically seen and are shown in Fig. 11.1A. These are: symmetrical hypertrophy of the muscular media **(M)**, extensive reduplication of the internal elastic lamina **(E)** and fibrotic thickening of the intima **(In)**. All these changes lead to reduction in diameter of the lumen.

Arterioles show a different type of wall thickening, sometimes referred to as *hyaline arteriolosclerosis* and shown in Fig. 11.1B. The normal layers of the wall become ill defined and are replaced by a homogeneous, eosinophilic (pink-stained) material called *hyaline* **(H)**, thought to consist of basement membrane-like material. This results in reduction in size of arteriolar lumina and may contribute to further hypertension. In the kidney, hypertensive vascular changes may lead to compromised renal blood supply with chronic ischaemic damage of the glomerulus *(hypertensive nephrosclerosis)*. This is further discussed in Ch. 15.

KEY TO FIGURES
E internal elastic lamina   **H** hyaline   **In** tunica intima   **M** tunica media   **P** proteinaceous material

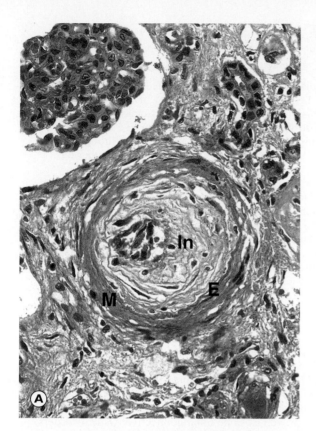

Fig. 11.2 Accelerated hypertension: kidney.
(A) Medium-sized artery (HP); **(B)** arteriole (HP).

Accelerated or *malignant hypertension* refers to a situation where the increase in blood pressure is of rapid onset and marked degree (systolic pressure >220 mmHg or diastolic pressure >120 mmHg). Under these circumstances muscular arteries develop severe thickening of the tunica intima **(In)** by proliferation of intimal cells. This gives the appearance of concentric lamellae ('onion skin' appearance), which encroach upon the arterial lumen as seen in Fig. 11.2A. In contrast to the findings in moderate hypertension, the tunica media **(M)** and internal elastic lamina **(E)** remain largely unchanged.

The impact of sudden and severe hypertension on arterioles is even more dramatic, as shown in Fig. 11.2B. The intimal cells undergo rapid proliferation (as in the muscular arteries), which is often complicated by disruption of the vessel wall, with leakage of plasma proteins, including fibrinogen, into and beyond the arteriolar wall. This change, known inaccurately as *fibrinoid necrosis*, is characterised by obliteration of the wall by intensely eosinophilic, amorphous, proteinaceous material **(P)**; the lumen is often completely occluded. Damage to the vessel wall may lead to thrombosis within the lumen.

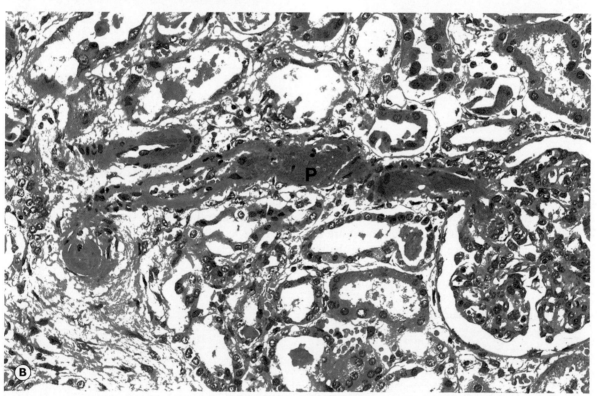

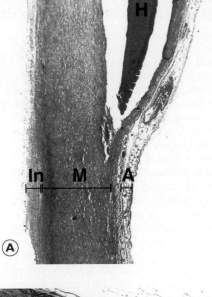

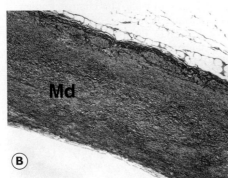

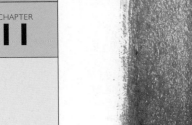

Fig. 11.3 Dissection of the aorta. (A) Aortic dissection (LP); **(B)** medial degeneration and loss of elastic fibres (Elastic van Gieson)(LP).

Aortic dissection most commonly affects the thoracic aorta (E-Fig. 11.1H), with the vast majority of cases associated with hypertension and a smaller number associated with connective tissue disorders (e.g. Marfan syndrome) (E-Fig. 11.1H). Dissection may occur in adults at any age, although it is most common in middle age, with males outnumbering females.

A laceration of the tunica intima (**In**) leads to tracking of blood into the tunica media (**M**). The plane of cleavage (dissection) is usually between the middle and outer thirds of the media, as in Fig. 11.3A; note the site of intimal laceration is not included in this field. The medial haematoma (**H**) then frequently bursts through the tunica adventitia (**A**) with rapidly fatal consequences.

The pathogenesis of dissection is poorly understood but some cases are associated with systemic hypertension and others with connective tissue disorders. Almost all cases exhibit a peculiar type of degeneration of the smooth muscle and elastic tissue of the tunica media known as *medial degeneration*. In medial degeneration, areas of the tunica media become replaced by acellular polysaccharide material (**Md**) and there is fragmentation and disruption of elastic fibres. This is shown in Fig. 11.3B. These features can be seen in the context of Marfan syndrome, as in this case, as well as some other connective tissue disorders.

Aneurysms

Abnormal dilatations of the heart or blood vessels are known as *aneurysms*. In clinical practice, aneurysms are most often encountered in relation to the aorta, ventricular wall of the heart or vessels of the base of the brain. In respect of aortic aneurysms, most are due to atherosclerosis, where the aortic wall is excessively thinned as a consequence of destruction of the tunica media. Table 11.1 lists the types of aneurysm, their aetiology and their most common sites of involvement. The main complications of an aneurysm are rupture, leading to haemorrhage, and thrombus formation, leading to occlusive or embolic phenomena (see Ch.9).

Table 11.1 Types of aneurysm.

Type	Common sites	Aetiology	Common effects of rupture
Atherosclerotic	Abdominal aorta	Weakening of tunica media owing to atheroma	Massive haemorrhage into retroperitoneum and peritoneal cavity
Saccular (Fig. 11.4)	Cerebral arteries	Developmental defects in tunica media and elastic laminae	Subarachnoid haemorrhage
Microaneurysms	Brain, retina	Hypertensive and diabetic small vessel disease	Brain and retinal haemorrhages
Mycotic (infective) aneurysms	Any arterial vessels	Destruction of tunica media by infected thrombus	Haemorrhage from affected vessel
Syphilitic (Fig. 5.11)	Ascending aorta	Damaged tunica media owing to syphilitic arteritis	Massive haemorrhage into mediastinum and thoracic cavity

KEY TO FIGURES
A tunica adventitia **AC** anterior cerebral artery **Ad** adventitia **C** communicating branch **E** internal elastic lamina **H** haematoma **In** tunica intima **M** tunica media **Md** medial degeneration **S** saccular aneurysm **W** wall of aneurysm

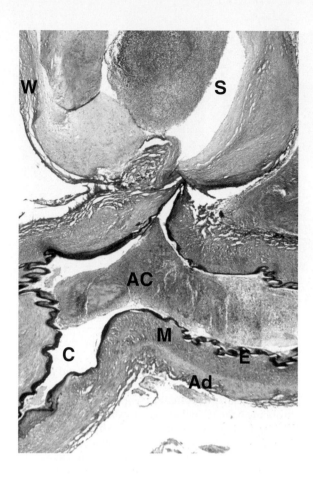

Fig. 11.4 Saccular aneurysm (Elastic van Gieson) (LP).

Saccular *(berry)* aneurysms are a characteristic type of aneurysm found in the cerebral circulation, particularly at junctions in the circle of Willis or at bifurcations of the major cerebral arteries (especially the middle cerebral). Saccular aneurysms most often manifest in middle age by rupturing to cause subarachnoid haemorrhage. These aneurysms are, however, an occasional incidental finding at all ages and are often multiple.

Fig. 11.4 illustrates a saccular aneurysm **(S)** arising from the anterior cerebral artery **(AC)** just proximal to the point where it gives rise to its anterior communicating branch **(C)**. The vessel has a normal tunica media **(M)**, adventitia **(Ad)** and internal elastic lamina **(E)** (elastin stains black with this staining method). Note that at the point of origin of the aneurysm, the tunica media is deficient. The wall of the aneurysm **(W)** is composed of loose fibrous intimal tissue and the lumen contains blood. There is no medial muscle or elastin in the aneurysm wall.

Inflammation of vessels (vasculitis)

Inflammation of the walls of blood vessels may occur in arteries *(arteritis)*, capillaries *(capillaritis)* or veins *(phlebitis, venulitis)*; the collective term is *vasculitis*. The classification of this group of disorders reflects an increasing understanding of the underlying pathogenic mechanisms.

■ **Direct infection:** Some cases of vasculitis arise from direct infection of the blood vessel wall, for example *syphilitic aortitis* (see Fig. 5.11) and *Aspergillus* infection.

■ **Damage to vessels:** Vascular injury and resulting inflammation may be caused by direct damage to vessels, such as mechanical trauma and radiation injury.

■ **Immunological:** The most common types of vasculitis are caused by a variety of immunological mechanisms, including:

  ■ The deposition of circulating immune complexes in the walls of blood vessels, as in *Henoch–Schönlein purpura* and *post-infectious glomerulonephritis.*

  ■ Direct damage to vessel walls by antibodies that react with endothelial cells *(Kawasaki's syndrome, systemic lupus erythematosus)* or glomerular basement membrane *(Goodpasture's syndrome).*

  ■ Vasculitides associated with *antineutrophil cytoplasmic antibody (ANCA)* such as *granulomatosis with polyangiitis* (previously known as Wegener's granulomatosis) and *microscopic polyarteritis* (Fig. 11.7).

■ **Idiopathic:** In some cases, the pathogenesis is unknown. In *giant cell arteritis* (Fig. 11.5) and *Takayasu's arteritis* the underlying process may be an abnormality of cell-mediated immunity. Another major type of vasculitis, *polyarteritis nodosa* (Fig. 11.6), probably belongs to the immunological group, but its aetiology remains unclear.

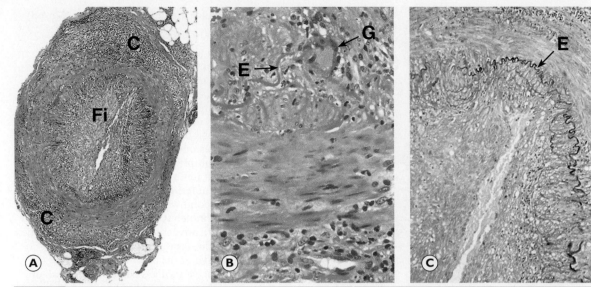

Fig. 11.5 **Giant cell arteritis. (A)** LP; **(B)** HP; **(C)** elastic stain (MP).

Giant cell arteritis is the commonest systemic vasculitis in adults. In the majority of cases, the medium-sized arteries of the head are involved (hence the alternative name ***temporal arteritis***), although involvement at other sites can occur, including the aorta. The pathogenesis is not known, with an immune-mediated reaction against the vessel wall believed to be responsible.

Histologically, multinucleated giant cells **(G)** are characteristic and tend to be arranged circumferentially, apparently in relation to degenerate fragments of the internal elastic lamina **(E)**. This is illustrated in Figs 11.5B and 11.5C. There is also an infiltrate of lymphocytes and plasma cells **(C)** in the vessel wall. Marked fibrous thickening **(Fi)** of the intimal layer, shown in Fig. 11.5A, may be complicated by thrombosis, which may produce acute blindness if the ophthalmic artery is affected. Occasionally, the involvement can be focal and giant cells may be elusive.

Giant cell arteritis often presents as localised throbbing pain or tenderness over the temporal artery in patients over the age of 50 years. Alternatively, it presents as more generalised pain involving the muscles of the pelvic and shoulder girdles in the condition known as ***polymyalgia rheumatica***. The diagnosis may be confirmed by temporal artery biopsy, although often treatment with immunosuppressive therapy (steroids) is commenced before biopsy because of the risk of ophthalmic artery involvement.

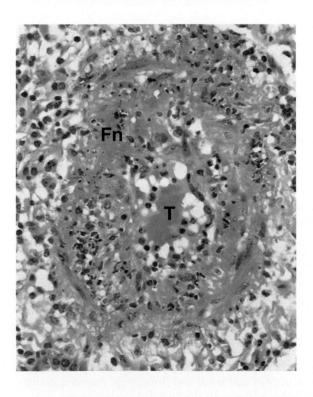

Fig. 11.6 **Polyarteritis nodosa (MP).**

Polyarteritis nodosa (PAN) is a systemic vasculitis affecting mainly medium and small muscular arteries of the kidneys, gut, heart, liver, peripheral nerves and brain. The typical features of an early lesion are shown in this high-power micrograph, where a segment of the vessel wall shows a necrotic area known as ***fibrinoid necrosis* (Fn)** associated with infiltration of the vessel wall with neutrophils. The lumen of the vessel contains fibrin thrombus **(T)**, giving rise to one of the common effects of vasculitis; ischaemia of the tissue supplied by the affected artery. In addition, the necrotic area of vessel wall may rupture during the healing phase when it is replaced by fibrous tissue and a small aneurysm may form. These small aneurysms appear as nodules on the affected vessels, hence the term ***nodosa***.

Apart from systemic symptoms such as fever, malaise, weakness and weight loss, the clinical presentation is extremely variable, depending on which tissues are involved. For example, kidney involvement may be manifest by pain, haematuria or proteinuria and heart involvement by angina, myocardial infarction or pericarditis. The disease is fatal if untreated, but most cases respond well to immunosuppressive therapy.

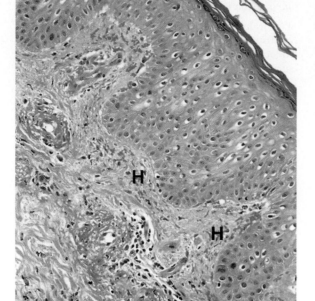

Fig. 11.7 Microscopic polyarteritis (MP).

Microscopic polyarteritis, also known as *leukocytoclastic vasculitis* or *hypersensitivity vasculitis*, arises in the context of an immune-mediated reaction to a wide range of precipitants, including drugs, tumour antigens and certain organisms. Typically, it is the smaller vessels that are affected, including arterioles, capillaries and venules, with involvement of the skin (where it causes palpable purpura), mucous membranes, kidneys, lungs and gastrointestinal tract. In contrast to PAN, microscopic polyarteritis causes haematuria, haemoptysis and bloody diarrhoea, rather than frank infarction or major haemorrhage.

Fig. 11.7 shows the typical features of microscopic polyarteritis. Neutrophils infiltrate the vessel walls **(V)**, which also show fibrinoid necrosis, and nuclear dust **(D)** (fragmented neutrophil nuclei/karyorrhexis) is commonly seen, hence the term leukocytoclastic.

Neutrophils, nuclear dust and haemorrhage **(H)** are seen in the surrounding dermis in this micrograph. As in any type of vasculitis, thrombosis of the affected vessels is common although it is not seen in this example.

Anti-neutrophil cytoplasmic antibody (ANCA), in particularly anti-MPO antibodies can be detected in the serum of approximately 70% of patients with microscopic polyarteritis. ANCA positivity is also found in most patients with *granulomatosis with polyangiitis (anti-PR3 subtype)* and may somehow directly cause the damage to blood vessel walls.

Malformations and tumours of blood vessels

There are a variety of malformations and tumours that arise from vascular channels. The commonest among these are *haemangiomas* (E-Fig. 11.2**G**), often regarded as hamartomas or developmental abnormalities (Fig. 11.8). Clinically, benign vascular malformations in the brain are of importance as there is a risk of spontaneous intracerebral haemorrhage. Often, such malformations are composed of both arterial and venous channels and are termed *arteriovenous malformations* (Fig. 11.9).

True neoplasms arising from blood vessels are rare and range from the benign *glomus tumour* (*glomangioma*; Fig. 11.10) to malignant tumours such as *Kaposi's sarcoma* (Fig. 11.11) and *angiosarcoma* (Fig. 11.12). Kaposi's sarcoma is associated with human herpesvirus 8 (HHV-8) infections and can be seen in patients with immunosuppression, e.g. secondary to HIV infection.

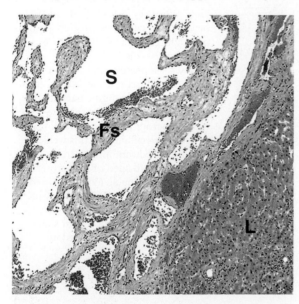

Fig. 11.8 Haemangioma (MP).

Benign tumours of vascular tissues most commonly occur in the skin and liver but may occur in any tissue. Many are present at birth or soon after and may be considered as hamartomas or developmental disorders. Haemangiomas are usually divided into *capillary* or *cavernous* types, the former composed of small capillary-sized spaces, the latter mainly of large, dilated vascular spaces.

Fig. 11.8 shows a typical *cavernous haemangioma* of the liver at low power. In the bottom right-hand corner is normal liver parenchyma **(L)**. The upper left half shows the haemangioma consisting of large vascular spaces **(S)**, some of which contain blood. These are lined by essentially normal endothelial cells, in contrast to angiosarcoma (Fig. 11.12), and separated by a fibrous stroma **(Fs)**. These tumours are common in the liver and are often found incidentally at autopsy or laparotomy.

KEY TO FIGURES

C lymphocytes and plasma cells   **D** nuclear dust   **E** internal elastic lamina   **Fi** fibrous thickening
Fn fibrinoid necrosis   **Fs** fibrous stroma   **G** giant cell   **H** haemorrhage   **L** liver parenchyma
S vascular space   **T** fibrin thrombus   **V** vessel wall

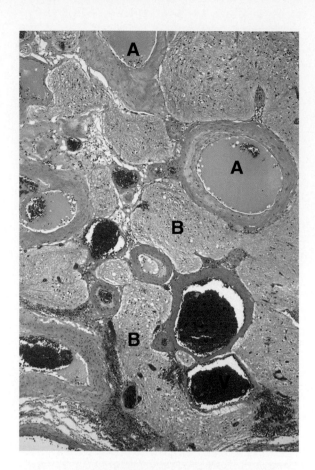

Fig. 11.9 Arteriovenous malformation (LP).

The brain is a clinically important site for vascular malformations, with resulting symptoms related to local mass effect, due to compression of the surrounding brain tissue, and haemorrhage. Commonest among the clinically significant vascular malformations encountered in the brain are arteriovenous malformations (AVMs). These lesions may arise anywhere in the vasculature of the CNS but are most often associated with superficial branches of the middle cerebral artery.

Macroscopically, AVMs typically appear as a tangle of worm-like vascular channels of varying sizes arising from vessels in the subarachnoid space and extending into superficial brain parenchyma. Occasional examples located exclusively in brain parenchyma may occur.

Histologically, as in this micrograph, AVMs are composed of numerous variably sized vascular channels ranging from thick-walled, recognisable arterial channels **(A),** with elastic fibres detectable on special stains, to thinner-walled, irregular venous channels **(V)**. Between these numerous vascular spaces is reactive brain parenchyma **(B)**. Often, this surrounding brain parenchyma contains evidence of previous haemorrhage in the form of macrophages containing haemosiderin pigment (not present in this field).

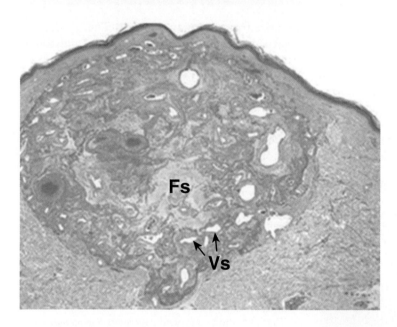

Fig. 11.10 Glomus tumour (LP).

Glomus bodies are specialised arteriovenous anastomoses in the dermis that have a role in temperature regulation through shunting blood away from the skin surface when exposed to cold temperatures. Benign tumours arising from the specialised smooth muscle of these glomus bodies are known as glomus tumours or glomangiomas. Although they are benign, they can be exquisitely painful, particularly if the affected region is immersed in cold water.

Macroscopically, they appear as small, raised, red/purple lesions, most commonly on the digits, particularly under the fingernails. In this low-power micrograph (Fig. 11.10), it can be appreciated that this well-circumscribed tumour, centred on the dermis, is formed of numerous small vascular spaces **(Vs)** separated by a fibrous stroma **(FS)** within which the glomus cells lie. These cells are typically round to cuboidal in shape and arranged around the tumour vessels.

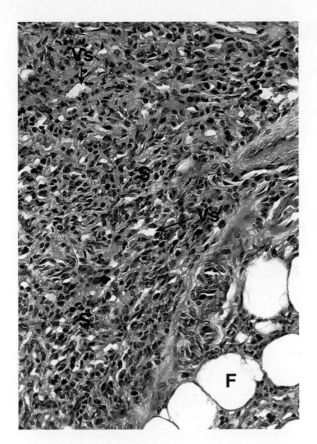

Fig. 11.11 **Kaposi's sarcoma (HP).**

Kaposi's sarcoma (KS) came to attention in the 1980s as an AIDS-defining illness. Subsequent investigations have identified ***human herpesvirus 8 (HHV-8)***, also known as ***KS-associated herpes virus***, as the aetiological agent in the vast majority of cases. Four variants are recognised: classic, immunosuppression/transplant-associated, endemic and AIDS-associated. Kaposi's sarcoma lesions are typically found on the skin as slightly raised, red/purple patches, although they may spread to other sites such as oral cavity, lymph nodes and gastrointestinal tract. As noted above, KS emerged as an important AIDS-defining illness in the 1980s. However, with the introduction of highly active antiretroviral therapy (HAART), KS is now relatively rare.

A typical lesion, illustrated here, consists of sheets of plump stromal cells **(S)** interspersed with irregular, slit-like vascular spaces **(Vs)**. A brisk mixed inflammatory cell infiltrate is typically present. The tumour is seen here infiltrating subcutaneous fat **(F)**. Extravasation of red blood cells, not seen here, is common.

Bacillary angiomatosis, caused by infection with *Bartonella species*, may appear very similar, except for the presence of numerous neutrophils and nuclear dust. This condition also occurs in the immunosuppressed patient but can be cured by antibiotic therapy.

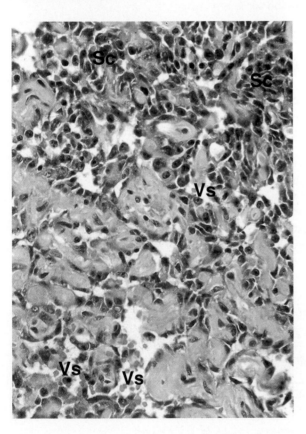

Fig. 11.12 **Angiosarcoma (HP).**

Angiosarcomas are rare, occurring most frequently in the skin, soft tissues, breast and liver, with approximately 50% arising in the head and neck. Those in the liver are associated with known carcinogens including arsenic (in some pesticides) and vinyl chloride. Those in the breast tissue may follow radiotherapy for breast cancer.

The typical appearance is of a raised, purple/red lesion on the face or scalp in the elderly. As the lesion enlarges, it may ulcerate and metastasise to local lymph nodes. On microscopy, angiosarcomas may display a variety of appearances ranging from tumours with numerous vascular spaces lined by plump, atypical endothelial cells to an undifferentiated spindle-celled tumour with few discernible vascular spaces.

In this example the malignant endothelial cells can be seen forming irregular branching vascular spaces **(Vs)** in some areas and solid sheets of cells **(Sc)** in other areas. Mitotic figures are common. The difference between these malignant endothelial cells and the benign endothelium lining vascular spaces in the haemangioma of the liver (Fig. 11.8) can be readily appreciated. Malignant tumours arising from the endothelium of the lymphatic system, ***lymphangiosarcomas*** are usually similar in appearance except for the absence of blood in the vascular spaces.

BASIC SYSTEMS PATHOLOGY ■ CARDIOVASCULAR SYSTEM

KEY TO FIGURES

A arterial channel   **B** brain parenchyma   **F** fat   **Fs** fibrous stroma   **S** stromal cells   **Sc** sheets of tumour cells   **V** venous channel   **Vs** vascular space

Diseases of the heart

Ischaemic heart disease

Of the diseases involving the heart, ischaemic heart disease is the most important in developed countries. In almost all cases, the cause of ischaemic heart disease is atherosclerosis of the coronary arteries, with or without accompanying thrombosis. Coronary artery atheroma and thrombosis are illustrated in Figs 8.5 to 8.7, and the stages of myocardial infarction are shown in Fig. 10.2.

> ### MYOCARDIAL INFARCTION
> A common consequence of coronary artery disease, myocardial infarction is a leading cause of morbidity and mortality in developed countries. Typical symptoms are of central chest pain, often described as tight or pressing, which may radiate to the left arm or jaw. A variety of symptoms, including nausea, vomiting, breathless and sweating, often accompany this chest pain.
>
> The clinical diagnosis of myocardial infarction rests on the demonstration of elevated levels of proteins released into the blood as a result of damaged myocytes *(troponin)*, combined with typical electrocardiographic changes. In some patients, especially those with diabetes mellitus, the typical chest pain can be absent and patients may present late with complications, the so-called 'silent' myocardial infarction.
>
> Treatment is directed towards establishing reperfusion of the ischaemic segment of myocardium as rapidly as possible to minimise the volume of infarcted tissue (see clinical box 'Angiography and stents' in Ch. 8).
>
> Complications of myocardial infarction include sudden death, arrhythmia, cardiac failure, ventricular rupture, rupture of papillary muscles with acute valve failure and mural thrombus with potential for thromboembolisation. Some of these complications may arise in the immediate aftermath of the infarction *(acute-phase complications)* and some may develop some time later.

Diseases of the heart muscle

The *cardiomyopathies* are disorders of the heart muscle resulting in disturbance of heart function (often described as systolic or diastolic dysfunction). A classification of cardiomyopathies is shown in Table 11.2. The abnormalities usually cause progressive cardiac failure, but sudden cardiac death caused by acute arrhythmia may be the first manifestation.

Other cardiomyopathies can be acquired, such as those seen in patients with alcoholism, severe vitamin deficiency (*beriberi*) or following an episode of myocarditis.

Some diseases of the heart muscle may be related to inherited enzyme deficiencies such as *Fabry disease* and *glycogen storage disorders*.

An infiltrative cardiomyopathy can be caused by deposition of *amyloid* (see Ch. 15) between the cardiac myocytes. This causes progressive cardiac failure due to a restriction of cardiac function.

Table 11.2 Classification and causes of cardiomyopathy.

Classification	Pathology	Aetiology
Dilated cardiomyopathy	Defective myocardial contractility leading to ventricular dilation and cardiac failure	Inherited, alcoholism, peripartum
Hypertrophic cardiomyopathy (E-Fig. 11.3**G**)	Hypertrophy of the interventricular septum leading to outflow obstruction	Inherited
Arrhythmogenic cardiomyopathy	Abnormal thinning of the right ventricular wall due to fibrosis and adipose tissue deposition	Inherited
Infiltrative/restrictive cardiomyopathy	Failure of the myocardium to relax due to abnormal infiltrate	Amyloidosis, others

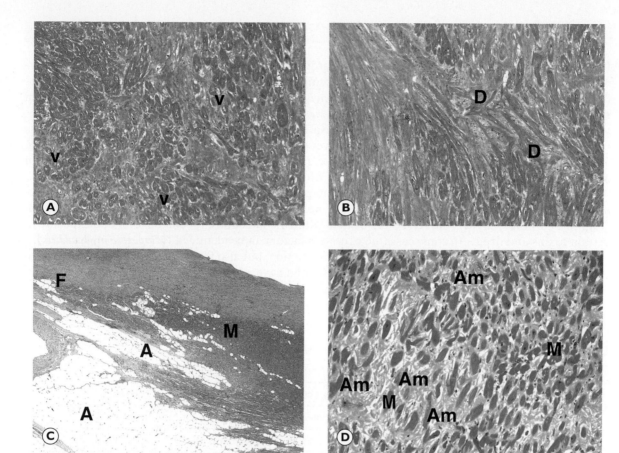

Fig. 11.13 **Cardiomyopathies. (A)** Hypertrophic cardiomyopathy (HP); **(B)** hypertrophic cardiomyopathy: myocyte disarray (HP); **(C)** arrhythmogenic cardiomyopathy (LP); **(D)** infiltrative cardiomyopathy (amyloid) (HP).

Cardiomyopathies are rare diseases of the heart muscle characterised by progressive loss of cardiac function. In the normal heart (E-Figs 11.4**H** and 11.5**H**) the cardiac myocytes contain small dark nuclei and the muscle fibres are orientated in a similar fashion. Compare this to Fig. 11.13A in which the cardiac myocytes contain hypertrophic muscle fibres, with enlarged nuclei. The muscle fibres show *vacuolar change* (**V**). In Fig. 11.13B, the muscle fibres are orientated in a haphazard manner, known as *myocyte disarray* (**D**). Hypertrophic cardiomyopathy (E-Fig. 11.3**G**) is associated with genetic mutations, often in the genes encoding *sarcomeric proteins* such as *troponin* or *myosin*.

The histological hallmarks of arrhythmogenic cardiomyopathy are infiltration of the myocardium by mature adipose tissue (**A**) admixed with fibrosis (**F**) (Fig. 11.13C). This condition tends to present in the right ventricle but, more recently, some left ventricular variants have been identified.

Arrhythmogenic cardiomyopathy is an important cause of *sudden cardiac death* in young people. It is associated with genetic mutations, particularly in genes encoding *desmosomal proteins* such as *plakophilin*.

Amyloid deposition is the most common cause of an infiltrative cardiomyopathy (Fig. 11.13D). In this condition, eosinophilic amyloid protein (**Am**), a fibrillary protein of approximately 10 nm in fibril diameter, is deposited between the cardiac myocytes (**M**). Amyloid is associated with a number of conditions including malignancy, chronic inflammatory disease and age. There are many subtypes of amyloid protein including *AL* (amyloid associated with light chain deposition), *AA* (amyloid associated with systemic inflammatory disease) and *ATTR* or *transthyretin*. These can be identified using tinctorial stains and immunohistochemistry as well as electron microscopy (see Ch. 15).

KEY TO FIGURE

A mature adipose tissue **Am** amyloid **D** disarray **F** fibrosis **M** cardiac myocytes **V** vacuolar change

BASIC SYSTEMS PATHOLOGY ■ CARDIOVASCULAR SYSTEM

Inflammation of the heart

Inflammation may affect the pericardium, myocardium or endocardium, either separately or concurrently. The causes are numerous, but the most common are ischaemia and infection. Most infections of the pericardium *(pericarditis)* and myocardium *(myocarditis)* are viral, whilst those of the endocardium *(endocarditis)* and valves *(valvulitis)* may be bacterial (Fig. 11.18) or fungal.

The main causes of pericarditis are summarised in Table 11.3. The histological features of most forms of acute pericarditis are virtually identical, whatever the cause, and are illustrated and discussed in Fig. 3.4. In tuberculous pericarditis, there is a chronic granulomatous response as described in Ch. 5. In malignant pericarditis, clumps of tumour cells are often mixed with the inflammatory exudate.

The term myocarditis implies inflammatory damage to the myocardium and, by common usage, usually excludes the acute inflammatory reaction to necrotic muscle fibres seen in myocardial infarction (Fig. 10.2). Primary myocarditis can be associated with viral infections, rheumatic fever and exposure to certain toxins and drugs. In some cases, no causative factor can be identified *(idiopathic myocarditis)*.

Endocarditis and valvulitis involve not only inflammation, but also thrombus deposition on the endocardium and/or valves. These are important diseases and have a high mortality rate, their clinical manifestations often resulting from embolic phenomena or from dysfunction of the valves.

Table 11.3 **Important causes of pericarditis.**

Cause	Aetiology	Frequency
Myocardial infarction	After transmural myocardial infarction	Common
Cardiac surgery	After surgical opening of pericardial sac	Common
Viral infections	Usually young adults. Coxsackie B virus most common	Common
Malignancy	Local invasion or metastatic tumour deposits	Uncommon
Uraemia	Renal failure	Uncommon
Bacterial infections	Secondary to lung infection, including TB	Uncommon
Rheumatic fever	Part of rheumatic pancarditis	Rare

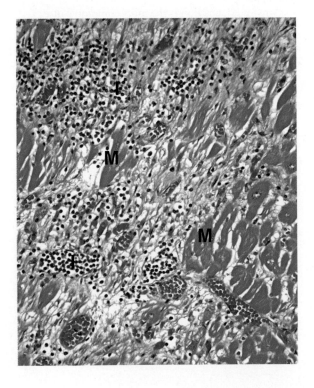

Fig. 11.14 **Viral myocarditis (HP).**

Myocarditis presents clinically with symptoms and signs reflecting inflammation or dysfunction of cardiac muscle. Hence, common presenting features include chest pain (stabbing in nature), tachycardia, arrhythmia, fever and cardiac failure. There are many causes, the commonest being as a consequence of viral infection, such as with Coxsackie A and B viruses. Other causes include bacteria, fungi and immune-mediated reactions, such as in systemic lupus erythematosus or as a drug hypersensitivity reaction.

Fig. 11.14 illustrates the appearances of a florid viral myocarditis identified at autopsy. There is a prominent lymphocytic inflammatory cell infiltrate **(I)** coursing between myocytes **(M)**, many of which are pale, granular and necrotic. The Dallas criteria for diagnosing myocarditis state that at least one focus of myocyte damage must be seen in order to diagnose myocarditis. In practice, due to the patchy nature of this condition, such foci can be difficult to identify.

Rheumatic fever

Rheumatic fever is a systemic inflammatory disease that, in susceptible individuals, follows several weeks after a *group A β-haemolytic streptococcal* throat infection. The systemic manifestations represent a disordered immunological response resulting in inflammation of connective tissues. All parts of the body may be involved, for example the joints and skin, with painful short-term consequences. Involvement of the heart is of great clinical importance because of potentially fatal acute myocarditis and endocarditis and the long-term consequences of chronic scarring of the heart valves (E-Fig. 11.6**G**).

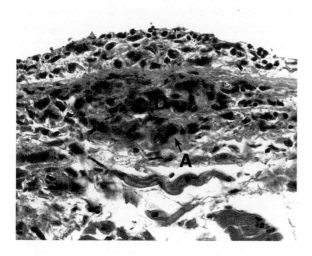

Fig. 11.15 Rheumatic carditis (HP).

The characteristic acute myocardial rheumatic lesion is the *Aschoff body* as shown in Fig. 11.15. The fully developed Aschoff body has a central, ill-defined area of degenerate material (**D**) surrounded by a mixed inflammatory cell infiltrate rich in T lymphocytes. Among these cells can often be seen a so-called *Anitschow myocyte* (**A**), recognised by its irregular, ribbon-like nucleus and extensive eosinophilic cytoplasm. Despite the name, these cells are considered to represent large modified macrophages. Aschoff bodies are found in the interstitial connective tissue of the myocardium, particularly near vessels in the subepicardial fibrous tissue and (as in this example) in the subendocardial connective tissue.

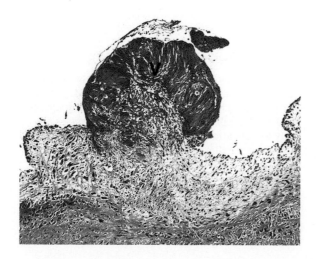

Fig. 11.16 Acute rheumatic endocarditis (MP).

The importance of acute rheumatic endocarditis relates to involvement of the heart valves (E-Fig. 11.7**G**), where endocardial roughening induces formation of fibrin and platelet thrombi. Fig. 11.16 illustrates part of a mitral valve leaflet affected by acute rheumatic endocarditis. A small thrombotic vegetation (**V**) has formed on the upper (atrial) surface of the valve leaflet at the site of the remnants of a large Aschoff body.

Chronic rheumatic valvular disease is the result of organisation and fibrous scarring of affected valves. This continues over many years with eventual thickening and distortion of the valve leaflets as well as the chordae tendineae. Such distortion commonly renders affected valves stenotic or incompetent.

KEY TO FIGURES
A Anitschow myocyte   **D** degenerate material   **I** inflammatory cells   **M** myocytes   **V** thrombotic vegetation

BASIC SYSTEMS PATHOLOGY ■ CARDIOVASCULAR SYSTEM

Valvulitis (endocarditis of valves)

The heart valves may become subject to a variety of vegetative lesions that have traditionally been described as forms of *endocarditis*. The primary phenomenon underlying all these conditions is the formation of thrombus on the valve leaflets or cusps.

As in the arterial system, roughening of the endocardial surface predisposes to thrombus formation (Ch. 9). This may occur when valve leaflets or cusps have been previously damaged by rheumatic fever or are congenitally abnormal. Thrombus formation may also follow autoimmune valve damage in systemic lupus erythematosus *(Libman–Sacks endocarditis)* and in the acute phase of rheumatic fever (Fig. 11.16). The most frequent type of valve thrombus, however, occurs in so-called *marantic endocarditis* (Fig. 11.17), in which warty, thrombotic vegetations develop on mitral and aortic valves. This phenomenon occurs in seriously ill patients, often those with widely disseminated malignancy, and is usually associated with a hypercoagulable state. Despite use of the term endocarditis in these conditions, inflammation is usually not a feature of the valve at the time of thrombus formation.

True valvular inflammation may arise, however, if these thrombotic vegetations on valves then become infected with bacteria, fungi or other organisms, conditions collectively referred to as *infective endocarditis*. Bacterial endocarditis tends to be divided into two clinicopathological patterns. In the first, traditionally known as *subacute bacterial endocarditis*, the thrombotic vegetations develop on previously damaged valves, which then become colonised by bacteria of low virulence such as *Streptococcus viridans*. Such organisms tend to reach the valves via a transient bacteraemia, for example following dental extraction. The major clinical consequences are those resulting from detachment of small thrombotic emboli, often infected, into the systemic circulation.

In the second type of bacterial endocarditis, known traditionally as *acute bacterial endocarditis* (Fig. 11.18 and E-Fig. 11.8**G**), thrombi form on previously normal valves and become infected by virulent organisms such as *Staphylococcus aureus*. In this case, the patient is usually already severely debilitated and septicaemic, for example from an infected urinary catheter, and the infecting organism is responsible for the septicaemia. In contrast with the subacute pattern, in the acute form the fulminating infection extends into the substance of the valve, causing tissue necrosis. Rapid destruction of the valve leaflet leads to valvular incompetence, with acute cardiac failure as the usual clinical outcome.

Fungal endocarditis, formerly rare, is now appearing more commonly as a complication of immunosuppressive therapy, intravenous drug abuse or AIDS. *Candida albicans* (Fig. 5.15) is the most common organism.

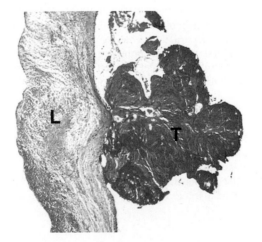

Fig. 11.17 **Marantic endocarditis (LP).**

Fig. 11.17 illustrates a mitral valve lesion of marantic (thrombotic, non-bacterial) endocarditis. Masses of thrombus **(T)** have developed on the superior surface of the valve leaflet **(L)**. Such thrombotic masses are only loosely attached to the underlying non-inflamed valve and are therefore readily detached, leading to major embolic consequences such as cerebral, renal and splenic infarction. In practice, this type of endocarditis is rarely diagnosed but is a common finding during autopsy.

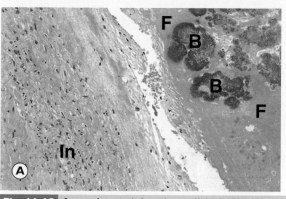

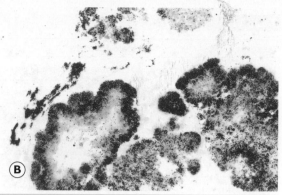

Fig. 11.18 Acute bacterial endocarditis (HP). (A) H&E; (B) Gram stain.

This example of *acute bacterial endocarditis* in Fig. 11.18 is taken from a patient who presented with acute heart failure following bacterial destruction of his aortic valve. In Fig. 11.18A, the fibrous tissue comprising the valve is seen at the lower left and is infiltrated by sparse inflammatory cells (**In**). In the upper right, there is a mass of eosinophilic fibrin (**F**) containing large colonies of purple-staining bacteria (**B**), in this case *Streptococcus bovis*.

Fig. 11.18B is from the same specimen and is stained with Gram stain. This demonstrates large quantities of Gram-positive, purple-staining streptococci embedded in the fibrin. This patient underwent an emergency aortic valve replacement and, with intravenous antibiotic treatment, made an excellent recovery.

Primary tumours of the heart

Whilst metastases to the pericardium and heart are not infrequent in the late stages of systemic malignancies, primary tumours of the heart are rare, the vast majority being benign. Of these, *myxomas* are the most common primary cardiac tumours occurring in adults (Fig. 11.19). In contrast, in children, the commonest primary tumours encountered are *rhabdomyomas*, which are often multiple, present in infancy and have a strong association with *tuberous sclerosis*. Other tumours that may arise in the heart include lipomas, fibromas and angiosarcomas.

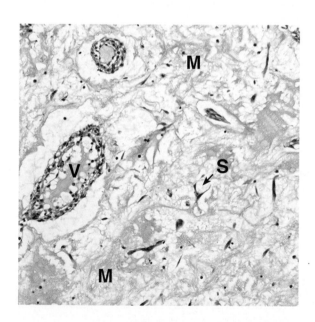

Fig. 11.19 Atrial myxoma (HP).

Atrial myxomas are the commonest primary tumours of the heart, with the overwhelming majority arising in the atria, particularly the left atrium. The cell of origin of these benign tumours is not known. A large proportion are sporadic in nature, although a small number (approximately 10%) arise as a manifestation of the autosomal dominant *Carney complex*. Symptoms are rather non-specific, with flu-like symptoms, outflow obstruction and embolic phenomena most common.

Macroscopically, myxomas appear as pedunculated, variably soft to firm masses, often arising in the region of the atrial septum. Histologically, they are formed of stellate tumour cells (**S**) and abnormal vascular channels (**V**) set in a myxoid matrix (**M**).

CARDIOVASCULAR SYSTEM

BASIC SYSTEMS PATHOLOGY

KEY TO FIGURES

B bacteria **F** fibrin **In** inflammatory cells **L** valve leaflet **M** myxoid matrix **S** stellate tumour cells **T** thrombus **V** abnormal vascular channel

Table 11.4 Chapter review.

Disorder	Main features	Figure
Hypertension	Abnormally raised blood pressure	
Essential hypertension	Walls of small muscular arteries thickened. Hyaline arteriosclerosis in arterioles.	11.1
Accelerated hypertension	Severe 'onion skin' thickening of tunica intima of small muscular arteries. Rapid proliferation of intima with accompanying fibrinoid necrosis.	11.2
Aortic dissection	Most commonly thoracic aorta. Medial haematoma forms following laceration of intima. Almost all cases show cystic medial necrosis.	11.3
Aneurysms	Variety of types summarised in Table 11.1	Table 11.1
Saccular (berry)	Develop from cerebral arteries. Manifest in middle age as common cause of non- traumatic subarachnoid haemorrhage.	11.4
Vasculitis	Classified by presumed aetiology as direct spread of infection, direct trauma to vessel, immune mediated or idiopathic	
Giant cell arteritis	Commonest systemic vasculitis in adults. Most often involves medium-sized vessels of head and neck. Cause unknown. Inflammatory cell infiltrate in vessel wall, including multinucleated giant cells.	11.5
Polyarteritis nodosa	Systemic vasculitis of small muscular arteries. Neutrophil-rich inflammatory cell infiltrate with associated fibrinoid necrosis of vessel wall. Small aneurysms may form in relation to weakened vessel wall.	11.6
Microscopic polyarteritis	Immune-mediated reaction to variety of agents. Typically, neutrophil infiltrate in walls of small vessels.	11.7
Tumours of blood vessels	Common forms benign. Rarer malignant forms.	
Haemangioma	Benign tumour of vessels subdivided as capillary or cavernous depending on size of vascular channels.	11.8
Arteriovenous malformation	Most often arise in association with superficial vessels of brain and may give rise to neurological symptoms and/or haemorrhage. Irregular vascular channels interspersed among reactive brain tissue.	11.9
Glomus tumour	Small, painful, raised lesion most commonly on the digits.	11.10
Kaposi's sarcoma	AIDS-defining lesion. Causative agent is HHV-8 in majority. Sheets of stromal cells interspersed with irregular vascular spaces.	11.11
Angiosarcoma	Approximately 50% arise in head and neck. Malignant. May metastasise to local lymph nodes. Atypical endothelial cells to undifferentiated spindle cells with irregular vascular spaces.	11.12
Ischaemic heart disease	See Ch. 8 (Atheroma) and Ch. 10 (Infarction)	
Cardiomyopathy	Myocardial dysfunction. Various causes, but many are genetically inherited.	Table 11.2, Fig. 11.13
Inflammation of the heart	May affect pericardium, myocardium, endocardium.	
Pericarditis	Inflammation of pericardium. Variety of causes.	3.4C
Myocarditis	Most often a viral aetiology, but may be bacterial, immune mediated, drug related or idiopathic. Inflammatory cell infiltrate between myocytes with myocyte destruction.	11.14
Rheumatic fever	Manifestation of systemic inflammatory disease following streptococcal throat infection. Rheumatic carditis: characteristic Aschoff bodies in myocardium, particularly subendocardial/subpericardial locations. Acute rheumatic endocarditis: inflammation of heart valves with formation of thrombotic vegetations.	11.15 11.16
Marantic endocarditis	Non-bacterial endocarditis most commonly associated with systemic illness (e.g. disseminated malignancy). Friable, thrombotic vegetations form on valves.	11.17
Acute bacterial endocarditis	Usually complicates systemic sepsis with virulent organism. Can arise on otherwise normal valve. Vegetation forms composed of fibrin containing colonies of causative organism.	11.18
Cardiac tumours	Primary cardiac tumours rare, with majority benign.	
Atrial myxoma	Benign tumour of unknown histogenesis. Small proportion autosomal dominant as part of Carney's complex. Stellate cells and atypical vascular spaces in a myxoid matrix.	11.19

12 Respiratory System

Diseases of the nose and pharynx

Allergic rhinitis (hay fever) commonly affects the nose, paranasal sinuses and nasopharynx and can predispose to *inflammatory nasal polyps* (Fig. 12.1). The *sinonasal (Schneiderian) papilloma* is particular to the nasal cavity and is usually unilateral (Fig. 12.2). Malignant tumours of the nasal passages and sinuses are rare, but *nasopharyngeal carcinoma* (Fig. 12.3) is of special interest because of its association with Epstein–Barr virus (EBV) infection.

Vocal cord polyps (laryngeal or singer's nodule) arise as smooth nodules on the surface of the true vocal cords, usually as a result of persistent inflammation (Fig. 12.4). The stratified squamous epithelium of the larynx may also contain a low risk HPV infection associated lesion, the *benign squamous papilloma.* Cigarette smoking and alcohol consumption predispose to the development of dysplasia and *invasive squamous cell carcinoma of the larynx.* (Fig. 12.5).

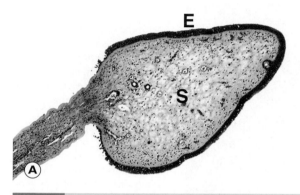

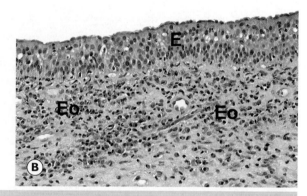

Fig. 12.1 Nasal polyps. (A) LP; (B) HP.

Nasal polyps are a consequence of chronic inflammation of the nasal mucosa (E-Fig. 12.1**H**), commonly infective or allergic in nature. Simple polyps of this type are generally bilateral and the finding of unilateral involvement suggests alternative diagnoses. There is marked oedema and engorgement of mucosal connective tissue and infiltration by chronic inflammatory cells. Eosinophils are prominent in allergic rhinitis.

In the low power view of a nasal polyp in Fig. 12.1A, note the grossly oedematous stroma (**S**) and stretched, but otherwise relatively normal, covering of respiratory type epithelium (**E**). As seen in Fig. 12.1B, the connective tissue contains an inflammatory cell infiltrate in which eosinophils (**Eo**) and plasma cells predominate. Eosinophils are also present in the surface respiratory epithelium.

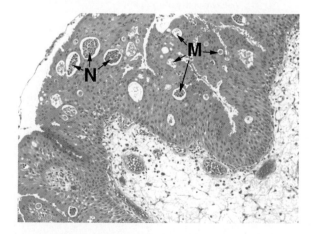

Fig. 12.2 Sinonasal (Schneiderian) papilloma (MP).

There are three main histological types of sinonasal papilloma: exophytic, inverted and oncocytic. The inverted and oncocytic subtypes are associated with a small risk of malignant transformation. These tumours are usually surgically resected.

Note the epithelial cells show eosinophilic, granular cytoplasm. The pseudostratified epithelium also contains mucin-filled cysts (**M**) and neutrophilic abscesses (**N**) characteristic of the sinonasal papilloma.

KEY TO FIGURES
E respiratory type epithelium   **Eo** eosinophils   **M** mucin-filled cysts
N neutrophilic abscesses   **S** oedematous stroma

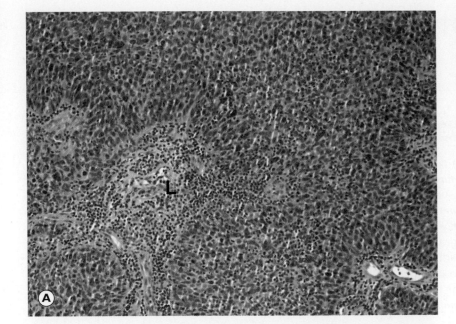

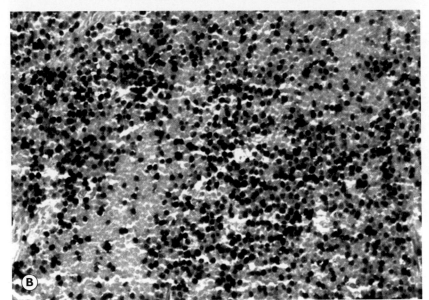

Fig. 12.3 Nasopharyngeal carcinoma. (A) MP; **(B)** in situ hybridisation (ISH) for EBV (MP).

In the nasal cavities and nasopharynx (E-Fig. 12.2**H**), most malignant tumours take the form of keratinising or non-keratinising squamous cell carcinomas (differentiated or undifferentiated). The undifferentiated group (illustrated) is associated with a dense, reactive lymphoid infiltrate in the stroma and is an example of a *lymphoepithelial carcinoma*.

Note the sheets of non-keratinising invasive carcinoma with abundant lymphoid cells **(L)** that are closely associated with the tumour. EBV is strongly associated with *nasopharyngeal carcinoma*, particularly the non-keratinising types. ISH techniques have been discussed in Ch. 1. EBV ISH (Fig. 12.3B) is more sensitive and specific than EBV immunohistochemistry and is a useful adjunct in the diagnosis of this tumour. The blue-black staining indicates positivity in the tumour cells. Furthermore, EBV negative nasopharyngeal carcinomas are associated with a worse prognosis than EBV positive tumours.

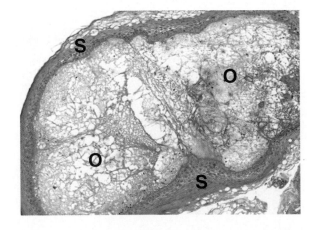

Fig. 12.4 Vocal cord polyp (LP).

Vocal cord polyps, also known as laryngeal or singer's nodules, are benign lesions which are common in smokers. They typically present as small (1–2 mm) smooth nodules on the true vocal cords. Histologically, the submucosa of the polyp is oedematous **(O)**, containing inflammatory cells and dilated vessels with a covering of stratified squamous epithelium **(S)**.

KEY TO FIGURES
C laryngeal cartilage **B** bone **K** keratinisation **L** lymphoid cells **O** oedematous submucosa
S stratified squamous epithelium

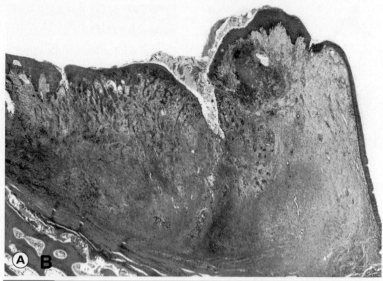
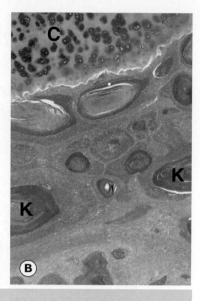

Fig. 12.5 **Squamous carcinoma of the larynx. (A)** LP; **(B)** MP.

Squamous cell carcinomas (SCC) form the vast majority of malignant tumours of the larynx (E-Fig. 12.3**H**), most commonly originating in the vocal cords but also occasionally arising in epiglottis, aryepiglottic folds and piriform fossae. SCCs of the larynx are generally keratinising in type and are often associated with overlying dysplastic surface epithelium.

Fig. 12.5A shows a low power view of a well differentiated SCC arising from the vocal cord. The section also shows part of the normal laryngeal wall including bone (**B**).

Fig. 12.5B from a moderately differentiated SCC shows invasion of the laryngeal cartilage (**C**). Note the infiltrating islands of tumour with central keratinisation (**K**).

Inflammatory diseases of the airways and lungs

The trachea and bronchi may become acutely inflamed due to infections by viruses or pyogenic bacteria to cause *acute tracheobronchitis* (Fig. 12.6). Bacterial infections of airways are frequently complicated by extension of inflammation into the surrounding lung parenchyma to cause a pattern of lung infection known as *bronchopneumonia* (Fig. 12.7), a common cause of illness and death in the debilitated and elderly. Another pattern of bacterial lung infection is *lobar pneumonia*, which involves a whole segment or lobe. In this setting, a more virulent bacterium such as the pneumococcus is usually involved and fit young people may be almost as susceptible as the elderly and debilitated. Lobar pneumonia illustrates many important principles of acute inflammation and the phenomenon of resolution and is discussed in Ch. 3 (Figs 3.3 and 3.7). In contrast, *tuberculosis* and *sarcoidosis* are classic examples of specific chronic inflammations and are discussed fully in Chs 4 and 5. Recurrent or persistent suppurative bacterial infections of bronchi may lead to irreversible dilatation of airways with marked thickening and chronic inflammation of the walls, a condition known as *bronchiectasis* (see Fig. 4.3). Abscess formation in the lungs is a serious complication of certain pneumonias, particularly *Staphylococcal* and *Klebsiella* pneumonias. Lung abscesses may also result from septic emboli causing infarction of the lung, bronchiectasis, bronchial obstruction (e.g. by tumour or foreign body) or as a complication of pulmonary tuberculosis.

The term *chronic obstructive pulmonary disease (COPD)* refers to conditions characterised by chronic or recurrent obstruction of air flow and includes chronic bronchitis and emphysema. Recurrent episodes of acute bronchitis or persistent, non-infective irritation of bronchial mucosa (e.g. as a result of cigarette smoking) may produce *chronic bronchitis* (Fig. 12.9), which is frequently associated with persistent dilatation of air spaces and destruction of their walls, a condition known as *emphysema* (Fig. 12.8). *Asthma* (Fig. 12.10) is a disorder of the airways characterised by reversible bronchoconstriction, often provoked by allergens in susceptible individuals, but also triggered by physical agents or infection. There is also increased secretion of bronchial mucus, leading to plugging of the bronchial lumina.

The massive capillary bed of the lungs makes them vulnerable to a variety of haemodynamic and other vascular disorders. Left ventricular failure results in engorgement of pulmonary capillaries and fluid transudation into the alveolar spaces causing *pulmonary congestion* and *oedema* (Fig. 12.11). Two other common vascular disorders of great clinical importance are *pulmonary embolism* and its sequel *pulmonary infarction*, illustrated in Figs 9.4 and 10.4 respectively.

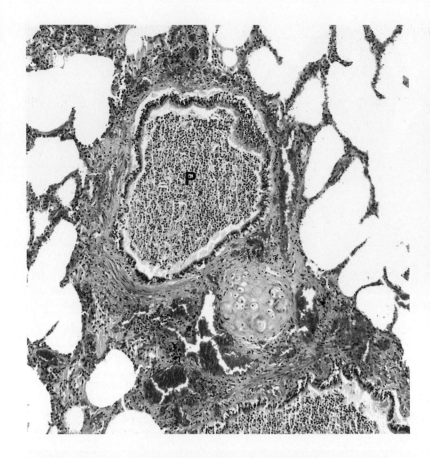

Fig. 12.6 Acute purulent bronchitis (MP).

Bacterial infections of the upper respiratory tract (E-Fig. 12.4**H**), often following a transient viral infection, tend to spread down the respiratory tract where they may produce an acute, purulent *tracheobronchitis* and *bronchiolitis*. The mucosa of the airways becomes acutely inflamed and congested and the smaller lobular bronchi and bronchioles become filled with purulent exudate (**P**) composed of protein rich fluid and numerous neutrophils. Strips of necrotic epithelium are often shed into the pus. The inflammatory process inhibits ciliary activity but promotes secretion of mucus, which, with the dead and dying neutrophils, pools in the airways and is coughed up as yellow-green sputum. In the early stages, the lung parenchyma is usually unaffected, but the alveolar spaces adjacent to the affected bronchioles often become filled with oedema fluid. In susceptible patients, this may then progress to *bronchopneumonia* (Fig. 12.7).

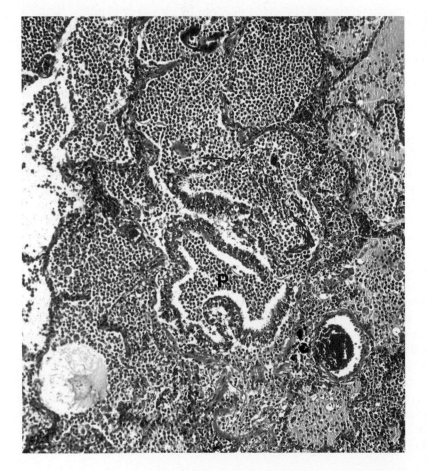

Fig. 12.7 Bronchopneumonia (MP).

Extension of bacterial infection from bronchioles into the surrounding lung parenchyma (E-Fig. 12.5**H**) leads to a patchy pattern of purulent pneumonic consolidation known as *bronchopneumonia*. This is in contrast to the involvement from the outset of a whole lobe or lobule, as occurs in *lobar pneumonia* (see Fig. 3.3) (E-Fig. 12.6**G**).

Each peribronchial focus of pneumonic consolidation has within it a small bronchus or bronchiole exhibiting the features of acute purulent bronchitis (**P**) (Fig. 12.6). As each focus of bronchopneumonia expands, it tends to merge with adjacent foci until the consolidation becomes confluent. Bronchopneumonia is a threat to the very young, elderly or those debilitated by pre-existing illness such as congestive cardiac failure or carcinomatosis and is a very common terminal event. No single organism is responsible, but *Streptococcus pneumoniae* and *Haemophilus influenzae* are the most common.

KEY TO FIGURES
B bullae **G** mucinous glands **In** chronic inflammatory cells **M** mucosal smooth muscle **P** purulent exudate

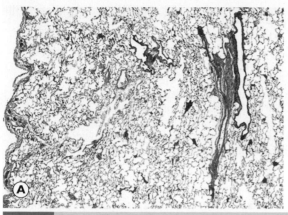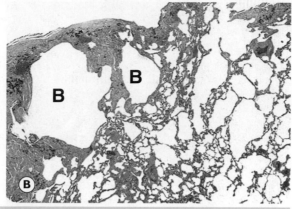

Fig. 12.8 **Pulmonary emphysema. (A)** Normal lung (LP); **(B)** emphysematous lung (LP).

Emphysema is a condition characterised by permanent enlargement of the respiratory spaces distal to the terminal bronchioles, accompanied by destruction of their walls. Comparison with normal lung (shown in Fig. 12.8A at the same magnification) demonstrates the marked increase in alveolar volume and consequent reduction in area of alveolar wall available for gaseous exchange in emphysema (Fig. 12.8B). This problem is compounded by the loss of elastic

'guy rope' support, which alveolar walls normally provide to the airways. As a result, the airways tend to collapse during expiration. Emphysema is often associated with recurrent or chronic infection of the airways *(chronic bronchitis)* and some degree of reversible airways obstruction caused by bronchospasm. In Fig. 12.8B, two small subpleural bullae **(B)** are present. These are common in emphysema and may rupture into the pleural space causing a *pneumothorax*.

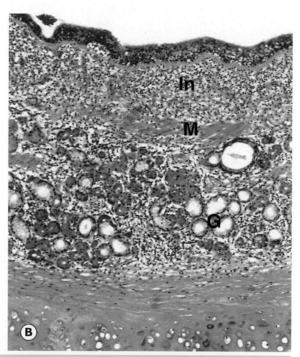

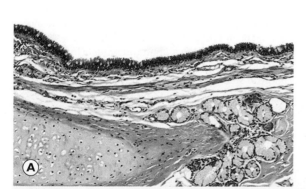

Fig. 12.9 **Chronic bronchitis. (A)** Normal bronchial wall (MP); **(B)** bronchial wall in chronic bronchitis (MP).

Chronic bronchitis is defined as excess sputum production on most days for at least 3 months in at least 2 consecutive years. Although well defined as a clinical term, pathological changes in chronic bronchitis are variable and relatively non-specific. Chronic irritation of the bronchial mucosa, either by tobacco smoke, atmospheric pollution or by repeated episodes of infection, induces chronic inflammatory and hyperplastic changes resulting in marked thickening of the bronchial wall. This feature is the main abnormality in cases of chronic bronchitis and is well illustrated in Fig. 12.9B when compared with the normal bronchial wall shown in Fig. 12.9A at the

same magnification. Three factors contribute to the increased thickness of the bronchial wall: infiltration of the submucosa by chronic inflammatory cells **(In)**, marked hypertrophy of mucosal smooth muscle **(M)** and marked hyperplasia of the mucous glands **(G)** with the production of copious mucus. In addition, the surface epithelium undergoes hyperplasia and often squamous metaplasia (not shown here). The consequent loss of ciliary activity then compounds the problem of excessive mucus production by destroying the 'mucociliary escalator' and provides an ideal environment for superimposed bacterial infection.

BASIC SYSTEMS PATHOLOGY ■ RESPIRATORY SYSTEM

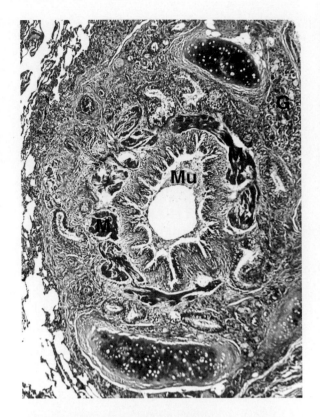

Fig. 12.10 Chronic asthma (MP).

Asthma is a common respiratory disorder characterised by instability of the smooth muscle of bronchiolar walls leading to *paroxysmal bronchoconstriction*. This results in diminution of airway diameter causing marked resistance to air flow, particularly on expiration. Clinically, there is shortness of breath, wheezing and cough. There are several aetiological and trigger factors for bronchospasm, including IgE-mediated hypersensitivity reactions to allergens, bacterial or viral infections, exertion, changes in air temperature and non-allergic sensitivity to specific environmental agents (often through occupational exposure). In severe asthma, reduction in bronchial diameter has three components: bronchospasm, mucosal oedema and luminal occlusion due to excessive mucus production. Single acute asthmatic attacks resolve with therapy leaving no apparent structural disorder. In chronic asthmatics, as in this example (Fig. 12.10), the bronchial walls become thickened via the process of *airway remodelling*. There is hypertrophy of smooth muscle (**M**), hyperplasia of submucosal mucous glands (**G**), protracted oedema of submucosa and marked infiltration by eosinophils. The bronchial lumen becomes obstructed by mucus (**Mu**) containing numerous eosinophils.

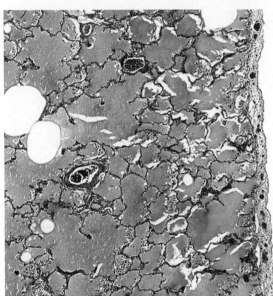

Fig. 12.11 Pulmonary oedema (LP).

Any condition in which the left ventricle or atrium fails to empty adequately increases pressure in the affected chamber, which is transmitted back to the pulmonary venous system and pulmonary capillaries. The pulmonary capillaries become dilated and congested with erythrocytes and the increased hydrostatic pressure results in *transudation* of plasma fluid into the alveolar spaces, causing pulmonary oedema.

As progressive cardiac failure is a terminal event in many diseases, pulmonary congestion and oedema are common post mortem findings. This condition also provides an ideal environment for the growth of pathogens of relatively low virulence, so superimposed bronchopneumonia is a common sequel (Fig. 12.7). Chronic pulmonary congestion, for example owing to mitral stenosis, may result in numerous small intra-alveolar haemorrhages followed by red cell lysis. Phagocytosis of released iron pigments, mainly haemosiderin, leads to the gross appearance known as *brown induration*.

Interstitial diseases of the lung

A wide range of pathogenic stimuli may cause interstitial lung inflammation, i.e. inflammation primarily involving the alveolar walls. This contrasts with the pneumonic or intra-alveolar inflammation seen in pneumonia.

Acute interstitial inflammation is often called *pneumonitis*. The clinical picture may be of catastrophic acute respiratory distress as seen in *adult respiratory distress syndrome (ARDS)*, which has a wide range of causes including viral and atypical pneumonias, shock, drugs and hypersensitivity reactions. Respiratory distress syndrome of premature infants (IRDS) is a similar phenomenon and both the adult and infant forms are characterised by the formation of hyaline membranes which line the alveolar walls (Fig. 12.12).

At the chronic end of the spectrum, interstitial lung disease usually presents as insidious onset of breathlessness secondary to *pulmonary fibrosis* (Fig. 12.13). The development of pulmonary fibrosis again may be due to a wide range of agents and may be preceded by an acute phase. The common causative factors are inorganic dusts such as silica, coal dust and asbestos, organic dusts such as mouldy hay in 'farmer's lung' and disorders of unknown cause such as *sarcoidosis* and *idiopathic pulmonary fibrosis* (see Fig. 4.5).

The disorders caused by inhalation of inorganic dusts are known as ***pneumoconioses*** and follow inhalation of mineral dusts (e.g. silica and asbestos), usually over a long period of industrial exposure, leading to fibrotic reactions in the lung. Inhalation of organic dusts (e.g. fungal spores and plant dusts) usually cause pulmonary fibrosis by the development of chronic allergic responses termed ***hypersensitivity pneumonitis***.

The end result of these diseases is the development of interstitial fibrosis in the lungs. Pulmonary fibrosis of this type results in thickening of the barrier between blood and air causing reduced gas transfer. As the disease progresses, these may cause pulmonary hypertension and respiratory failure may develop. In most of these diseases, there are few clues to the causative agent when the fibrosis is well developed. Exceptions to this rule include ***silicosis*** (Fig. 12.14), which has a distinctive pattern of fibrosis, ***asbestosis*** (Fig. 12.15) where the presence of plentiful asbestos bodies is diagnostic and ***sarcoidosis*** where characteristic granulomas may be seen (see Fig. 4.8).

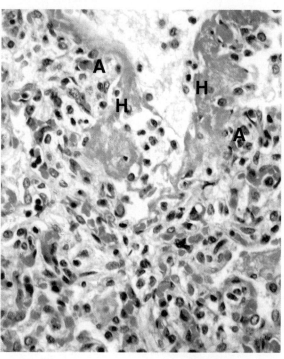

Fig. 12.12 Diffuse alveolar damage (HP).

At the very acute end of the spectrum of interstitial lung diseases, the histological appearances of the lung are characterised by the formation of ***hyaline membranes*** **(H)**, which represent accretions of protein and necrotic cell debris upon the alveolar surface of the alveolar walls **(A)**. The other name sometimes used for this condition is ***diffuse alveolar damage (DAD)***. Characteristically, the alveolar walls are thickened owing to a mixed inflammatory infiltrate, oedema, congestion of capillaries and haemorrhage. In combination with the hyaline membranes, this greatly inhibits gaseous exchange and results in respiratory failure. Occasionally, there are characteristic histological features of a particular aetiological agent such as caseating granulomas in miliary TB (see Fig. 5.6) or nuclear inclusion bodies in cytomegalovirus infection (see Fig. 5.13).

In most cases, the histological appearance is non-specific and a careful history is important in defining the cause. In premature infants (IRDS), the cause is a deficiency of pulmonary surfactant. In adults, there is a wide variety of causes, but the common factor is widespread damage to capillary endothelial cells and/or alveolar lining cells.

This condition is often fatal but may resolve completely with treatment or progress to pulmonary fibrosis.

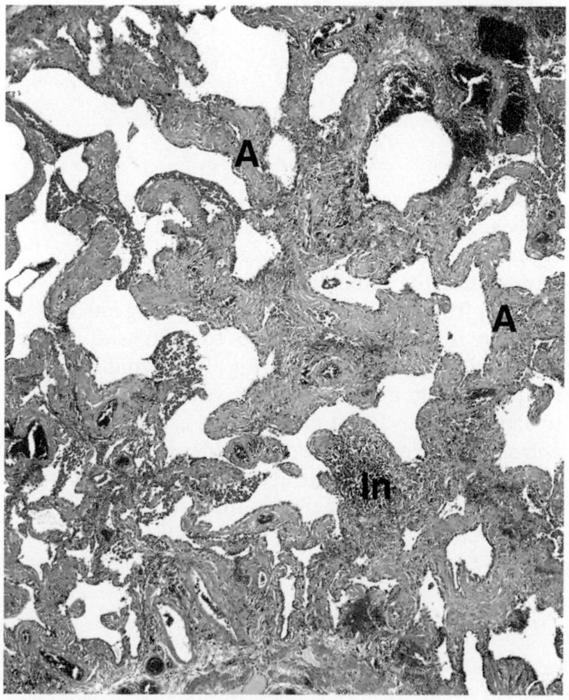

Fig. 12.13 Pulmonary fibrosis (LP).

This condition may represent the end stage of acute diffuse alveolar damage or of subacute disease as in hypersensitivity pneumonitis. Often, however, the condition presents with insidious breathlessness and lung biopsy shows established pulmonary fibrosis. As seen in Fig. 12.13, the alveolar walls **(A)** are markedly thickened because of the deposition of collagen. There is a variable chronic inflammatory infiltrate **(In)** consisting mainly of lymphocytes. In addition, the alveolar epithelium consists mainly of type II pneumocytes. When no aetiological factors can be established from the biopsy and careful recording of the clinical history, the condition is called ***idiopathic pulmonary fibrosis***. The histological pattern associated with this diagnosis is described as ***usual interstitial pneumonitis***, as in this case. In other cases, there may be distinctive histological features such as granulomas in sarcoidosis and asbestos bodies in asbestosis. Some cases are associated with a significant clinical history such as exposure to particular drugs, for example bleomycin-induced pulmonary fibrosis. In the late stages, the normal lung parenchyma may be densely fibrotic with macroscopically visible spaces. In this situation, it is known as ***honeycomb lung***.

RESPIRATORY SYSTEM

BASIC SYSTEMS PATHOLOGY

KEY TO FIGURES
A alveolar wall   **G** mucinous glands   **H** hyaline membranes **In** inflammatory infiltrate   **M** smooth muscle   **Mu** mucus

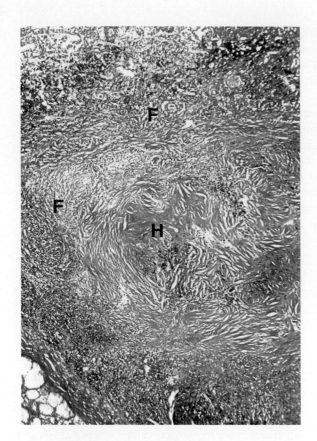

Fig. 12.14 Silicosis (MP).

Silicosis is a form of pneumoconiosis that tends to occur in miners and others with industrial exposure to silica dusts. Initially, the inhaled silica particles are phagocytosed by macrophages that accumulate in clumps, very occasionally forming granuloma-like masses. The presence of silica-laden macrophages excites a vigorous focal fibrotic reaction resulting in the formation of nodules of collagenous tissue. The centre of each focus becomes progressively acellular and hyaline (**H**) and is surrounded by a variable zone of more cellular fibrous tissue (**F**), exhibiting a relatively sparse chronic inflammatory cell infiltrate in which black, carbon-laden macrophages abound. Usual histological methods do not reveal the presence of silica; it can, however, be demonstrated as refractile particles by polarised light microscopy. As the process continues, the fibrotic nodules may coalesce, resulting in widespread pulmonary fibrosis.

Silicosis is the most common of the pneumo-conioses. Other examples are asbestosis (Fig. 12.15) and berylliosis in which the inhaled particles excite a giant cell granulomatous reaction similar to that seen in sarcoidoses (see Fig. 4.8).

All of the clinically significant inorganic dust diseases of the lung lead to progressive fibrosis with respiratory failure and diminished gaseous exchange. Disruption of the pulmonary microvasculature may lead to pulmonary hypertension.

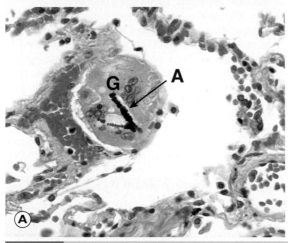
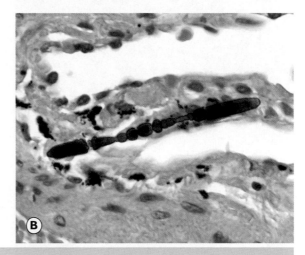

Fig. 12.15 Asbestosis. (A) HP; (B) HP.

Asbestos, a complex silicate, occurs in the form of long needle-like or serpentine fibres. The needle-like forms are more pathogenic and, when inhaled into the lung parenchyma, they become coated with proteinaceous material to form segmented ***asbestos bodies***. The presence of asbestos fibres excites a macrophage and giant cell response, which ultimately leads to fibrosis in a similar manner to that of silicosis (Fig. 12.14). The major fibrotic lesions initially occur in the subpleural zone of the lower lobes. Fig. 12.15A shows an alveolar space containing a giant cell (**G**) in which there are typical asbestos bodies (**A**).

The brownish colour of the asbestos bodies derives from the incorporation of haemosiderin in the proteinaceous coat. Fig. 12.15B shows the beaded appearance of this encrusted iron at higher magnification, with a very fine central core representing the actual fibre.

Apart from its tendency to produce lung fibrosis, exposure to asbestos predisposes to neoplastic change. ***Mesotheliomas*** of the pleura (Fig. 12.25) and less often the peritoneum may occur many years after exposure to asbestos. This latent period often exceeds 20 years and so disease usually occurs in older patients, long after the period of industrial exposure. Asbestos exposure also greatly increases the risk of lung carcinomas, especially in cigarette smokers.

KEY TO FIGURES
A asbestos body   **F** fibrous tissue   **G** giant cell   **H** hyaline centre

Genuinely benign lung tumours are rare. Most bronchial adenomas are in fact *carcinoid tumours* arising from lung neuroendocrine cells (Fig. 12.22). These may be locally invasive and occasionally metastasise. Their histological appearance is similar to well differentiated neuroendocrine tumours in the gastrointestinal tract (see Fig. 13.13).

The great majority of primary malignant tumours of the lung are carcinomas that arise in the bronchi and are thus often called *bronchogenic carcinomas*. Carcinogens in cigarette smoke are the major aetiological agents. Other less important factors include exposure to radiation, asbestos (especially when combined with smoking), as well as other minerals such as nickel and chromium. Air pollution and genetic predisposition are other possible factors. Occasionally, tumours may arise in a pre-existing lung scar.

Bronchogenic carcinomas are of various histological types, but in broad terms they are divided into two main groups: *small cell carcinoma* (Fig. 12.17) and *non–small cell carcinomas*. The current World Health Organization (WHO) Classification of lung tumours further divides non–small cell lung carcinomas into histological sub-groups, including squamous cell carcinoma (Fig. 12.18), non-mucinous adenocarcinoma (Figs 12.19 and 12.20), mucinous adenocarcinoma and large cell carcinoma (Figs 12.21 and Table 12.1). There are further subcategories of tumours, the commonest of which are listed in Fig. 12.16. The term non-small cell carcinoma, not otherwise specified (NOS), can be used in small biopsies where there are no morphological or immunohistochemical features of a specific tumour subtype. Neuroendocrine tumours of the lung are also discussed in Fig. 12.22. It should also be noted that mixtures of these tumour types can occur, most often in the form of adenosquamous carcinoma. Metastatic tumours, usually blood-borne from distant organs, are also very common in the lungs (see Figs 7.16 and 12.23).

The pleura is the site of an uncommon but fatal tumour known as malignant mesothelioma (Fig. 12.25). Mesothelioma occurs almost exclusively in those exposed to asbestos.

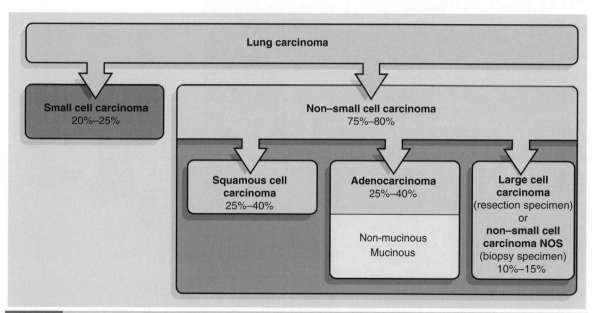

Fig. 12.16 **Relative frequencies and main histological subtypes of bronchogenic carcinoma.**

Accurate classification of bronchial carcinomas is important to ensure the most effective treatments are offered to the patient. The term 'non–small cell carcinoma' encompasses groups of tumours with different histological appearances and associated molecular signatures, for which there are emerging targeted therapies. In general, small cell carcinoma is widely disseminated at the time of presentation and so it is treated primarily by systemic chemotherapy. In contrast, non–small cell tumours are more likely to be localised and are usually treated using combinations of surgery and chemotherapy or radiotherapy in the first instance.

There is geographical variation both in the incidence of lung cancer and also in the relative frequency of different histological types. This is reflected in the range of figures provided here for some tumour types. Lung adenocarcinoma is now more frequent than squamous carcinoma within the United States, but squamous carcinoma remains the most common diagnosis in Europe at present. It has been suggested that these trends may reflect changes in patterns of cigarette smoking, but further epidemiological study is required. Adenocarcinoma is less strongly associated with cigarette smoking and many of the lung cancers that occur in non-smokers are of this type.

DIAGNOSIS OF LUNG CARCINOMA

The diagnosis of lung carcinoma is usually first suspected due to symptoms such as weight loss, breathlessness and *haemoptysis*, often in patients who are cigarette smokers. Initial investigation typically involves obtaining a chest radiograph, followed by more detailed imaging using other modalities such as computed tomography scanning. If a lung mass is identified, formal diagnosis is usually made on the basis of small amounts of material obtained by minimally invasive techniques such as bronchoscopic biopsy or radiologically guided needle biopsy for peripherally situated lung masses. This is because management of lung carcinoma is highly dependent upon initial classification of histological type. During bronchoscopy, samples for cytological examination are often obtained, as well as small biopsies, because bronchial washings and brush cytology samples can allow retrieval of cells from sites that are not visible or accessible for biopsy. This means that both cytological and histological techniques have complementary roles in the pathological diagnosis of lung cancer. Cytological preparations are illustrated here alongside the biopsy findings for comparison.

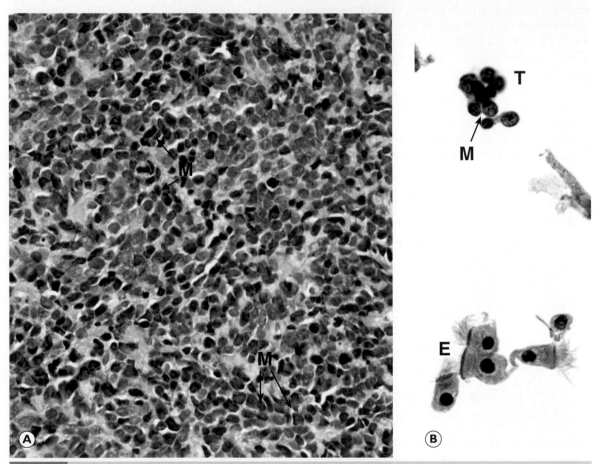

Fig. 12.17 **Small cell carcinoma. (A)** Biopsy (HP); **(B)** cytology (Papanicolaou stain, HP).

Small cell carcinoma, previously termed oat cell carcinoma, is an important and highly malignant tumour that most commonly arises centrally within the lung. As seen at high magnification in Fig. 12.17A, the old name derives from the supposed resemblance of the small, tightly packed, darkly stained, ovoid tumour cells to oat grains. In areas, the cells appear crushed and there is brisk mitotic and apoptotic activity. In clinical practice, immunohistochemical staining is commonly used to confirm this diagnosis, revealing evidence of *neuroendocrine differentiation*.

These tumours rapidly and extensively invade the bronchial wall and surrounding parenchyma and may compress and invade nearby pulmonary veins. Early lymphatic and blood-borne spread is a feature of these tumours. Small cell tumours have the worst prognosis of all bronchogenic carcinomas because, although they are the most responsive to chemotherapy, they almost always relapse early.

Apart from their local and metastatic effects, these tumours may also secrete peptide hormones, such as antidiuretic and adrenocorticotrophic hormones *(ectopic hormone secretion)* giving rise to various *tumour-related endocrine and paraneoplastic syndromes*. Fig. 12.17B shows typical bronchial cytology of small cell carcinoma. The tumour cells **(T)** have scant cytoplasm and hyperchromatic nuclei and show nuclear moulding **(M)**. Some normal bronchial epithelial cells **(E)** are also present for comparison.

KEY TO FIGURES
B bronchus   **E** bronchial epithelial cells   **K** keratinisation   In infiltration   **M** moulding of nuclei
T tumour cells

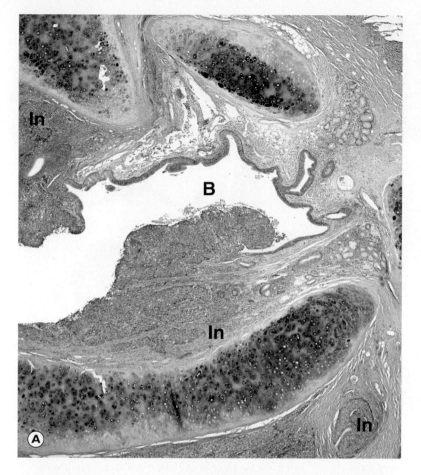

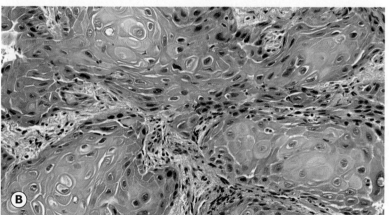

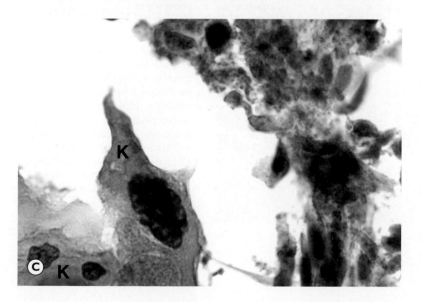

Fig. 12.18 Squamous cell carcinoma of bronchus. (A) Biopsy (LP); **(B)** biopsy (MP); **(C)** cytology (Papanicolaou stain, HP).

Squamous cell carcinoma usually arises in the main bronchi or their larger branches (E-Fig. 12.7**G**), close to the lung hilum and often in an area of epithelium which has previously undergone *squamous metaplasia*, for example as a result of cigarette smoking. Bronchial mucosa adjacent to tumours frequently shows evidence of *squamous dysplasia*. Fig. 12.18A shows a centrally arising carcinoma which protrudes into the lumen of a large bronchus **(B)** *(endobronchial)*, as well as infiltrating **(In)** the surrounding parenchyma. Eventually, such tumours tend to obstruct the involved airway as well as spreading via local lymphatics to regional lymph nodes. These tumours have the typical features of squamous cell carcinoma, but vary widely in degree of differentiation.

At one end of the spectrum is the well differentiated keratinising type as illustrated in Fig. 7.3, where the likeness to normal stratified squamous epithelium is evident and there is formation of keratin in areas. Fig. 12.18B shows a moderately differentiated squamous cell carcinoma. There is no keratinisation in this example, but the tumour is still recognisably squamous, forming islands of large, eosinophilic cells with central whorling and with intercellular bridges *(desmosomes)* between the cells. At the other end of the spectrum are poorly differentiated tumours in which squamous characteristics, such as desmosomes, are difficult to identify and are seen only at high magnification (see Fig. 7.3). Some tumours are so poorly differentiated that squamous features cannot be seen by light microscopy and these tumours are classified as *large cell carcinomas* (Fig. 12.21).

Well differentiated squamous cell carcinomas are readily identifiable using cytological methods. Fig. 12.18C shows numerous large, highly atypical squamous cells with evidence of cytoplasmic keratinisation. Keratin **(K)** appears orange in colour when stained by the Papanicolaou method. Comparison of these images with those of Fig. 12.17 highlights the difference in cell size.

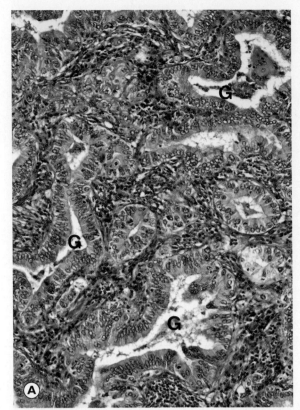

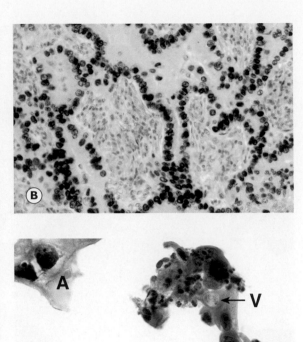

Fig. 12.19 **Adenocarcinoma of the lung. (A)** Acinar pattern with H&E stain (MP); **(B)** biopsy with staining for TTF-1 (MP); **(C)** cytology (Papanicolaou stain, HP).

Adenocarcinomas tend to arise more peripherally in the lung and have a particular predilection for old areas of scar tissue, such as healed tuberculosis. Adenocarcinoma of the lung is not as closely linked with cigarette smoking as other primary lung tumours.

Adenocarcinoma is divided into non-mucinous and mucinous subtypes. There are different architectural patterns of non-mucinous adenocarcinoma that are associated with outcome and therefore these are usually described in the pathology report. Acinar pattern shown in Fig. 12.19A with gland formation **(G)** and papillary pattern are of intermediate grade whereas solid and micropapillary patterns are associated with a worse prognosis. Most tumours show a mixture of architectural patterns.

Mucinous adenocarcinoma is composed of columnar cells with abundant intracytoplasmic mucin or goblet type cells and often involves both lungs at presentation.

Fig. 12.19B illustrates specific immunohistochemical staining for ***thyroid transcription factor-1 (TTF-1)***, which is strongly expressed in the nuclei of most primary lung adenocarcinomas. This can be useful in diagnostic practice (Table 12.1).

In the cytological preparation shown in Fig. 12.19C, note the groups of large adenocarcinoma cells **(A)** with prominent nucleoli and cytoplasmic vacuoles **(V)** containing mucin. These contrast with occasional normal ciliated bronchial epithelial cells **(E)**.

Very poorly differentiated variants of adenocarcinoma are included in the category of large cell undifferentiated carcinoma (Fig. 12.21).

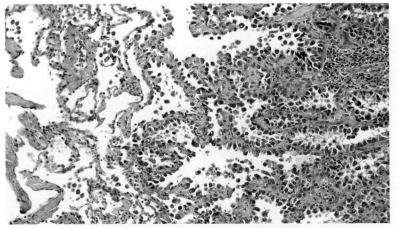

Fig. 12.20 **Lepidic pattern (MP).**

Previously known as bronchioloalveolar carcinoma, this is now regarded as an architectural pattern of non-mucinous adenocarcinoma, which is associated with a more favourable prognosis. The characteristic feature is that the malignant cells grow along the alveolar walls. The non-neoplastic alveolar walls on the left are somewhat fibrotic and inflamed. Small tumours composed of purely lepidic pattern glands are termed ***adenocarcinoma in situ***.

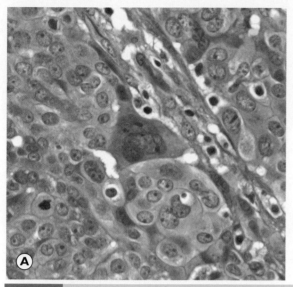 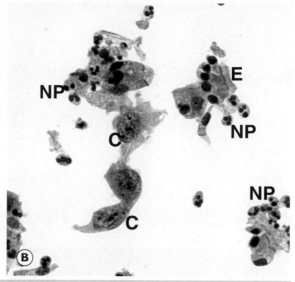

Fig. 12.21 Large cell carcinoma. (A) Biopsy (HP); **(B)** cytology (HP).

Large cell carcinoma is defined as an undifferentiated carcinoma with no discernible features of either squamous or glandular differentiation by light microscopy. These tumours consist of large, anaplastic epithelial cells growing in islands and sheets. By definition, no evidence of keratinisation, intercellular bridges or intracytoplasmic mucin is seen (Fig. 12.21A). The whole tumour from a resection specimen must be examined by light microscopy to be diagnosed as large cell carcinoma. If these features are seen in a biopsy specimen, it is described as *non-small cell*

carcinoma NOS as biopsies only sample a tiny part of the tumour and other diagnostic features may be apparent in the resection specimen or following immunohistochemistry (see below).

Fig. 12.21B shows large, undifferentiated malignant cells (**C**). In contrast to those seen in the previous examples of squamous carcinoma and adenocarcinoma, these cells lack any evidence of specific differentiation. Normal ciliated bronchial epithelial cells (**E**) are present and there are scattered neutrophil polymorphs (**NP**).

Table 12.1 Subtyping of non-small cell (NSC) lung carcinoma by immunohistochemistry.

Tumour type	TTF1	Napsin	p40	CK5/6
Adenocarcinoma	+	+	–	–
Adenocarcinoma	+	–	–	–
Squamous cell carcinoma	–	–	+	+
Squamous cell carcinoma	–	–	+	–
Non–small cell carcinoma (not otherwise specified)	–	–	–	–

The majority of lung cancers are diagnosed using a combination of biopsy and cytology as described above. Acquiring biopsy tissue is therefore important to subtype the tumour accurately and to provide material for molecular testing (see clinical box 'Molecular aspects of lung cancer'). Non–small cell carcinomas are broadly subdivided into squamous cell carcinoma or adenocarcinoma on the basis of the histological features described earlier. Some of these tumours are very poorly differentiated and do not show the diagnostic light microscopy features but, at a cellular level, will express proteins associated with these histological types.

A panel of immunohistochemical markers (see Ch. 1) can be used to detect these proteins and favour a histological type. This has led to an increase in patients being able to access targeted therapies for specific tumour types. The table above summarises a typical panel of markers used for diagnosis: + denotes a positive marker and – denotes a negative marker. TTF1 and Napsin are expressed in adenocarcinomas, whereas these markers are usually negative in squamous cell carcinoma, which expresses p40 and CK5/6.

KEY TO FIGURES

A adenocarcinoma cells   **C** undifferentiated malignant cells   **E** bronchial epithelial cells   **G** glandular formations   **NP** neutrophil polymorphs   **V** cytoplasmic vacuole

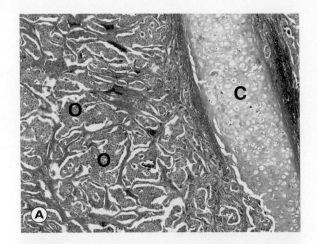

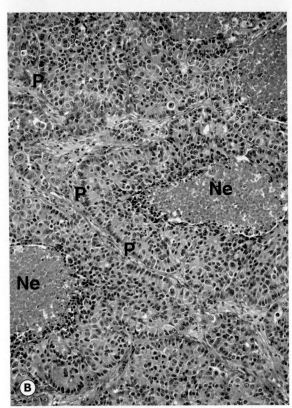

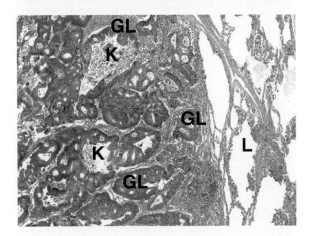

Fig. 12.22 **Neuroendocrine tumours. (A)** Carcinoid tumour LP; **(B)** large cell neuroendocrine carcinoma MP.

Neuroendocrine tumours of the lung are classified into four main types. The commonest of these, *small cell carcinoma*, is illustrated in Fig. 12.17. The other types are *carcinoid tumour (CT)*, *atypical carcinoid tumour (ACT)* and *large cell neuroendocrine carcinoma (LCNEC)*.

Carcinoid tumours typically present in younger patients as a polypoid endobronchial mass. They show similar histological features to their counterparts in the GI tract and pancreas. As seen in Fig. 12.22A, carcinoids are well differentiated tumours composed of organoid nests **(O)** and trabeculae of uniform cells with granular *(salt and pepper)* chromatin. There are very few mitoses and there is no evidence of necrosis. A tumour can be seen infiltrating around the bronchial cartilage **(C)**. Carcinoids are usually surgically resected and have an excellent prognosis, although they are generally regarded as low grade malignant due to their propensity to metastasise, particularly to lymph nodes. ACT (not illustrated), shows features of a well differentiated neuroendocrine tumour but with a higher mitotic rate than CT and/ or small areas of necrosis. Prognosis is worse than CT with higher rates of metastasis.

Contrast the appearances in Fig. 12.22A with those of the highly malignant LCNEC in Fig. 12.22B. The tumour cells are arranged in nests and islands and have abundant, rather granular cytoplasm. Central zones of necrosis **(Ne)** are also commonly seen and the tumour cell nuclei show peripheral palisading **(P)**. As the tumour is poorly differentiated, immunohistochemical staining may be useful in confirming this diagnosis. Demonstrating neuroendocrine differentiation is important in planning therapy, since these patients may benefit from specific types of chemotherapy.

Fig. 12.23 **Lung metastasis.**

Fig. 12.23 shows a metastatic deposit of colonic adenocarcinoma (see also Fig 7.16). The lungs are a common site for metastatic disease, which are typically multiple and bilateral. Note the malignant glands **(GL)** infiltrating the lung tissue **(L)** and forming a garland or rim around central areas of 'dirty' necrosis composed of karyorrhectic debris **(K)**.

Adenocarcinoma in the lung, particularly if showing a mucinous or enteric phenotype, should be distinguished from a metastasis from another primary site using immunohistochemical staining. In this case, the tumour would stain positively with colorectal markers (CK20, CDX2) and would be negative for lung adenocarcinoma markers (TTF1, Napsin). Wedge resection or lobectomy for pulmonary metastases is now a surgical option in a number of metastatic cancers, particularly if solitary.

KEY TO FIGURES
C bronchial cartilage   **G** separate green and orange signals   **GL** Malignant glands   **K** karyorrhectic debris   **L** lung parenchyma   **P** peripheral palisading   **N** normal fused yellow signal   **Ne** necrosis   **O** neuroendocrine tumour nests   **P** peripheral palisading   **T** tumour cell nuclei

MOLECULAR ASPECTS OF LUNG CANCER

Recently, molecular tests have been introduced into the routine pathological assessment of lung cancer specimens. Particular histological subtypes harbour molecular signatures, which, if detected, allow specific targeted therapies to be used. Three of these tests are outlined briefly although the repertoire of molecular tests available is likely to increase over the next few years, particularly with the introduction of next generation sequencing (see Ch. 1).

* ***EGFR mutation***: *Epidermal growth factor receptor (EGFR)* mutations are the commonest driver mutations in lung adenocarcinoma and are associated with a poor prognosis. The mutation is typically found in tumours in young women, Asian ethnicity, light or never smokers and those with lepidic or micropapillary growth patterns. The *EGFR* gene codes for a cell surface protein tyrosine kinase receptor, which binds to EGF and activates downstream pathways (RAS/ PI3K) involved in cell replication and cell death. Mutation of the gene causes dysregulation of these pathways and is a key event in the development of lung cancer. Patients with certain *EGFR* mutations show an improved survival with specific tyrosine kinase inhibitors that block EGFR activity. *EGFR* mutations are most commonly detected by a PCR-based test for mutations in exons 18 to 21.

* ***ALK rearrangements***: *Anaplastic lymphoma kinase (ALK)* gene rearrangements are most commonly associated with adenocarcinomas and are almost mutually exclusive with EGFR and KRAS mutations. Similar to *EGFR* mutations, *ALK* rearrangements are more common in younger patients who are light or never smokers. The most frequent abnormality is *EML4-ALK* fusion as a result of an inversion on the short arm of chromosome 2. *ALK* fusions are most commonly detected via fluorescence in situ hybridisation (FISH; see Fig. 12.24). Patients with ALK rearrangements show improved outcome with ALK inhibitors.

* ***PD-1/PD-L1***: Programmed death-1 is an immune checkpoint protein on the surface of cytotoxic T cells. Non-small cell lung cancers express PD-Ligand 1 and can bind with T lymphocytes to impair function and therefore suppress the immune response to the tumour. Immune checkpoint inhibitor drugs (usually monoclonal antibodies) bind to PD-1 or PD-L1 and allow the immune system to recognise and destroy the tumour cells, although the immune system is highly complex and there are often other pathways and signals at play. Immunohistochemistry for PD-L1 expression is now routinely used to assess possible tumour response to specific immunomodulatory drugs. PD-L1 testing is also likely to be used in other tumour types such as melanoma, genitourinary cancers and gastrointestinal cancers.

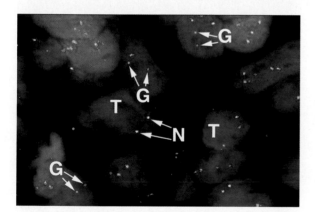

Fig. 12.24 FISH for ALK gene rearrangements.
(Courtesy of Mr Thomas Kerr)

FISH is a common molecular technique and the basics of the test are introduced in Ch. 1. Fig. 12.24 shows lung adenocarcinoma tumour cell nuclei (**T**) viewed under a fluorescence microscope. The labelled ALK region of chromosome 2 (known as 2p23) normally shows overlapping green and orange signals, giving a yellow signal (**N**). When there is a rearrangement present, the signals break apart and separate green and orange signals can be seen (**G**). The number of nuclei with an abnormal signal are counted and, if >50% are present, this is regarded as a positive test.

BASIC SYSTEMS PATHOLOGY ■ RESPIRATORY SYSTEM

EFFUSIONS

An accumulation of fluid within the pleural cavity is termed *pleural effusion*. Similar collections of fluid can also occur within the other serous cavities, described as *ascites* within the peritoneal cavity or as *pericardial effusion* when within the pericardium.

Such collections of fluid are divided into two broad groups on the basis of their protein content. *Transudates* have low protein content and their formation reflects altered hydrostatic or colloid osmotic pressures *(Starling forces)*. Common causes include congestive cardiac failure and hypoalbuminaemia. In contrast, *exudates* have high protein content and, in broad terms, are a result of damage to the integrity of the microvasculature, allowing leakage of plasma proteins across capillary walls. The causes of exudates are diverse but include infection, infarction, inflammation and malignancy.

Cytological examination of fluid from effusions is frequently used in clinical practice, often as a means of guiding further investigation. Malignant cells can be identified in such samples and the type of tumour can often be determined by a combination of morphological examination and use of immunostaining. Distinguishing carcinoma cells from reactive mesothelial cells and from malignant mesothelioma can be extremely challenging.

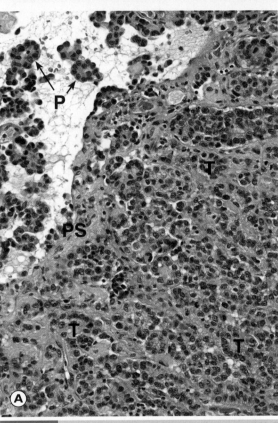
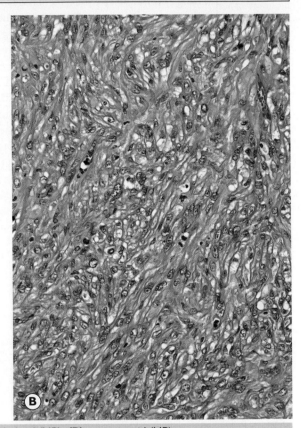

Fig. 12.25 **Malignant mesothelioma of pleura. (A)** Epithelioid (HP); **(B)** sarcomatoid (HP).

The pleura is frequently involved in secondary spread of tumours such as bronchial and breast carcinoma. Involvement of the pleura by tumour usually gives rise to a *pleural effusion* (see clinical box 'Effusions').

Primary malignant tumours of the pleura, known as *mesotheliomas* (E-Fig. 12.8**G**) because of their origin from mesothelial cells, are rare but of great interest since they are related to exposure to asbestos, often in the distant past. Even more rarely, mesotheliomas arise from the peritoneum and these are also often associated with a history of asbestos exposure. Pleural mesothelioma forms a dense sheet of tumour over the pleural surface, often encasing the lung in a hard, white shell. Mesothelioma may extend into the lung parenchyma but, more frequently, the tumour invades through the tissues of the chest wall, often at sites of previous biopsy or chest drain insertion. Metastatic spread is uncommon.

Fig. 12.25A shows pleura that are involved by a malignant mesothelioma with an *epithelioid* growth pattern. The tumour can be seen to involve the pleural surface **(PS)**, where it adopts a papillary architecture **(P)**, as well as infiltrating in a tubular, gland-like pattern **(T)**. This may be difficult to distinguish from metastatic adenocarcinoma. Most mesotheliomas have both epithelioid components and sarcomatoid spindle cell components. Mesotheliomas of this type are said to be *mixed or biphasic*. Occasionally, one pattern predominates. Fig. 12.25B shows a different area of the same tumour illustrated in Fig. 12.25A. In this field, the tumour is composed of plump spindle-shaped cells with no epithelioid elements. Both the epithelioid and spindle-cell components of this tumour exhibit the pleomorphism characteristic of malignancy.

KEY TO FIGURES
P papillary architecture   **PS** pleural surface   **T** tubular architecture

Table 12.2 **Chapter review.**

Disorder	Main Features	Figure
Nose, nasopharynx and larynx		
Nasal polyps	Oedematous, polypoid respiratory mucosa with vascular congestion, numerous eosinophils and plasma cells.	12.1
Sinonasal (Schneiderian) papilloma	Three main types (inverted, exophytic, oncocytic). Small risk of malignant transformation.	12.2
Nasopharyngeal carcinoma	Various types including keratinising squamous, non-keratinising squamous and undifferentiated carcinoma. EBV association.	12.3
Vocal cord polyp	Small, smooth nodule(s) on the vocal cords. Oedematous submucosa covered with stratified squamous epithelium.	12.4
Laryngeal carcinoma	Mostly squamous and well differentiated, strongly associated with smoking and alcohol consumption.	12.5
Inflammatory lung disease		
Acute purulent bronchitis	Purulent exudate within lumina of bronchi and bronchioles, some surrounding oedema in parenchyma.	12.6
Bronchopneumonia	Extension of purulent material into alveolar spaces around bronchi, may become confluent (compare with lobar pneumonia, Fig. 3.3).	12.7
Emphysema	Abnormal permanent dilatation of airspaces with reduced alveolar area for gas exchange, peripheral bullae may form.	12.8
Chronic bronchitis	Clinical definition, histological changes include thickened bronchial wall due to inflammation, smooth muscle and bronchial gland hyperplasia.	12.9
Asthma	Paroxysmal bronchoconstriction, no acute changes but when chronic, smooth muscle hyperplasia, hypersensitivity pneumonitis	12.10
Pulmonary oedema	Alveolar spaces filled with fluid transudate due to altered Starling forces. May be foci of alveolar haemorrhage with haemosiderin in macrophages.	12.11
Interstitial lung disease		
Hyaline membrane disease	Result of diffuse alveolar damage (DAD). Fibrin within alveolar exudate forms hyaline membranes. May be fatal, resolve or progress to fibrosis.	12.12
Pulmonary fibrosis	Deposition of collagen within alveolar walls, reducing gas exchange. Many causes, end stage of DAD and hypersensitivity pneumonitis.	12.13
Silicosis	Inorganic dust deposition resulting in collagenous scars with hyaline centre and surrounding fibrosis. Silica visible on polarisation.	12.14
Asbestosis	Complex silicate causing fibrosis in lower lobes, often subpleural. Asbestos bodies formed due to protein and iron encrustation.	12.15
Tumours of lung and pleura		
Small cell carcinoma	Highly malignant but chemosensitive. Small cells with little cytoplasm showing nuclear moulding.	12.17
Squamous cell carcinoma	Central tumours arising from squamous metaplasia and dysplasia. Endobronchial growth may cause obstruction.	12.18
Adenocarcinoma	More often peripheral, some associated with scars. Glandular formations, often with mucin formation.	12.19, 12.20
Large cell carcinoma (or non-small cell carcinoma NOS)	No evidence of clear line of differentiation following light microscopy and immunohistochemistry.	12.21
Neuroendocrine tumours of lung	Carcinoid tumour, atypical carcinoid and large cell neuroendocrine tumour with evidence of neuroendocrine differentiation.	12.22
Lung metastases	Usually multiple and bilateral. Solitary lung lesions should be distinguished from a metastasis.	12.23
Malignant mesothelioma	Important association with asbestos. Epithelioid and spindle cell components. Spreads along pleural surfaces.	12.25

13 Gastrointestinal system

Introduction

The alimentary system includes the mouth and its associated salivary glands, the oesophagus, stomach, small and large bowels, appendix and anus. The function of the alimentary tract is the ingestion, digestion and absorption of nutrients, along with the storage and expulsion of waste products. A wide range of congenital and acquired diseases may affect all parts of the tract.

Diseases of the oral tissues and salivary glands

The mouth and associated structures can be involved in a wide variety of disease states that may be loosely divided into three categories. First, many systemic diseases, particularly dermatological conditions, exhibit oral manifestations, e.g. *lichen planus* (see Fig. 21.7) and *syphilis* (see Fig. 5.11). Second, all oral tissues may be subject to acute or chronic inflammatory states, the most common being dental caries and its sequelae, *periapical abscess* formation and periodontal disease (i.e. inflammation of the gums). Of more general interest is inflammation of the salivary glands leading to *chronic sialadenitis* (Fig. 13.3). Third, many benign and malignant tumours may arise in the oral tissues, the most common being *squamous cell carcinomas* of the lips, oral mucosa, tongue and oropharynx (Fig 13.1 and 13.2). A wide range of salivary tumours, both benign (Figs 13.4 and 13.5) and malignant (Fig 13.6 and 13.7), can arise in both major and minor salivary glands. A fascinating but fairly esoteric range of benign and malignant tumours arises in the jaws.

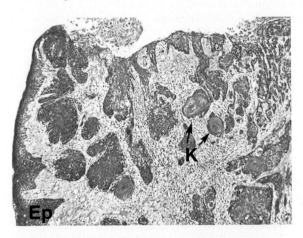

Fig. 13.1 Carcinoma of the tongue (LP).

Malignant tumours of the mucosa of the lips, tongue, cheeks and gums are almost invariably squamous cell carcinomas. They tend to be well differentiated and metastasise to regional lymph nodes (see Fig. 7.13). Fig. 13.1 illustrates a squamous carcinoma involving the tongue (E-Fig. 13.1000**H**). The tumour has arisen from adjacent normal stratified squamous epithelium **(Ep)** and has deeply infiltrated the tongue. It exhibits keratin pearl formation **(K)**. These tumours are usually preceded by dysplasia of the epithelium (see Figs 7.1 and 17.7) that may be identifiable clinically as thickened white patches *(leukoplakia)* or reddish patches *(erythroplakia)* of mucosa.

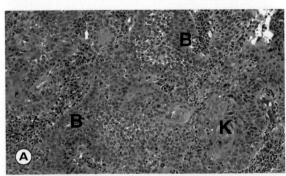
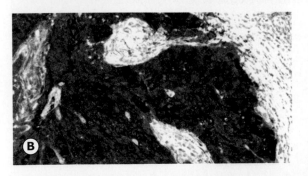

Fig. 13.2 Oropharyngeal squamous cell carcinoma.
(A) H&E (MP); **(B)** immunohistochemical staining for p16 (MP).

Oropharyngeal squamous cell carcinomas (OPSCC) are associated with *high risk HPV types*, similar to squamous cell carcinomas in the anogenital region (see Ch. 17). Many of these tumours arise in the tonsils and are associated with an improved outcome compared to HPV negative tumours. HPV positive tumours typically present in a younger population and the tumours often display basaloid morphology. This is illustrated in Fig. 13.2A where much of the tumour is composed of small dark cells **(B)** with areas of abrupt keratinisation **(K)**.

Determination of HPV status in OPSCC is essential for diagnostic and staging purposes. A wide range of tests is available, using molecular techniques such as in situ hybridisation (ISH) and polymerase chain reaction (PCR). High risk HPV infection causes upregulation of p16 protein expression. Strong p16 expression can be detected by immunohistochemical methods as illustrated in Fig. 13.2B. Note the strong positive brown staining of both the nuclei and the cytoplasm of the tumour cells.

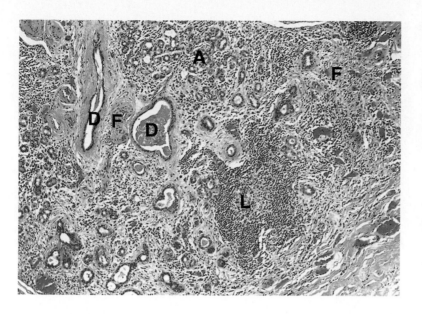

Fig. 13.3 **Chronic sialadenitis (LP).**

Prolonged obstruction of a large salivary gland duct by a calculus *(sialolith)* results in chronic inflammation and acinar atrophy in the gland, termed *chronic sialadenitis*. Fig. 13.3 is from the submandibular gland (E-Fig. 13.2 **H**), the gland most frequently involved. Two salivary duct branches **(D)** are dilated, with periductal fibrosis **(F)** and infiltration by lymphocytes and formation of lymphoid follicles **(L)**. The surrounding secretory acini **(A)** are markedly atrophic and the interstitial spaces have become expanded by fibrous tissue **(F)**.

INFLAMMATION OF THE SALIVARY GLANDS

Sialadenitis may also be caused by viral infections (most commonly mumps), bacterial infections (*Staphylococcus aureus* and *Streptococcus viridans*), autoimmune disease *(Sjögren's syndrome)* and **sarcoidosis**, as well as other rarer causes such as IgG4 disease. A dry mouth due to dehydration, drugs or Sjögren's syndrome also predisposes to bacterial sialadenitis, as do calculi as mentioned above.

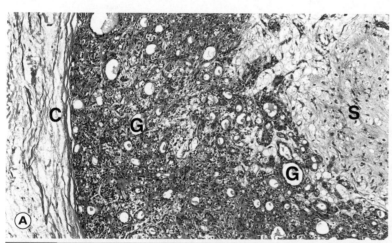
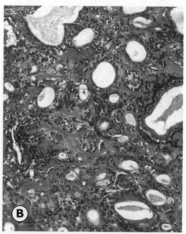

Fig. 13.4 **Pleomorphic adenoma of the salivary glands. (A)** Typical pleomorphic form (MP); **(B)** monomorphic variant: basal cell adenoma (HP).

The most common salivary gland tumour is the *pleomorphic adenoma*, formerly known as *mixed salivary tumour*. The latter term was acquired from the histological appearance of columns and islands of benign epithelial cells, separated by loose myxoid connective tissue stroma in which areas resembling cartilage may be found. Pleomorphic adenomas occur most commonly in the parotid gland. They are usually encapsulated but irregular in shape; in the parotid gland, this leads to difficulty in achieving total excision (bearing in mind the course of the facial nerve) and local recurrence can occur. Pleomorphic adenomas are benign, but very rarely malignant change may supervene after many years, called carcinoma ex pleomorphic adenoma. Fig. 13.4A demonstrates

the typical features of benign pleomorphic adenomas, namely a strongly staining neoplastic epithelial element with glands **(G)** and a pale blue-stained, loose connective tissue stroma **(S)**, somewhat resembling cartilage. Note that the tumour is circumscribed by a thin fibrous capsule **(C)**.

Much less commonly, salivary adenomas are entirely composed of the glandular epithelial component and contain none of the myxomatous stromal component that often dominates the picture in the typical pleomorphic salivary adenoma; this variant is described as a *basal cell adenoma* and an example is shown in Fig. 13.4B.

KEY TO FIGURES

A acini   **B** basaloid tumour cells   **C** capsule   **D** duct   **Ep** epithelium   **F** fibrosis/fibrous tissue
G gland   **K** keratinisation   **L** lymphoid follicle   **S** stroma

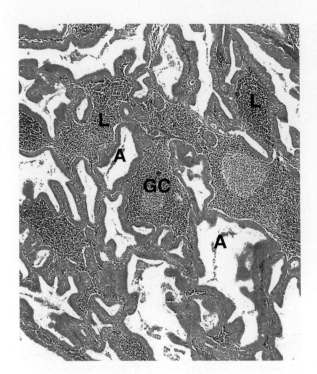

Fig. 13.5 **Warthin's tumour (MP).**

This unusual benign tumour occurs almost exclusively in and around the parotid gland; it commonly arises in middle-aged and older men and mostly in smokers.

The tumour, which is often cystic, is composed of large glandular acini **(A)** embedded in dense lymphoid tissue **(L)** in which typical germinal centres **(GC)** are often seen. The glandular element consists of a surface layer of tall columnar epithelium, rather resembling that of large salivary ducts, overlying a layer of cuboidal cells.

The histogenesis of this tumour is not understood, but the glandular element may represent hamartomatous salivary duct tissue within lymph nodes in and around the parotid gland. Warthin's tumour is also known as ***adenolymphoma*** or ***papillary cystadenoma lymphomatosum***, but the former may give an erroneous impression of malignancy and Warthin's tumour is the preferred term.

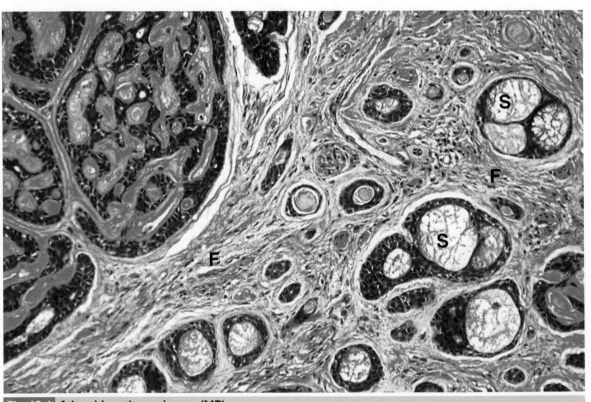

Fig. 13.6 **Adenoid cystic carcinoma (MP).**

An important malignant tumour of salivary tissue is ***adenoid cystic carcinoma***. This tumour is seen most often in the submandibular and sublingual glands and also in the minor salivary glands.

Histologically, it has a characteristic cribriform (sieve-like) appearance owing to the presence of small spaces **(S)** in a mass of tightly packed tumour cells. The tumour cells are arranged in clumps and cords, separated by a fibrous stroma **(F)**, which may exhibit a marked degree of hyalinisation.

These tumours are locally invasive and prone to recurrence following surgical excision. Spread to regional lymph nodes is frequent and wide local spread is common, although the rate of growth is often slow. Perineural invasion, which is often extremely painful, is a common feature of this tumour.

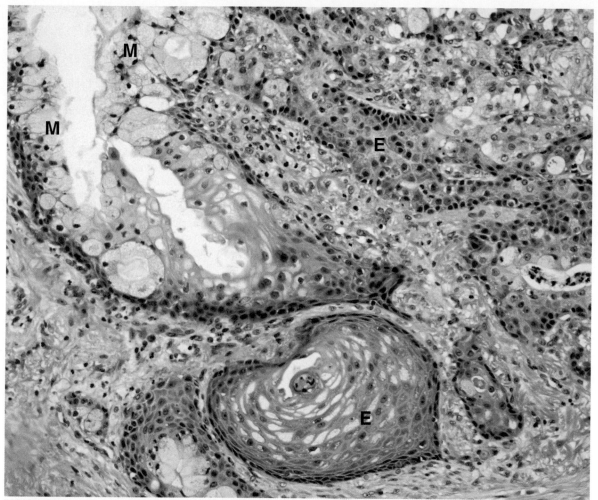

Fig. 13.7 Mucoepidermoid carcinoma (MP).

Mucoepidermoid carcinoma is the most common malignant tumour of salivary gland, but is still relatively rare, comprising about 15% of all salivary gland tumours. As the name indicates, the tumour consists of a mixture of squamous (epidermoid) **(E)** and glandular (muco) elements **(M)**. Intermediate cells with both squamous and glandular features can also be identified.

These tumours most often occur in the parotid gland but may also arise in the minor salivary glands. They may be low, intermediate or high grade. Low grade tumours pursue an indolent course with local invasion while high grade tumours are locally invasive and may metastasise.

Other malignant tumours of the salivary glands include acinic cell tumour, epithelial myoepithelial carcinoma, secretory carcinoma and many others. Molecular techniques are of increasing importance in the diagnosis and classification of salivary gland tumours.

As in almost every other tissue or organ in the body, always consider whether a mass lesion could be a metastasis from a primary malignant tumour at another site. Also, lymphoma can arise in or spread to almost any organ. The most common lymphoma arising in the salivary glands is of the mucosa associated lymphoid tissue (MALT) lymphoma type and usually occurs on a background of chronic inflammation.

Oesophageal diseases

Infections of the oesophagus are rare in healthy individuals, but in debilitated or immunosuppressed patients, infection with herpes simplex virus (see Fig. 5.12) or *Candida albicans* (see Fig. 5.15) can occur. The lower oesophagus frequently becomes inflamed as a result of gastric acid reflux, producing either *oesophagitis* or sometimes *chronic peptic ulceration*, analogous to that seen in the stomach and duodenum (see Figs 4.2 and 13.10). This condition is known as *gastro-oesophageal reflux disease* (*GORD* or *GERD*, depending on how you spell oesophagus). In response to reflux of acid, the squamous mucosa of the lower oesophagus may undergo metaplastic transformation into a form of glandular epithelium similar to that seen in the stomach or small intestine. This metaplastic condition is termed *Barrett's oesophagus* (Fig. 13.8).

KEY TO FIGURES

A acinus **E** epidermoid (squamous) elements **GC** germinal centre **F** fibrous stroma **L** lymphoid tissue **M** mucous (glandular) elements **S** spaces in tumour cell masses

BASIC SYSTEMS PATHOLOGY ■ GASTROINTESTINAL SYSTEM

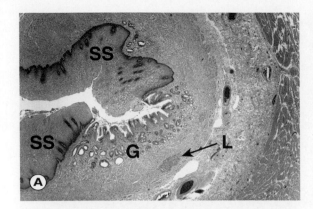

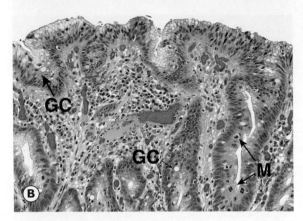

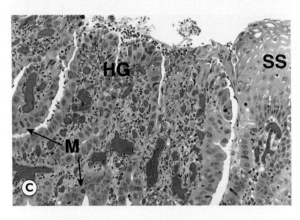

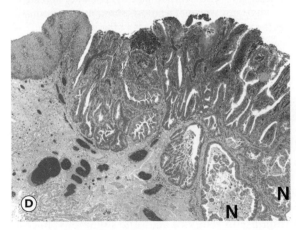

Fig. 13.8 Barrett's oesophagus. **(A)** No dysplasia (LP); **(B)** low grade dysplasia (HP); **(C)** high grade dysplasia (HP); **(D)** invasive adenocarcinoma (LP); **(E)** invasive adenocarcinoma (HP).

Fig. 13.8A shows a transverse section of the lower oesophagus (E-Fig. 13.3**H**) in which there is an abrupt transition from stratified squamous epithelium **(SS)** to metaplastic glandular epithelium **(G)**. An infiltrate of lymphocytes and plasma cells with occasional lymphoid aggregates **(L)** is seen. Chronic inflammation is commonly found in this condition. The detail of the glandular epithelium cannot be seen at this magnification but it generally consists of a mucous secreting glandular mucosa, similar to that of gastric cardia (E-Fig. 13.4 **H**). The goblet cells that characterise intestinal metaplasia are often found in a patchy distribution so some biopsies may miss them. By definition, glandular epithelium found within the oesophagus (as opposed to within a hiatus hernia) is diagnostic of *Barrett's oesophagus*.

At high magnification in Fig. 13.8B, glands with goblet cells **(GC)**, indicating intestinal metaplasia, are seen with associated *low grade dysplasia*. Low grade dysplasia is characterised by enlargement, crowding and disorganisation of the epithelial cell nuclei and increased mitotic activity **(M)**. This can be difficult to differentiate from the reactive changes in inflamed mucosa. If a clear determination cannot be made, the biopsy is classified as indefinite for dysplasia to signal the need for follow up and repeat biopsy.

In Fig. 13.8C, *high grade dysplasia* **(HG)** is shown at high power. There is adjacent surface squamous epithelium **(SS)**. The pleomorphism and hyperchromasia of the glandular epithelial cell nuclei is easily appreciated and there are prominent mitotic figures **(M)**. The presence of high grade dysplasia in biopsies from Barrett's oesophagus is a very worrying feature and some patients may already have invasive *oesophageal adenocarcinoma*.

Fig 13.6D and 13.8E illustrate invasive oesophageal adenocarcinoma, arising from high grade dysplasia. This example is from the same patient as Fig. 13.8C. In this case, the initial biopsies demonstrated high grade dysplasia and a subsequent specimen revealed invasive adenocarcinoma. The malignant glands have complex architecture and some include central 'dirty' necrosis **(N)**, similar to that seen in colorectal carcinoma (see Fig. 13.24). Atypical mitotic figures **(AM)** are easily seen and the nuclei are highly pleomorphic.

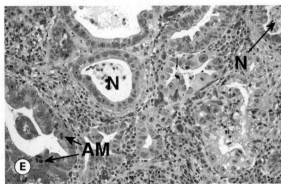

KEY TO FIGURES
AM atypical mitoses **G** glandular mucosa **GC** goblet cell **HG** high grade dysplasia
L lymphoid aggregate **M** mitotic figures **N** dirty necrosis **SS** stratified squamous epithelium

CARCINOMA OF THE OESOPHAGUS

The most common oesophageal neoplasm used to be **squamous cell carcinoma**, which is similar to squamous cell carcinomas at other sites (see Figs 7.3 and 17.8). However, the incidence of **adenocarcinomas** arising in Barrett's oesophagus at the lower end of the oesophagus is increasing and comprises almost 50% of oesophageal carcinomas in developed countries. Both adenocarcinoma and squamous cell carcinoma of the oesophagus have a very poor prognosis. The lower oesophagus may also be involved by local spread of adenocarcinoma of the upper stomach.

Patients with longstanding GORD/GERD are at risk of developing adenocarcinoma of the oesophagus. The sequence of events appears to be oesophagitis → Barrett's oesophagus without dysplasia → low grade dysplasia → high grade dysplasia → invasive carcinoma. High grade dysplasia is a premalignant condition and oesophagectomy often reveals co-existing superficially invasive carcinoma. Because of the grim prognosis of oesophageal carcinomas, Barrett's oesophagus is usually regularly monitored by endoscopy and biopsy. High grade dysplasia and superficially invasive carcinomas can be locally resected or ablated by photodynamic therapy (PDT), laser therapy or other means before reaching an advanced stage.

Diseases of the stomach

Gastritis

Inflammation of the stomach is termed *gastritis* and may be divided into acute and chronic forms.

■ **Acute gastritis** may be associated with the use of aspirin or other non-steroidal anti-inflammatory drugs (NSAIDs) and excessive alcohol consumption and also occurs in severely debilitated patients. It may present with nausea and vomiting but is also an important cause of haematemesis. Although not uncommon, acute gastritis rarely requires biopsy.

■ **Chronic gastritis** can be divided into distinct subtypes, each of which has particular histological features (Fig. 13.9):

– **Chronic infection:** *Helicobacter pylori* is the usual infective agent.

– **Chronic chemical gastritis** (also known as **reactive** or **reflux gastritis**) is associated with reflux of bile or alkaline duodenal secretions into the stomach, especially following surgical procedures, and with chronic alcohol consumption or with use of gastrotoxic drugs such as NSAIDs.

– **Chronic autoimmune gastritis** is associated with autoantibodies to various components of gastric parietal cells and with pernicious anaemia.

■ Less common causes include **Crohn's disease**, **graft-versus-host disease** and **gastric outlet obstruction**.

Peptic ulceration

The histological details of chronic peptic ulceration in the stomach are described in Ch. 4 (see Fig. 4.2). Acid-induced necrosis of the gastric wall, the acute inflammatory response, organisation, granulation tissue formation and fibrous scarring occur concurrently. *H. pylori* infection is almost always present in chronic duodenal ulceration and most cases of chronic gastric ulceration (E-Fig. 13.5**G**) and must be eradicated for permanent healing. The outcome of this dynamic process depends on which is the dominant element, i.e. the damaging stimulus or the attempts of the body to heal the damage.

There are three main complications of chronic peptic ulceration:

■ **Perforation:** If tissue destruction outstrips attempts to confine or repair it, the process may extend rapidly through the wall, leading to perforation (Fig. 13.10A).

■ **Haemorrhage:** Tissue necrosis may extend deeply enough to involve the wall of a large artery. This is most common in long-standing chronic gastric ulcers on the posterior wall, in the region of the left gastroepiploic artery. This vessel tends to become incorporated in the fibrous scar on the serosal aspect of a chronic gastric ulcer and may then be eroded during a subsequent acute exacerbation of ulceration (Fig. 13.10B). This may produce torrential haemorrhage, presenting as *haematemesis* and/or *melaena*, which may be fatal.

■ **Obstruction:** Persistent attempts at repair lead to progressive fibrous scarring, which undergoes shrinkage and ultimately causes distortion and thickening of the wall of the viscus, commonly at the lower end of the oesophagus or in the pyloric region of the stomach. The narrowing may cause *stricture* formation with partial or even complete obstruction of the lumen. When the ulcerative process is still active, obstruction may be compounded by inflammatory oedema of the mucosa surrounding the ulcer.

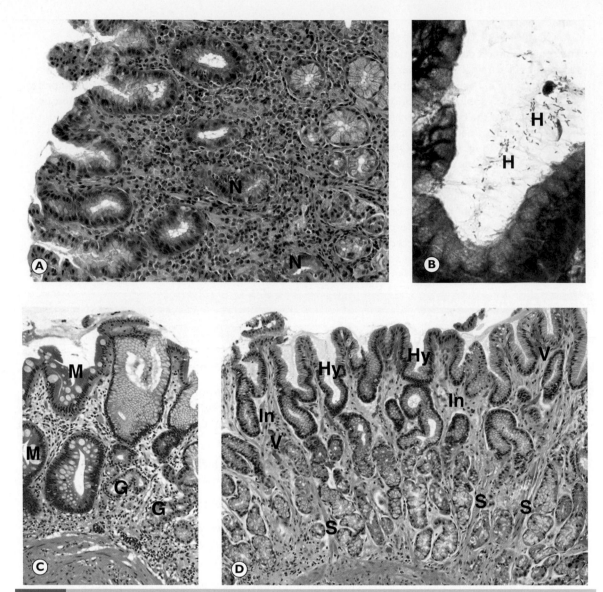

Fig. 13.9 Chronic gastritis. (A) *H. pylori* infection (MP); **(B)** *H. pylori* infection (Cresyl violet) (HP); **(C)** autoimmune gastritis (MP); **(D)** chemical gastritis (MP).

H. pylori infection is the most common cause of chronic gastritis, typically affecting the mucosa of the antrum, but extending to the body of the stomach in some cases (pangastritis). The histological features, as shown in Fig. 13.9A, include a mixed inflammatory infiltrate in the lamina propria with neutrophils, plasma cells, lymphocytes and eosinophils. Typically, neutrophils **(N)** are seen infiltrating the epithelium of the gastric glands: this is often described as ***active, chronic gastritis***, indicating a combination of acute and chronic inflammation. ***Intestinal metaplasia*** is quite common in association with this type of gastritis and it may lead to dysplasia (Fig. 13.11). In intestinal metaplasia, the gastric epithelial cells are replaced with goblet cells and columnar absorptive cells typical of the small intestine. *H. pylori* organisms can sometimes be seen in routine H&E preparations, but a range of special stains will highlight the organisms. The Cresyl violet stain shown in Fig. 13.9B at high magnification demonstrates the *H. pylori* organisms **(H)** in the

mucus layer at the surface of the epithelium. Bacterial invasion of the mucosa is not a feature.

In contrast, autoimmune-type chronic gastritis primarily affects the body of the stomach (E-Fig. 13.6**H**). As seen in Fig. 13.9C from the gastric body, the histological features include atrophy of the gastric glands with loss of parietal cells. The glands **(G)** are small and the mucosa is thinned. The lamina propria is infiltrated mainly with lymphocytes and plasma cells, and intestinal metaplasia **(M)** is a prominent feature. Chronic autoimmune gastritis in its late stages is often termed ***chronic atrophic gastritis***. Chemical or reactive gastritis, as shown in Fig. 13.9D, is characterised by inflammation of the superficial mucosa with a scanty infiltrate of inflammatory cells **(In)** (lymphocytes and plasma cells). The gastric glands show hyperplasia of the foveolae of the glands **(Hy)**, the part of the gland where cell division occurs and, characteristically, the lamina propria is oedematous with marked vasodilatation **(V)**. Spurs of smooth muscle **(S)** branch from the muscularis mucosae into the lamina propria.

KEY TO FIGURES
A artery **Ex** inflammatory exudate **F** fibrous scar tissue **G** glands **H** *H. pylori* organisms
Hy foveolar hyperplasia **In** inflammatory cells **M** intestinal metaplasia **MP** muscularis propria
Mu mucosa **N** neutrophils **S** smooth muscle spurs **SM** submucosa **V** vasodilatation

COMPLICATIONS OF CHRONIC GASTRITIS

Chronic gastritis is very common and, in untreated patients, was often associated with the development of peptic ulceration and its complications (see Fig. 13.10). However, the recognition and treatment of *H. pylori* infection as well as the widespread use of **proton pump inhibitors (PPIs)** to reduce gastric acid secretion, has greatly changed the incidence of serious complications. Gastric adenocarcinoma, which is usually preceded by intestinal metaplasia and dysplasia (see Figs 13.11 and 13.12) is known to have a strong association with *H. pylori* gastritis but may also occur with any other form of chronic gastric inflammation. *H. pylori* is also associated with gastric lymphoma (MALT lymphoma) (see Fig. 16.7).

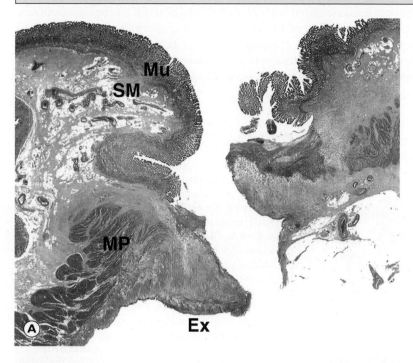

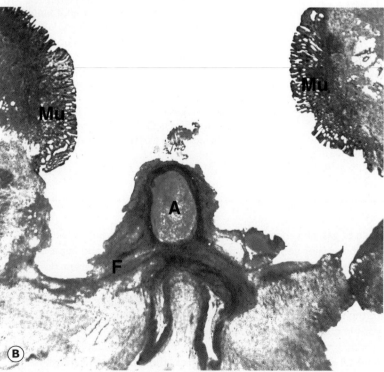

Fig. 13.10 Complications of peptic ulceration. (A) Perforated gastric ulcer (LP); **(B)** bleeding gastric ulcer (LP).

Perforation of peptic ulcers has become less common with the advent of effective medical treatment for gastritis and peptic ulcer. It results in discharge of gastric contents into the peritoneal cavity with resulting ***acute peritonitis***. In the perforated gastric ulcer shown in Fig. 13.10A, tissue necrosis has extended through the full thickness of the wall, with complete destruction of the mucosa **(Mu)**, submucosa **(SM)** and muscle layers **(MP)**. Peritonitis is manifested by an acute inflammatory exudate **(Ex)** on the serosal surface of the stomach. The margins of the perforated ulcer are lined by necrotic tissue, beneath which is a zone of acute inflammation, similar to that found in the floor of a more chronic ulcer (see Fig. 4.2). There is no evidence of fibrous granulation tissue or fibrous scar since the destructive process has been too acute. Perforations such as this occur most commonly in peptic ulcers in the first part of the duodenum but also occur in the stomach, as in this example.

Haemorrhage from erosion of a large artery in the base of an ulcer may occur in untreated chronic gastric ulcers as shown in Fig. 13.10B. Note the eroded artery **(A)** trapped in the fibrous scar tissue **(F)** forming the floor of the ulcer. Part of the arterial wall is undergoing necrosis as a result of acid attack and massive haemorrhage will follow.

Gastric neoplasia

By far the most common malignant tumours of the stomach are *adenocarcinomas* (90%–95%). These may assume a variety of gross morphological forms, including *malignant ulcers* with heaped-up edges, *fungating polypoid tumours* or *diffuse infiltration* of the wall *(linitis plastica)*, giving rise to the so-called *leather bottle stomach*. Gastric adenocarcinomas are classified histologically as *intestinal type* (Fig. 13.12A and B), often arising on a background of intestinal metaplasia and dysplasia, or *diffuse type* (Fig. 13.12C and D). *Gastric lymphoma* (see Fig. 16.7) and *neuroendocrine tumours* (previously known as *carcinoid tumours*) (Fig. 13.13) make up a small percentage of stomach malignancies. Both adenocarcinoma and gastric lymphoma are associated with *H. pylori* infection. Of the benign tumours, gastric adenomas comprise only a small proportion of gastric polyps, most of which are inflammatory or regenerative. Mesenchymal tumours occur in the stomach and other parts of the gastrointestinal tract including lipomas, leiomyomas and *gastrointestinal stromal tumours (GIST)* (Fig. 13.14), which are mainly found in the gastrointestinal tract; rare examples occur at other sites such as the mesentery, the retroperitoneum and the pelvis.

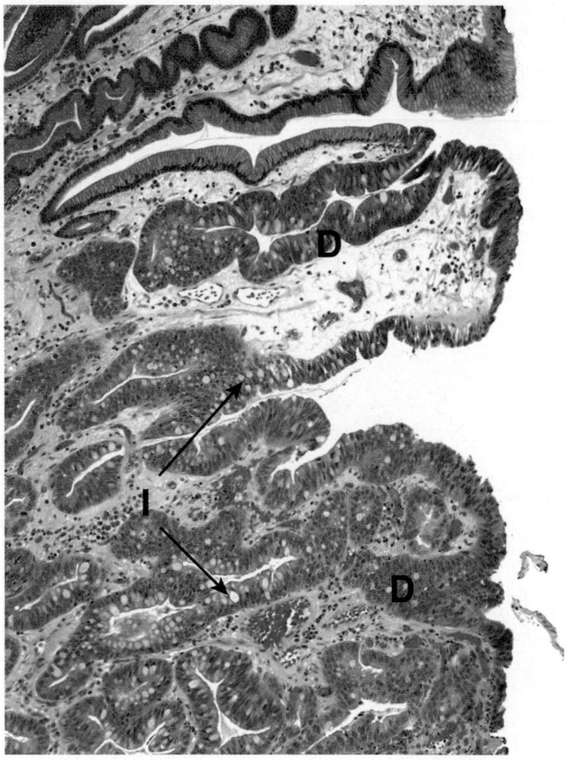

Fig. 13.11 Gastric dysplasia (MP).

Dysplasia is defined as an epithelial change with many similarities (morphological and molecular) to invasive carcinoma, but which does not breach the basement membrane of the epithelium. In the stomach, dysplasia goes by many names including *carcinoma in situ*, *non-invasive neoplasia*, *intraepithelial neoplasia* and *category 4 lesions*, depending on which classification is in use. Dysplasia may arise in association with longstanding chronic gastritis of any type. Generally, the sequence of events seems to be gastric atrophy, intestinal metaplasia, low then high grade dysplasia and finally invasive carcinoma, usually of intestinal type. However the individual steps in this progression remain to be elucidated. Fig. 13.11 shows *high-grade dysplasia* (D) of the gastric mucosa, arising on a background of *intestinal metaplasia* (I). There is marked irregularity of the glands with nuclear enlargement, hyperchromasia and crowding of the epithelial cells. There is little evidence of mucus production by epithelial cells and cellular polarity (basal alignment of nuclei) is completely lost. Note the similarity to dysplasia in Barrett's oesophagus (see Fig. 13.8). The importance of detecting gastric dysplasia is that treatment can prevent progression to gastric carcinoma.

GASTRIC CARCINOMA

There are large differences in incidence of gastric cancer in different parts of the world. As well as different rates of *H. pylori* infection, the other major aetiological factor appears to be diet and in particular high consumption of smoked and salted foods. Diffuse type carcinomas seem to have different risk factors and, unlike the intestinal type, are not thought to be associated with preceding inflammation, atrophy, metaplasia or dysplasia. Carcinoma of the stomach may be staged histologically as *early* or *late*, with early carcinomas infiltrating into the submucosa but not into the muscularis propria. Early gastric carcinomas have an excellent prognosis in contrast to late gastric carcinomas.

In patients with advanced gastric carcinoma, a variety of conventional chemotherapeutic agents may be used. A small but important subset of these tumours over-express the *HER-2* gene and these patients may benefit from treatment with drugs targeting the her-2 protein, similar to those used in the management of breast carcinoma (see Ch. 18). *HER-2* amplification status can be determined on biopsies of the tumour, using immunohistochemical methods and/or fluorescence in situ hybridisation (FISH). This testing allows therapy to be tailored for individual patients and avoids unnecessary, potentially toxic treatments in patients who will not benefit from them.

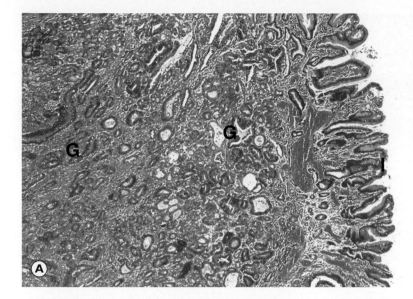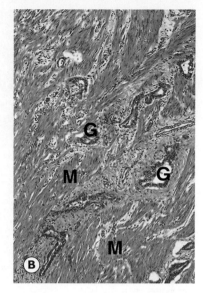

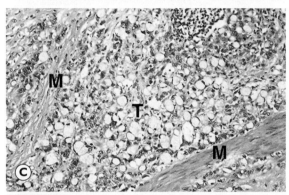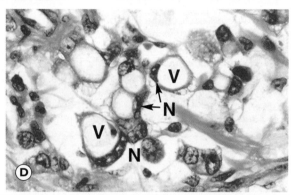

Fig. 13.12 **Gastric carcinoma. (A)** Intestinal type adenocarcinoma (LP); **(B)** intestinal type adenocarcinoma (MP); **(C)** diffuse type adenocarcinoma (MP), **(D)** diffuse type adenocarcinoma (HP).

Gastric adenocarcinomas of the **intestinal type** are well or moderately differentiated and usually form a polypoid tumour mass or an ulcer with heaped-up edges. As mentioned above, this type of gastric carcinoma is usually preceded by gastric dysplasia and its precursors (Fig. 13.11). The low power view in Fig. 13.12A shows irregular malignant glands **(G)** infiltrating the gastric wall beneath a dysplastic mucosa with focal intestinal metaplasia. Deeper in the gastric wall in Fig. 13.12B, malignant glands **(G)** are seen infiltrating the muscularis propria **(M)**.

Diffuse type gastric carcinomas are poorly differentiated adenocarcinomas with little or no discernible gland formation. This pattern tends to take the form of a diffuse infiltration of the stomach wall starting as a flat localised area of infiltration, but in advanced cases giving rise to *linitis plastica* or *leather bottle stomach* (E-Fig. 13.7**G**). In Fig. 13.12C, the tumour cells **(T)** can be seen forming a diffuse sheet infiltrating between bundles of smooth muscle in the muscularis propria **(M)**. At high power in Fig. 13.12D, the tumour includes many *signet ring cells*, so named because the cytoplasm is occupied by a mucin-filled vacuole **(V)** pushing the nucleus **(N)** to the periphery of the cell. If the tumour consists of more than 50% of signet ring cells overall, it is called a signet ring carcinoma. These tumours are generally more poorly differentiated than the intestinal type. Some gastric carcinomas produce large amounts of extracellular mucin giving rise to *mucinous adenocarcinomas* (see Fig. 7.5).

KEY TO FIGURES
D high grade dysplasia **G** malignant glands **I** intestinal metaplasia **M** muscularis propria
N nucleus **T** tumour cells **V** mucin vacuole

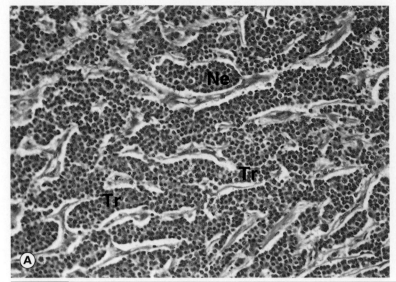

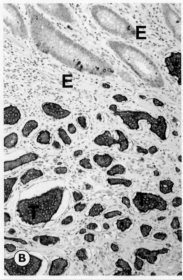

Fig. 13.13 **Gastrointestinal well differentiated neuroendocrine tumour. (A)** H&E (MP); **(B)** chromogranin (HP).

These tumours are found in the appendix, small intestine, rectum, stomach and colon, in that order of frequency, and in many other sites such as pancreas and lung (see Fig. 12.22). The behaviour of neuroendocrine tumours ranges from benign to malignant, depending on site of tumour, size, depth of invasion into the wall of the gut and mitotic activity. They may secrete a variety of hormone products such as *serotonin (5-HT),* which may cause *carcinoid syndrome*.

In well differentiated neuroendocrine tumours, the tumour cells form nests **(N)** and trabeculae **(Tr)** as in Fig. 13.13A, glandular structures or diffuse sheets of cells. The cells characteristically are small and uniform with round nuclei, stippled chromatin and pinkish granular cytoplasm.

Immunohistochemical staining will often reveal the hormone products within the cells as in Fig. 13.13A of duodenal mucosa, where tumour cells **(T)** have been stained for *chromogranin A*, a protein associated with the secretory granules. Note also the positive staining of normal neuroendocrine cells scattered in the adjacent normal duodenal epithelium **(E)**. Note that the wider group of neuroendocrine neoplasms also includes aggressive, high grade tumours such as *small cell carcinoma* (see Fig. 12.17).

NEUROENDOCRINE TUMOURS OF THE GASTROINTESTINAL TRACT

These tumours can arise at various sites and they are usually well differentiated. They may secrete a range of hormone products, typically including **5-HT (serotonin)** and other vasoactive compounds. These products can cause clinical vasomotor symptoms described as *carcinoid syndrome*. In the past, the term *carcinoid tumour* was used for all of these tumours, reflecting the fact that they have some similarities to conventional carcinomas, but their behaviour can be difficult to predict. This nomenclature has been by replaced by a classification system that aims to reflect the likely biological behaviour and prognosis of the tumours. The criteria for classification vary at different sites in the GI tract but the terms used range from *well differentiated neuroendocrine tumour* through to *poorly differentiated neuroendocrine carcinoma*, the latter having aggressive biological behaviour and a poorer prognosis. For gastrointestinal tumours, the term carcinoid tumour alone should be avoided as this fails to convey the relevant prognostic information. In contrast, this term is still used for well differentiated tumours in the lung, with more aggressive variants described as atypical carcinoid tumours (see Ch. 12).

KEY TO FIGURES
E neuroendocrine cell   **F** fascicle   **N** nest of tumour   **S** spindle cells   **T** tumour cells   **Tr** trabeculae

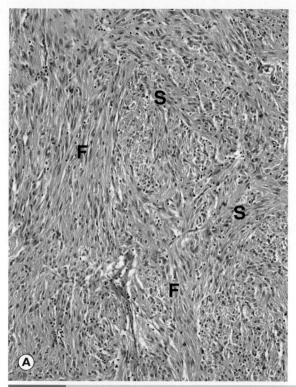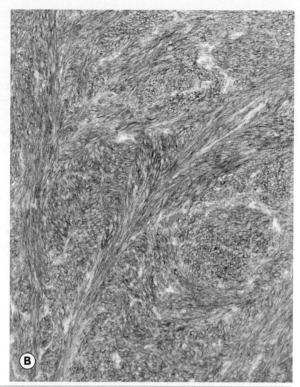

Fig. 13.14 **Gastrointestinal stromal tumour.** **(A)** H&E (MP); **(B)** immunohistochemistry for CD117 (MP).

Gastrointestinal stromal tumours (GISTs) are a specific type of mesenchymal tumour found mainly in the gastrointestinal tract. Previously, many of these tumours were misdiagnosed as leiomyomas, neurofibromas, Schwannomas and leiomyosarcomas. However, although instances of the above tumours do occur in the gastrointestinal tract, the majority of these tumours turn out to be GISTs. GISTs are thought to be derived from the interstitial cells of Cajal or a precursor cell. One of the key features of these tumours is that they are positive for *CD117 (c-kit)* (>95%) and may also be positive for DOG1, CD34 and smooth muscle actin

(SMA) by immunohistochemical staining. They are composed of spindled, epithelioid or pleomorphic cells that may resemble smooth muscle or nerve sheath tumours. The cells may be arranged in fascicles, nests or sheets, with variable amounts of collagen in the stroma. Fig. 13.14A shows a typical GIST with spindle cells **(S)** arranged in randomly orientated fascicles **(F)**. The histological features, however, can be very variable and immunostaining for CD117 and CD34 is important to confirm the diagnosis. Positive immunostaining for CD117 of the same tumour is shown in Fig. 13.14B.

MOLECULAR BIOLOGY AND SPECIFIC TREATMENTS FOR GISTS

GISTs have a wide spectrum of clinical behaviour. About a quarter of gastric GISTs and half of small intestinal GISTs are malignant. The most useful pathological features that predict malignant behaviour are site, size of tumour and high mitotic rate. Most are treated by complete excision but, where this is not possible, treatment with a specific monoclonal antibody, imatinib, is indicated. c-kit is a membrane receptor protein for stem cell factor. When stem cell factor binds to c-kit, it is activated and acts as a tyrosine kinase, an enzyme that activates other intracellular proteins by phosphorylation of the amino acid tyrosine. Mutations in c-kit lead to constitutional activation of this signalling pathway, resulting in cell proliferation and, in time, formation of tumours. Imatinib is a tyrosine kinase inhibitor and so blocks the activity of the mutated c-kit protein. Most GISTs are responsive to imatinib initially, although with time many become resistant and the tumour recurs. A small proportion of tumours have no c-kit mutation but have activating mutations in a very similar cell surface receptor/tyrosine kinase enzyme, called platelet derived growth factor receptor-α (PDGFR α); this acts, and is treated, in the same way.

Diseases of the small intestine and appendix

Inflammation of the small intestine due to self-limiting infections is very common but rarely biopsied. *Giardiasis* (see Fig. 5.19) is a common infective cause of inflammation in some countries and is often diagnosed on biopsy. Other inflammatory conditions affecting the small intestine include *coeliac disease* (Fig. 13.15) and *Crohn's disease* (Fig. 13.16). *Appendicitis* (Fig. 13.17) is extremely common and is a classic example of acute inflammation.

Primary tumours of the small intestine and appendix are very rare, with the exception of *neuroendocrine tumours* (Fig. 13.13) and *lymphomas*, which may be MALT lymphomas (see Fig. 16.7), enteropathy-associated or occasionally of Burkitt lymphoma type (see Fig. 16.8). Neuroendocrine tumours occur in the appendix, as do rare *adenomas*. Although broadly similar in appearance to colonic adenomas, these mucin-producing tumours (called *low grade* or *high grade appendiceal mucinous neoplasms*) often distend the appendix, producing the macroscopic appearance of a *mucocoele*. If tumours of this type rupture, mucin and neoplastic mucin-secreting epithelium may be released into the peritoneal cavity, causing a form of mucinous ascites called *pseudomyxoma peritoneii*. Rarely, these tumours may become frankly malignant.

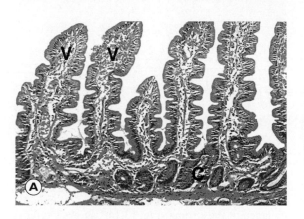

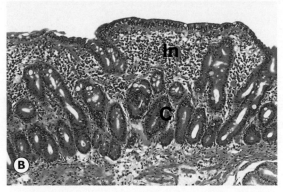

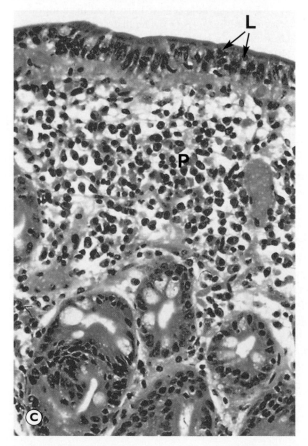

Fig. 13.15 **Coeliac disease (gluten-sensitive enteropathy). (A)** Normal jejunal mucosa (MP); **(B)** atrophic jejunal mucosa (MP); **(C)** atrophic jejunal mucosa (HP).

Hypersensitivity to gluten (a constituent of wheat, rye and barley) gives rise to *coeliac disease (gluten sensitive enteropathy, coeliac sprue)*, a condition in which the patient's own immune system damages the small bowel mucosa. Clinically, this results in a malabsorption syndrome with very variable symptoms, including weight loss, anaemia and *steatorrhoea* (diarrhoea containing unabsorbed lipid) in severe cases.

The diagnosis is usually confirmed by endoscopic biopsy of the proximal small intestine. Fig. 13.15A shows normal mucosa with villi **(V)** and short crypts **(C)**. In coeliac disease, as shown in Fig. 13.15B, there is infiltration of the duodenal mucosa by inflammatory lymphocytes and plasma cells **(In),** loss of villi *(villous atrophy)*, and hyperplasia (elongation) of crypts **(C)**. The result is a flat small bowel mucosa. At high power, Fig. 13.15C shows the preponderance of plasma cells **(P)** in the lamina propria with the typical increase in *intraepithelial lymphocytes* **(L)**. These lymphocytes are mainly T cells and represent a cell-mediated immune reaction to gluten. Specific antibodies to various antigens are also a characteristic indication of a humoral component to the aberrant immune response.

KEY TO FIGURES
C crypts **G** granuloma **In** inflammatory cells **L** intraepithelial lymphocytes **SM** submucosa
P plasma cells **U** ulcer **V** villus

CHRONIC INFLAMMATORY BOWEL DISEASE

Chronic inflammatory bowel disease is a group of conditions including *Crohn's disease* and *ulcerative colitis*. These are chronic inflammatory conditions of unknown aetiology with a typically relapsing course. Both conditions may lead to surgical removal of large parts of the bowel. Other conditions may mimic these two diseases such as diverticulosis-related colitis, radiation colitis and ischaemic colitis. Infections, including TB, must also be ruled out before a diagnosis of chronic inflammatory bowel disease is made. Ulcerative colitis and Crohn's disease can occasionally be very difficult to differentiate from each other clinically and pathologically and often the distinction can only be made at the time of colectomy. Unlike ulcerative colitis, Crohn's disease may affect any part of the gastrointestinal tract, so diagnostic difficulty only arises when disease is limited to the colon and rectum. In this situation, the term *indeterminate colitis* may be used until there is enough information for a definitive diagnosis; thus the term indeterminate colitis does not indicate a specific disease, only that there is idiopathic chronic inflammatory bowel disease that cannot yet be fully classified. The distinction is important, as different treatment options are appropriate for the different conditions. Both ulcerative colitis and Crohn's disease may have extra-intestinal manifestations such as arthritis, sacroileitis and sclerosing cholangitis. Both may be associated with the development of adenocarcinoma of the bowel, but this risk is particularly high in long-standing ulcerative colitis.

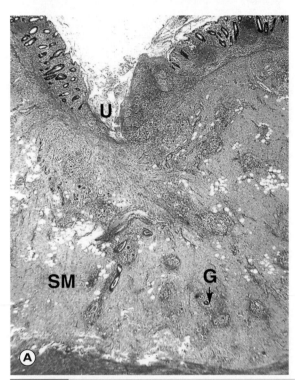

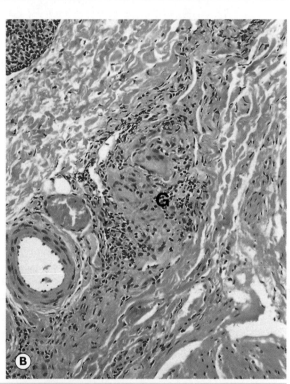

Fig. 13.16 **Crohn's disease. (A)** Fissured ulcer (MP); **(B)** Crohn's granuloma (HP).

Crohn's disease is a chronic inflammatory disease of unknown aetiology. It mainly involves the small intestine (E-Fig. 13.8**H**), especially terminal ileum, but quite often affects large bowel and anus and occasionally parts of the upper gastrointestinal tract. When restricted to the colon, it may be confused clinically with *ulcerative colitis* (see Fig. 13.18) and, in the anus, with anal fissures and fistulae. Crohn's disease is characteristically patchy in distribution, affecting short segments with lengths of normal bowel in between *(skip lesions)*. As shown in Fig. 13.16A, the affected segments of small intestine show gross thickening of the wall, mainly because of marked oedema and inflammation of the submucosa **(SM)**. This oedema produces the typical 'cobblestone' macroscopic appearance of the mucosa, in which domed areas of swollen mucosa and submucosa are criss-crossed by linear depressions caused by narrow *fissured ulcers*. A typical fissured ulcer **(U)** can be seen here. Fissured ulcers may extend into and even through the muscularis propria, giving rise to *fistulae* (abnormal

connections) between different parts of the bowel or between the bowel and bladder, vagina or even the skin surface. Fig. 13.16A also demonstrates two other characteristic features of Crohn's disease. First, the inflammatory changes are *transmural* (i.e. affect all layers from mucosa to serosa). Second, non-caseating granulomas **(G)**, often containing giant cells, may be found in all layers. A granuloma in the submucosa is shown at higher magnification in Fig. 13.16B. The granulomas in Crohn's disease resemble those seen in sarcoidosis (see Fig. 4.8). Granulomas such as these may also be found in lymph nodes draining the affected segment of bowel. The result of longstanding transmural inflammation is widespread fibrosis, which may cause the characteristic strictures seen in Crohn's disease (E-Fig. 13.9**G**), leading to bowel obstruction. Patients who have repeated operations to remove segments of small bowel may eventually develop short bowel syndrome, characterised by malabsorption and rapid intestinal transit time.

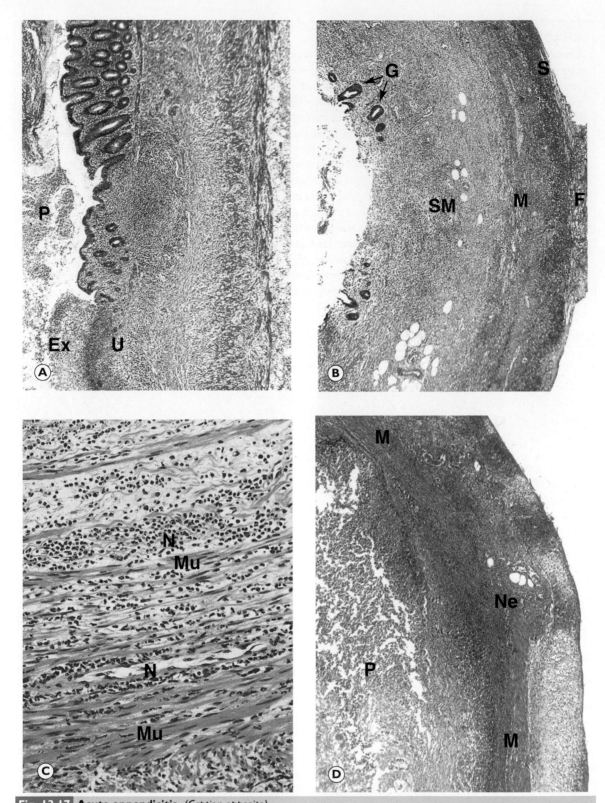

Fig. 13.17 **Acute appendicitis.** *(Caption opposite)*

DIFFERENTIAL DIAGNOSES OF THE ACUTE ABDOMEN
A range of intra-abdominal diseases may present with features similar to those of acute appendicitis.
These include mesenteric adenitis, gallstone disease, kidney and ureteric stones, acute urinary tract
infections, ectopic pregnancy, acute salpingitis, ovarian cysts and tumours, diverticular disease, inflamed
Meckel's diverticulum and perforation of gastric and duodenal ulcers. Careful history taking, examina-
tion and targeted investigation is essential.

Acute inflammation of the appendix (E-Fig. 13.10**H**).Is one of the most common surgical emergencies and is a typical example of acute inflammation (see Ch. 3). The earliest change, shown in Fig. 13.17A, is ulceration of the mucosa **(U)** with an overlying acute fibrinopurulent inflammatory exudate **(Ex)** and a purulent exudate **(P)** within the lumen. At this stage, the patient may experience vague central abdominal pain. As the condition progresses, the inflammation spreads through all layers of the wall of the appendix and the mucosal ulceration becomes more extensive (Fig. 13.17B). Few of the original mucosal glands **(G)** now remain intact and large numbers of neutrophils have infiltrated through the submucosa **(SM)** and muscle layer **(M)** to the serosa **(S)**, where at one point a fibrinous exudate **(F)** is beginning to form on the peritoneal surface. This *peritonitis*, involving the parietal peritoneum in the right iliac fossa, is responsible for the classic clinical features of acute appendicitis, with localisation of the pain to the right iliac fossa. The peritoneal exudate often spreads to cover most of the serosal surface of the appendix and the mesoappendix, even though the point at which the inflammation spreads through the appendix wall may remain localised. At high power, Fig. 13.17C shows the acute inflammatory infiltrate in the muscular layer of the wall of the appendix; the inflammatory infiltrate consists mainly of neutrophils **(N)**. The smooth muscle fibres **(Mu)** are separated by inflammatory oedema. Severe continuing inflammation of the appendix wall often leads to extensive necrosis of the muscle layer *(gangrenous appendicitis)*, which predisposes to perforation of the appendix with more widespread peritonitis. This feature can be seen in Fig. 13.17D where the muscle layer **(M)** is identifiable up to a point where it has undergone necrosis **(Ne)**. Perforation of the appendix is imminent and will almost certainly take place at this site. The pus **(P)** that fills the lumen will then be discharged into the peritoneal cavity, leading to a more severe and extensive peritonitis, which is infective. In the absence of appropriate treatment, the complications of perforation may ensue, including appendiceal abscess, subdiaphragmatic abscess, septicaemia, shock and death.

Diseases of the large intestine

The colon and rectum are subject to various viral, bacterial and parasitic infections that are usually short-lived and readily diagnosed by microbiological methods; important exceptions are *amoebic colitis* (see Fig. 5.22), and various infections in immunosuppressed individuals, which are often diagnosed in biopsy specimens. Of great importance is chronic inflammatory bowel disease, i.e. *ulcerative colitis* (Fig. 13.18) and Crohn's disease. Other causes of chronic diarrhoea include *microscopic colitis* (Fig. 13.19), radiation-induced colitis, ischaemic colitis and diverticulitis-associated colitis among others. Raised intraluminal pressure in the colon, probably as a result of a low residue diet, may lead to saccular herniation of mucosa through the muscle layers of the bowel wall; the diverticula so formed may become inflamed, giving rise to *diverticulitis* (Fig. 13.25), which may have serious sequelae. The large intestine may undergo infarction, either as a result of mesenteric artery occlusion by thrombus or embolus, or, more commonly, by venous infarction following hernial strangulation or *volvulus* (see Fig. 10.5).

Colonic polyps are very common. By far the most common is the *hyperplastic polyp* (Fig. 13.20), a benign lesion typically seen in the left colon and thought to have no malignant potential. Less common non-neoplastic polyps include *inflammatory pseudopolyps* as seen in ulcerative colitis (Fig. 13.18A) and polypoid hamartomas such as *Peutz-Jeghers' polyps*. Neoplastic benign polyps can be divided into two main groups: *conventional adenomas* and *serrated lesions*. The first of these groups is characterised by typical epithelial dysplasia and these lesions are well recognised as an important precursor of colorectal adenocarcinoma via the traditional *adenoma–carcinoma sequence*. These conventional adenomas are further classified according to their architecture as *tubular*, *villous* and *tubulovillous adenomas* (Fig. 13.21) and may show low or high grade epithelial dysplasia, reflecting their likely malignant potential. *Serrated lesions* (Fig 13.22 and 13.23). are a distinct group of polyps with some similarities in appearance to hyperplastic polyps, having star-shaped, irregular crypt outlines. The role of these lesions in colorectal carcinogenesis has been established more recently as these lesions generally lack typical cytological dysplasia. They are associated with specific defects in DNA mismatch repair and are linked to cancers in which there are high levels of *microsatellite instability* (see Ch. 1). Nomenclature for the polyps within this group continues to evolve but important subtypes include the *sessile serrated lesion* (sometimes called *sessile serrated polyp* or *sessile serrated adenoma*), the *sessile serrated lesion with dysplasia* and the *traditional serrated adenoma* (which shares some features of conventional adenoma but with serrated crypt architecture).

Malignant tumours of the colon and rectum are very common and almost all are *adenocarcinomas* (Fig. 13.24); most appear moderately differentiated with a clearly defined glandular pattern. The anal canal, lined by squamous epithelium, is occasionally the site of *squamous cell carcinoma* identical to squamous cell carcinomas at other sites (see Fig. 7.3), although local invasion of the anal canal by adenocarcinoma of the lower rectum also occurs.

KEY TO FIGURES
Ex inflammatory exudate   **F** fibrinous exudate   **G** glands   **M** muscularis propria   **Mu** smooth muscle fibres   **N** neutrophils   **Ne** necrosis   **P** pus   **S** serosa   **SM** submucosa   **U** ulceration

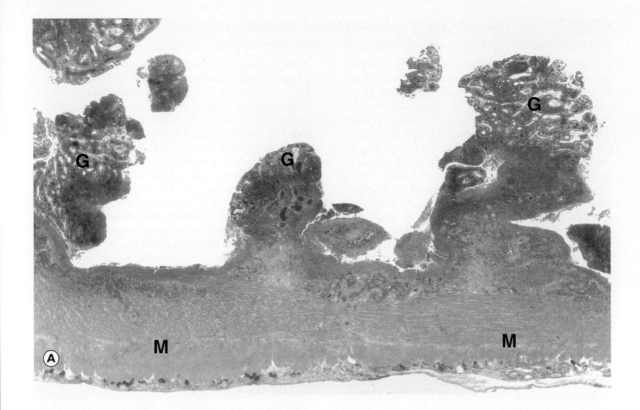

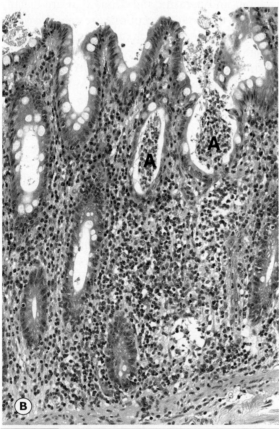

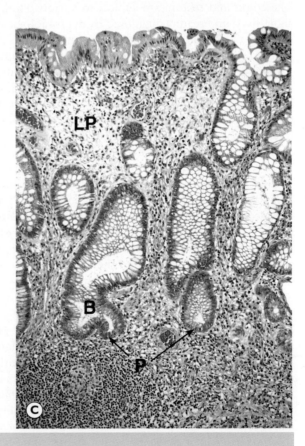

Fig. 13.18 **Ulcerative colitis.** *(Caption opposite)*

KEY TO FIGURES

A crypt abscess **B** branched crypt **C** collagen band **G** colonic glands **In** inflammation in lamina propria **L** intraepithelial lymphocytes **LP** lamina propria **M** muscularis propria **P** Paneth cell metaplasia

Fig. 13.18 Ulcerative colitis. (A) Active disease with pseudopolyp formation (LP); **(B)** acute disease (HP); **(C)** quiescent phase disease (HP). *(Illustrations opposite)*

Ulcerative colitis is a chronic relapsing inflammatory disease of unknown cause affecting the large bowel (E-Fig. 13.11**H**). The disease always involves the rectum but often extends proximally to involve the whole colon. It is sometimes accompanied by systemic features such as anaemia, arthritis and uveitis.

In active disease, there is acute inflammation of the mucosa with neutrophils accumulating in the lamina propria and in the lumina of the colonic glands (crypts) to form *crypt abscesses*; ulceration of the mucosa occurs, but the ulcers are superficial rather than fissured as in Crohn's disease (see Fig. 13.16). In severe cases, ulceration may develop extensively throughout the length of the colon as shown in Fig. 13.18A (E-Fig. 13.12**G**). Note that ulceration has destroyed much of the mucosa and submucosa in this field, leaving isolated islands of non-ulcerated mucosa, which is swollen by acute and chronic inflammatory changes; some of the colonic glands **(G)** remain. Non-ulcerated areas such as this project above the surrounding ulcerated areas to produce *inflammatory pseudopolyps*. Despite the severity and extent of the inflammation and ulceration, the changes are mainly confined to the mucosa and submucosa. The muscularis propria **(M)** is not involved. The inflammatory changes are rarely transmural, a useful

distinguishing feature from Crohn's disease. Fig. 13.18B illustrates features indicative of acute-on-chronic inflammatory activity, namely the presence of crypt abscesses **(A)** in the glands, depletion of mucus-containing goblet cells and the presence of neutrophils, as well as chronic inflammatory cells, in the lamina propria.

During quiescent periods between acute exacerbations, the mucosa damaged by earlier severe inflammation or ulceration shows mixed features of chronic inflammation and attempts at restitution. Fig. 13.18C shows a mucosal biopsy taken during a quiescent phase. The lamina propria **(LP)** is infiltrated by lymphocytes, plasma cells and eosinophils. The colonic glands usually show reduction in the numbers of mucin-secreting goblet cells (although that is not a major feature in this example) and there is mild reactive change in the epithelial cells. The crypts are shortened and often branched **(B)**. Paneth cell metaplasia **(P)** may be seen. Repeated episodes of inflammation, ulceration and epithelial regeneration may lead to dysplastic change in the constantly irritated epithelium. This factor may contribute to the high incidence of colonic adenocarcinoma arising in patients with a long history of ulcerative colitis.

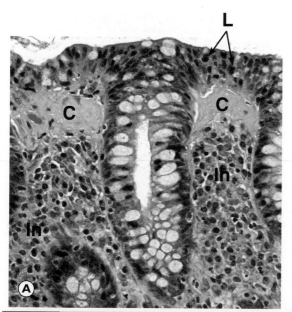

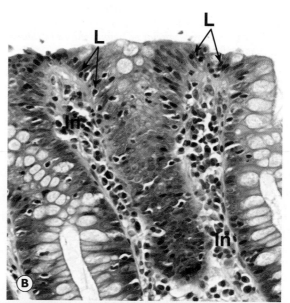

Fig. 13.19 Microscopic colitis. (A) Collagenous colitis (HP); **(B)** lymphocytic colitis (HP).

Microscopic colitis is the collective term for *collagenous* and *lymphocytic colitis*, conditions that typically cause watery, non-bloody diarrhoea with a normal-appearing bowel at colonoscopy. The two conditions have similarities but their exact relationship and aetiologies are unknown. There is a connection with autoimmune disease and coeliac disease in particular, and also with certain drugs, including H$_2$-receptor antagonists and non-steroidal anti-inflammatory drugs (NSAIDs). *Collagenous colitis*, found mainly in middle-aged and elderly women, is shown in Fig. 13.19A. It is characterised by a band of collagen **(C)** deposited immediately below the epithelial basement membrane. There is also inflammation **(In)** of the lamina

propria with occasional inflammatory cells and erythrocytes trapped within the collagen band. The surface epithelium contains increased numbers of intraepithelial lymphocytes **(L)**. The changes may be patchy throughout the colon and are generally least prominent in the distal colon and rectum.

Lymphocytic colitis, shown in Fig. 13.19B, occurs in both men and women and generally affects the whole colon. Typically, there is a marked increase in intraepithelial lymphocytes **(L)** in both the surface epithelium and glands, with degenerative change in the surface epithelium. There is also an inflammatory infiltrate **(In)** the lamina propria. The changes are similar to collagenous colitis, but without the collagen band.

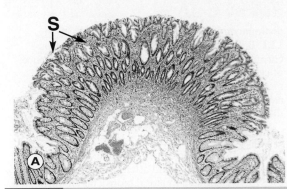

Fig. 13.20 **Hyperplastic polyp. (A)** LP; **(B)** MP.

Hyperplastic (metaplastic) polyps are very common in the large bowel. They are usually small, often multiple and occasionally bleed. They may coexist with neoplastic polyps and malignant tumours but most do not have malignant potential. An exception is the rare hereditary *hyperplastic polyposis syndrome*; these patients may develop invasive adenocarcinoma. At low

magnification, Fig. 13.20A shows a typical hyperplastic polyp, composed of crypts with a characteristic 'saw tooth' outline **(S)**; this is also seen at medium power in Fig. 13.20B. Apart from mild crowding, i.e. hyperplasia, the epithelial cells lining the crypts are very similar in appearance to normal colonic epithelium and exhibit no evidence of dysplasia.

Fig. 13.21 **Colonic adenomatous polyps. (A)** Tubular adenomas: polyposis coli (LP); **(B)** villous adenoma (MP); **(C)** tubulovillous adenoma (LP); **(D)** low grade tubular adenoma (MP); **(E)** low grade villous adenoma (HP); **(F)** high grade dysplasia (HP); **(G)** invasive adenocarcinoma in polyp (LP). *(Illustrations opposite)*

Classic adenomatous polyps (as distinct from the serrated type) in the large bowel show three main histological patterns: *tubular adenoma*, *villous adenoma* and *tubulovillous adenoma*.

Tubular adenomas are by far the most common type and usually have a pedicle or stalk of normal tissue connecting to the bowel wall (E-Fig. 13.13**G**). The adenoma consists of dysplastic colonic epithelium arranged in branched tubular glands. When seen with the naked eye, these tumours have a smooth or slightly bosselated surface. Tubular adenomas may be solitary or multiple. In one heritable condition known as *familial adenomatous polyposis (FAP)*, numerous tubular adenomas develop throughout the colon with a high rate of progression to adenocarcinoma. Fig. 13.21A shows two tubular adenomas **(T)** in a segment of colon from a patient with FAP. Note the darkly stained adenomatous masses connected to the underlying mucosa by stalks, which merely represent extensions of the normal mucosa and submucosa.

Villous adenomas, which are much less common, are usually sessile, that is to say they arise from a broad base (E-Fig. 13.14**G**). They are composed of narrow, frond-like outgrowths of epithelial cells supported by a delicate connective tissue stroma giving a papillary appearance both histologically and with the naked eye. A typical sessile villous adenoma is illustrated in Fig. 13.21B.

Tubulovillous adenomas exhibit intermediate features and contain at least 25%–50% villous architecture. In the example shown in Fig. 13.21C,

note that the stalk is covered by normal colonic-type mucosa that contrasts markedly with the densely staining dysplastic epithelium of the adenoma. Cytologically, all three types of adenoma show varying degrees of *dysplasia* ranging from low grade (Figs 13.21D and E) up to high grade (Fig. 13.21F).

Fig. 13.21E shows a high power view of low grade dysplasia in a colonic villous adenoma. The cells are enlarged and crowded with elongated, pseudostratified nuclei, increased nuclear to cytoplasmic ratio, and increased mitotic activity (see Fig. 7.13). Note in Figs 13.21D and E that the glandular architecture remains highly organised in low grade dysplasia. Fig. 13.21E shows high grade dysplasia, characterised by more complex gland architecture **(C)**, forming a cribriform (net-like) pattern with greater nuclear atypia and focal intraluminal necrosis **(N)**. By definition, adenomas exhibit no evidence of invasive carcinoma. However, although classified as benign, all adenomas have the potential to develop invasive adenocarcinoma. This occurs more frequently in villous adenomas than in the other types and is more likely with increasing size and high grade dysplasia.

Fig. 13.21G shows a very low magnification view of a large villous adenoma **(V)** in a resection specimen with invasive adenocarcinoma arising within it. Note the irregularly shaped malignant glands **(G)** that infiltrate the stalk of the polyp and extend into the underlying submucosa. This invasive adenocarcinoma had given rise to several lymph node metastases, which were identified within the colectomy specimen.

KEY TO FIGURES
C complex gland architecture   **G** malignant glands   **N** necrosis   **S** saw tooth outline   **T** tubular
adenoma   **V** villous adenoma

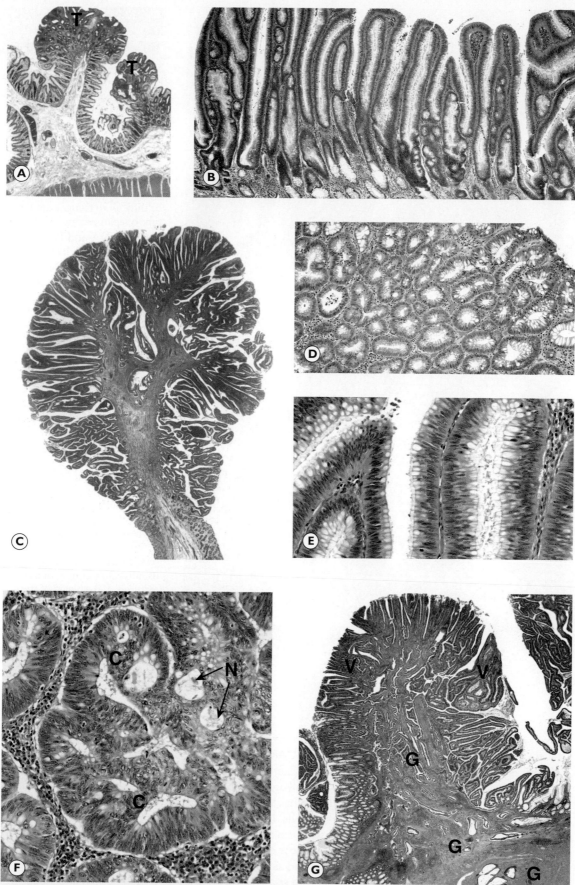

Fig. 13.21 **Colonic adenomatous polyps.** *(Caption opposite)*

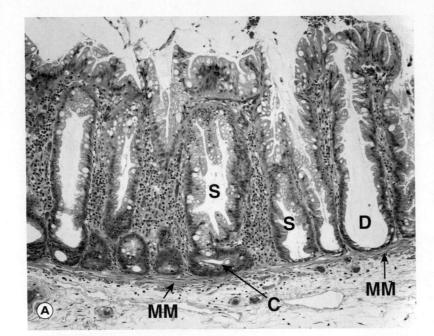

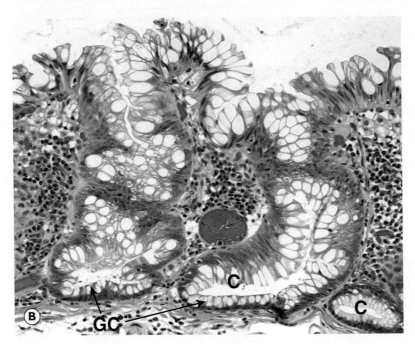

Fig. 13.22 **Serrated polyps.**
(A) Sessile serrated lesion (LP);
(B) sessile serrated lesion (HP).

Sessile serrated lesions are a relatively recently recognised type of polyp that appear quite similar to hyperplastic polyps (Fig. 13.20), having irregularly shaped, saw-tooth crypts with star-shaped outlines **(S)**. There is often a thick layer of mucus over the surface of the lesion and they can therefore be difficult to recognise at the time of colonoscopy. As shown in Fig 13.22A and B, they differ architecturally from hyperplastic polyps as the crypts typically appear dilated at their bases **(D)** and they may have branched L-shaped or inverted T-shaped forms, with some crypts **(C)** running parallel to the muscularis mucosae **(MM)**. Another typical histological feature is 'inverted maturation', illustrated in Fig. 13.22B. This term describes the fact that sessile serrated lesions often have numerous goblet cells **(GC)** in the bases of the crypts. This differs from other polyps and from normal mucosa as this part of the crypt would usually be the site of cell division. Taken together, all of these features are described as 'architectural dysplasia' but sessile serrated lesions do not usually show conventional cytological dysplasia of the sort illustrated in Fig. 13.21. The rare lesions which do show these architectural changes as well as cytological dysplasia are currently described using the term *sessile serrated lesion with dysplasia*.

MOLECULAR PATHWAYS TO COLORECTAL CARCINOMA

The recognition and investigation of various hereditary colorectal cancer syndromes such as familial adenomatous polyposis (FAP), hereditary non-polyposis colon cancer (HNPCC, also known as Lynch syndrome) and hyperplastic polyposis syndrome has led to huge advances in the understanding of the development of adenocarcinoma in the large bowel. It has long been understood that adenomas may develop into adenocarcinomas through the stepwise accumulation of genetic mutations. In the case of typical adenomas, the first step seems to be the loss of both copies of the *APC* gene. Individuals with FAP already have one copy of this gene inactivated as a germ line mutation (the 'first hit' according to Knudson's hypothesis; see Ch. 7); individuals with sporadic carcinomas must lose both copies to develop disease. Activation of the oncogene *KRAS* is also an early event, as is inactivation of *P53*.

A second, more recently discovered, pathway is the **serrated pathway**. In this pathway, serrated polyps with increasing degrees of dysplasia develop into invasive adenocarcinoma. Other characteristic features include increased DNA methylation and high levels of microsatellite instability (MSI-H) due to mutations in mismatch repair genes. This is a fast-advancing field and further pathways and subtypes of carcinoma are under investigation. Apart from the intrinsic fascination of these mechanisms, they may prove useful in determining optimal methods of treatment for different types of adenocarcinoma.

MOLECULAR DIAGNOSTIC TECHNIQUES IN COLORECTAL CARCINOMA

Around 15% of colorectal carcinomas show defects in their DNA mismatch repair machinery, either due to a germ line mutation in a mismatch repair gene (as seen in **Lynch syndrome**, an inherited disease associated with a high risk of colorectal and other malignancies, also known as **hereditary non-polyposis colorectal cancer, HNPCC**) or, in sporadic cases, due to epigenetic mechanisms such as *MLH1* gene promoter hypermethylation. These sporadic cases often also harbour a *BRAF* mutation.

These mutations can be detected using immunohistochemical methods (see Ch. 1), which demonstrate loss of expression of the protein products of the mismatch repair genes. The gene *MLH1* is paired with *PMS2* and the gene *MSH2* with *MSH6* and hence their loss of staining usually occurs in pairs (E-Fig. 13.15**H**). A molecular test for microsatellite instability can also be performed, with tumours described as 'MSI-high' or 'unstable' for a positive result.

Until recently, testing by clinical geneticists has typically been used to identify patients with Lynch syndrome/HNPCC but there is now growing recognition that a subset of sporadic cancers can have MSI and this is associated with a more favourable prognosis. It is therefore recommended that all colorectal cancer patients have their tumours tested, not only to check for Lynch syndrome but also to identify the cases with sporadic MSI, who have a better outcome but respond less well to 5-fluorouracil based chemotherapy regimens.

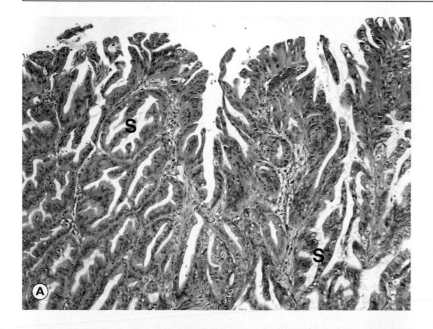

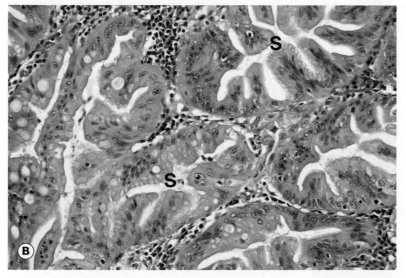

Fig. 13.23 Serrated polyps.
(A) Traditional serrated adenoma (LP); **(B)** traditional serrated adenoma (HP).

Traditional serrated adenomas are quite rare polyps that combine the presence of star-shaped, irregular crypt architecture alongside typical adenomatous dysplasia, similar to that seen in typical tubular and villous adenomas.

The low power image in Fig. 13.23A highlights the saw-tooth outlines of the crypts **(S)** but, in contrast to hyperplastic polyps and sessile serrated lesions, the lining epithelium shows obvious hyperchromasia due to enlarged, atypical nuclei. This dysplastic epithelium is shown at higher magnification in Fig. 13.23B. Note that the nuclei are large and vesicular and show pseudo-stratification, similar to that seen in conventional tubular and villous adenomas (see Fig. 13.21).

KEY TO FIGURES
C horizontal crypts **D** dilated crypt base **GC** goblet cells **MM** muscularis mucosae **S** saw tooth outline

TARGETED THERAPIES FOR COLORECTAL CANCER

As described above, cancers with microsatellite instability respond poorly to chemotherapy using conventional 5-FU based regimens. *BRAF* sequencing is part of the molecular test for MSI as it identifies spontaneous mutations and is also a poor prognostic marker. Testing for mutations in *EGFR* and *KRAS* is also useful in guiding therapy and predicting prognosis. Patients with mutations in *KRAS* are typically treated with standard chemotherapy, whilst those with wild-type *KRAS* benefit from the addition of antibody-based drugs such as cetuximab that act to inhibit the epidermal growth factor receptor.

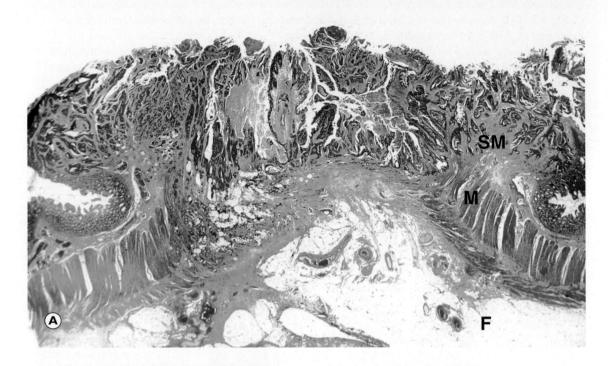

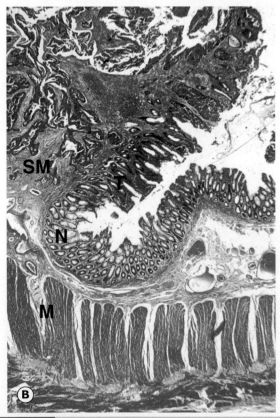

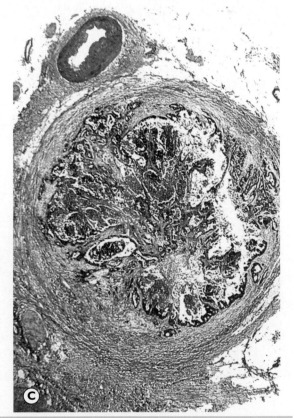

Fig. 13.24 **Adenocarcinoma of the colon.** *(Caption opposite)*

Fig. 13.24 Adenocarcinoma of the colon. (A) Invasive tumour (LP); (B) edge of lesion in (A) (MP); (C) invasion of vein (MP). *(Illustrations opposite)*

Adenocarcinoma of the large intestine is a common malignant tumour, arising most frequently in the sigmoid colon and the rectum. There are three common macroscopic patterns of growth; tumours may consist of a central ulcer with raised margins, some tumours may infiltrate the entire circumference of the bowel forming an annular stricture, or they may develop as a protuberant cauliflower-like (exophytic) mass, most commonly seen in the caecum and proximal colon (E-Fig. 13.16**G**).

Fig. 13.24A shows an ulcerated adenocarcinoma of the rectum; the tumour has infiltrated deeply through the submucosa (**SM**), muscularis propria (**M**) and out into the mesorectal fat (**F**). Fig. 13.24B shows the raised, everted edge of this tumour at higher magnification. There is an abrupt transition between normal rectal mucosa (**N**) and the malignant tumour epithelium (**T**). In this area, the tumour has infiltrated into the submucosa (**SM**), but not the muscularis propria (**M**). Fig. 13.24C shows a vein in the serosa of the colon; it is filled with colonic adenocarcinoma, which is growing along it as a solid cord. Venous invasion of this sort is associated with a high risk of tumour spread to the liver. The tumour cells pass via the portal venous system and may lodge in the liver

microcirculation where they give rise to new metastatic deposits of adenocarcinoma (see Fig. 7.16).

The prognosis of colonic and rectal carcinomas depends on a number of factors, the most important being tumour *stage* as assessed by the depth of invasion of the bowel wall, the presence of lymph node and distant metastases and evidence of tumour invasion into veins and lymphatics. Staging is vital for optimal management of all tumours. *Dukes' classification* has been in general use for staging colorectal carcinomas since 1932. This system, initially applied to rectal tumours only, divides tumours into three stages designated A to C. In *Dukes' stage A*, the tumour is confined to the bowel wall. If the tumour extends into the pericolic fat, it is classified as *Dukes' stage B* and the presence of metastases in lymph nodes automatically classifies it as *Dukes' stage C*. However, the more detailed TNM staging system is often used in conjunction with or instead of the Dukes' classification. In addition, features such as grade, circumferential margin involvement, venous invasion and number of positive lymph nodes are used to help determine whether additional chemotherapy is required.

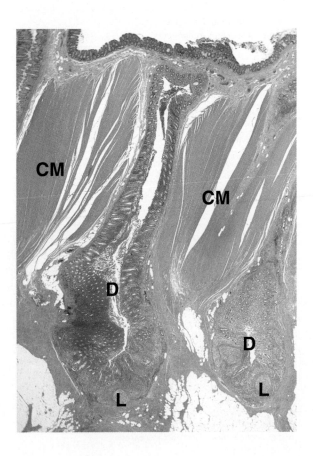

Fig. 13.25 Diverticular disease (LP).

Diverticular disease is a common condition in the elderly; it may involve any part of the colon although the sigmoid colon is the most frequently and most severely affected part.

The normal muscular wall of the colon consists of an inner circular layer and a discontinuous outer longitudinal layer represented by the *taeniae coli*. Diverticula are formed by herniation of pouches of colonic mucosa (**D**), including mucosal lymphoid tissue (**L**), through unsupported areas of the circular muscle between the taeniae coli. The diverticula bulge towards the serosal surface and often contain faecal material (E-Fig. 13.17**G**). This probably results from abnormally high intraluminal pressure associated with low residue diets and subsequent constipation. A characteristic histological feature is marked hypertrophy of the circular muscle layer (**CM**).

Acute inflammation, *diverticulitis*, may develop following obstruction of the narrow neck of a diverticulum. Complications include acute haemorrhage, perforation, peritonitis, paracolic abscess formation and fistula formation with other viscera such as bladder and vagina. Diverticulosis-associated colitis may mimic ulcerative colitis but tends to be localised to the area adjacent to the openings of the diverticula.

KEY TO FIGURES
CM circular muscle layer   **D** diverticulum   **F** perirectal fat   **L** lymphoid tissue   **M** muscularis propria   **N** normal rectal mucosa   **SM** submucosa   **T** tumour

Table 13.1 Chapter review.

Disorder	Clinical presentation	Main features	Figure
Mouth and oropharynx			
Squamous cell carcinoma	Non-healing ulcer, erythro-plakia, leukoplakia	Nests of epithelial cells with eosinophilic cytoplasm, intercellular bridges, squamous pearls, keratinisation	13.1
HPV-associated oropharyngeal carcinoma	Often tonsillar ulcer or mass Younger age group; associated with high risk HPV; better prognosis.	Typically basaloid squamous cell carcinoma with small, dark cells and abrupt keratinisation. *P16* positive	13.2
Salivary glands			
Sialadenitis	Pain and swelling, often after food if there is a calculus Mainly submandibular	Chronic inflammatory cell infiltrate, fibrosis, atrophy of gland tissue	13.3
Pleomorphic adenoma	Painless swelling, mainly parotid	Mixed epithelial and connective tissue components	13.4A
Basal cell adenoma	Painless swelling, often male smokers, mainly parotid	Epithelial cells forming nests, trabeculae and glands	13.4B
Warthin's tumour	Painless swelling, may be cystic, almost exclusively parotid	Glandular element consisting of tall columnar cells with lymphoid tissue, including reactive germinal centres	13.5
Adenoid cystic carcinoma	Initial painless swelling, later nerve pain	Epithelial cells arranged in cribriform pattern with hyalinised, fibrotic stroma, perineural invasion common	13.6
Mucoepidermoid carcinoma	Painless swelling, usually parotid or minor glands	Mixed squamous and glandular (mucus- producing) components	13.7
Oesophagus			
Barrett's oesophagus	Heartburn	Metaplastic glandular (intestinal) epithelium at lower end of oesophagus	13.8A
Dysplasia	Heartburn	Atypical epithelial cells with pleomorphic nuclei, architectural distortion, increased mitotic activity	13.8B and C
Carcinoma	Obstruction, dysphagia	May be squamous cell carcinoma or adenocarcinoma	Like 7.3 Like 13.8D and E
Stomach			
Chronic gastritis – *H. pylori* associated	Dyspepsia, haemorrhage	Chronic inflammation of lamina propria with neutrophils infiltrating glands, *H. pylori* in surface mucus	13.9A and B, 4.2
Chronic gastritis – autoimmune type	Megaloblastic (macrocytic) anaemia	Atrophic body of stomach with reduction or absence of parietal cells, intestinal metaplasia	13.9C
Chronic gastritis – reflux or chemical type	Dyspepsia, haemorrhage	Foveolar hyperplasia of glands with saw tooth outline, minimal inflammation, smooth muscle bundles in lamina propria	13.9D
Peptic ulceration (E-Fig. 13.5**G**)	Dyspepsia, haemorrhage, perforation	Discontinuity of epithelial surface with necrotic slough, granulation tissue and fibrosis lining the defect	13.10
Gastric dysplasia	Dyspepsia	Atypical epithelial cells with pleomorphic nuclei, architectural distortion, increased mitotic activity	13.11
Gastric carcinoma – intestinal type	Dyspepsia, weight loss abdominal pain, anaemia	Atypical invasive glands with atypical epithelial cells, mucus production	13.12A and B
Gastric carcinoma – diffuse type (E-Fig. 13.7**G**)	Dyspepsia, weight loss abdominal pain, anaemia	Malignant signet ring cells forming sheets with no gland formation (linitis plastica appearance)	13.12C and D

Table 13.1 Chapter review—cont'd.

Disorder	Clinical presentation	Main features	Figure
Small intestine			
Coeliac disease	Anaemia, weight loss, steatorrhoea	Blunting/flattening of small bowel villi, increased lymphocytes and plasma cells in the lamina propria, increased intraepithelial lymphocytes, crypt hyperplasia	13.15
Giardiasis	Diarrhoea, steatorrhoea	Mucosa normal or inflamed with villous atrophy, sickle-shaped parasitic *Giardia lamblia* organisms on epithelial surface	5.19
Appendix			
Acute appendicitis	Right iliac fossa pain, fever, vomiting	Ulceration of mucosa, transmural acute inflammatory infiltrate	13.17
Enterobius vermicularis (pinworm)	Incidental finding	Pinworm sections seen within lumen of appendix	5.24
Large intestine			
Microscopic colitis (lymphocytic and collagenous colitis)	Watery, non-bloody diarrhoea with normal colonoscopy	Subtle inflammation of lamina propria, increased lymphocytes and apoptotic bodies in epithelium, subepithelial collagen band n collagenous subtype	13.19
Ulcerative colitis (E-Fig. 13.12**G**)	Bloody diarrhoea, pain, fever, toxic megacolon	Inflammation and ulceration of mucosa, crypt abscesses, distortion of crypt architecture	13.18
Diverticular disease (E-Fig. 13.17**G**)	Altered bowel habit, pain in left iliac fossa, rectal bleeding, often asymptomatic	Herniation of mucosa through muscularis propria with surrounding inflammation and fibrosis	13.25
Hyperplastic polyp	Incidental finding, bleeding	Polypoid glandular lesion with saw tooth architecture but no dysplasia	13.20
Tubular adenoma (E-Fig. 13.13**G**)	Incidental finding, bleeding	Polyp, usually with stalk, glandular architecture with variable dysplasia	13.21A
Villous adenoma (E-Fig. 13.14**G**)	Incidental finding, bleeding	Polyp, usually sessile, villous architecture with variable dysplasia	13.21B
Tubulovillous adenoma	Incidental finding, bleeding	Polyp, glandular and villous architecture with variable dysplasia	13.21C
Serrated lesions	Incidental finding, bleeding	Polypoid glandular lesion with saw tooth architecture and variable dysplasia	13.22, 13.23
Adenocarcinoma (E-Fig. 13.16**G**)	Haemorrhage, obstruction, anaemia	Invasive glands with atypical epithelial cells, mucus production, 'dirty' necrosis in lumina	13.24
Various sites throughout GI tract			
Gastrointestinal stromal tumour (GIST)	GI haemorrhage, mass lesion, incidental finding, usually stomach or small intestine	Mainly spindle cells in collagenous stroma, less commonly epithelioid or pleomorphic	13.14
Neuroendocrine tumour	Usually incidental finding, commonly appendix, or small bowel obstruction, rarely carcinoid syndrome	Small uniform cells with round nuclei, stippled chromatin and pinkish, granular cytoplasm. High grade forms include small cell carcinoma	13.13
Crohn's disease (E-Fig. 13.9**G**)	Diarrhoea, weight loss, obstruction, fistula formation, usually small bowel/colon but can affect mouth to anus	Transmural inflammation, granulomas, fibrosis, fissuring ulceration, skip lesions	13.16

14 Liver and pancreaticobiliary system

Disorders of the liver

The liver is affected by a wide range of disorders, the most important of which are listed below. The liver performs many different metabolic functions and liver disease produces diverse clinical symptoms and signs. The pathophysiology of the more common symptoms and signs is described in Table 14.1.

■ **Acute hepatic necrosis** has been described in Ch. 2. This usually results from exposure to certain drugs or poisons or occurs as part of a fulminant viral infection.

■ **Acute hepatitis** has many causes. It may resolve or become persistent *(chronic hepatitis)*.

■ **Chronic hepatitis** is diagnosed when biochemical manifestations of liver cell damage have persisted for more than 6 months. It may eventually progress to cirrhosis.

■ **Cirrhosis** is the end stage of various types of liver disease in which there is liver cell loss and architectural distortion over a long period. It is characterised by destruction of normal liver architecture, which is replaced by regenerative nodules of hepatocytes separated by bands of fibrous tissue. There may be evidence of continuing active damage to liver cells. Eventually, liver function is impaired or fails totally *(chronic liver failure)*. The distortion of vascular architecture leads to *portal hypertension.* Various different types of cirrhosis are illustrated and discussed in Fig. 14.5.

■ **Malignant disease** frequently involves the liver, most commonly as metastatic spread, especially from primary lesions in the gut, breast and lung (see Fig. 7.16). Less frequently, the liver becomes diffusely infiltrated in haematolymphoid malignancies such as Hodgkin and non-Hodgkin lymphomas.

■ **Primary malignancy** of the liver, *hepatocellular carcinoma* (Fig. 14.7), is uncommon and most often arises where there is pre-existing cirrhosis.

■ **Right-sided cardiac failure** involves the liver when raised venous pressure is transmitted to the central hepatic venules, resulting in congestion of the sinusoids with blood. Hepatocytes in the centrilobular area (zone 3 of the liver acinus) may then undergo atrophy or even frank necrosis.

■ **Inborn errors of metabolism**, often reflecting single gene defects, can result in the abnormal accumulation of various metabolites within hepatocytes. These are known as *storage diseases* and include *glycogen storage diseases*, *mucopolysaccharidoses*, *lipidoses*, *haemochromatosis* (Fig. 14.6) and *Wilson's disease.* Liver biopsy may be useful in the diagnosis of such disorders.

Table 14.1 Clinical features of hepatobiliary diseases and their pathophysiology.

Sign/Symptom	Clinical feature	Mechanism
Jaundice	Yellow discolouration of tissues owing to bile pigments	Failure of metabolism or excretion of bile
Bleeding	Easy bruising and prolonged clotting time of blood	Failure of hepatic synthesis of clotting factors
Oedema	Swelling of dependent parts owing to extracellular accumulation of water	Failure of hepatic synthesis of albumin resulting in reduced plasma oncotic pressure
Ascites	Fluid in peritoneal cavity	Low serum albumin and portal hypertension
Gynaecomastia	Enlarged male breasts	Failure to detoxify endogenous oestrogens
Encephalopathy	Altered consciousness, lack of coordination, may lead to coma	Failure to detoxify ammonia and excitatory amino acids which result from protein breakdown
Haematemesis and/or melaena	Vomiting blood and passing blood	Bleeding from oesophageal varices or per rectum owing to portal hypertension

KEY TO FIGURES
C Councilman bodies   **H** hydropic degeneration   **In** inflammatory cells

Acute inflammation of the liver

Hepatocytes (E-Fig. 14.1**H**), with their high degree of metabolic activity, are readily disturbed by toxins and demonstrate the histological cellular responses known as ballooning, fatty change and necrosis as described in Ch. 2. Acute inflammation of the liver parenchyma is usually marked by focal accumulation of inflammatory cells, usually in relation to necrotic hepatocytes. The exception to this is in the formation of **hepatic abscesses**, which usually develop either as a result of bacterial infections from the biliary tract or from a septic focus in the abdomen drained by the portal venous system to the liver.

Acute hepatitis is a general term for inflammation of the liver parenchyma, which can then be further classified according to aetiology. The four most important groups of conditions causing acute hepatitis are:

■ **Viral hepatitis:** This is illustrated in Fig. 14.1 and its various subtypes are outlined in Table 14.2.

■ **Toxins:** Alcohol is the most common hepatic toxin (Fig. 14.2).

■ **Drugs:** Hepatitis may be caused by the anaesthetic gas halothane, particularly after repeated exposure. Isoniazid, a drug commonly used in the treatment of tuberculosis, results in acute hepatitis in a small proportion of cases. Many other drugs occasionally cause hepatitis.

■ **Systemic infections:** Infections caused by *Leptospira* and *Toxoplasma* usually involve the liver as part of disseminated disease. Other systemic infections may cause multiple minute infective lesions as in bacterial septicaemia and miliary tuberculosis (see Fig. 5.7).

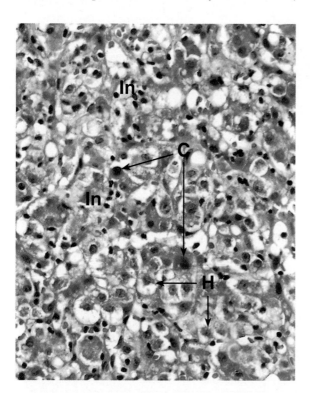

Fig. 14.1 **Acute viral hepatitis (HP).**

The viral agents causing acute hepatitis all produce a similar histological picture in the acute phase.

There is widespread swelling and ballooning of hepatocytes owing to hydropic degeneration (**H**) and this progresses to focal or **spotty necrosis** throughout the lobule. The areas of necrosis are identified by aggregates of inflammatory cells (**In**) surrounding eosinophilic (pink stained) bodies called **Councilman bodies** (**C**), representing the cytoplasm of necrotic liver cells. The Kupffer cells are very active and, within portal tracts, there are increased numbers of chronic inflammatory cells (not illustrated here).

In time, regeneration of the dead hepatocytes occurs. In hepatitis A and E, complete resolution is the rule, but in hepatitis B, C and D, activity may persist or the disease may progress to chronic hepatitis (Fig. 14.3).

Rare cases of viral hepatitis occur in which there is massive liver necrosis instead of the focal type seen here. This is particularly seen with hepatitis E in pregnancy. Such fulminant cases are usually fatal.

Table 14.2 **Viral causes of hepatitis.**

Virus Type	Mode of transmission	Acute hepatitis	Chronic hepatitis	Chronic carrier	Notes
Hep A	Faecal-oral	Yes	No	No	Mild, self-limiting (rarely fulminant)
Hep B	Blood, saliva, semen	Yes	Yes	Yes	Transmission - needle sharing, sexual, transfusion
Hep C	Blood, saliva, semen	Yes	Yes	Yes	Transmission - needle sharing, sexual, transfusion
Hep D	Blood, saliva, semen	Yes	Yes	Yes	Only in association with hepatitis B
Hep E	Faecal-oral	Yes	No	No	Usually mild, self-limiting (rarely fulminant)

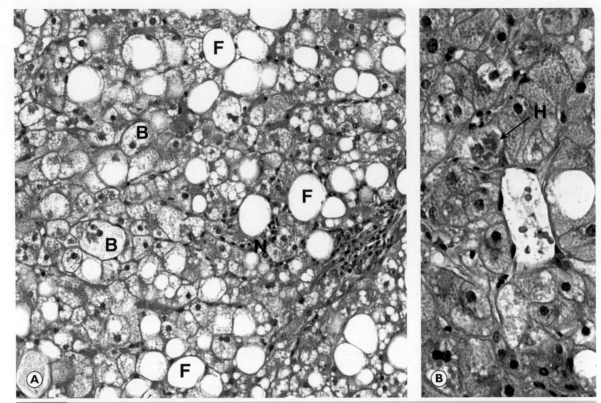

Fig. 14.2 **Alcoholic hepatitis. (A)** MP; **(B)** HP.

Alcohol is a potent hepatotoxin when taken in large quantities and liver changes occur even after isolated bouts of heavy drinking. Early evidence of metabolic injury to the hepatocytes is the appearance of *steatosis* or *fatty change* (F), manifest by the accumulation of lipid in the form of large cytoplasmic vacuoles within some hepatocytes, usually displacing the nucleus to one side (see Fig. 2.4). With more severe metabolic disruption, the hepatocytes undergo hydropic degeneration (see Fig. 2.5) and become swollen and vacuolated, an appearance described as *ballooning degeneration* (B). In some cases, the metabolic disruption may be irreversible and some hepatocytes undergo necrosis. The location of necrotic hepatocytes (N) is marked by foci of neutrophils and lymphocytes. This is illustrated at high magnification in Fig. 14.2B. Some hepatocytes accumulate an eosinophilic material, derived from cytokeratin intermediate filaments, termed *Mallory's hyaline* (H). This material forms irregular cytoplasmic globules, usually near the

nucleus, and stains a glassy pink colour, which is slightly darker than the normal cytoplasm. The hepatocytes around the centrilobular veins appear to be most vulnerable to alcohol toxicity and, in some individuals, delicate fibrosis may be seen around the central veins and perivenular hepatocytes.

With prolonged alcohol abuse, there is progressive fibrosis because of hepatocyte necrosis and regeneration of liver cells and this can develop into alcoholic cirrhosis (Fig. 14.5A). Fatty change, alcoholic hepatitis and hepatic cirrhosis may all occur in the same individual. Some individuals develop recurrent alcoholic hepatitis and are likely to proceed to cirrhosis, whilst others may develop cirrhosis insidiously with no preceding episodes of acute hepatitis. Reversible fatty change may occur in a healthy individual after a single drinking binge. The presence of fatty change in a known alcoholic is an indicator of continuing alcohol intake.

NON-ALCOHOLIC FATTY LIVER DISEASE
This is a relatively common disorder that closely resembles alcoholic liver disease, but which occurs in the absence of excessive alcohol intake. It is often diagnosed incidentally due to the discovery of deranged liver function tests upon routine blood testing. Patients may have no symptoms or clinical signs of liver disease at the time of diagnosis. It is thought that this process may account for a large proportion of patients who present with cirrhosis or end-stage liver disease without any preceding history of overt liver pathology (a pattern of disease often referred to as *cryptogenic cirrhosis*).

Of interest, epidemiological studies suggest that non-alcoholic fatty liver disease is very prevalent in developed country populations and it is strongly associated with other common metabolic disorders such as obesity, dyslipidaemia, impaired glucose tolerance and non-insulin dependent diabetes mellitus. Like alcoholic liver disease, there is a spectrum of pathological changes from simple steatosis through *non-alcoholic steatohepatitis* (known as *NASH*) to eventual hepatic fibrosis and cirrhosis. Clearly, given the morphological similarity to alcohol-related liver disease, this diagnosis can only be made after correlation of the clinical and pathological findings.

KEY TO FIGURES
B ballooning degeneration   **F** fatty change   **H** Mallory's hyaline   **N** necrosis

When inflammation of the liver continues without improvement for 6 months or more, the condition is described as *chronic hepatitis*. Conventionally, this term excludes chronic inflammation of the liver caused by alcohol, bacterial agents and biliary obstruction. The main causes of chronic hepatitis are summarised below:

■ **Viral infection**
  – *Hepatitis B*: chronic hepatitis occurs in ~ 5%–10% of cases (but ~80% if hepatitis D superinfection)
  – *Hepatitis C*: chronic hepatitis occurs in ~85% of cases
  – Other hepatitis viruses
■ **Autoimmune disease**
  – *Autoimmune hepatitis*
    • Usually occurs in middle-aged women
    • Positive serum auto-antibodies (anti-nuclear antibodies, anti-smooth muscle antibodies)
    • Often associated with other auto-immune diseases, e.g. rheumatoid arthritis, thyroid disease.
  – *Primary biliary cirrhosis*
    • Usually occurs in middle aged women
    • Positive anti-mitochondrial antibodies in most patients
    • Autoimmune destruction of intrahepatic bile ducts
    • Despite name, cirrhosis occurs only with end-stage disease
  – *Primary sclerosing cholangitis*
    • Usually young or middle-aged, more common in men
    • Strongly associated with inflammatory bowel disease
    • Fibrous obliteration of intrahepatic and extrahepatic bile ducts
■ **Toxic/metabolic**
  – *Wilson's disease*: disorder of copper metabolism with CNS effects *(hepatolenticular degeneration)*
  – *α1-Antitrypsin deficiency*: protease inhibitor deficiency causing chronic lung and liver damage
  – *Drug-induced hepatitis*: many causes and various histological patterns

Histologically, chronic hepatitis is characterised by:
■ The presence of inflammatory cells (mainly lymphocytes) in portal tracts (E-Fig. 14.2 **H**) or scattered within the liver lobules, or both.
■ Necrosis of hepatocytes, either concentrated upon the *limiting plate* of hepatocytes around the portal tracts (*interface hepatitis*, previously called *piecemeal necrosis*) or scattered within the liver lobules (*lobular hepatitis*, previously called *spotty necrosis*), or both.
■ The presence of fibrosis, either in the portal tracts, or extending from the portal areas into the adjacent parenchyma as short septa, or forming 'bridges' across the lobular structure, causing architectural distortion.
■ Assessment of these features can be used to determine how active the disease is (*grade* of chronic hepatitis) and how far the disease has progressed (*stage* of disease). The general principles of grading and staging are outlined below.

STAGING AND GRADING OF CHRONIC HEPATITIS

Various scoring systems have been devised for grading and staging hepatitis. These aim to give information about appropriate treatment and likely disease prognosis. In this context, **grade** is used to reflect the severity of any ongoing inflammation or necrosis. The extent of such damage can be assessed within portal areas and within the liver lobule. When there is significant inflammation, drug treatment may be initiated to reduce continuing liver damage and to prevent the development of progressive disease with fibrosis.

Stage is a means of assessing the degree of damage to the connective tissue framework of the liver. Fibrosis tends to begin within the portal areas and fine septa then extend out into the parenchyma. Eventually, if disease continues to progress, bands of collagen form between adjacent portal tracts, dividing the liver parenchyma into distorted nodules and culminating in **cirrhosis**.

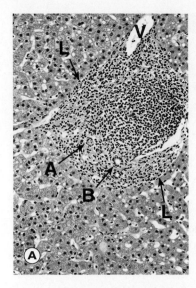

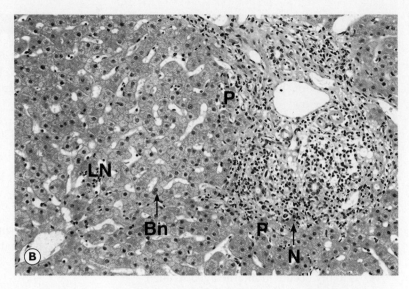

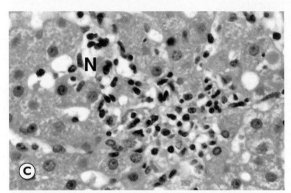

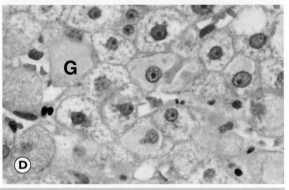

Fig. 14.3 **Chronic hepatitis.** **(A)** LP; **(B)** MP; **(C)** HP; **(D)** HP.

Fig. 14.3A shows inflammation confined to a portal tract. The periportal hepatocytes, called the *limiting plate* **(L),** show no necrosis. The bile duct **(B),** the artery **(A)** and vein **(V)** are easily seen. This corresponds to low grade disease. In contrast, Fig. 14.3B shows higher grade disease. Inflammation and necrosis extend out from the portal tract to involve periportal hepatocytes **(P),** which show necrosis **(N).** This pattern is described as *interface hepatitis.* In addition to changes around the portal tract, there is necrosis of individual hepatocytes in the liver lobule **(LN),** a feature described as *lobular hepatitis.* This is shown in Figs 14.3B and C. Regeneration of liver cells may be seen, reflected in binucleate cells **(Bn)** or liver cell plates two cells wide. In more severe cases, liver cell necrosis and inflammation may become confluent

to form bands of *bridging necrosis* extending between adjacent portal tracts.

If disease progresses, there is fibrosis in the liver, with continued liver cell regeneration that ultimately leads to cirrhosis.

In chronic hepatitis caused by hepatitis B virus, the cytoplasm of hepatocytes may assume a pale pink, *ground-glass* appearance **(G),** seen in Fig. 14.3D, caused by accumulation of viral proteins. In hepatitis C infection, lymphoid follicles and focal fatty change may be a clue to diagnosis.

Previous classifications have used the terms chronic persistent and chronic aggressive hepatitis. These are no longer used. Current classifications define chronic hepatitis in terms of aetiology and histological grade.

CHRONIC VIRAL HEPATITIS
On a global scale, chronic viral hepatitis is an important public health problem. Both hepatitis B and hepatitis C may give rise to symptomatic chronic hepatitis or to an asymptomatic carrier state. Normally, when hepatitis B is acquired in adulthood, the risk of chronic viral carriage is around 1%–10%. In the developing world, transmission of hepatitis is commonly from mother to child *(vertical transmission)*. This is important because when infection occurs at the time of childbirth, chronic carriage will occur in 90%–95% of cases. These patients may develop chronic liver fibrosis with eventual cirrhosis. Cirrhosis is a major risk factor for the development of *hepatocellular carcinoma* and in some areas where hepatitis B infection is highly prevalent, hepatocellular carcinoma (a rare tumour in most developed countries) is the most common form of malignancy.

KEY TO FIGURE
A artery   **B** bile duct   **Bn** binucleate cell   **C** chronic inflammation   **D** bile ductules   **F** fibrosis
G ground glass hepatocytes   **Gr** granuloma   **L** limiting plate   **LN** lobular necrosis   **N** necrosis
P periportal hepatocytes   **V** vein

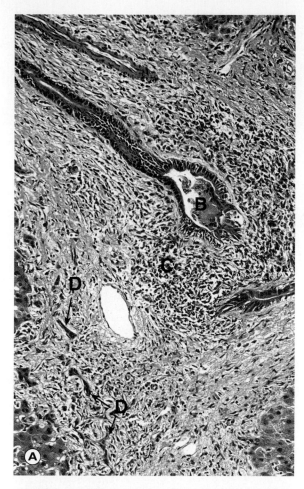

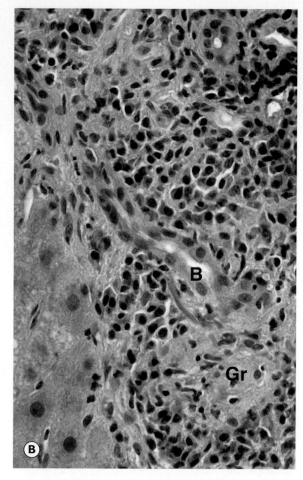

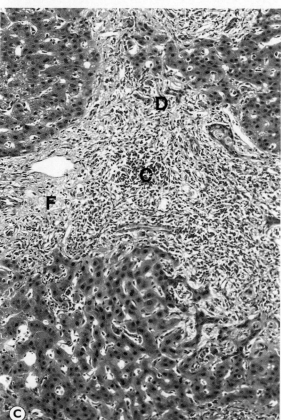

Fig. 14.4 **Primary biliary cirrhosis. (A)** Early lesion (MP); **(B)** granuloma (HP); **(C)** later lesion (MP).

Primary biliary cirrhosis is a chronic inflammatory disease of the liver in which destructive inflammatory changes are centred primarily on bile ducts (E-Fig. 14.3**H**). The earliest changes are seen in the epithelium of the larger bile ducts **(D)** as shown in Fig. 14.4A. There is vacuolation of the epithelial cells and infiltration of the wall and surrounding tissues by lymphocytes. A characteristic feature at this stage is the formation of *histiocytic granulomas* **(Gr)** in relation to damaged bile ducts, illustrated in Fig. 14.4B. Portal tracts then become expanded by chronic inflammatory cells **(C)**.

As seen in Fig. 14.4C, the inflammatory cells extend from the portal tracts into the liver parenchyma, resulting in *interface hepatitis* (previously called *piecemeal necrosis*), occurring along the limiting plate in a manner similar to chronic hepatitis (Fig. 14.3). As liver cells are destroyed, the portal tracts also become expanded by fibrosis **(F)**. Large bile ducts are no longer visible, having been destroyed. At the periphery of the portal tracts, there is proliferation of small bile ductules **(D)**, which do not appear to be canalised. This feature is best seen in Fig. 14.4A.

If primary biliary cirrhosis proceeds unchecked, true cirrhosis develops (Fig. 14.5). Note that this disease is referred to as primary biliary cirrhosis even in its earlier stages when there is no evidence of cirrhotic change.

BASIC SYSTEMS PATHOLOGY ■ LIVER AND PANCREATICOBILIARY SYSTEM

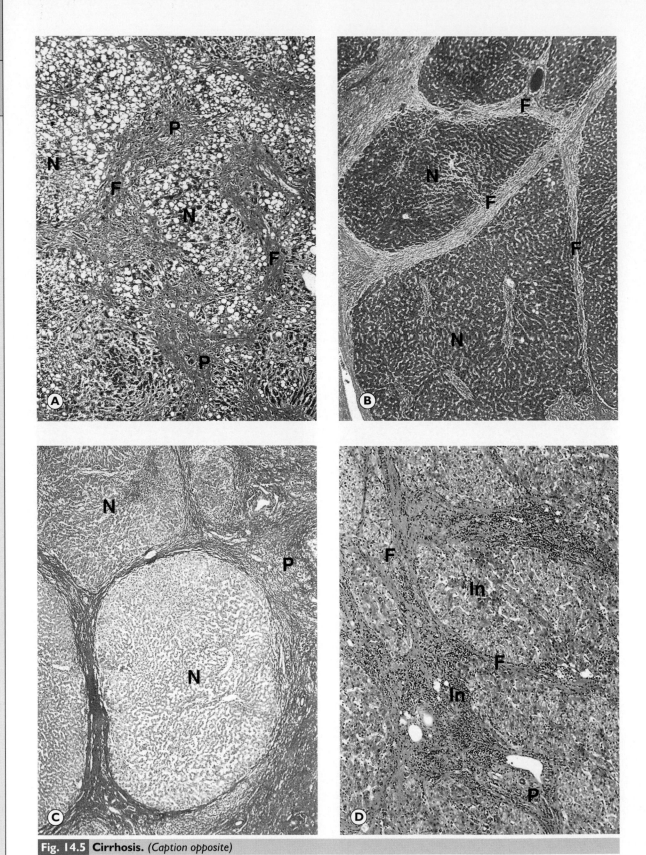

Fig. 14.5 Cirrhosis. *(Caption opposite)*

KEY TO FIGURES
F fibrous tissue   **In** inflammation   **N** nodule   **P** portal area

Fig. 14.5 Cirrhosis. **(A)** Alcoholic cirrhosis **(MP)**; **(B)** cryptogenic cirrhosis **(MP)**; **(C)** cryptogenic cirrhosis (van Gieson stain) **(MP)**; **(D)** cirrhosis due to progressive chronic hepatitis **(MP)**. *(Illustrations opposite)*

Cirrhosis is the end result of continued damage to liver cells from a great many causes. It is characterised by wholesale disruption of the liver architecture (E-Fig. 14.4**H**) with the formation of nodules of regenerating liver cells separated by fibrous bands. There are two main effects of this altered liver architecture and cellular damage, namely disordered hepatocyte function (Table 14.1) and disturbance of blood flow through the liver from portal vein to hepatic vein.

The effect of vascular obstruction within the liver is an increase in portal venous pressure termed *portal hypertension*. Anastomoses open up between the portal circulation and the systemic venous system, resulting in large, dilated veins called *varices*. The most important site of *varices* is in the lower oesophagus, but they can occur elsewhere. These dilated thin-walled veins are liable to rupture and this is a common fatal event in patients with cirrhosis.

The classification of cirrhosis is based on the disease that caused the underlying liver damage. The most important causes are chronic alcohol abuse, chronic hepatitis and biliary cirrhosis (primary and secondary to obstruction). In a small percentage of cases, no underlying disease can be found. This is known as *cryptogenic cirrhosis* (see clinical box 'Non-alcoholic fatty liver disease').

The diagnosis of cirrhosis is confirmed by percutaneous liver biopsy. Histological examination is directed towards identifying the nature of any underlying disease process, as well as establishing evidence of cirrhosis. In Fig. 14.5A, the features of cirrhosis are broad fibrous bands **(F)** connecting portal areas **(P)** and intervening nodules **(N)** of liver cells showing marked fatty change. This is an example of alcoholic cirrhosis. Fig. 14.5B shows a typical cirrhotic pattern, with bands of fibrous tissue **(F)** disrupting the lobular architecture. Here, there is no inflammation,

fatty change or specific features. If there are also no clinical pointers to the aetiology, this is classified as cryptogenic cirrhosis. Fig. 14.5C is from the same patient, this time stained using the van Gieson method, which emphasises the fibrosis (stained red).

Cirrhosis following progressive chronic hepatitis is illustrated in Fig. 14.5D. The portal tracts **(P)** contain large numbers of chronic inflammatory cells and, in some areas, these inflammatory cells spill over the limiting plate into nodules of hepatocytes. There are also focal areas of inflammation **(In)** in the liver parenchyma. The portal tracts show evidence of fibrosis and fibrous bands **(F)** containing chronic inflammatory cells have formed bridges between adjacent portal areas. These features are characteristically seen in the more active forms of chronic hepatitis (Fig. 14.3).

Once fibrous tissue has been deposited, cirrhosis has traditionally been viewed as a virtually irreversible process, but there is emerging evidence that, in some cases, treatment that achieves control of the underlying liver disease may result in some restitution of the liver architecture. Repeated liver biopsy can be used to monitor progress.

Older classifications of cirrhosis grouped the diseases according to the size of the regenerative nodules seen at post-mortem or laparotomy. In *macronodular cirrhosis*, (E-Fig. 14.5**G**) large nodules up to several centimetres in diameter are present. *Micronodular cirrhosis* is characterised by small and uniform regenerative nodules up to 1 cm in diameter. Whilst it is useful to describe macroscopic features, this classification does not help in assessing disease type or progression. In active cirrhosis, as seen in Fig. 14.5D, there is evidence of continuing damage to liver cells, whereas in inactive cirrhosis there is no evidence of continuing liver damage.

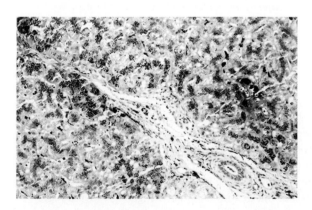

Fig. 14.6 Haemochromatosis (Perls' stain) **(MP)**.

Haemochromatosis is a condition characterised by excessive deposition of iron in the tissues. It is due to an inherited defect of iron transport such that excessive iron is absorbed from a normal diet. Pathologically, excessive iron is deposited in many tissues, especially myocardium, liver, adrenal glands, pancreas and synovial joints. Hepatic involvement causes cirrhosis. As seen in Fig. 14.6, liver cells accumulate enormous amounts of iron, which are stained blue by Perls' stain. Excessive iron may also be stored in the liver in conditions where frequent blood transfusion is required. This is termed *secondary haemosiderosis*.

CLINICAL FEATURES OF IRON OVERLOAD

Genetic haemochromatosis is an autosomal recessive disorder that occurs due to a single amino acid substitution within the protein encoded by the *HFE* gene. Clinical presentation tends to be earlier in men than in women because normal menstrual blood loss in premenopausal females reduces the extent of iron deposition within the tissues and so exerts a degree of physiological control. The diagnosis may be first suspected due to deranged liver function tests, but other clinical signs include skin pigmentation and the development of diabetes mellitus due to chronic pancreatic damage. These features gave rise to the old clinical description of haemochromatosis as *bronzed diabetes*, a term that serves as a useful aide memoir.

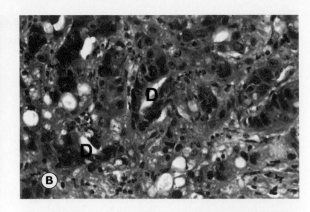

Fig. 14.7 **Hepatocellular carcinoma. (A)** MP; **(B)** HP; **(C)** HP.

In developed countries, primary carcinoma of the liver is a relatively uncommon condition compared with metastatic tumours from other sites. On a worldwide basis, the incidence of *hepatocellular carcinoma* (often confusingly called *hepatoma*) (E-Fig. 14.6**G**) is closely related to the prevalence of hepatitis B virus infection. In some parts of Africa, it accounts for up to 40% of all cancers, while in Europe and the USA it only accounts for around 2%. Cirrhosis from any cause also predisposes to the development of hepatocellular carcinoma. These tumours are associated with rapid clinical progression and average survival from diagnosis is only around 6 months. The tumour may form a single massive nodule, multiple small nodules, or exhibit a diffuse infiltrating pattern. Fig. 14.7A shows normal hepatocytes **(H)** on the left and malignant hepatocytes **(T)** on the right.

Sometimes, poorly differentiated tumours form irregular duct-like structures **(D)** as shown in Fig. 14.7B and may resemble metastatic adenocarcinoma. In this situation, immunohistochemical staining may be helpful (see clinical box 'Metastatic tumour in the liver').

In contrast, very well differentiated hepatocellular carcinomas may produce well-formed ducts **(D)** and even secrete bile **(B)** as shown in Fig. 14.7C.

Alpha-fetoprotein (αFP) is secreted by a large proportion of hepatocellular carcinomas and is a useful tumour marker.

METASTATIC TUMOUR IN THE LIVER

The liver is commonly affected by metastatic malignant tumours, particularly metastatic carcinomas. For this reason, *staging* of most newly diagnosed malignant tumours involves biochemical testing of liver function, as well as careful radiological assessment to identify any evidence of tumour deposits. When such tests do reveal mass lesions, percutaneous liver biopsy may sometimes be undertaken to confirm the diagnosis histologically. More often, liver biopsy is used when a patient is found to have multiple tumour deposits in the liver but without any known primary site of tumour. In this setting, the pathologist plays a vital role in confirming the diagnosis of malignancy and in investigating the likely site of origin of the tumour.

The pathological examination of a liver biopsy that is obtained from a mass lesion begins with assessment of a routine H&E stained section to confirm whether the biopsy has successfully targeted the tumour mass. If a tumour is present, it is then necessary to decide whether it could be a primary liver tumour, either a hepatocellular carcinoma or possibly a benign liver lesion such as a haemangioma (see Fig. 11.8). If it is a metastatic malignant tumour, it is necessary to determine the type of tumour, e.g. carcinoma, melanoma, lymphoma, etc. Immunohistochemical staining is useful but is always guided by the histological appearance on H&E staining.

Metastatic adenocarcinoma is very common and immunostaining can help to distinguish likely sites of origin such as colon, lung, breast, etc. This allows the pathologist to direct further investigation of the patient. Sometimes, confirming a diagnosis in this way is sufficient to guide further management, allowing immediate treatment of the tumour with appropriate chemotherapy and avoiding the need for further biopsy.

Disorders of the biliary system

Cholestasis is the term applied to accumulation of bile within the liver. This is illustrated in Fig. 14.8. Gallbladder disease is a common surgical problem in developed countries and is often associated with stone formation and chronic obstruction of the cystic duct leading to *chronic cholecystitis* (Fig. 14.9). *Cholesterolosis* describes the deposition of cholesterol and other lipids within the lamina propria of the gallbladder. This is commonly seen in cholecystectomy specimens and is illustrated in Fig. 14.10. Primary carcinoma of the gallbladder is very rare (Fig. 14.11). Tumours of the biliary system are relatively rare and usually take the form of highly malignant adenocarcinomas known as *cholangiocarcinomas* (Fig. 14.12).

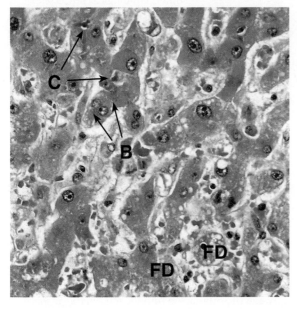

Fig. 14.8 Cholestasis (HP).

Cholestasis, or accumulation of bile within the liver, is a consequence of obstruction to bile flow. This may occur in the extrahepatic biliary tree (most commonly as a result of gallstones), in the intrahepatic biliary tree because of destruction of bile ducts (as in primary biliary cirrhosis) or at the level of the hepatocytes owing to failure to secrete bile. The latter is a common feature of liver cell damage from any cause or may be a reaction to certain drugs.

In all types of cholestasis, there is accumulation of bile (**B**) within the hepatic parenchyma. In ductal obstruction, there are also plugs of bile within the canaliculi (E-Fig. 14.7**H**) (**C**). Hepatocytes containing bile show *feathery degeneration* (**FD**) where the cytoplasm becomes foamy.

Acute biliary obstruction predisposes to the development of bacterial infection in the stagnant bile, a very serious condition called *ascending cholangitis*. Long standing obstruction of the biliary tract may result in *secondary biliary cirrhosis*.

Fig. 14.9 Chronic cholecystitis (LP).

Many gallbladders (E-Fig. 14.8**H**) containing stones are removed surgically because of abdominal pain. *Gallstones* are formed from the constituents of bile and may be composed of cholesterol, bile pigments or a mixture of these. In broad terms, they occur due to an imbalance in the ratio of these normal bile constituents. This is well illustrated by the frequent occurrence of pigment stones in patients with chronic *haemolytic anaemia*. Excess breakdown of erythrocytes results in increased excretion of the haem breakdown products bilirubin and biliverdin in bile. These then precipitate to form dark, crystalline gallstones, which may cause biliary obstruction.

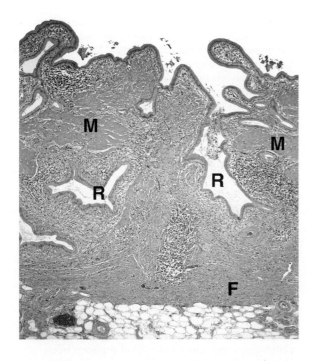

On histological examination, there is low grade chronic inflammation with marked muscle hypertrophy (**M**) and an infiltrate of lymphocytes and plasma cells in the submucosal layer. Irregular gland-like mucosal pockets extend deep into and beyond the thickened muscle layer and are known as *Rokitansky–Aschoff sinuses* (**R**).

Outside the muscle layer, there is fibrosis (**F**) and mild chronic inflammation beneath the serosa. If bile becomes inspissated and concentrated within the gallbladder, it may cause an acute chemical cholecystitis with many neutrophils and often extensive haemorrhage within the gallbladder wall.

KEY TO FIGURES
B bile   **C** canalicular bile plugs   **D** duct-like structure   **F** fibrosis   **FD** feathery degeneration
H normal hepatocytes   **M** muscle hypertrophy   **R** Rokitansky-Aschoff sinuses   **T** malignant tumour cells

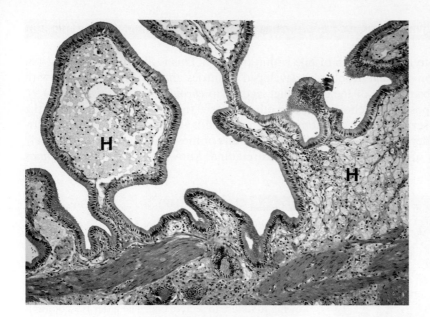

Fig. 14.10 Cholesterolosis (MP).

Fig. 14.10 shows accumulation of foamy, lipid-laden histiocytes (H) within the lamina propria of the gallbladder. Macroscopic examination of the mucosa reveals many tiny flecks of yellow upon a background that may be red and congested or green-stained with bile pigments. This appearance (like so many other pathological processes!) is likened to food and is termed *strawberry gallbladder*. Cholesterolosis often co-exists with cholesterol gallstones and probably reflects the presence of increased cholesterol levels within the bile. It is commonly seen in cholecystectomy specimens.

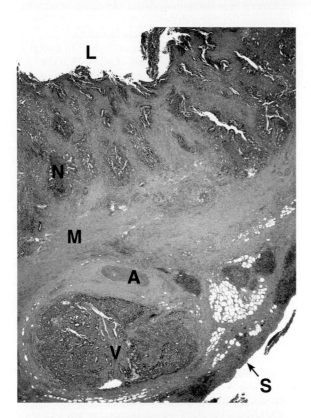

Fig. 14.11 Carcinoma of gallbladder (LP).

Carcinoma of the gallbladder usually occurs in the elderly. Fig. 14.11 shows a moderately differentiated adenocarcinoma, which invades through the full thickness of the gallbladder wall, from the lumen (L) to the serosal surface (S). The wall is replaced by adenocarcinoma with a glandular pattern. There are zones of necrotic debris (N) within the islands of infiltrating tumour cells. Invasion has occurred through the submucosa into the muscularis propria (M) of the gallbladder and beyond into the outer serosa (S). In addition, there is a tumour within a large vein (V) in the subserosa. An adjacent muscular artery (A) is visible.

Gallbladder carcinoma is often seen to arise from surface epithelium that has undergone intestinal metaplasia and subsequent dysplasia. Similar carcinomas can also occur in the intrahepatic and extrahepatic bile ducts (intrahepatic and extrahepatic *cholangiocarcinomas*, Fig. 14.12). These tumours tend to cause early obstructive jaundice, but tumours in the gallbladder rarely cause obstruction to the bile flow and therefore usually present late in the disease or are identified incidentally at the time of cholecystectomy. Gallbladder carcinoma frequently infiltrates directly into the liver, often rendering the tumour inoperable.

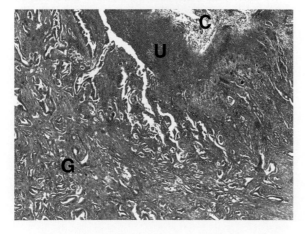

Fig. 14.12 Extrahepatic cholangiocarcinoma (MP).

Cholangiocarcinomas can arise throughout the biliary tree, including the common bile duct and hepatic ducts. Conditions that result in persistent inflammation of the bile ducts increase the risk of developing cancer, including primary sclerosing cholangitis and parasite infestation. These tumours often show similar histological features to pancreatic and gallbladder adenocarcinomas. Fig. 14.12 shows a cholangiocarcinoma of the distal common bile duct. Note the malignant infiltrating glands (G) arising from the common bile duct (C), which is also ulcerated (U) and inflamed.

Pancreatitis

Inflammation of the pancreas (E-Fig. 14.9**H**) (pancreatitis) may present in acute or chronic form. *Acute pancreatitis* is thought to occur as a result of inappropriate activation of pancreatic enzymes, which causes autodigestion of the pancreas and triggers an inflammatory cascade, which can result in necrosis both within the pancreas itself and in extra-pancreatic adipose tissues. Alcohol excess and gallstones are by far the two most common causes in western countries (Table 14.3). Acute pancreatitis can range from a mild, self-limiting illness to severe pancreatitis with shock and multi-organ failure due to extensive necrosis and haemorrhage. Immediate complications of acute pancreatitis include infection, haemorrhage and shock. Long-term complications include *pseudocyst* formation as a result of resolution of large areas of necrosis and chronic pancreatitis. *Chronic pancreatitis* is characterised by fibrotic replacement of the pancreas. Alcohol excess is the commonest cause of chronic pancreatitis, which is frequently associated with intractable epigastric pain and pancreatic insufficiency. Chronic pancreatitis is also a risk factor for *pancreatic cancer* (Fig. 14.14).

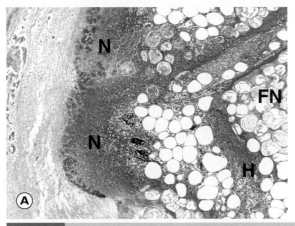
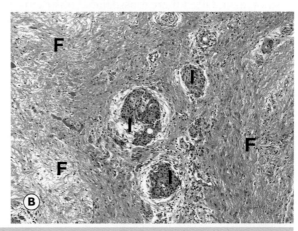

Fig. 14.13 **Pancreatitis. (A)** Acute (MP); **(B)** chronic (MP).

In acute pancreatitis, the pancreas typically appears oedematous and pale (E-Fig. 14.10**G**). There is often associated fat necrosis, which can be recognised as multiple chalky white flecks throughout the peripancreatic and omental fat. If the pancreatitis is severe, there is often widespread necrosis and interstitial haemorrhage due to vascular injury. Thrombosis of the splenic artery can also occur. Note the widespread necrosis (**N**) in Fig. 14.13A. The adipose tissue is also necrotic (**FN**) with a surrounding inflammatory reaction including histiocytes (**H**). Contrast these appearances and those of the normal pancreas to chronic pancreatitis in Fig. 14.13B. The histological hallmark is replacement fibrosis (**F**) throughout the gland with atrophy of predominantly the exocrine component (E-Fig. 14.11**G**). The pancreatic ducts are often dilated containing inspissated proteinaceous material (not shown here). In Fig. 14.13B, the exocrine tissue has been completely replaced by fibrosis leaving only the islets of Langerhans (**I**). In other types of chronic pancreatitis, such as autoimmune, there is often a dense associated chronic inflammatory infiltrate rich in lymphocytes and plasma cells.

Table 14.3 **Causes of acute pancreatitis**

Alcohol (commonest)	Genetic • Inherited mutations of trypsinogen function
Biliary tract disease • Gallstones (commonest) • Malignancy	Metabolic • Hyperlipidaemia/triglyceridaemia • Hypercalcaemia
Drugs • Steroids • Azathioprine • Diuretics • NSAIDs • ACE inhibitors	Autoimmune • Including IgG4 related diseases
Infections • Mumps • Coxsackie virus • CMV	Miscellaneous • Sphincter of Oddi dysfunction • Scorpion bite

KEY TO FIGURES
A artery   **C** common bile duct   **F** fibrosis   **FN** necrotic fat   **G** malignant glands   **H** lipid-laden histiocytes   **I** islets of Langerhans   **L** lumen   **M** muscularis propria   **N** necrosis   **S** serosa   **U** ulcer **V** vein with tumour

Pancreatic cancer

Pancreatic ductal adenocarcinomas (PDAC) arise from the pancreatic ductal epithelium and are of great importance because of their insidious manner of growth, often remaining undetected until an advanced stage (Fig. 14.14). Other primary malignant tumours of the pancreas can arise from the acinar structures *(acinic cell carcinoma)* or the islets of Langerhans *(neuroendocrine tumours)*. Neuroendocrine tumours of the pancreas show similar histological features to their counterparts in the gastrointestinal (GI) tract (see Fig 13.13) and are assessed in a similar fashion. Like GI neuroendocrine tumours, most pancreatic tumours are non-functioning; however, some produce excess hormone products including insulin *(insulinoma)* and glucagon *(glucagonoma)*. Other uncommon tumours that can involve the pancreas include metastases and lymphoma.

Most PDACs arise in the head of the gland where they tend to obstruct the common bile duct, thus presenting with obstructive jaundice. Tumours arising in the body and tail of the pancreas are very difficult to detect clinically and are often at an advanced stage at diagnosis. Histologically, PDACs are composed of glandular elements resembling the ductal structures in the gland, usually with marked surrounding desmoplasia. Often there is associated obstructive chronic pancreatitis. Precursor lesions include mucin-producing cystic neoplasms (Fig. 14.15) and *Pancreatic Intraepithelial Neoplasia (PanIN)*, which is a form of dysplasia in the pancreatic ducts (Fig. 14.14).

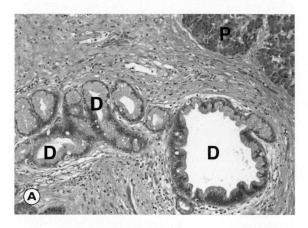
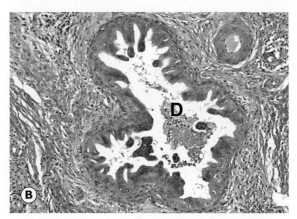
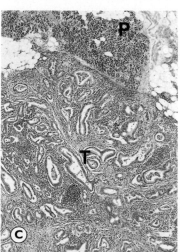
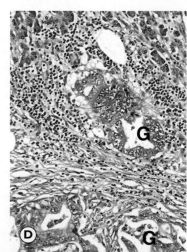
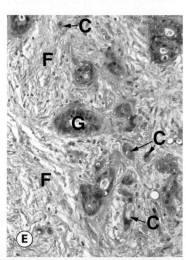

Fig. 14.14 Pancreatic neoplasia. (A) PanIN1A (MP); **(B)** PanIN3 (MP); **(C)** pancreatic ductal adenocarcinoma (LP); **(D)** moderately differentiated (HP); **(E)** poorly differentiated (MP).

In *PanIN,* the ducts are lined by tall mucinous columnar cells showing varying degrees of dysplasia, which are graded as mild with low risk of progression to invasive cancer (PanIN1A or B), moderate (PanIN2) or severe (PanIN3). All grades of PanIN are known to harbour similar genetic mutations to pancreatic cancer.

PanIN1 is illustrated in Fig. 14.14A in which there is a mucinous lining of the ducts **(D)**, rather than biliary type non-mucinous epithelium. Compare this to PanIN3 in Fig. 14.14B in which the duct displays a micropapillary architecture and there is marked

cytological atypia, akin to severe dysplasia/carcinoma in situ at other sites (see Fig. 7.2). Fig. 14.14C shows a tumour **(T)** with normal pancreas **(P)** on the upper right. At higher magnification in Fig. 14.14D, the tumour shows a pancreaticobiliary pattern, with marked variation in the size and shape of the neoplastic glands **(G)**.

Fig. 14.14E shows a more poorly differentiated tumour with infiltrating malignant glands **(G)** and single cells **(C)** in a markedly desmoplastic stroma **(F)**. Macroscopically, the tumours are often hard and white due to this stromal reaction.

CLINICAL ASPECTS OF PANCREATIC CANCER
Pancreatic tumours are usually diagnosed by a combination of radiology (CT scan and/or MRI), endoscopic ultrasound and cytological assessment (FNA of pancreas or common bile duct brushings). PDAC is usually treated with a combination of chemotherapy and surgery. A **Whipple's procedure** or **pancreato-duodenectomy** is usually required to remove tumours in the head of pancreas along with the gallbladder, a portion of duodenum, common bile duct and associated lymph nodes. Many centres now perform pylorus-preserving surgery to preserve the outflow function of the stomach. Unfortunately, only a small proportion (10%–15%) of patients with PDAC are suitable for surgical intervention due to advanced tumour stage at diagnosis or poor medical fitness to withstand the stresses of such a major operation.

Cystic lesions of the pancreas

Cystic lesions are often detected incidentally following imaging for another condition. There are a variety of different types of cystic lesion that can involve the pancreas, listed in Table 14.4. The commonest cyst in the pancreas is the **pseudocyst**, so-called because it is devoid of an epithelial lining. Pseudocysts arise as a complication of pancreatitis. True cysts of the pancreas contain an epithelial lining. There are two types of mucinous cyst associated with a risk of invasive PDAC and therefore are usually followed up and treated surgically when any worrying features arise. These are **intraductal papillary mucinous neoplasms (IPMN)** and **mucinous cystic neoplasms (MCN)** and are described in Fig. 14.15.

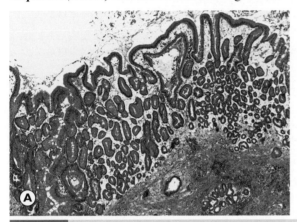
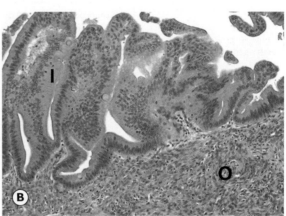

Fig. 14.15 **Pancreatic mucinous cysts. (A)** Intraductal papillary mucinous neoplasm (IPMN) (LP); **(B)** mucinous cystic neoplasm (MCN) (MP).

IPMNs are multilocular cystic lesions lined by mucin producing epithelium, which involve the pancreatic ductal system and can show a range of dysplastic changes. Endoscopically, mucin is often seen extruding from the ampulla of Vater. IPMNs most commonly involve the head of the gland. IPMN can be classified according to the part of the ductal system involved, i.e. main duct or side branch, and by the type of epithelial lining of the cyst, which can be intestinal, gastric (as shown in Fig. 14.15A) or pancreaticobiliary type. Approximately a third of patients with IPMN will also harbour an invasive cancer, therefore it is important that the cyst and associated pancreatic tissue is thoroughly sampled in any resection specimen.

MCNs (Fig. 14.15B) are almost exclusively found in women and are also associated with invasive cancer. MCNs are usually found in the tail of the gland, are macrocystic and do not communicate with the ductal system. The cyst is lined by mucin producing epithelium, which can also show various grades of dysplasia. In Fig. 14.15B, there is an intestinal type epithelium **(I)** with low grade dysplasia, similar to a low grade adenoma in the colon. The histological hallmark is the presence of an ovarian type fibrous stroma **(O)**. IPMN and MCN are usually treated by surgical resection due to the risk of associated invasive cancer.

Table 14.4 **Classification of pancreatic cystic lesions.**

True cysts: Neoplastic	**Mucinous:** mucinous cystic neoplasm intraductal papillary mucinous neoplasm **Non-mucinous:** serous cystadenoma
True cysts: Non neoplastic	Lymphoepithelial cyst Epidermoid cyst Congenital cyst
Other	Cystic degeneration of pancreatic ductal adenocarcinoma, neuroendocrine tumour, metastasis or acinar cell carcinoma Pseudocyst

KEY TO FIGURES
C single infiltrating malignant cells   **D** ducts   **F** desmoplastic stroma   **G** malignant gland   **I** intestinal type epithelium   **O** ovarian type stroma   **P** pancreas   **T** tumour

BASIC SYSTEMS PATHOLOGY ■ LIVER AND PANCREATICOBILIARY SYSTEM

Table 14.5 Chapter review.

Disorder	Main features	Figure
Inflammatory liver diseases		
Acute hepatitis	Cloudy swelling, fatty change, liver cell necrosis- various causes May resolve or persist as chronic hepatitis	14.1
Viral hepatitis	Hepatotropic viruses (A,B,C,D,E, etc.) or others (CMV, EBV, HSV, etc.) Hep A and E faecal-oral transmission, no chronicity or carrier state Hep B (D) and C blood borne, chronic hepatitis and carrier states	14.1
Alcoholic liver disease	Steatosis: fat droplets in hepatocytes Steatohepatitis: ballooning degeneration, neutrophils, Mallory's hyaline. Fibrosis/cirrhosis- initially perivenular and pericellular collagen	14.2
Non-alcoholic fatty liver disease	Same morphological spectrum as alcoholic liver disease Association with obesity, dyslipidaemia, NIDDM	Like 14.2
Chronic hepatitis	Persisting more than 6 months, various causes Portal/interface/lobular inflammation (grade) Extent of fibrosis (stage)	14.3
Primary biliary cirrhosis	Early autoimmune damage to bile ducts with granuloma formation Later interface hepatitis, ductular proliferation and progressive fibrosis	14.4
Cirrhosis	Diffuse process, end stage of chronic liver damage Formation of regenerative nodules divided by fibrous bands	14.5
Haemochromatosis	Defect of HFE gene, iron overload with deposition in liver, heart, endocrine organs, joints and skin Progressive cirrhosis	14.6
Liver tumours		
Haemangioma	Benign proliferation of blood vessels in the liver Common incidental finding on imaging	11.8
Hepatic metastases	Usually carcinoma, especially GI tract (portal drainage), breast, lung. Tendency to be multiple.	7.16
Hepatocellular carcinoma	Primary malignant tumour arising from hepatocytes- may secrete bile. Serum alpha-fetoprotein useful serum marker. Often single nodule.	14.7
Biliary disease		
Cholestasis	Extrahepatic or intrahepatic obstruction to bile flow. Plugs of bile in liver canaliculi. Feathery degeneration of hepatocytes.	14.8
Chronic cholecystitis	Usually due to gallstones- cholesterol, pigment or mixed types. Chronic scarring, muscle hypertrophy, Rokitansky-Aschoff sinuses.	14.9
Cholesterolosis	Deposition of lipid-laden histiocytes in lamina propria. Gross appearance of 'strawberry gallbladder'.	14.10
Gallbladder carcinoma	Uncommon, usually elderly patients. Origin from surface intestinal metaplasia and dysplasia. Presents late, often liver infiltration.	14.11
Cholangiocarcinoma	Adenocarcinoma arising in intrahepatic or extrahepatic bile ducts. Typically causes intense fibrous stromal reaction.	14.12
Pancreatic disease		
Acute pancreatitis	Gallstones and alcohol main risk factors. Pancreatic enzymes cause tissue damage and necrosis. High risk of multi-organ failure.	14.13A
Chronic pancreatitis	May follow repeated episodes of acute pancreatitis. Commonly alcohol related. Scarring and loss of gland tissue. Back pain, risk of diabetes.	14.13B
Pancreatic adenocarcinoma	Usually head of pancreas, insidious growth. Presents late with obstructive jaundice. Poor prognosis.	14.14
Pancreatic endocrine tumours	Origin from islet cells. Resemble carcinoid tumours seen at other sites. Uncommon. Named for secretory product, e.g. insulinoma, glucagonoma.	13.13
Pancreatic cystic lesions	Often incidental finding. Broadly divided into non-neoplastic and neoplastic. MCN and IPMN associated with pancreatic adenocarcinoma.	14.15

15 Urinary system

Introduction

The *urinary tract* comprises the kidneys, pelvicalyceal systems, ureters, bladder and urethra. The kidney is responsible for excretion of the waste products of metabolism, the waste products being excreted in the form of an aqueous solution called *urine*. Urine passes from the kidneys into the pelvicalyceal systems and thence via the ureters to the bladder, which acts as a reservoir. Urine is held in the bladder by a series of muscular sphincters until sufficient volume has accumulated. Relaxation of the sphincters and contraction of smooth muscle in the bladder wall allows the urine to be voided to the exterior through the urethra *(micturition)* at a convenient time.

The kidney

The kidney is divided into two main anatomical divisions, the *cortex* and *medulla* (E-Fig. 15.1H). Disorders of the kidney may affect either of these zones, but diseases affecting one part will often have secondary effects on the other component. Disorders may arise from a wide range of pathological causes, many of which are common in other organ systems (e.g. infections, tumours, drug reactions, vascular disorders). However, the kidney is unusual in that it is much more prone to immunological disorders than most other organs. Vascular diseases such as hypertension, diabetes mellitus and vasculitis may also have profound effects on renal function. Disorders of the kidney can be conveniently divided into categories according to which structural component of the kidney is primarily affected:

Glomerulus (E-Fig. 15.2H)

■ *Glomerulonephritis (GN)* of various types, most of which are due to deposition of immunoglobulins and/or complement components (collectively called *immune complexes*) within the glomerulus (Figs 15.2 to 15.7).

■ *Vasculitis:* strictly speaking, this is a vascular disorder, but some forms affect the glomerular capillaries giving the clinical and pathological appearances of a GN. (Fig. 15.3)

■ *Ischaemia:* common systemic diseases, including hypertension and diabetes mellitus, as well as a range of thrombotic and embolic conditions may cause glomerular injury.

■ *Disorders involving deposition of material in the glomerulus*

  – *Diabetes mellitus:* deposition of abnormal glycosylated proteins causes irreversible structural and functional abnormalities in the glomerulus (Fig. 15.9).

  – *Amyloidosis:* deposition of amyloid proteins in the glomerulus alters the structure and therefore the function of the glomerulus (Fig. 15.10).

■ *Congenital and structural abnormalities:* some inherited conditions result in abnormal glomerular structure and function; an example is the condition thin basement membrane disease.

Tubules and interstitium (E-Fig. 15.3H)

■ *Acute tubular necrosis (ATN)* is usually due to profound hypotension causing ischaemic damage to tubular epithelial cells. Some forms of drug toxicity may give rise to similar appearances.

■ *Interstitial nephritis (AIN)* is an important cause of acute renal failure and is most often due to drug hypersensitivity.

■ *Infections* including acute and chronic *pyelonephritis*, renal abscess and TB.

■ *Mechanical obstruction* of the ureters or bladder may lead to *hydronephrosis* and recurrent infection.

Blood vessels

■ *Hypertension* causes marked changes to both large and small renal vessels. The changes of benign/essential hypertension and accelerated/malignant hypertension are discussed in Fig. 15.15.

■ *Thrombotic microangiopathy* is a pattern of vascular damage that results in intravascular thrombosis due to endothelial cell injury. It is typically seen in association with haemolytic anaemia, thrombocytopenic purpura and often renal failure. Although many of the pathological changes are due to damage to the microcirculation, especially the glomerular capillaries, thrombosis also occurs in larger vessels.

■ *Vasculitis* may affect larger vessels as well as glomerular capillaries, but the main manifestations are usually glomerular.

■ *Diabetes mellitus* is an important metabolic disease that has profound vascular effects, affecting both large vessels and the microvasculature.

Clinical patterns of renal injury

Damage to one component of the kidney inevitably damages the other parts. Severe reversible damage to any of the above components of the kidney may lead to *acute renal failure* or *acute kidney injury (AKI)*. Some conditions are reversible, e.g. some types of AKI and most cases of acute diffuse proliferative GN, but many lead to progressive damage. In cases with progressive damage, there will be some degree of permanent renal impairment and a proportion of these will develop *chronic renal failure*, a condition that was invariably fatal until the advent of renal dialysis and kidney transplantation.

■ *Acute renal failure:* Abrupt cessation of activity of the nephrons usually presents initially as a marked fall in urine production *(oliguria)*, which may even be total *(anuria)*. This is accompanied by a rapid rise in serum urea and creatinine levels. Disturbances of fluid and electrolyte balance soon follow, particularly a rise in the serum potassium level and metabolic acidosis.

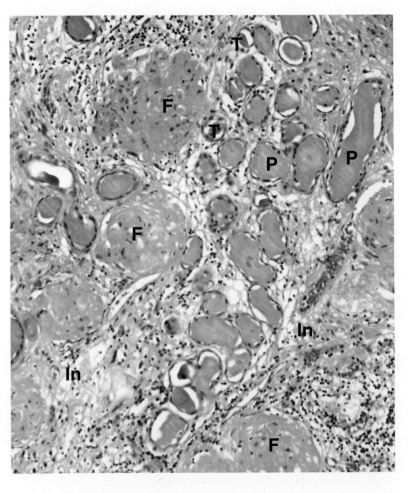

Fig. 15.1 End-stage kidney (MP).

Many kidney diseases, whatever the underlying cause, may progress to chronic renal failure. Macroscopically, the kidneys are usually found to be small and firm with symmetrical thinning of the cortex and poor demarcation of cortex from medulla. This condition is known as the *end-stage kidney*. In both gross and histological appearance, there is often little clue to the original renal pathology. In the cortex, the non-functioning or *obsolescent* glomeruli are replaced by avascular, acellular fibrous material *(fibrosis)* **(F)**, shown in Fig. 15.1. The cortical tubules **(T)** also become shrunken and atrophic and the expanded interstitial spaces **(In)** undergo fibrosis; some atrophic tubules may become cystically dilated with *casts* of inspissated proteinaceous material **(P)**, which is highly eosinophilic (pink-staining) and resembles thyroid follicles, thus often called *thyroidisation*.

KEY TO FIGURES
F fibrosis of glomerulus   **In** interstitial space   **P** protein cast   **T** tubule

■ **Chronic renal failure**: Progressive retention of nitrogenous metabolites causes a slow rise in serum creatinine levels due to insufficient glomerular filtration. Concomitant failure of tubular function produces widespread abnormalities in biochemical homeostasis, including salt and water retention, metabolic acidosis and other electrolyte imbalances, particularly hyperkalaemia.

Diseases of the glomerulus

Glomerular disorders arise from a variety of causes; the two major causes being *immunological* (including disorders confined to the kidney and some systemic diseases) and *metabolic* (the most important being diabetes mellitus). It is confusing to many students that there is not a direct one-to-one relationship between a

Table 15.1 Clinical syndromes associated with glomerular disease.

Syndrome	Clinical features	Histological changes	Associated disease
Acute nephritis	Haematuria, Hypertension, Uraemia (↑BUN) Oedema (often periorbital), Oliguria or anuria	Hypercellular glomerulus with obstructed capillary loops	Acute post-infective GN IgA nephropathy/Henoch-Schönlein purpura SLE
Nephrotic syndrome	Proteinuria (3.5 g/24 h), Hypoalbuminaemia, Oedema, Hyperlipidaemia	Changes to the structure of the glomerular filtration mechanism, including the GBM and/or podocytes	Diabetes mellitus Amyloidosis Minimal change nephropathy Focal segmental glomerulosclerosis Membranous nephropathy SLE
Mixed nephritic–nephrotic syndrome	Features of both nephritic and nephrotic syndromes	Both cellular proliferation and GBM alterations	Membranoproliferative GN (mesangiocapillary GN) SLE
Asymptomatic haematuria	Periodic dark-coloured urine or microscopic haematuria	Proliferation of glomerular cells or structural abnormalities of GBM	IgA nephropathy Thin basement membrane disease SLE
Asymptomatic proteinuria	Proteinuria	Early stages of the changes in the GBM seen in the nephrotic syndrome	Early phases of all of the conditions which cause nephrotic syndrome

ROLE OF RENAL BIOPSY

The introduction of safe and reliable techniques of percutaneous needle biopsy of the kidney has greatly increased knowledge about the natural history of renal diseases, particularly by elucidating the underlying lesion early in the course of glomerular diseases when treatment might be applied effectively. It is of limited value in chronic renal failure when the kidney is shrunken and histological changes are non-specific, i.e. **end-stage kidney** (Fig. 15.1). Renal biopsy is also frequently used in the assessment of renal transplants to detect the presence of transplant rejection, drug toxicity and a number of other conditions that may cause reduced function of the graft. Maximum information is obtained from a needle biopsy of renal tissue using a combination of the following methods:

■ **Light microscopy**, including special stains to define glomerular structures

■ **Electron microscopy** to show the presence and precise location of immune complexes, which appear as irregular deposits of electron-dense material **(dense deposits)**, and other deposits such as amyloid, diabetic changes, structural changes to the glomerular basement membrane (GBM) and podocytes.

■ **Immunofluorescence microscopy** to localise and identify the class of immunoglobulins and complement components.
The immunofluorescence and electron microscopic patterns of immune complex deposition can be vital to differentiate between different types of GN, which have similar patterns of glomerular damage by light microscopy. Examples include:

■ **IgA nephropathy:** granular deposits of IgA in the mesangium

■ **Membranous nephropathy:** granular deposits of IgG and complement on the epithelial side of the GBM

■ **Goodpasture's syndrome:** linear deposits of IgG along the GBM

■ **Systemic lupus erythematosus (SLE):** deposits of most classes of immunoglobulin and many complement components at any site in the glomerulus
Interpretation of a renal biopsy also requires information about the clinical history, physical examination and other investigations to arrive at a correct diagnosis. For example, a membranous pattern of GN might be idiopathic, related to use of certain drugs (e.g. gold, penicillamine) or may be part of the spectrum of SLE (Class V lupus nephritis).

BASIC SYSTEMS PATHOLOGY ■ URINARY SYSTEM

particular mechanism of damage and a particular histological appearance and/or clinical syndrome. In fact, most causes of glomerular damage will give rise to one of several clinical presentations, summarised in Table 15.1, along with the diseases with which they are most commonly associated. Acute and chronic renal failure are described above and may supervene in any of the above conditions. For example, an individual with a severe nephritic syndrome may progress quickly to acute renal failure or an individual with undiagnosed diabetes mellitus, who has had undetected proteinuria for some time, may first be diagnosed with chronic renal failure.

Glomerulonephritis

Most types of GN are caused by immune complex deposition in the glomerulus. This applies to *primary GN*, where the condition is confined to the kidney (e.g. *membranous nephropathy*, *membranoproliferative GN*), and to diseases with a systemic component (e.g. *Goodpasture's syndrome*, *SLE*, *Henoch-Schönlein purpura*).

The site of immune complex deposition is dependent on the size of the complexes, which is in turn dependent on the type of antigen and on the class of immunoglobulin produced, i.e. the host response. The antigen may be either a normal component of the body (a *self antigen* as in Goodpasture's) or an *external antigen* such as a bacterial product (as in *post-streptococcal GN*). Immune complexes may be deposited from the circulating blood or may be formed in situ. In the latter situation, the complexes may involve intrinsic glomerular antigens (basement membrane components in Goodpasture's) or antigens that have been deposited there from the circulation (e.g. DNA in the case of SLE). An important exception to this rule is minimal change nephropathy where the podocytes are thought to be damaged by a cell-mediated immune response, rather than by immune complex deposition.

Whatever the mechanism of damage to the glomerulus, the various immunological insults alter the structure and therefore the function of the glomerulus and ultimately of the nephron as a whole.

In response to damaging stimuli, the glomerulus appears to react in one or more of the following ways:

■ Swelling and/or proliferation of the normally flat endothelial cells lining the glomerular capillaries

■ Proliferation of the epithelial cells investing the outer surface of the glomerular capillary tuft (the podocytes (E-Fig. 15.4**H**) and the cells lining Bowman's capsule *(crescent formation)*

■ Thickening of glomerular basement membranes (E-Fig. 15.5**H**)

■ Proliferation of the cells of the mesangium and excessive production of acellular mesangial material

These reactions give rise to various histological patterns of GN, which can be identified by light microscopy. This is then put together with the immunofluorescence and electron microscopy findings, clinical history and other investigations to come to a definitive diagnosis. As in many other areas of histopathology, good communication between pathologists and clinicians is vital to arrive at an accurate diagnosis, which is essential for appropriate treatment.

Patterns of GN may be described as:

■ *Diffuse:* affecting all glomeruli

■ *Focal:* affecting some glomeruli

■ *Global:* the entire glomerulus is abnormal

■ *Segmental:* only part of the glomerulus is abnormal

We shall now consider some specific examples of GN, reviewing the typical histological and immunofluorescence patterns and their associated clinical presentations. As indicated in Table 15.1, some diseases may present clinically in several different ways, with nephritic or nephritic features or even combinations of these.

For convenience, we shall begin with disorders which typically give rise to acute nephritic features (*acute diffuse proliferative GN*; Fig. 15.2 and *necrotising GN*; Fig. 15.3) followed by those with mixed patterns of haematuria and proteinuria (*mesangial proliferative GN*; Fig. 15.4 and *membranoproliferative GN*; Fig. 15.5) and then important causes of nephrotic syndrome (*membranous GN*; Fig. 15.6, *focal segmental glomerulosclerosis*; Fig. 15.7 and *minimal change disease*; Fig. 15.8).

At the end of this section on glomerular diseases, we shall consider the typical changes of diabetes mellitus in the kidney (Fig. 15.9) and the features of renal amyloidosis (Fig. 15.10). It is worth bearing in mind that primary GN is a relatively rare disease, whilst diabetes and hypertension together account for the bulk of clinically important renal dysfunction in developed counties; in the developing world, toxins and infections are also very important factors in the burden of chronic renal disease.

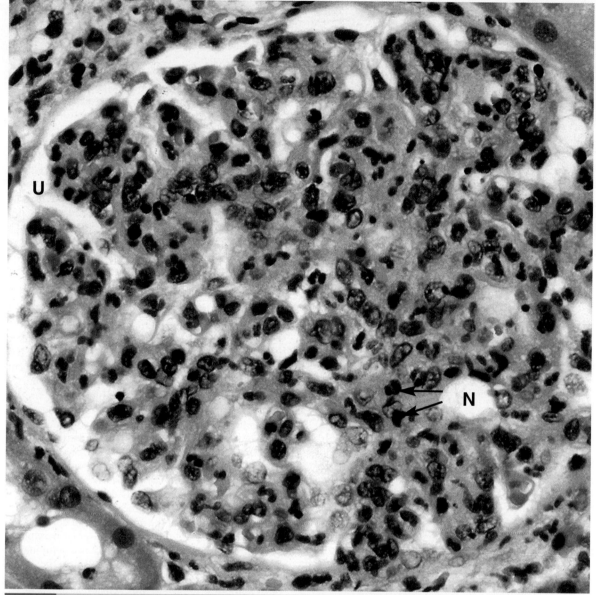

Fig. 15.2 | **Acute diffuse proliferative ('endocapillary') glomerulonephritis (HP).**

This form of global and diffuse GN most commonly occurs in children and often follows a streptococcal throat infection. It is also commonly referred to as ***post-streptococcal GN*** for this reason. Other possible underlying infections include bacterial endocarditis, pneumococcal pneumonia, hepatitis B or C, HIV and many others. Glomerular cellularity (E-Fig. 15.2**H**) is markedly increased due to swelling and proliferation of endothelial and mesangial cells and infiltration by neutrophils (**N**). The capillary lumina are blocked by cells but the urinary space (**U**) remains clear, as there has been no proliferation of epithelial cells. The obstruction of glomerular capillary lumina diminishes glomerular filtration and causes leakage of erythrocytes; hence this condition usually presents with haematuria, transient hypertension and oedema, i.e. acute nephritis. Immunofluorescence microscopy reveals granular deposits of IgG and complement on the glomerular basement membranes and in the mesangium and, on electron microscopy, there are characteristic large sub-epithelial deposits known as 'humps'. A similar pattern of glomerular damage may occur rarely in SLE without preceding infection (Class IV lupus nephritis).

KEY TO FIGURES
N neutrophils   **U** urinary space

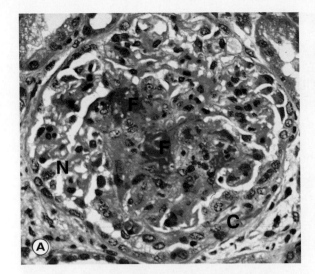

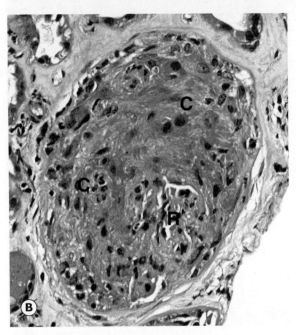

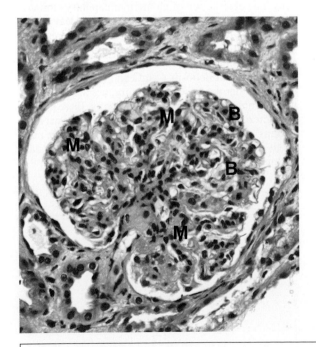

Fig. 15.3 Necrotising GN. (A) Segmental necrotising GN (HP); **(B)** glomerular crescent (HP).

As described above, glomerular disease, which is focal and segmental, affects only a proportion of the glomeruli (focal) and only part of each glomerulus (segmental). Fig. 15.3A shows a segmental necrotising GN in which a segment of the glomerular tuft becomes necrotic with infiltration by neutrophils and deposition of fibrin (**F**). Adjacent segments are normal (**N**) or nearly normal (depending on the underlying disease). Segmental necrosis is often associated with proliferation of epithelial cells of Bowman's capsule, which may progress to frank crescent formation. An early crescent (**C**) is seen here. This pattern of GN is found in a range of settings, including acute exacerbations of IgA nephropathy, systemic vasculitis, SLE (Class III lupus nephritis) and some cases of Goodpasture's syndrome. Segmental necrotising lesions may heal by fibrosis, leaving a lesion very similar to focal segmental glomerulosclerosis (FSGS; see Fig. 15.7). As in many cases, the immunofluorescence microscopy is vital to make the diagnosis: in IgA nephropathy, mesangial IgA (and usually C3) deposits are found, in Goodpasture's there is linear deposition of IgG around the GBM, in SLE all classes of immunoglobulin and several complement components are detected. Continued proliferation of a crescent may obliterate the glomerular tuft as seen in Fig. 15.3B, leading to irreversible glomerular destruction and subsequent nephron atrophy. In this example, the tiny glomerular remnant (**R**) is surrounded by a large crescent (**C**). Large numbers of crescents are associated with rapidly progressive renal failure, often called *rapidly progressive GN* (a clinical but not a pathological term). This is characteristic of *Goodpasture's syndrome* where autoantibodies are formed that react with the α3 subchain of collagen type IV, present in glomerular and alveolar basement membranes. These individuals experience pulmonary haemorrhage as well as renal failure. Where the renal lesion occurs in the absence of lung disease, the condition is known as *anti-glomerular basement membrane disease.* A large crescent as shown here heals as a globally sclerosed glomerulus.

Fig. 15.4 Mesangial proliferative GN (HP).

This diffuse and global pattern of glomerular damage is characterised by increased mesangial matrix and cellularity (**M**) without basement membrane abnormality (**B**). This pattern of glomerular damage is typical of *IgA nephropathy* and the related condition *Henoch-Schonlein purpura (HSP).* Both may present with asymptomatic haematuria or acute nephritis. The renal changes of HSP are identical to those in IgA disease but, in HSP, there is a vasculitic skin rash and gastrointestinal and joint involvement. Immunofluorescence staining reveals deposits of IgA in the mesangium and there are corresponding mesangial dense deposits by electron microscopy. Acute exacerbations of IgA nephropathy may develop segmental necrotising GN (Fig. 15.3A) and even occasionally crescents (Fig. 15.3B). Healing of these lesions leads to secondary focal segmental glomerulosclerosis (Fig. 15.7). Other conditions that have a mesangial proliferative pattern (but different immunological and electron microscopy findings) are resolving acute diffuse proliferative GN (Fig. 15.2) and SLE (Class II).

KEY TO FIGURES
B normal glomerular basement membrane   **C** crescent   **D** double contour basement membrane
F fibrin   **M** increased mesangial matrix and cellularity   **N** normal glomerular segment   **R** glomerular remnant

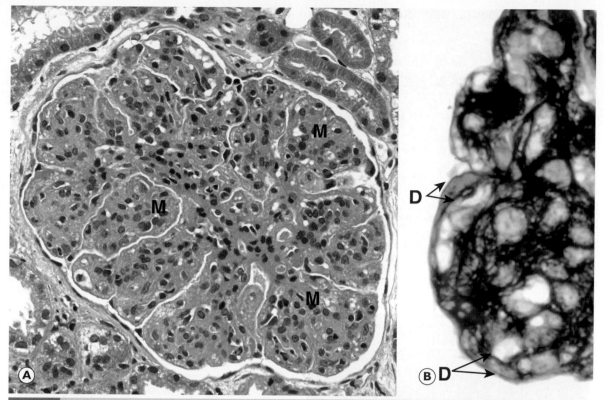

Fig. 15.5 Membranoproliferative (mesangiocapillary) glomerulonephritis. **(A)** (HP); **(B)** methenamine silver (HP).

This diffuse and global pattern of GN may be either idiopathic or secondary. The clinical presentation is either nephrotic syndrome or mixed nephrotic–nephritic syndrome. Idiopathic membranoproliferative GN (MPGN) is conventionally subdivided into types I, II and III, all having a similar appearance by light microscopy but different findings by immunofluorescence and electron microscopy (EM).

Readily visible, as in Fig. 15.5A, is the expansion and increased cellularity of each segment of the glomerulus, producing an exaggerated lobular appearance. The characteristic feature is reduplication of the glomerular basement membranes with interposition of mesangial cells between the two layers. This is seen in Fig. 15.5B, which is stained with a special method to demonstrate the double contour **(D)** of the glomerular basement membrane. There is increased mesangial cellularity and matrix **(M)**. White blood cells also infiltrate the glomerulus and there is often mild endothelial cell proliferation. In MPGN type I, EM shows dense deposits composed of C3 (and IgG in some cases) in the subendothelial position. Type II MCGN varies in light microscopic appearance but is characterised by deposition of a ribbon of dense material

of in the glomerular basement membrane, giving rise to the alternative name of **dense deposit disease**. Type III MPGN is rare, with subepithelial deposits and basement membrane spikes on EM.

This traditional classification is based upon morphology and electron microscopy, rather than understanding of the underlying disease process. Further elucidation of the mechanism of disease has transformed our understanding and we now know that some of these patients have an abnormality affecting the complement cascade, giving rise to so-called **C3 nephropathy** (see clinical box 'The spectrum of C3 nephropathy').

Secondary MPGN is one of the patterns of renal disease in SLE (class IV lupus nephritis), where it may have additional features, including immunoglobulin deposits in all parts of the glomerular basement membrane and in the mesangium, 'wire-loop lesions', a mixed pattern of immunoglobulins and complement deposition, as well as superimposed membranous or segmental patterns of GN. This pattern of GN may also occur in individuals with hepatitis B or C, cryoglobulinaemia and other conditions.

THE SPECTRUM OF C3 NEPHROPATHY: DENSE DEPOSIT DISEASE AND C3 GLOMERULONEPHRITIS

This new classification affecting MPGN is based upon immunofluorescence findings. If immunoglobulins are identified as well as C3, the disease is viewed as immunoglobulin-mediated and is still defined as MPGN type I or type III, depending upon the location of the immune complexes. In contrast, those cases with **isolated C3** in the glomerulus fall within the category of **C3 nephropathy**. Morphological and EM patterns vary and almost any pattern of glomerular damage can occur in C3GN, although MPGN is most common. All cases formerly called MPGN type II or **dense deposit disease** are now known to fall within this spectrum, as do a proportion of those previously classified as types I or III (now called **C3 glomerulonephritis** or **C3GN**).

We now know that these patients have various congenital or acquired abnormalities affecting the **alternative pathway** of complement activation, some of which can be detected by serological tests or by genetic screening. Testing should be offered whenever the renal biopsy findings are of glomerulone-phritis with dominant C3. Traditionally, renal outcomes in patients with MPGN were quite varied and some groups, including those with dense deposit disease, had a high chance of recurrence in transplant-ed kidneys. As well as conventional immunosuppressant drugs, there are now emerging targeted thera-pies such as anti-C5 antibodies, which may modify the underlying disease process in some patients.

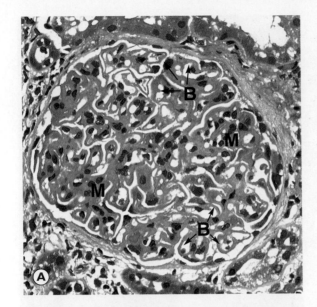

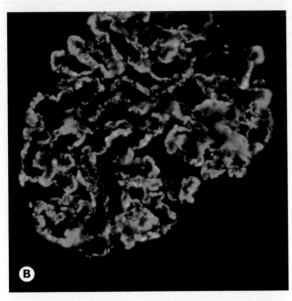

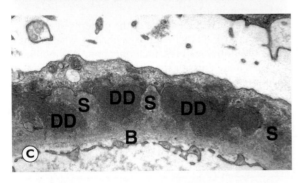

Fig. 15.6 Membranous nephropathy. **(A)** H&E (HP); **(B)** IgG immunofluorescence (HP); **(C)** EM.

Membranous nephropathy is a diffuse global pattern of glomerular injury where damage to the glomerular basement membrane leads to proteinuria and, often, the nephrotic syndrome. *Primary* or *idiopathic membranous nephropathy* accounts for about 85% of cases. An identical pattern of injury, known as *secondary membranous nephropathy*, may arise in individuals with malignant tumours elsewhere in the body (5%–10% of cases), individuals taking certain drugs (gold, penicillamine, captopril and non-steroidal anti-inflammatory drugs) and in certain infections (hepatitis B and C, malaria). A third important category is the autoimmune disease SLE, which can give rise to almost any pattern of glomerular damage (Table 15.1); this pattern is known as lupus nephritis Class V.

In membranous nephropathy, immune complexes are deposited on the epithelial side of the glomerular basement membrane (subepithelial deposits). These deposits induce elaboration of additional basement membrane material between the deposits, giving rise to the pathognomonic 'spikes' on the outer surface of the basement membrane, which can be seen with the silver stain by light microscopy or by electron microscopy, as shown in Fig. 15.6C. By light microscopy (Fig. 15.6A), the glomerular basement membranes **(B)** appear thick, eosinophilic and sometimes slightly refractile. There is no associated endothelial or epithelial (podocyte) proliferation, although there may be a slight increase in mesangial material **(M)** in severe and long-standing cases. The immune complexes in most cases of membranous nephropathy consist of IgG and complement (C3). Obviously, the antigen in the immune complexes will depend on the underlying cause (e.g. DNA in SLE, viral antigens in hepatitis, probably self-antigens in the idiopathic form).

Fig. 15.6B shows the characteristic immunofluorescence pattern of membranous nephropathy. An antibody specific for IgG and labelled with fluorescein is incubated with a section of kidney. The antibody binds to IgG deposited in the kidney. This micrograph demonstrates IgG as bright green fluorescent granular deposits incorporated on the epithelial surface of the glomerular basement membranes. Fig. 15.6C is a high-power electron micrograph of a glomerular basement membrane **(B)** with additional spikes **(S)** of basement membrane material on the epithelial side (E-Fig. 15.5 **H**). Between the spikes, dense deposits (immune complexes) **(DD)** are easily identified. The presence of the immune complexes probably activates complement, which, by means of the membrane attack complex, damages the glomerular basement membrane and allows leakage of protein.

KEY TO FIGURES

B glomerular basement membrane **DD** dense deposit **M** mesangial matrix **S** spike **Sc** sclerosis

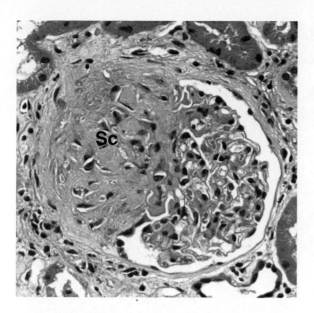

Fig. 15.7 Focal segmental glomerulosclerosis (HP).

Focal segmental glomerulosclerosis (FSGS) may occur as an idiopathic GN or as secondary segmental sclerosing lesions as described in Fig. 15.3. In addition, almost any lesion that causes marked loss of nephrons may induce secondary FSGS. The histological lesion in all of these situations is similar. Segments of some glomeruli are replaced by fibrosis (sclerosis) **(Sc)**. Hyalinosis, the deposition of plasma proteins to give a bland eosinophilic mass, is also commonly a feature of these lesions, although it is not demonstrated in this example. Some authorities believe that idiopathic FSGS is related to minimal change disease (Fig. 15.8). Certainly, both are characterised by negative immunofluorescence and 'fusion' of podocyte foot processes on EM. However, the case remains to be proven.

FSGS is characterised by proteinuria and often full-blown nephrotic syndrome. This pattern of disease may be seen in SLE (class III lupus nephritis).

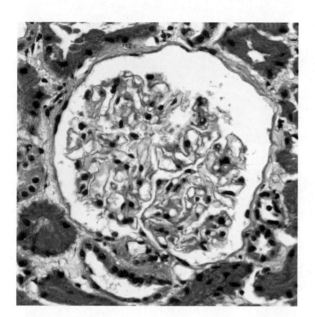

Fig. 15.8 Minimal change disease (HP).

Minimal change disease may occur at any age but is much more common in children. It presents with nephrotic syndrome without haematuria and usually without impairment of renal function, i.e. there is no increase in serum creatinine or urea. Some cases present after an upper respiratory tract infection and it is thought that cell-mediated immunity may be the mechanism of glomerular damage. Most patients recover with no treatment but some require immunosuppression and a few relapse after withdrawal of immunosuppression. As the name implies, the glomeruli appear almost normal on light microscopy (as seen here). Immunofluorescence (IF) is negative. Examination of the glomeruli by electron microscopy demonstrates alterations in the structure of the podocyte foot processes that are 'fused' or 'effaced', i.e. the foot processes form a continuous layer along the urinary side of the basement membrane. This is a non-specific change found in various types of glomerular damage, including FSGS, so only if it occurs in conjunction with normal light microscopy and negative IF can it be said to confirm minimal change disease.

OUTCOMES OF GLOMERULAR DISORDERS

The renal disorders in which the major abnormality involves the glomerulus may subside spontaneously or with treatment. However, if they progress, glomerular blood flow is obstructed, glomerular filtration ceases and the tubules associated with affected glomeruli become involved; thus many nephrons may cease to function. When sufficient nephrons have been affected, the clinical features of the disease gradually progress to chronic renal failure.

By way of illustration, a patient with the nephrotic syndrome caused by diabetic glomerular disease may slowly develop the features of chronic renal failure as individual nephrons are destroyed. In contrast, a patient who initially presents with the acute nephritic syndrome caused by a rapidly progressive GN with extensive crescents (Fig. 15.3) may quickly progress to acute renal failure. As the glomeruli are rapidly destroyed by the disease process this becomes irreversible.

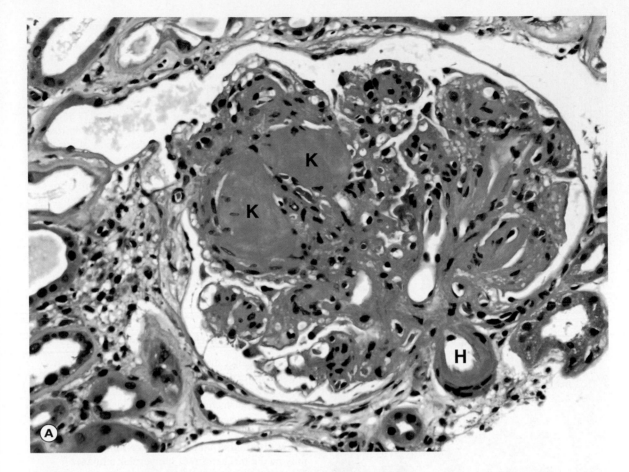

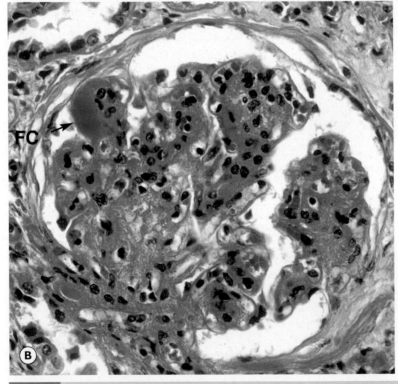

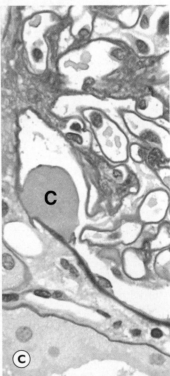

Fig. 15.9 **Diabetic glomerulosclerosis.** *(Caption opposite)*

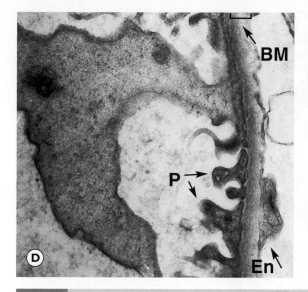

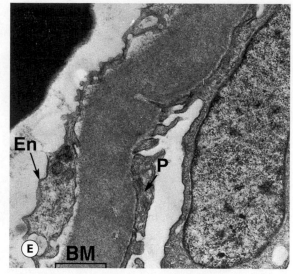

Fig. 15.9 **Diabetic glomerulosclerosis. (A)** Nodular glomerulosclerosis (HP); **(B)** diffuse glomerulosclerosis (HP); **(C)** capsular drop (PAS) (HP); **(D)** normal glomerular basement membrane (EM); **(E)** diabetic basement membrane (EM). *(Illustrations (A), (B) and (C) opposite)*

In diabetes mellitus, renal disease may occur in several ways. People with diabetes have an increased predisposition to the development of renal infections such as pyelonephritis (Fig. 15.11) and papillary necrosis (Fig. 15.14), which may cause acute renal failure. There is also a tendency to severe large vessel atherosclerosis increasing the risk of renal ischaemia and infarction.

Longstanding diabetes mellitus may result in characteristic changes to the glomeruli *(diabetic glomerulosclerosis)*. Among the early glomerular changes is a uniform and homogeneous thickening of the glomerular capillary basement membrane. This is best seen by electron microscopy as in Fig. 15.9E with the normal shown for comparison in Fig. 15.9D. In both micrographs note the glomerular capillary basement membrane **(BM)** invested by thin endothelial cell cytoplasm **(En)** on the inner aspect and by epithelial cell (podocyte) foot processes **(P)** externally. In diabetes, the basement membrane may be up to four or five times normal thickness.

Later, there is an increase in mesangial matrix, the latter often segmental and localised to produce characteristic acellular *Kimmelstiel-Wilson nodules*, often with compressed mesangial cell nuclei pushed to their periphery. This is called *nodular diabetic glomerulosclerosis* and is shown in Fig. 15.9A; note the Kimmelstiel-Wilson nodules **(K)**.

In another pattern, the mesangial matrix increase is diffuse and global, not segmental and nodular,

producing the change called *diffuse diabetic glomerulosclerosis*, illustrated in Fig. 15.9B. Both patterns may occur in the same kidney and nodule formation may be superimposed upon the diffuse change within the same glomerulus. In both patterns, there is escape of plasma protein across the thickened, but leaky, glomerular basement membrane into the urinary space. Occasionally, inspissated protein may be deposited on the outer surface of the glomerular tuft forming *fibrin caps* **(FC)** as seen in Fig. 15.9B or on the inner surface of Bowman's capsule forming *capsular drops* **(C)** as seen in Fig. 15.9C.

A characteristic feature of diabetic renal disease is *hyalinisation* of arterioles similar to that seen in hypertension (Fig. 15.15), but characteristically affecting both afferent and efferent arterioles. This arteriolar hyalinisation **(H),** seen in association with nodular diabetic glomerulosclerosis in Fig. 15.9C, may also extend into the vascular hilum of the glomerulus. The combination of arterial atherosclerosis and arteriolar hyalinisation progressively reduces the blood flow to the glomeruli; thus chronic ischaemic changes, such as hyalinisation of glomeruli and periglomerular fibrosis, are common associated findings in diabetic renal disease.

The initial glomerular basement membrane changes result in proteinuria and even the nephrotic syndrome, but with progressive diabetic glomerulosclerosis and chronic ischaemic nephron atrophy, the features of chronic renal failure supervene.

KEY TO FIGURES
BM glomerular basement membrane   **C** capsular drop   **En** endothelial cell cytoplasm   **FC** fibrin cap   **H** hyalinised arteriole   **K** Kimmelsteil-Wilson nodule   **P** podocyte foot process

BASIC SYSTEMS PATHOLOGY ■ URINARY SYSTEM

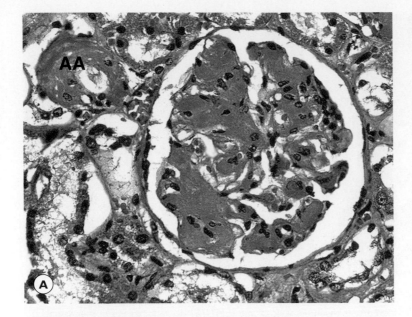

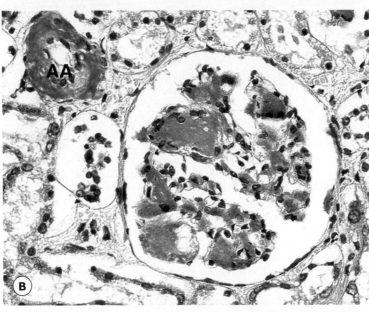

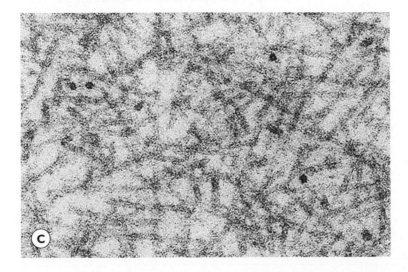

Fig. 15.10 **Renal amyloidosis.**
(A) H&E (HP); **(B)** sirius red (HP);
(C) EM.

The kidneys are the organs most commonly involved by *systemic amyloidosis* (see Ch. 16) (E-Fig. 15.6) renal failure is one of the most serious clinical complications, accounting for the majority of deaths from the disease. These sections are from an autopsy specimen, taken from a woman with a 20-year history of rheumatoid arthritis.

Amyloid deposition usually begins in the glomerular mesangium and around capillary basement membranes, leading to progressive obliteration of capillary lumina, destruction of glomerular endothelial, mesangial and podocyte cells and, eventually, complete replacement of the glomerulus by a confluent mass of amyloid. Concurrently, the walls of renal arterioles and arteries may become infiltrated by amyloid, causing impairment of the blood supply to the glomerulus. Interstitial spaces between renal tubules may also become infiltrated, further compromising tubular function. With H&E staining in Fig. 15.10A, amyloid appears as a homogeneous eosinophilic (pink) material, difficult to distinguish from collagen or hyaline deposition. Staining methods such as Congo red or Sirius red, as in Fig. 15.10B, readily distinguish amyloid, which stands out as red-stained material. In this case, amyloid is present in the glomerulus and in the wall of an affected afferent arteriole **(AA)**. Amyloid of the kidney usually presents with proteinuria, often severe enough to produce the *nephrotic syndrome*. Increasing amyloid deposition leads to glomerular ischaemia and tubular atrophy and chronic renal failure supervenes.

Electron microscopy is a useful method for detection of amyloid in tissues. Fig. 15.10C shows a portion of thickened glomerular basement membrane. The amyloid is seen to have a fibrillar ultrastructure, each fibril being composed of the precursor peptide arranged as finer filaments of a β-pleated sheet. In this instance, the amyloid was deposited as a result of long-standing rheumatoid disease and was presumably of the serum amyloid A protein type.

The tubules and interstitium may be primarily damaged as a result of hypovolaemic shock, by inorganic and organic toxins or as the result of infection. In hypovolaemic states and intoxication, tubular epithelial cells may exhibit marked cytoplasmic degenerative changes or frank necrosis leading to the pathological term *acute tubular necrosis* (Fig. 15.12) and producing the clinical syndrome of acute renal failure. Tubular epithelial cells have considerable powers of recovery and regeneration and acute renal failure may be reversible under such circumstances if the patient can be sustained in the interim by dialysis and other supportive measures.

Another increasingly important cause of tubulo-interstitial disease is drug toxicity giving rise to *interstitial nephritis* (Fig. 15.13). In this condition, a large number of drugs have been implicated including certain antibiotics, non-steroidal anti-inflammatory drugs, thiazide diuretics and proton pump inhibitors. Onset may be acute or chronic. There is a mixed inflammatory infiltrate in the interstitium in which eosinophils may be prominent. Tubular damage occurs and the condition may proceed to chronic renal failure.

Infections of the kidney include acute and chronic pyelonephritis and tuberculosis (see Ch. 5). Acute suppurative bacterial infections of the kidney (*pyelonephritis*) usually follow ascending infection from the lower urinary tract, particularly when there is obstruction to urinary outflow such as in benign prostatic hyperplasia or pressure from the fetus in pregnancy; in such cases, coliform organisms (such as *Escherichia coli* and *Proteus* species) are the most frequent infecting agents. Infection may also spread to the kidney by the haematogenous route during episodes of bacteraemia. Acute pyelonephritis may be complicated by the development of papillary necrosis (Fig. 15.14) or pus accumulation in a dilated, obstructed pelvicalyceal system (*pyonephrosis*). Acute pyelonephritis is illustrated in Fig. 15.11. Tuberculous infection of the kidneys and lower urinary tract may also arise by similar routes of spread.

Patients with urinary reflux or obstruction are prone to develop recurrent pyelonephritis Repeated attacks lead to scarring and after many episodes the kidney becomes coarsely scarred, a phenomenon termed *chronic pyelonephritis*.

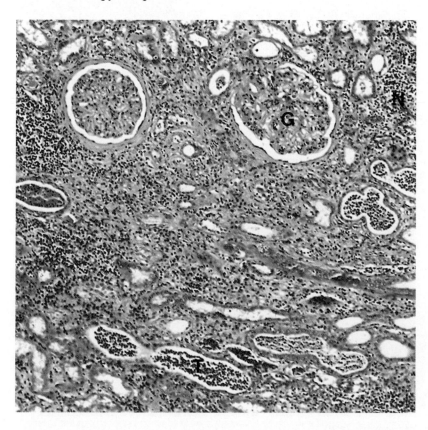

Fig. 15.11 **Acute pyelonephritis (MP).**

Fig. 15.11 illustrates established acute pyelonephritis. There is extensive infiltration of the kidney by small dark-staining neutrophil polymorphs (N), which are also seen filling dilated tubules (T). Abscess formation may ensue and, in untreated cases, multiple abscesses may merge to produce larger abscesses. These may discharge into the pelvicalyceal system to produce *pyonephrosis* or through the capsule into perinephric fat to produce a *perinephric abscess*. Note that the glomeruli (G) are spared.

With time and repeated episodes or persisting infection, the renal parenchyma becomes permanently damaged and replaced by fibrous tissue. Eventually, the features are of end-stage kidney with loss of glomeruli as well as tubules.

KEY TO FIGURES
AA afferent arteriole   **G** glomerulus   **N** neutrophil polymorphs   **T** dilated tubule

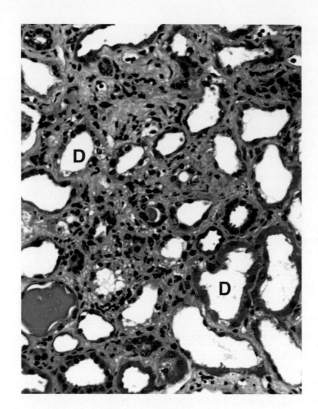

Fig. 15.12 Acute tubular necrosis (MP).

Acute tubular necrosis is a fairly common cause of acute renal failure. One of the most common underlying causes is acute ischaemia caused by hypotension. A fairly small drop in the circulating volume in an elderly person with compromised circulation, e.g. due to dehydration after an episode of vomiting and diarrhoea, may lead to acute renal failure. A renal biopsy is sometimes necessary to determine the cause and to prevent unnecessary treatment, although the majority of cases resolve without intervention. Supportive measures are usually all that is required to allow the renal tubules to regenerate.

The term necrosis is actually a misnomer as frank necrosis is seldom seen. The changes may be quite subtle in the early stages but in established ATN, as in Fig. 15.12, the tubules are dilated (D) with flattening of the epithelium. This is usually most prominent in the proximal convoluted tubules, which have the highest oxygen requirement. The epithelium at higher magnification (not shown) can be seen to have lost the brush border and plasma membrane infoldings that allow the proximal convoluted tubules to perform their function. As recovery progresses, mitotic figures become apparent in the regenerating epithelium and then the specialised features of the epithelium are restored.

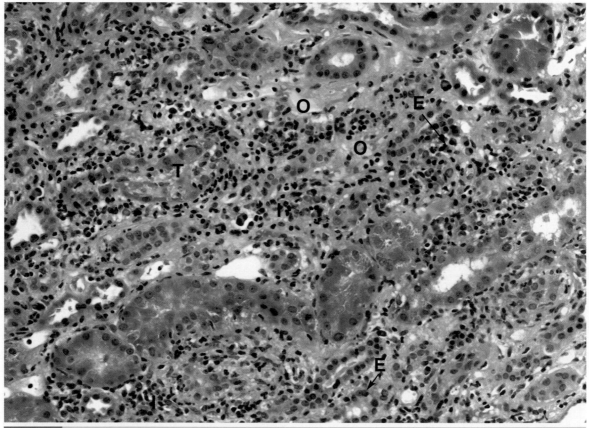

Fig. 15.13 Acute tubulo-interstitial nephritis (MP).

Interstitial nephritis most commonly occurs as an adverse hypersensitivity reaction to drugs, including antibiotics, non-steroidal anti-inflammatory agents and others. It often presents with features of systemic illness, including fever, rash and eosinophilia, with varying degrees of renal impairment. The pattern on renal biopsy is of interstitial oedema (O). There is infiltration by eosinophils (E) and mononuclear inflammatory cells (I) in the spaces between the tubules. There may be foci of tubulitis (T), where inflammatory cells invade beneath the tubular basement membrane. Treatment is supportive, including withdrawal of the offending drug.

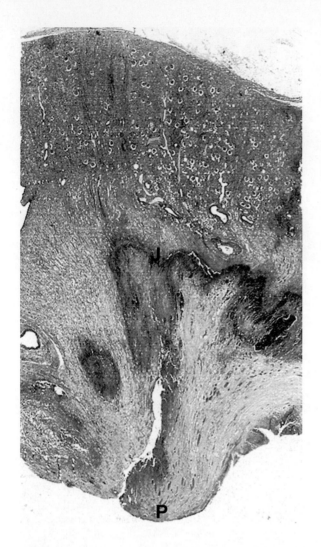

Fig. 15.14 **Renal papillary necrosis (LP).**

Fig. 15.14 shows the condition known as *papillary necrosis* or *necrotising papillitis*. At the earliest stage, there is coagulative necrosis of the tip of the papilla **(P)**, with preservation of ghost-like outlines of the papillary tubules and collecting ducts. This is followed by a neutrophil inflammatory response at the junction **(J)** between normal and necrotic papilla. This largely disappears at a later stage when the necrotic papilla separates and is shed. There may also be calcification.

This condition, which is probably ischaemic in nature, often occurs in association with acute infection of the urinary parenchyma and pelvicalyceal system, particularly when accompanied by an obstructive pathology affecting the lower urinary tract. It may also be seen with or without overt infection in diabetic nephropathy and in analgesic nephropathy (E-Fig. 15.7**G**).

If there is sudden loss of many papillae, the patient may develop acute renal failure.

Vascular disorders

The kidney is especially vulnerable to the effects of arterial hypertension as illustrated in Figs 11.1 and 11.2, and irreversible damage to nephrons may result either acutely from accelerated (malignant) hypertension or progressively over a period of years in benign (essential) hypertension.

Hypertensive nephrosclerosis resulting from benign (essential) hypertension is illustrated in Fig. 15.15. Malignant or accelerated hypertension causes a different pattern of renal damage, similar to the changes seen in acute *scleroderma*, and may result in acute renal failure. In reality, hypertension cannot be neatly divided into essential and accelerated types; individuals who have had mild hypertension for many years may progress quite suddenly to very high blood pressures that put eyesight, kidneys and other organs at severe risk. This is especially the case where the individual has underlying renal disease that progresses. Other individuals may develop accelerated hypertension out of the blue.

Various forms of vasculitis may also affect the kidney, including *polyarteritis nodosa* (see Fig. 11.6) and those associated with *antineutrophil cytoplasmic antibody (ANCA)* such as *granulomatosis with polyangiitis* (previously known as Wegener's granulomatosis) and *microscopic polyarteritis* (see Fig.11.7).

Small *infarcts* of the renal cortex are common in patients with the above vascular disorders. They are usually seen as incidental findings in kidneys removed for other reasons (e.g. tumours). The infarcts are usually seen as wedge-shaped pale scars with the base abutting the renal capsule, although they may be seen in any stage of infarction (see Fig. 10.1). In kidneys with extensive infarcts, the cortical surface is pitted and the kidney is shrunken. In rare cases, abrupt interruption to the blood supply, such as renal artery thrombosis, may lead to renal cortical infarction where the entire renal cortex undergoes coagulative necrosis. The renal medulla is much more resistant to ischaemia.

KEY TO FIGURES
D dilated tubules   **E** eosinophil   **I** mononuclear inflammatory cells   **J** junction between normal and necrotic tissue   **O** interstitial oedema   **P** renal papilla   **T** tubulitis

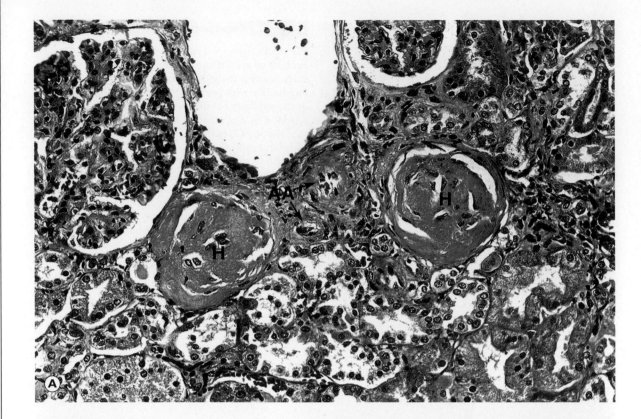

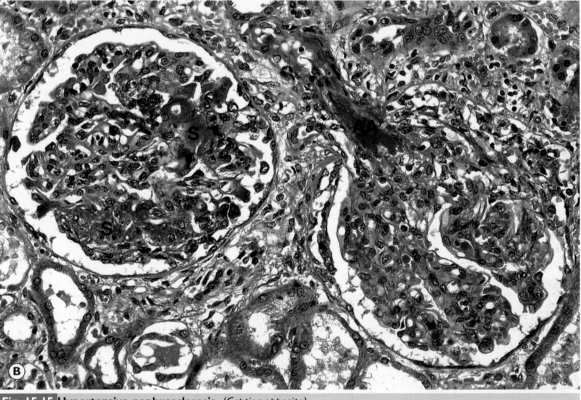

Fig. 15.15 **Hypertensive nephrosclerosis.** *(Caption opposite)*

KEY TO FIGURES
AA afferent arteriole   **H** hyalinised sclerosed glomerulus   **S** segment of glomerulus

Fig. 15.15 Hypertensive nephrosclerosis. **(A)** Benign hypertensive nephrosclerosis (HP); **(B)** malignant hypertensive nephrosclerosis (HP). *(Illustrations opposite)*

The vessel changes in systemic hypertension have been discussed and illustrated in some detail in Figs 11.1 and 11.2. The kidney is particularly vulnerable to the damaging effects of these vessel changes and renal failure is an important complication of untreated hypertension. The pathological changes in the kidney depend on the severity and rate of progress of the hypertension.

In *benign (essential) hypertension*, the hypertension is of gradual onset and progression, with only moderately elevated diastolic pressure. Large and medium-sized renal arteries show marked thickening of their walls by a combination of medial hypertrophy, elastic lamina reduplication and fibrous intimal thickening: this is shown in Fig. 11.1A. The arterioles show hyaline thickening of their walls as seen in Fig. 11.1B These changes reduce the calibre of all renal afferent vessels and the resulting chronic ischaemia leads to progressive *sclerosis (hyalinisation)* of the glomerulus and subsequent disuse atrophy of the tubular component of the nephron.

Fig. 15.15A shows a group of glomeruli, two of which have become converted into hyaline, amorphous, pink-staining masses (**H**) as a result of chronic ischaemia owing to hyalinisation of the walls of their afferent arterioles (**AA**); the other glomeruli are as yet unaffected. Slowly progressive loss of functioning nephrons may eventually lead to chronic renal failure and the morphological state known as end-stage kidney (Table 15.1).

In contrast, in *malignant (accelerated) hypertension*, where the rise in blood pressure is rapid and severe, the arterial and arteriolar changes are different. Large and medium-sized arteries may show only concentric thickening of the intima by loose, rather myxomatous, fibroblastic tissue as seen in Fig. 11.2A and there is no elastic lamina reduplication or significant medial hypertrophy. Small arteries may show marked concentric fibroblastic intimal thickening ('onion-skin' lesion) so that the lumen is often virtually obliterated. Arterioles frequently show patchy acute necrosis of their walls with the accumulation of amorphous, brightly eosinophilic, proteinaceous material *(fibrinoid)* in the damaged walls; this is shown in Fig. 11.2B. This change is known as *fibrinoid necrosis*.

In the kidney, as seen in Fig. 15.15B, this often affects the afferent arterioles (**AA**) at the glomerular hila and may extend into the glomerular tuft to affect some segments (**S**) of the glomerular capillary network. The onset of small vessel changes is acute and may produce an abrupt reduction in blood supply to the nephrons, often producing glomerular micro-infarction and acute tubular necrosis. The effect is to produce a catastrophic reduction in glomerular filtration and the patient may develop acute oliguric or anuric renal failure. Not infrequently, the patient with longstanding benign hypertension may suddenly develop an accelerated phase and the histological changes in the kidney may be those of mixed benign and malignant nephrosclerosis.

Pathology of renal transplantation

Renal transplantation has become a routine treatment for chronic renal failure in many countries. The transplant recipient is freed from a life of regular dialysis with a consequent improvement in quality of life. The function of the transplanted kidney may however be affected by a number of factors in the days, weeks and months following transplantation. The most important of these include:

- **Acute tubular necrosis**: this is identical to acute tubular necrosis from other causes (Fig. 15.12). The major factor here is the 'cold ischaemic time', i.e. the length of time between harvesting of the kidney and re-establishment of vascular perfusion in the donor. Supportive measures may be needed in the immediate post-transplantation phase but usually this will resolve.
- **Rejection** (see Fig. 15.16)
- **Drug toxicity**: routinely used immunosuppressive agents, such as ciclosporin A and related compounds (the calcineurin inhibitors), may have a range of effects on the kidney. Histologically, there may be changes in the tubules and/or the blood vessels. Exquisite control of dosage and sometimes transfer to a different agent will usually control this problem.
- **Infection**: transplant recipients require immunosuppression to prevent rejection of the graft and this makes them susceptible to a range of infections.
- **Recurrent GN**: this is more likely to be a problem months to years after transplantation than in the early stages.

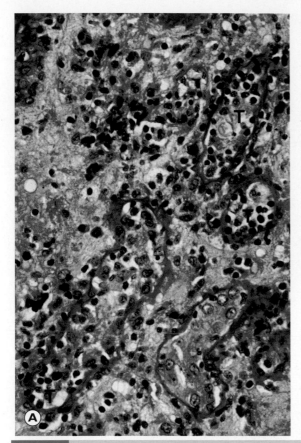

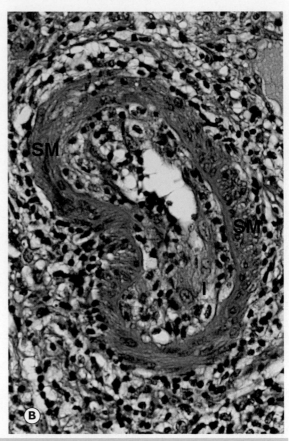

Fig. 15.16 **Renal transplant rejection. (A)** T cell mediated rejection, Type I (MP); **(B)** T cell mediated rejection Type II (HP).

Rejection of a transplanted kidney (or other organ) depends mainly on the degree of *human leukocyte antigen (HLA)* mismatch between donor and recipient. Obviously, transplantation between identical twins has the best chance of success, but this is rarely feasible. Tissue typing is routinely carried out on potential donors to identify recipients with the closest HLA match.

The *Banff classification* (originally designed by a panel of renal pathologists in Banff in Canada) is a semi-quantitative method for assessing rejection. Various features of rejection are graded numerically and the scores combined to classify according to the type and degree of severity of rejection. The classification is regularly reviewed and updated.

The Banff classification recognises several categories of rejection, the two most important of which are *T-cell-mediated rejection* and *antibody mediated rejection,* both of which may have acute and chronic phases. Acute rejection occurs within days to months after transplantation while chronic rejection may take years. Both T-cell and antibody mediated rejection may occur at the same time and some of the histological features overlap. Fig. 15.16 illustrates the most common variant of renal transplant rejection, T-cell-mediated rejection. Acute T-cell-mediated rejection, Banff Type I, is shown in Fig. 15.16A. The interstitium is infiltrated by lymphocytes that are also seen within the tubular epithelium *(tubulitis)* **(T)**. Tubulitis represents a cell-mediated immune response

directed against donor tubular epithelial cells and results in destruction of tubules. The glomeruli are generally not affected in the acute phase.

Acute T-cell-mediated rejection Types II and III manifest as a T-cell immune response against vascular endothelial cells. The typical features of Type II T-cell mediated rejection shown in Fig. 15.16B include infiltration of the vascular endothelium by inflammatory cells and swelling and proliferation of endothelial cells, a pattern known as *intimal arteritis* **(I)**. The smooth muscle of the wall of the artery **(SM)** is relatively unaffected. When there is inflammation of the full thickness of the vessel wall or fibrinoid necrosis, this is classified as type III acute T-cell mediated rejection. As the condition becomes chronic, there is intimal thickening owing to fibrosis and proliferation of myointimal cells.

Antibody mediated rejection may show a variety of histological changes including acute tubular, vascular and glomerular changes. Key features are the presence of the complement component C4d on the endothelium of peritubular capillaries (demonstrated by immunostaining techniques) and the presence of circulating specific anti-donor antibodies in the recipient's blood.

Chronic rejection is characterised by a combination of the above changes with tubular atrophy and interstitial fibrosis and loss of glomeruli. Unchecked chronic rejection will inexorably proceed to end-stage kidney.

KEY TO FIGURES

A adipose tissue   **I** intimal arteritis   **M** smooth muscle cells   **N** tumour cell nest   **S** oedematous stroma   **SM** smooth muscle of artery wall   **T** tubulitis   **V** blood vessels

A range of benign and malignant tumours occurs in the kidney and many are unique to the kidney. Benign tumours include *papillary adenoma*, a fairly common incidental finding in nephrectomy specimens, *oncocytoma*, illustrated in Fig. 15.17, and *angiomyolipoma*, shown in Fig. 15.18.

The most common and important malignant renal tumour in adults is *renal cell carcinoma*. Several subtypes are recognised and some of the more common variants are illustrated in Fig. 15.19. One of its important methods of spread is by venous invasion, typically giving rise to 'cannon ball' lung metastases and often bone metastases.

Our understanding of renal tumour pathology has been transformed in recent years by the use of new molecular techniques. Classification is now based upon a combination of histological appearances, immunohistochemical findings and the presence of typical genetic changes in certain tumour types. For example, papillary renal cell carcinomas typically show gains of chromosomes 7 and/or 17, as well as loss of the Y chromosome. These new investigative techniques have also revealed a range of rare but important hereditary renal cell carcinomas.

The kidney is the site of an important malignant tumour of children, *nephroblastoma* or *Wilms' tumour* (Fig. 15.20); this is an example of a *'small round blue cell tumour'* and is of embryological origin.

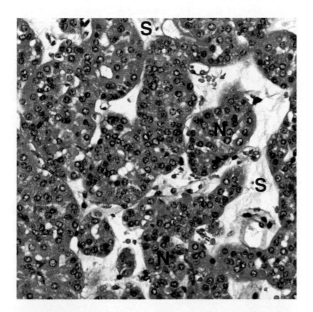

Fig. 15.17 Oncocytoma (HP).

Oncocytoma is a fairly common benign renal neoplasm. Macroscopically, the tumour is a mahogany brown colour with a well-defined margin (E-Fig. 15.8**G**). It arises in the renal cortex. There is often a central, irregular, fibrotic scar, which may be identifiable radiologically. Necrosis and haemorrhage are very rare, in contrast to renal cell carcinoma.

Microscopically, the tumour is composed of small regular round cells arranged in nests (**N**) as shown in Fig. 15.17. The cell nests are separated by an oedematous stroma (**S**). There is little cellular pleomorphism and minimal if any mitotic activity. The cells have abundant granular eosinophilic cytoplasm, resulting from the very large numbers of mitochondria that pack the cytoplasm.

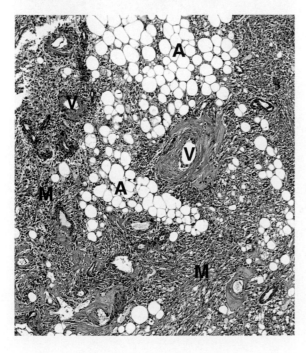

Fig. 15.18 Angiomyolipoma (LP).

This is an uncommon but important tumour of the kidney, consisting of a mixture of abnormal blood vessels (**V**), sheets of smooth muscle cells (**M**) and adipose tissue (**A**). The smooth muscle cells often have an epithelioid appearance, i.e. they are round to ovoid in shape with plentiful eosinophilic or clear cytoplasm. Most angiomyolipomas are benign but a few, usually with atypical histological features, may behave in a malignant fashion. This tumour is very common in patients with *tuberous sclerosis* and is often multiple in these patients. Angiomyolipomas also occur in the liver and rarely at other sites.

Angiomyolipomas belong to a group of esoteric tumours called *PEComas*, supposedly derived from Perivascular Epithelioid Cells. This group includes a variety of rare tumours occurring at many anatomical sites, which are all immunoreactive for a combination of melanocyte markers (HMB45 and MelanA) and smooth muscle markers (actin and/or desmin). This group includes the clear cell ('sugar') tumour of the lung and other sites.

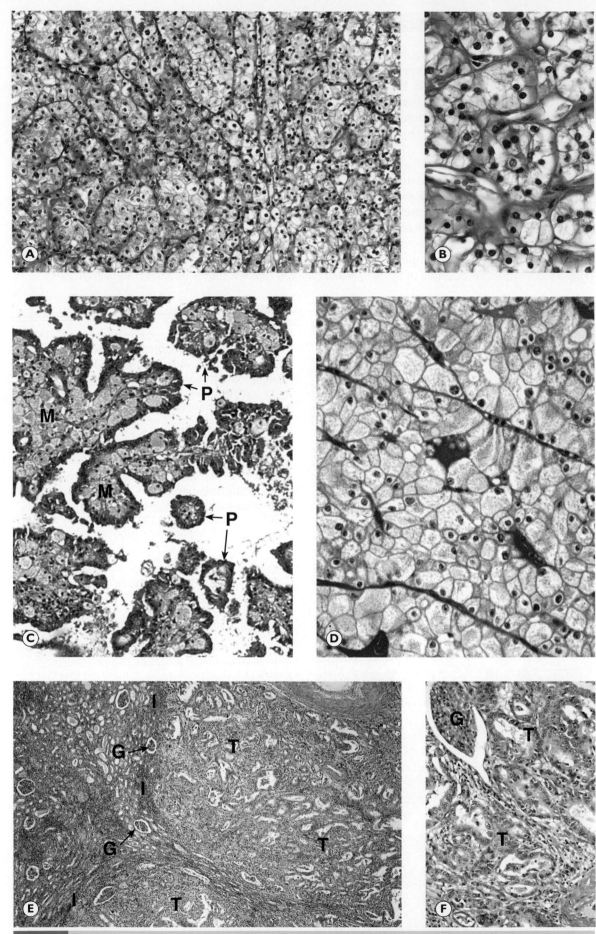

Fig. 15.19 Renal cell carcinoma. *(Caption opposite)*

The most common primary malignant tumour of the kidney is the ***renal cell carcinoma*** derived from renal tubular epithelium. Renal cell carcinoma may be subclassified according to histological and cytogenetic criteria. All types of renal cell carcinoma may present with one or more of the classic triad of signs: haematuria, flank pain and a palpable mass. However, many of these tumours come to medical attention after being detected on imaging studies carried out for other reasons. A few renal cell carcinomas are hereditary and some are found in ***von Hippel-Lindau syndrome***, in association with cerebellar and retinal haemangioblastomas. However, the great majority of cases are sporadic. The major variants of renal cell carcinoma are:

- **Clear cell carcinoma:** This is by far the most common type and generally has the worst prognosis. As seen in Figs 15.19A and B, the tumour cells are large and polygonal in shape and the cytoplasm is clear because of the accumulation of cytoplasmic glycogen and lipid. In other areas of the tumour, the cytoplasm is granular and pink-staining, more closely resembling the tubular epithelium from which these tumours are derived.
- **Papillary carcinoma:** The next most common variant, this tumour is composed of papillary structures as shown in Fig. 15.19C. The tumour is often surrounded by a thick fibrous capsule and there is typically extensive necrosis and haemorrhage. Microscopically, the tumour consists of papillary structures **(P)** surrounded by a layer of cuboidal to columnar malignant epithelial cells. The papillary cores are often packed with foamy macrophages **(M)**. Other areas may have tubular architecture.

- **Chromophobe carcinoma:** This tumour consists of sheets of malignant epithelial cells with pale cytoplasm (as in Fig. 15.19D) and prominent cell boundaries that resemble plant cells. Note the difference between this tumour and clear cell carcinoma in Fig. 15.19B.
- **Collecting duct carcinoma:** This is a rare but highly aggressive tumour arising in the distal collecting ducts of the renal medulla. It is composed of irregular, infiltrating tubules composed of pleomorphic cells with prominent nucleoli. Typically, there is a prominent stromal desmoplastic reaction with associated inflammation **(I)**, as shown at low power in Fig. 15.19E. Tumour infiltrates between normal structures and glomeruli **(G)** are clearly seen adjacent to the malignant tubular structures **(T)**. This is shown at higher magnification in Fig. 15.19F.
- **Sarcomatoid carcinoma** (not illustrated): This is not a separate subtype of tumour but rather a pattern that may be found in combination with any of the other types of renal cell carcinoma. As suggested by the name, the tumour cells resemble sarcoma. The presence of this pattern confers a worse prognosis.

Clear cell carcinoma typically forms a well-defined yellow mass with cystic change and areas of haemorrhage (E-Fig. 15.9**G**). It tends to breach the walls of intrarenal venous tributaries and to grow as solid cords along the lumen of the renal vein towards and into the inferior vena cava. From here, venous emboli spread tumour deposits to the lung, producing typical isolated *'cannon ball secondaries'*. Renal carcinoma also has a particular propensity for metastasis to bone and brain.

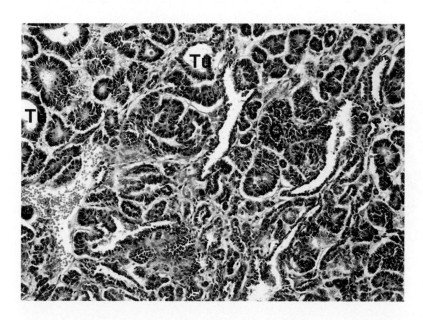

Fig. 15.20 **Nephroblastoma (MP).**

This is one of the most common malignant tumours of infants and children (E-Fig. 15.10**G**) and is believed to originate from embryonic renal blastema. It is composed of a mixture of primitive and undifferentiated cells **(C)** and tubular structures **(Tu)**, resembling primitive renal tubules; occasionally, structures resembling immature glomeruli are also found. There are many histological variants of this tumour, some of which contain primitive tissue cells such as skeletal muscle precursors (rhabdomyoblasts).

KEY TO FIGURES

C undifferentiated cells   **G** normal glomeruli   **I** inflammation   **M** foamy macrophages   **P** papillary structures   **T** malignant tubules   **Tu** primitive tubular structures   **V** blood vessel

The most important disorders of the lower urinary tract are infection and neoplasia. Infections are common, but usually remain confined to the bladder *(cystitis)*; ascending spread into the ureters and pelvicalyceal systems may result in renal parenchymal involvement *(acute pyelonephritis)* as shown in Fig. 15.11. Persistent or repeated infection in the urinary tract predisposes to the development of urinary stones *(calculi)*, particularly in the bladder and pelvicalyceal systems. Infections of the urethra *(urethritis)* are commonly sexually transmitted, often involving the organisms *N. gonorrhoeae* and *Chlamydia*.

The pelvicalyceal system, ureters and bladder are lined by a specialised epithelium known as *transitional epithelium (urothelium)* (E-Fig. 15.11**H**). Malignant tumours of the urothelium, known as transitional cell or urothelial carcinomas (Fig. 15.22), are common and are of particular interest because of the possible role of chemical carcinogens such as aniline dyes in their pathogenesis. Urothelial carcinomas may be either invasive or non-invasive. Most of the deeply invasive tumours are high-grade carcinomas. Malignant tumours are probably preceded by the development of urothelial dysplasia and carcinoma in situ (Fig. 15.21). Benign tumours include *transitional cell papillomas* and *inverted papillomas*.

Classification and grading of transitional cell neoplasms is complex and continues to evolve. The traditional WHO 1973 system recognised benign papillomas as well as transitional cell carcinomas of grades 1, 2 and 3. This system has some limitations as the criteria for these categories are not very well defined and a large proportion of tumours tend to be classified as grade 2. Also, some tumours that are now known to behave in a benign fashion are classified as grade 1 carcinomas. The newer WHO/ISUP 2004 system uses the term *papillary urothelial neoplasm of low malignant potential (PUNLMP)* for these very low grade tumours with likely benign behaviour and it splits the remaining malignant tumours into low grade and high grade groups. The two systems do not directly correspond. Despite the limitations described above, the old 1973 WHO classification remains in widespread use as a validated and reproducible system, but now it is used alongside the newer WHO/ISUP 2004 system as these are thought to provide the best prognostic information when applied in conjunction. This is illustrated in Table 15.2.

Table 15.2 Classification of urothelial tumours.

WHO 1973 classification	WHO/ISUP 2004 classification
Papilloma	Papilloma
Transitional cell carcinoma Grade 1	Papillary urothelial neoplasm of low malignant potential (PUNLMP)
	Low-grade urothelial carcinoma
Transitional cell carcinoma Grade 2	
Transitional cell carcinoma Grade 3	High-grade urothelial carcinoma

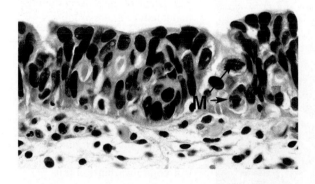

Fig. 15.21 Bladder carcinoma in situ (HP).

Carcinoma in situ of the urinary bladder is characterised by replacement of normal epithelium by cells indistinguishable from those seen in high grade urothelial carcinoma. The epithelial cells are enlarged and crowded, with enlarged hyperchromatic nuclei and prominent mitotic figures **(M)**, one of which is near the epithelial surface. The architecture of the epithelium appears disorganized and chaotic. The epithelium is not thickened and this area might, at cystoscopy, merely appear reddened. Urothelial carcinoma in situ may be found in isolation or in association with papillary urothelial carcinoma (Fig. 15.22). These lesions are likely to progress to invasive carcinoma.

KEY TO FIGURES
BV blood vessels   **M** mitotic figures   **S** stroma   **SM** smooth muscle   **T** tumour

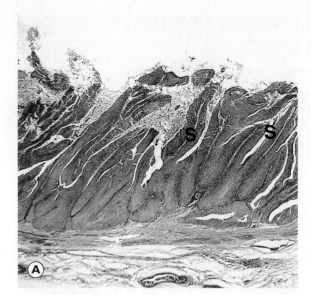

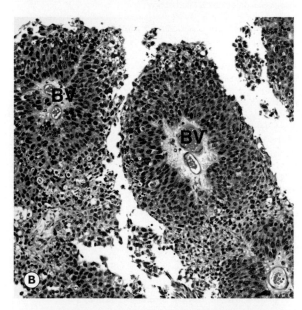

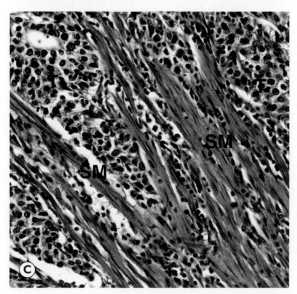

Fig. 15.22 Urothelial (transitional cell) carcinoma. **(A)** Low grade (LP); **(B)** high grade (LP); **(C)** high grade (HP).

Urothelial (transitional cell) carcinomas (TCC) are common. All are regarded as malignant despite the fact that many show no evidence of invasion when first detected. Fig. 15.22A shows a low grade urothelial carcinoma (TCC grade 1) with frond-like papillary outgrowths from the urothelial surface with a slender connective tissue stroma **(S)** supporting the layers of neoplastic cells which are enlarged and disorganised compared to normal urothelium.

In high grade urothelial carcinomas (TCC grade 3), there may also be a surface papillary component as shown in Fig. 15.22B. At high magnification, the blood vessels **(BV)** in the connective tissue stroma of the papillary cores are obvious. The covering epithelium is thickened, with crowded, atypical urothelial cells, which fail to mature towards the surface. High grade urothelial carcinomas may have no papillary component but instead form a sessile ulcerated plaque. High grade tumours, as shown in Fig. 15.22C, may invade deeply into the bladder wall. In advanced stage tumours, the tumour cells **(T)** infiltrate between smooth muscle bundles **(SM)** of the detrusor muscle, indicating a poor prognosis.

Urothelial carcinomas (E-Fig. 15.12**G**) are frequently multifocal in origin and there is a strong link between their development and exposure to certain industrial chemicals such as aniline dyes. Cigarette smoking has also been causally linked with the development of urothelial carcinomas.

The prognosis of urothelial carcinomas depends on their location, the grade of the tumour, and the extent of local invasion when the tumour is first detected. The cytology of urothelial carcinomas is shown in more detail in Fig. 7.4. Occasionally, squamous carcinomas may develop in the bladder from metaplastic epithelium associated with chronic inflammation by a stone or parasitic infection (schistosomiasis, see Fig. 5.23). Rarely, adenocarcinoma arises from embryological urachal remnants in the dome of the bladder or from intestinal metaplasia of the urothelium at other sites (usually secondary to chronic inflammation).

Table 15.3 Chapter review.

Site	Disorder	Main pathological features	Figure
Kidney: glomerular disorders	End-stage kidney	Sclerosed glomeruli, atrophic tubules, interstitial fibrosis	15.1
	Acute diffuse proliferative GN	Enlarged hypercellular glomeruli, infiltration by neutrophils, obstructed capillary loops	15.2
	Necrotising GN	Necrosis of glomerular tuft, may be segmental, may be associated with crescent formation	15.3
	Mesangial proliferative GN	Expanded mesangium with increased mesangial cells	15.4
	Membranoproliferative (mesangiocapillary) GN	Hypercellular, hyperlobular glomeruli with double contour GBM	15.5
	Membranous nephropathy	Thickened GBM, 'spikes' (silver stain)	15.6
	Focal segmental glomerulosclerosis	Idiopathic or secondary to segmental necrosis or nephron loss. Segment of tuft replaced by fibrosis	15.7
	Minimal change disease	Normal light microscopy and immunofluorescence, 'fused' podocyte foot processes on electron microscopy	15.8
	Diabetic nephropathy	Diffuse and nodular glomerulosclerosis, hyalinised arterioles, capsular drops, fibrin caps, thickened GBM	15.9
	Renal amyloidosis	Deposition of insoluble fibrillar protein in glomerulus and vessel walls, stains with Congo and Sirius red	15.10
Kidney: interstitial disorders	Acute pyelonephritis	Infiltration of interstitium and tubules by neutrophil polymorphs. May form abscesses and pyonephrosis	15.11
	Acute tubular necrosis	Dilated renal tubules with flattened 'simplified' epithelium, vacuolation and fragmentation of tubular cell cytoplasm	15.12
	Acute tubulo-interstitial nephritis	Often due to drug hypersensitivity. Interstitial oedema with eosinophils and mononuclear cells. Focal tubulitis	15.13
	Renal papillary necrosis	Infarction of renal papilla with inflammation at edge of infarcted area	15.14
Kidney: vascular disorders	Essential hypertension	Hypertrophied arteries with fibroelastic intimal thickening, sclerosed glomeruli	15.15A
	Accelerated hypertension	Fibrinoid necrosis of arterioles, 'onion-skin' intimal thickening of medium and large sized arteries, vascular thrombosis, acute ischaemia of glomeruli	15.15B
Kidney: transplant rejection	Acute T-cell mediated rejection	Inflammation of tubules (tubulitis) and interstitium (type I) Inflammation of arteries (intimal arteritis, transmural arteritis, fibrinoid necrosis of artery wall (types II and III))	15.16
Kidney: tumours	Oncocytoma	Brown tumour macroscopically, often with central scar. Nests of bland epithelial cells with round nuclei and eosinophilic granular cytoplasm	15.17
	Angiomyolipoma	Mixture of abnormal blood vessels, smooth muscle cells and adipose tissue. Most are benign	15.18
	Renal cell carcinoma	Clear cell: cells have clear cytoplasm Papillary: papillary epithelial structures with foamy macrophages in papillary cores Chromophobe: cells with pale-stained cytoplasm and prominent cell borders Collecting duct: infiltrating tumour with desmoplasia	15.19
	Nephroblastoma	Primitive undifferentiated cells, tubular structures	15.20
Bladder	Carcinoma in situ	Flat lesion consisting of highly atypical epithelial cells with mitotic figures and no maturation of cells towards the surface	15.21
	Urothelial carcinoma (transitional cell carcinoma)	Papillary structures covered by abnormal urothelial cells. High grade lesions may form solid ulcerated plaque. Graded as high or low (and/or 1, 2, 3)	15.22

16 Lymphoid and haematopoietic systems

Functions of the lymphoreticular system

The lymphoreticular system is composed of various organs and tissues which facilitate the interaction of lymphocytes with cells of monocyte–macrophage lineage in the generation of immune responses. The main organs and tissues of the system are the thymus (E-Fig. 16.1**H**), spleen (E-Fig. 16.2**H**), lymph nodes, bone marrow and mucosa- associated lymphoid tissue (MALT), such as tonsils (E-Fig. 16.3**H**) and Peyer's patches of the gut (E-Fig. 16.4**H**).

Lymphocytes are produced in the bone marrow. Their number is selectively expanded, mainly in lymph nodes (E-Fig. 16.5**H**), in response to specific immunological requirements. Many lymphoid cells circulate through peripheral tissues via blood and lymphatic vessels in a constant search for antigens.

The monocyte–macrophage system includes tissue macrophages (histiocytes), which are found in virtually every organ. These become activated following tissue damage and, together with monocytes recruited from the blood, act as phagocytic cells in the process of organisation (see Ch. 2). These cells also process antigen for presentation to T lymphocytes. Some tissues include a population of specialised dendritic antigen-presenting cells that have a role in initiating specific immune responses.

We will consider disorders affecting some of the main organs of the haematolymphoid system as follows:

■ **Lymph nodes**

– reactive processes

– metastatic tumours

– primary tumours (lymphoma).

■ **Bone marrow**

– abnormalities of haematopoiesis

– metastatic tumours

– myeloma

– leukaemia and lymphoma

– myeloproliferative and myelodysplastic processes.

Reactive disorders of lymph nodes

The lymphoreticular system is remarkably labile and quickly responds to the presence of infective agents or foreign material in the activation of an immune response. There are two main patterns of immune response:

■ The *cell-mediated response*: This involves the activity of T lymphocytes that are either directly or indirectly cytotoxic.

■ The *humoral response*: This involves the activation of B lymphocytes, which differentiate into antibody-secreting plasma cells; interaction of antibody with antigen leads to destruction or inactivation of the antigen.

Lymphadenopathy (lymph node enlargement) is a common consequence of infection and other immune reactions. Various different histological appearances can occur. These are determined by the nature of the immune stimulus and the patient's capacity to mount an immune response. In broad terms, three main patterns of non-specific lymphadenopathy are recognised which reflect reaction and expansion of different constituent areas of the lymph node (Fig. 16.1):

■ follicular hyperplasia

■ paracortical hyperplasia

■ sinus hyperplasia/sinus histiocytosis.

Some infections and other immune stimuli give rise to more specific patterns of lymphadenopathy which can allow the pathologist to suggest a particular aetiology. Examples include the finding of multiple minute granulomas in cases of toxoplasmosis, granulomatous lymphadenitis with caseous necrosis in tuberculosis (see Ch. 5) and follicular lysis in HIV infection (see Ch. 5).

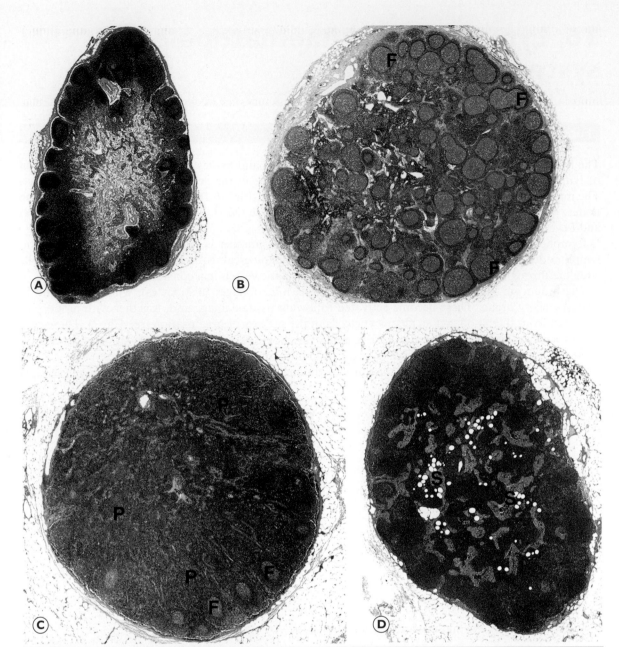

Fig. 16.1 **Reactive hyperplasia of lymph nodes. (A)** Normal lymph node (LP); **(B)** follicular hyperplasia (LP); **(C)** paracortical hyperplasia (LP); **(D)** sinus hyperplasia (LP).

Damage to or inflammation of any tissue may excite a reactive response in the draining lymph nodes. The three basic patterns of response, follicular hyperplasia, paracortical hyperplasia and sinus hyperplasia, may be seen separately or in combination, depending upon the nature of the stimulus. A low power image of a normal lymph node is included in Fig. 16.1A for comparison, showing small, peripherally located follicles (**F**) in the cortex.

In *follicular hyperplasia*, illustrated in Fig. 16.1B, there is an increase in number and size of cortical lymphoid follicles. This reflects a B-cell (humoral) response and results in the production and clonal expansion of antibody secreting plasma cells.

In *paracortical (parafollicular) hyperplasia*, seen in Fig. 16.1C, there is expansion of the T-cell parafollicular zone (**P**) with small, inconspicuous B-cell follicles (**F**) pushed to the periphery of the node beneath the capsule. This pattern is commonly seen in response to viral infection.

In *sinus hyperplasia* or *sinus histiocytosis*, shown in Fig. 16.1D, there is no great increase in the lymphoid component of the node, but the medullary sinuses (**S**) are extremely prominent due to dilatation and hyperplasia of histiocytic cells lining the sinuses. This reaction is seen in nodes draining tissues from which endogenous particulate matter such as lipid is released. A common example is necrotic tumour.

KEY TO FIGURES
F follicle   **GC** germinal centre   **N** necrosis   **P** paracortex   **S** medullary sinus   **SS** subcapsular sinus
T tumour

This is less common than reactive lymphadenopathy, but is also a frequent finding in clinical practice. Although primary malignant tumours of the lymphoid system are the main focus of this section, it is important to recognise that metastatic spread of other tumours such as carcinoma and malignant melanoma (E-Fig. 16.6**G**) to lymph nodes is a regular occurrence (see Fig. 7.13 and Fig. 16.2), and this possibility must therefore always be considered before suggesting a diagnosis of lymphoma.

Lymphoma is a primary tumour of lymphoid tissue. This group of disorders is divided into two broad categories on the basis of the cell types present:

■ *Non-Hodgkin lymphoma* (NHL) may be derived from B or T lymphocytes.

■ *Hodgkin lymphoma* (HL), previously known as Hodgkin's disease, is characterised by the presence of *Reed–Sternberg* cells.

Lymphoma usually presents with involvement of a group of lymph nodes and may then spread to involve multiple nodal groups, as well as other haematolymphoid organs such as bone marrow and spleen. NHL may arise in other organs or tissues such as skin, gut, thyroid, brain, salivary gland, lung and testis. Classification of lymphoma is complex and will be considered in the next section.

Other constituent cells of the lymph node may rarely proliferate and so give rise to lymphadenopathy. One example is a group of disorders known as *Langerhans' cell histiocytosis.* This condition has previously been known as *histiocytosis X* and by a range of eponymous designations, reflecting different patterns and severities of disease (*Letterer–Siwe, Hand–Schüller–Christian disease,* etc.). It is characterised by proliferation of histiocytic cells, which resemble the Langerhans' antigen-presenting cells found in normal skin and lymph nodes. There is a spectrum of severity, ranging from benign and localised to disseminated and rapidly fatal disease, which can involve skin, viscera, bone marrow and lymph nodes.

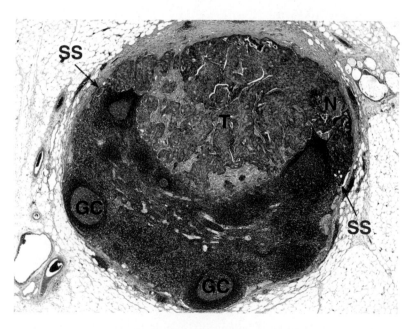

Fig. 16.2 **Metastatic colonic carcinoma in lymph node (LP).**

This micrograph shows a mesenteric lymph node from a patient with colonic adenocarcinoma (see Fig. 13.24). Carcinoma cells invade into lymphatic channels draining the primary tumour and gain access to the regional lymph nodes through the *afferent lymphatic channels*. These malignant cells enter the *subcapsular sinus* (**SS**) of the lymph node and may settle at this site where they can proliferate to form a secondary tumour mass.

A new deposit (**T**) typically resembles the primary lesion. Here, the features are those of colonic adenocarcinoma. There are areas of necrosis (**N**) with the tumour. Reactive follicles with germinal centres (**GC**) are seen within the lymph node.

LYMPH NODE SAMPLING AND EXAMINATION IN COMMON CANCERS
Examination of lymph nodes draining many malignant tumours is a routine part of the pathological assessment of tumour *stage* (the extent of disease spread, important in planning treatment and in predicting likely prognosis). The surgeon will usually excise not only the main tumour mass for examination, but also any associated groups of regional lymph nodes that drain the site of the primary mass, e.g. axillary lymph nodes in breast carcinoma, hilar and mediastinal nodes in lung cancer.

On occasion, the pathologist may receive a lymph node that contains metastatic tumour from a patient who is not already known to have pre-existing malignant disease. In this setting, examination of the metastatic deposit, often with use of special staining techniques such as immunohistochemistry, may allow the pathologist to suggest a likely site of origin of the tumour and so guide further investigation and management of the patient.

Lymphoma classification

Division of lymphomas into non-Hodgkin and Hodgkin types reflects important differences in both clinical behaviour and tumour morphology.

Non-Hodgkin lymphomas (NHLs) form a large and diverse group of diseases, all of which are malignant, despite the suffix -oma. The main features common to this group are listed below:

■ Presentation is usually with painless lymphadenopathy.

■ Disease may appear to be localised to one nodal group or may be widely disseminated, with generalised lymphadenopathy and involvement of other organs.

■ Biopsy is usually performed to establish the diagnosis and to allow classification.

■ Definitive classification involves assessment of cell morphology, immunophenotype and molecular/cytogenetic features.

■ A number of forms of NHL show characteristic chromosomal abnormalities that are useful in diagnosis and, in some instances, in assessing prognosis.

■ Most tumours are derived from a clonal proliferation of B or T lymphocytes and may be broadly divided into low- and high-grade types.

■ B-cell lymphomas are considerably more common than T-cell types.

■ B-cell lymphomas may arise at extranodal sites, most commonly within mucosa-associated lymphoid tissue (MALT), and these behave differently from nodal lymphomas.

■ T-cell lymphomas most frequently occur in skin and may present as a disease termed *mycosis fungoides.*

Hodgkin lymphoma (HL) is less common (Fig. 16.13)

■ Whilst most cases of NHL are widespread at the time of diagnosis, HL may be localised to a single nodal group.

■ Spread is predictable, usually by involvement of contiguous nodal groups and with dissemination to liver, spleen and bone marrow only late in disease.

■ The neoplastic cells (Reed–Sternberg cells and variants) often form only a small proportion of the mass, with a prominent reactive haematolymphoid cell population forming the bulk.

■ Extranodal involvement is uncommon.

THE IMPORTANCE OF TUMOUR TYPE IN CLINICAL MANAGEMENT
Hodgkin lymphoma (HL) usually spreads by orderly involvement of contiguous nodal groups and staging of this disease is therefore very important in planning patient management. Whilst non-Hodgkin lymphoma generally requires systemic treatment with chemotherapy, the earlier stages of HL can often be treated effectively by localised irradiation of the affected nodal groups.

Various systems have been devised for the *classification* of haematolymphoid tumours. Classification of tumours is necessary to allow recognition of those that have similar features and facilitates improved prediction of behaviour, prognosis and response to treatment. Most earlier systems were based primarily upon the morphological appearances of the tumour cells, dividing lymphomas on the basis of architecture into *diffuse* (sheets of cells with no pattern of organisation) versus *follicular* (arranged in nodules resembling the follicles of a normal node), on the basis of cell size into small cell and large cell types (broadly reflecting low-grade or high-grade behaviour), or on the basis of similarities to normal constituent cells within the lymph node (e.g. centrocytes, centroblasts, immunoblasts, etc). Although these classification systems were useful in allowing certain subtypes of lymphoma to be described and identified, it is now recognised that morphology alone is imperfect and is insufficient to allow reliable separation of some entities that appear histologically similar but behave differently.

The development of immunohistochemical staining methods and of newer molecular techniques has revolutionised the practice of haematolymphoid pathology. The most recent internationally recognised system of classification is that of the *World Health Organization (WHO)*. This system uses a combination of clinical, morphological, immunohistochemical and molecular techniques to recognise subgroups of lymphoma with shared characteristics. The WHO classification includes a very large number of entities, but only those that are common or that illustrate an important pathophysiological concept will be considered here (Fig. 16.3).

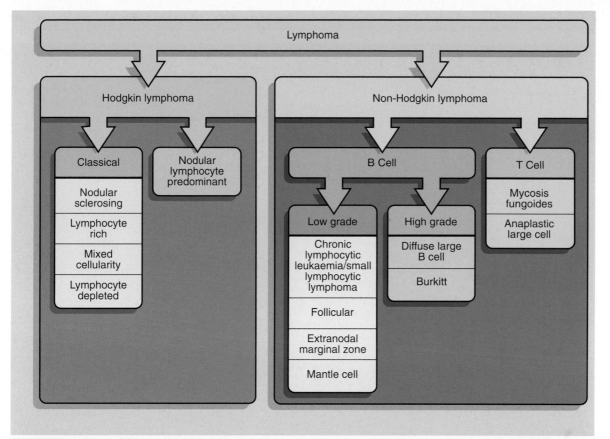

Fig. 16.3 Simplified classification chart of entities to be considered.

An approach to lymph node examination in clinical practice

In clinical practice, the diagnostic pathologist first considers the *architecture* of the involved lymph node and notes the *cytological features* of the constituent cells, including cell size, nuclear shape, the presence, type and position of nucleoli and the amount and distribution of cytoplasm. This initial assessment guides the selection of appropriate immunohistochemical stains which can identify whether the tumour is of B or T cell lineage, as well as other markers which characterise specific subtypes of lymphoma (see Fig. 16.10).

This examination is often sufficient to achieve a diagnosis but may be supplemented, particularly in difficult cases, by *molecular investigations*. Molecular studies can confirm *clonality* of the cell population where there is uncertainty about whether a lymphoid cell population is reactive or neoplastic (by showing that all tumour cells have the same immunoglobulin or T cell receptor gene rearrangement) or can be used to look for non-random chromosomal translocations that characterise a particular tumour type, e.g. a t(8;14) translocation is typically present in cases of Burkitt lymphoma.

All of these findings should then be correlated with the clinical and radiological information so that an appropriate plan can be formulated for optimal patient management. From the pathologist's point of view, this may involve further staging of the tumour by sampling of tissue from other sites, e.g. bone marrow biopsy, or by the assessment of subsequent biopsies for residual disease following treatment. Some newer therapies use specific molecular targeting systems and in some instances, pathological examination to look for immunopositivity within the tumour is needed to predict whether a certain drug will be effective, e.g. rituximab targets the CD20 antigen of B cell tumours and so will lack efficacy in CD20 negative tumours. In addition to their diagnostic value, some markers also provide important prognostic information. For example, high grade B cell NHL may be divided into distinct prognostic and therapeutic groups using a combination of immunohistochemical and molecular methods (see clinical box 'WHO classification of lymphoid neoplasms').

WHO CLASSIFICATION OF LYMPHOID NEOPLASMS
The most recent revision of this classification emphasises the importance of combining clinical, histological, immunohistochemical and genetic features to allow reliable recognition and diagnosis of disease. This is essential so that all pathologists use the same, reproducible criteria to diagnose disease and therefore we know that we can make meaningful observations regarding how different groups of tumours behave and respond to treatment. Advances in molecular diagnostic methods have been used to refine and subclassify some tumour groups, aiming to give better prognostic information and guide treatment. An example of this is seen in the revised classification of high grade B cell non-Hodgkin lymphomas, where rearrangements of the *MYC, BLC2* and *BLC6* genes are now used diagnostically to define aggressive 'double hit' and 'triple hit' subtypes of the disease.

B cell non-Hodgkin lymphoma

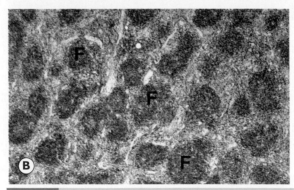

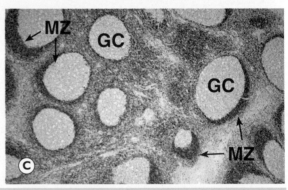

Fig. 16.4 **Follicular lymphoma. (A)** H&E of lymph node with follicular lymphoma (LP); **(B)** immunohistochemical stain for bcl-2 in follicular lymphoma (LP); **(C)** immunohistochemical stain for bcl-2 in normal reactive node (LP).

This is a common form of B cell lymphoma that tends to occur in middle-aged and older adults and presents as painless lymphadenopathy. These tumours are derived from germinal centre B cells and usually have a nodular or *follicular* architecture **(F)** (Fig. 16.4A) The cells are a mixture of small centrocyte-like cells and larger centroblast-like cells. Although most tumours are low grade, an increasing proportion of centroblastic cells indicate more aggressive behaviour. The tumour cells show a similar pattern of immunopositivity to normal germinal centre B cells. Most cases are characterised by a specific chromosomal abnormality, t(14;18), which juxtaposes the immunoglobulin heavy chain *(IGH)* gene on chromosome 14 with the gene for the anti-apoptotic protein *BCL-2* on chromosome 18. Because IgH is expressed in normal mature B cells, this chromosomal rearrangement results in over-expression of bcl-2 protein within the tumour cells and so these cells effectively avoid the normal pathway of apoptotic destruction. In normal reactive lymph nodes, the cells of the mantle zone **(MZ)** are bcl-2 positive but germinal centre cells **(GC)** are bcl-2 negative (Fig. 16.4C). In contrast, strong bcl-2 positivity is characteristically seen within the neoplastic follicles **(F)** in follicular lymphoma (Fig. 16.4B).

KEY TO FIGURE
F follicle   **GC** germinal centre   **M** mitotic figure   **MZ** mantle zone   **P** prolymphocytes   **PC** proliferation centre

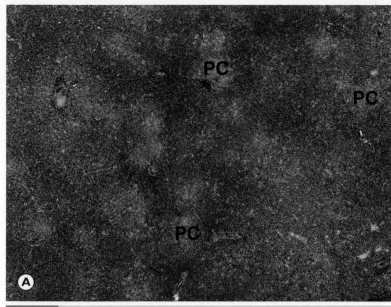

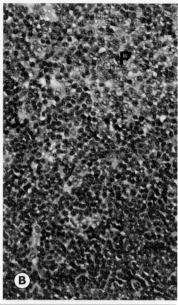

Fig. 16.5 Chronic lymphocytic leukaemia/small lymphocytic lymphoma. (A) LP; (B) HP.

This is a common form of NHL usually seen in older adults. As the name suggests, there is a spectrum of disease from a predominantly leukaemic form, in which there is extensive marrow involvement (Fig. 16.16) and the malignant cells circulate in peripheral blood, through to a lymphoma of the same morphology and immunophenotype, which lacks any significant circulating component and is characterised by lymphadenopathy. Many patients have some degree of lymphadenopathy, but the term small

lymphocytic lymphoma is used only in the absence of circulating atypical lymphocytes. As shown in Fig. 16.5B, this is a low grade lymphoma composed of sheets of small, mature B lymphocytes with varying numbers of slightly larger prolymphocytes **(P)**. These larger cells tend to be arranged in aggregates termed **proliferation centres (PC)**, which give a characteristic appearance of vague nodularity on low power examination (Fig. 16.5A). These areas appear paler and are sometimes referred to as **pseudofollicles**.

LOW GRADE B CELL LYMPHOMAS

Various forms of low grade B cell lymphoma can appear very similar on routine histology. Immunohistochemistry allows us to distinguish many of the common subtypes. For example, chronic lymphocytic leukaemia/ small lymphocytic lymphoma cells are typically CD5 and CD23 positive, whilst mantle cell lymphomas are typically CD5 and cyclin D1 positive but are CD23 negative. Immunohistochemical stains are always used as a panel in this setting because individual markers may be misleading or unhelpful if interpreted in isolation. The features must also be correlated with clinical and molecular findings.

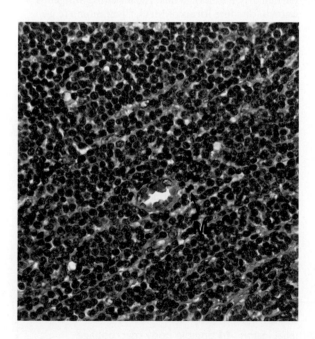

Fig. 16.6 Mantle cell lymphoma (MP).

This is a relatively uncommon lymphoma but it is considered as part of the differential diagnosis in cases of small B cell lymphoma and is important as its behaviour is significantly more aggressive than other morphologically similar tumours. Mantle cell lymphoma usually occurs at extranodal sites, particularly within the gastrointestinal tract and may present with the clinical pattern of **lymphomatous polyposis**. Morphologically, it may have a diffuse pattern as shown here or may be vaguely nodular, occasionally adopting a mantle zone pattern of infiltration around reactive germinal centres. As shown in Fig. 16.6, the cells are slightly larger than those of the other lymphomas discussed thus far and mitotic figures **(M)** are more frequent. Positive nuclear staining with cyclin D1, a protein involved in regulation of cell cycle, is characteristically seen in this tumour. There is usually an associated t(11;14) translocation, juxtaposing the *BCL-1* locus with the *IGH* gene and accounting for the over expression of cyclin D1.

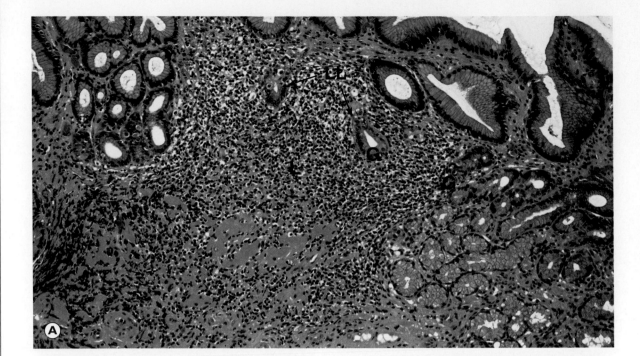

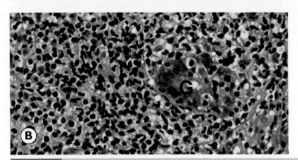

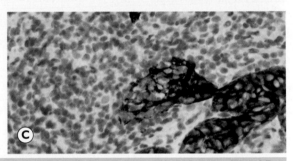

Fig. 16.7 **Gastric biopsy involved by extranodal marginal zone (MALT) lymphoma. (A)** H&E (MP); **(B)** H&E (HP); **(C)** cytokeratin immunostaining (HP).

The term *MALToma* is most commonly used to refer to this group of low-grade B-cell lymphomas. These occur at *extranodal sites* such as stomach, salivary gland, thyroid gland, lacrimal gland and lung, arising from the mucosa-associated lymphoid tissue (MALT) at these sites. The cells show morphological and immunophenotypic features similar to those of a subset of mature B cells found within the normal nodal marginal zone. These are unusual, indolent tumours, which, unlike most other NHLs, tend to remain localised for long periods and may even regress in some circumstances. MALT lymphomas usually arise on a background of chronic inflammation and, in cases where the cause of this inflammatory process is remediable, such as *Helicobacter pylori* associated gastritis, the tumour may regress following treatment of the underlying condition.

It appears that chronic antigenic stimulation initially results in polyclonal B-cell activation and proliferation as part of the normal immune response. Over time, continuing proliferation may result in accumulation of genetic aberrations and, later in the disease process, a smaller number of B-cell

clones are identifiable *(oligoclonality)*. Ultimately, a *monoclonal* infiltrate emerges, presumably due to selective pressures. At this point, some tumours may still regress if the initiating stimulus is removed; however, other tumours do not and, in these cases, specific chromosomal translocations are often present, particularly t(11;18). Whilst the initiating antigen is known for some forms of MALT lymphoma (e.g. *Helicobacter* gastritis, *Chlamydia* conjunctivitis), there are other chronic inflammatory disorders which are known to predispose to MALT lymphoma (e.g. Hashimoto's thyroiditis, Sjögren's syndrome) for which the initiating antigen remains elusive.

Histologically, this gastric biopsy shows an infiltrate of small lymphoid cells **(L)** (Fig. 16.7A) which characteristically form *lymphoepithelial lesions* **(LL)** by migrating into normal glandular epithelium **(G)**. In Fig. 16.7B, small lymphocytes are seen at higher magnification within the epithelium of a damaged gastric gland **(G)**. Immunohistochemical staining with an epithelial cell marker (Fig. 16.7C) may be used to highlight residual, partially destroyed glands and this can be helpful in diagnosis.

KEY TO FIGURES

G gastric gland   **L** lymphoid infiltrate   **LL** lymphoepithelial lesion   **M** tingible body macrophage
MF mitotic figure   **MP** muscularis propria   **P** peritoneal surface   **SM** submucosa   **V** villi

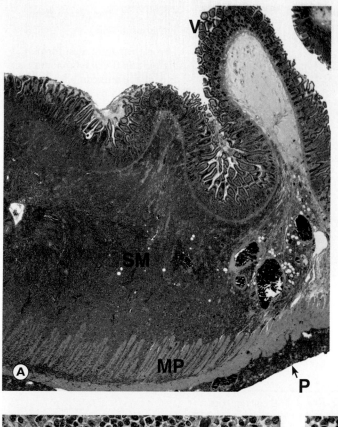
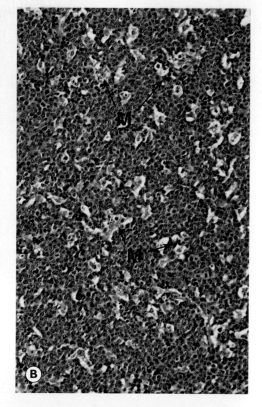
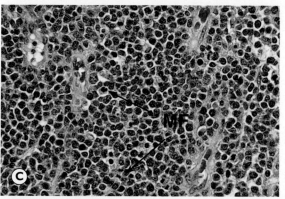
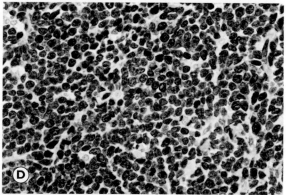

Fig. 16.8 **Burkitt lymphoma. (A)** H&E of small intestine with Burkitt lymphoma (LP); **(B)** H&E of small intestine with Burkitt lymphoma (MP); **(C)** H&E of small intestine with Burkitt lymphoma (HP); **(D)** immunostaining for cell proliferation using Ki67 (HP).

Although this is a relatively uncommon disease in industrialised countries, it is frequent in parts of Africa and illustrates certain pathophysiological concepts. The form of this disease that is typically seen in sub-Saharan Africa is known as **_endemic Burkitt lymphoma_**. This usually occurs in children and is closely associated with Epstein–Barr virus (EBV) infection. Sporadic and HIV-associated forms of the disease are less closely correlated with EBV. African Burkitt lymphoma typically affects the mandible or certain visceral organs, whilst the non-endemic form most frequently affects the ileocaecal area as shown in Fig. 16.8A and may present with symptoms of intestinal obstruction (E-Fig. 16.7**G**) or visceral perforation.

Histologically, the tumour is composed of sheets of intermediate sized lymphoid cells, which have an extremely high rate of proliferation. At low magnification (Fig. 16.8A), tumour cells are seen

to infiltrate through the full thickness of the wall of the terminal ileum, from the surface villi **(V)** of the mucosa, through the submucosa **(SM)**, muscularis propria **(MP)** and serosa to reach the peritoneal surface **(P)**.

Characteristically, there are sheets of tumour cells with intervening **_tingible body macrophages_** **(M)** which produce a **_'starry sky'_** appearance (Fig. 16.8B). These cells contain apoptotic debris due to the very high rate of tumour cell turnover (Fig. 16.8C). This high proliferation rate is one of the defining features of Burkitt lymphoma. Numerous mitotic figures **(MF)** are seen and immunostaining to identify cells in cell cycle (using the antibody Ki67) shows that virtually 100% of tumour cells are proliferating (Fig. 16.8D). Most cases have a typical t(8;14) translocation, juxtaposing the _c-MYC_ gene with the immunoglobulin heavy chain gene.

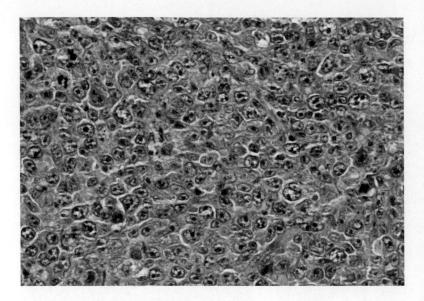

Fig. 16.9 Diffuse large B-cell lymphoma (HP).

This is the commonest form of high-grade B-cell lymphoma and, as the name implies, it is characterised by a *diffuse* (sheet-like) infiltrate of large B cells (Fig. 16.9). The morphology of these cells is very variable, but they may resemble the centroblasts or immunoblasts seen in normal lymph nodes. Some diffuse large B-cell lymphomas arise in patients known to have a previous low-grade B-cell lymphoma such as chronic lymphocytic leukaemia (CLL)/small lymphocytic lymphoma (SLL) or follicular lymphoma and can be shown by molecular methods to be clonally related to these tumours. This is termed *high-grade transformation* and is associated with a poor prognosis.

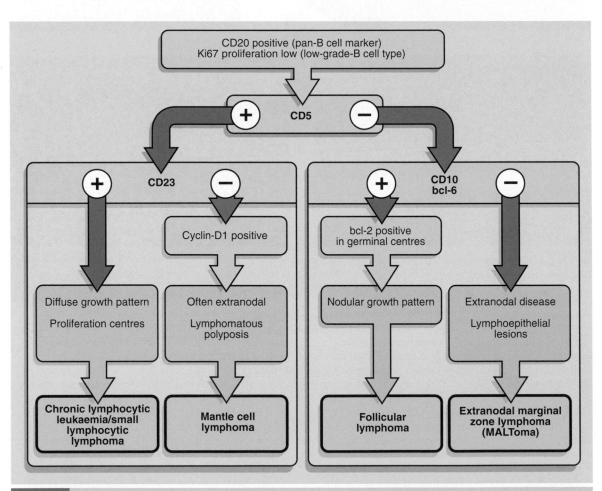

Fig. 16.10 Example of basic immunohistochemical approach to differential diagnosis.

This chart illustrates a simplified scheme for use of immunohistochemistry in the differential diagnosis of low-grade B-cell NHLs. It is important to note that these stains are never used in isolation and that their selection is guided by the morphological appearance of the lymph node. Occasional tumours show atypical patterns of immunoreactivity and interpretation must therefore always be in the context of the clinical setting, the histological appearance of the tumour and the results of ancillary investigations such as molecular testing. This chart need not be learned but aims to illustrate the general approach of the diagnostic pathologist to interpretation of immunohistochemical staining.

T-cell non-Hodgkin lymphoma

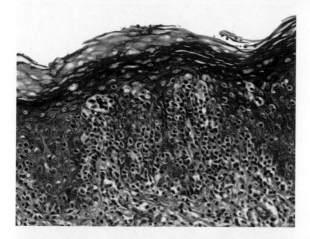

Fig. 16.11 Mycosis fungoides (MP).

This form of T-cell lymphoma involves the skin and tends to have an indolent course. It presents as persistent, scaling, erythematous lesions, which are flat initially, but gradually progress through stages described as *patch*, *plaque* and *tumour*. Systemic spread can occur late in the disease process. Early disease may mimic inflammatory disorders such as psoriasis, both clinically and pathologically. Fig. 16.11 shows the early plaque stage of the disease. Atypical, small lymphocytes, often with complex infolding of their nuclear membranes (described as *cerebriform*) infiltrate the epidermis, but without evidence of *spongiosis* (oedema within the epidermis); this is termed *epidermotropism*.

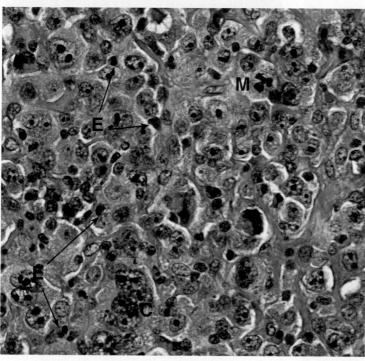

Fig. 16.12 Anaplastic large cell lymphoma (HP).

As the name suggests, this is a tumour that is composed of large, highly atypical cells. These cells usually have irregularly shaped, convoluted nuclei and tend to be of T-cell lineage. In this example in Fig. 16.12, the cells have multiple large nucleoli and there is an atypical tripolar mitotic figure (**M**). Fairly numerous eosinophils (**E**) are seen, as well as an occasional bizarre tumour giant cell (**GC**).

Most cases of anaplastic large cell lymphoma are characterised by the occurrence of a specific chromosomal rearrangement that affects the *anaplastic lymphoma kinase (ALK)* gene. The effects of this abnormality can be identified by immunohistochemical staining for ALK-1 (see Fig. 12.24). This is an important prognostic marker.

CLINICAL FEATURES OF SOME T-CELL NON-HODGKIN LYMPHOMAS

Some other types of T-cell lymphoma are of particular clinical interest. **Enteropathy-associated T-cell lymphoma** is seen in some patients who present with symptoms of **malabsorption**. Clinically, there is **steatorrhoea** (fatty diarrhoea due to failure of absorption of dietary lipid), often associated with anaemia and various vitamin deficiencies. This presentation closely resembles coeliac disease (gluten-sensitive enteropathy, see Fig. 13.15), but patients fail to respond to dietary gluten restriction and it is thought that the disorder known as **refractory coeliac disease** or **refractory sprue** is a precursor of overt lymphoma. In its earliest stages, the histological features of this disease also resemble coeliac disease, but the intraepithelial lymphocytes have an abnormal immunophenotype and sensitive molecular techniques can demonstrate clonality of the intraepithelial lymphoid cells. Over time, this may evolve into an aggressive lymphoma that often forms multiple tumour masses in the small intestine. Patients may then present with features of small intestinal obstruction or even with acute peritonitis due to perforation through a necrotic tumour mass.

A later section in this chapter deals with bone marrow disease and with leukaemias, including **acute lymphoblastic leukaemia (ALL)**. As we have previously noted, leukaemia and lymphoma are not always entirely distinct entities and the same tumour may produce either a solid tissue mass or may diffusely involve bone marrow, giving rise to a leukaemic picture. Most ALL presents as childhood leukaemia and is derived from precursor B lymphoblasts. The T-cell form of ALL is less frequent but usually occurs in adolescent boys, forming a mediastinal lymphomatous mass involving the thymus (the site of normal T-cell maturation). These patients may therefore present with symptoms related to compression of vital structures within the mediastinum such as the superior vena cava

KEY TO FIGURES
E eosinophil   **GC** tumour giant cell   **M** atypical mitotic figure

Hodgkin lymphoma

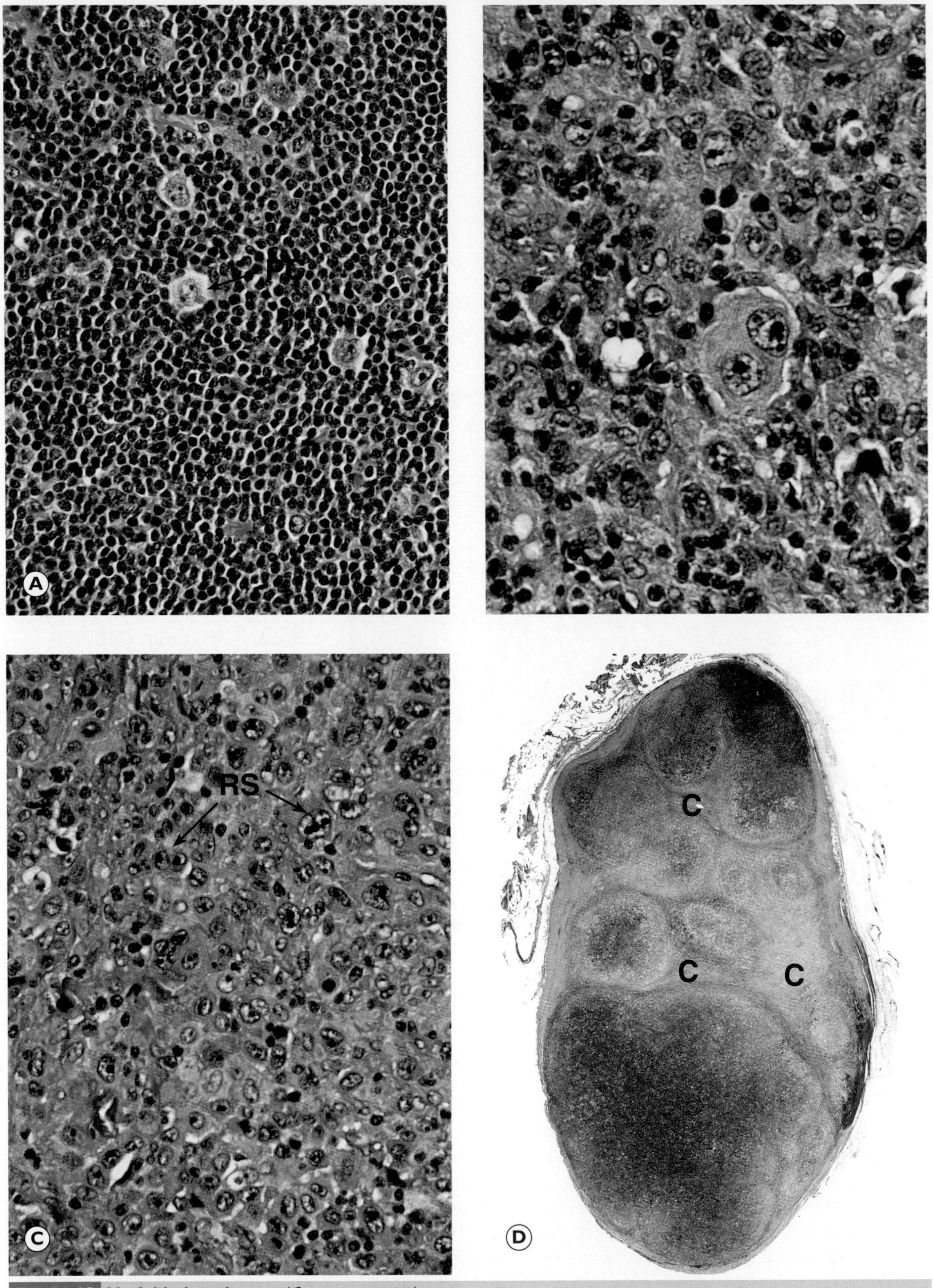

Fig. 16.13 **Hodgkin lymphoma.** *(Caption opposite)*

THE REED–STERNBERG CELL AND ITS VARIANTS

These large cells are essential for diagnosis of Hodgkin lymphoma (HL). The classical form has two nuclei or a single bi-lobed nucleus with two prominent, inclusion-like, eosinophilic nucleoli, usually as large as normal small lymphocytes. This gives rise to the appearance of 'owl's eyes'. **Mononuclear** variants appear similar but have a single nucleus. **Lacunar cells** are associated with nodular sclerosing HL and have a folded nucleus with surrounding pale, delicate cytoplasm. This cytoplasm is often disrupted during histological processing, leaving the nucleus within a clear space (the lacuna). **Lymphohistiocytic variants (L&H cells)** are also known as **'popcorn' cells** as they have abundant cytoplasm and highly convoluted nuclei, resembling popcorn kernels. These are found in nodular lymphocyte predominant HL.

Fig. 16.13 **Hodgkin lymphoma. (A)** Nodular lymphocyte predominant pattern (HP); **(B)** mixed cellularity pattern (HP); **(C)** lymphocyte depleted pattern (HP); **(D)** nodular sclerosing pattern (LP). *(Illustrations opposite)*

Nodular lymphocyte predominant Hodgkin lymphoma is distinct from the classical forms of the disease. This entity was described more recently and the Reed–Sternberg cell variants in this type are known to be activated B lymphocytes. These cells show a different pattern of immunohistochemical staining from Reed–Sternberg cells in the other *(classical)* forms of the disease and this subtype may be difficult to differentiate from some forms of B-cell NHL. This disease has an excellent prognosis and is illustrated in Fig. 16.13A. Reactive lymphocytes make up the bulk of the tissue in affected nodes and form extensive sheets within which are scattered relatively few mononuclear Reed–Sternberg cells. These cells are also termed 'popcorn' cells **(PC)** because of the lobulated contour of their nuclei. *Classical lymphocyte rich Hodgkin lymphoma* is not illustrated but appears morphologically similar and immunostaining is required to separate these disorders.

Mixed cellularity Hodgkin lymphoma is shown in Fig. 16.13B. Here, classic Reed–Sternberg cells (RS cells) **(RS)** are mixed with a variable population of reactive cells including lymphocytes **(L)**, histiocytes **(H)**, eosinophils **(E)**, neutrophils **(N)** and plasma cells.

The type with the worst prognosis is *lymphocyte depleted Hodgkin lymphoma*. This is illustrated in Fig. 16.13C. Affected nodes are replaced by sheets of large pleomorphic cells, which are Reed–Sternberg cell variants, with only a few classic RS cells **(RS)**. Lymphocytes **(L)** and other reactive cells are scanty.

Most commonly, HL destroys the normal architecture of the lymph node completely, producing a homogeneous appearance in which no trace of the original cortico-medullary demarcation and follicular pattern remains. However, one form of Hodgkin disease, the *nodular sclerosing* pattern seen in Fig. 16.13D, results in the deposition of broad irregular bands of pink-staining collagenous fibrous tissue **(C)** which separates the cellular Hodgkin tumour mass into islands, imparting a nodular appearance to the cut surface of the node. The nodular sclerosing pattern is associated with a good prognosis if diagnosed at an early stage.

Conventionally, the histological subtype of HL has been an important indicator of prognosis, with better outcomes in variants with few RS type cells and a larger proportion of reactive cells (such as lymphocyte predominant and lymphocyte rich) and therefore the worst prognosis in lymphocyte depleted disease, where RS cells are very numerous. Modern management has considerably reduced these differences in outcome between histological subtypes and it is now possible to achieve complete cure of HL. Tumour *stage* is now the primary determinant of prognosis. There is, however, a tendency for the lymphocyte predominant type to present with localised disease (excellent prognosis) while the lymphocyte depleted type typically presents with disseminated disease (poor prognosis).

Bone marrow disease

The bone marrow spaces between the trabeculae of spongy bone are occupied by adipose tissue with intervening collections of haematopoietic cells which are responsible for the production of red blood cells, white blood cells and platelets (E-Fig. 16.8**H**). These cell lines are derived from a reservoir of *hae-matopoietic stem cells*, which differentiate into the various specialised cell lines in response to specific growth factors. The bone marrow is able to respond rapidly to increased demands for the various blood cells by increased proliferative activity of the precursor and stem cells.

The main diseases involving the bone marrow are:

- abnormalities of haematopoiesis
- metastatic tumours
- myeloma
- leukaemia and lymphoma
- myeloproliferative and myelodysplastic processes.

Haematopoietic disorders

Disorders of haematopoiesis are common, but are largely outside the scope of this book. Cytological examination of smear preparations of aspirated bone marrow and histological examination of trephine biopsy specimens of bone marrow form an important method of investigating some diseases.

Most *anaemias* (lack of red cells) are the result of lack of iron, vitamin B_{12} or folate or are due to excessive red cell breakdown (haemolytic anaemia). One type (leukoerythroblastic anaemia) is due to destruction of the haematopoietic tissue by tumour or fibrosis and histological examination of a bone marrow biopsy is vital to establish the diagnosis.

KEY TO FIGURES
C collagen **E** eosinophil **H** histiocyte **L** lymphocyte **N** neutrophil **PC** 'popcorn' cells **RS** Reed–Sternberg cell

Metastatic tumour in bone marrow

The bone marrow is a common site for blood-borne metastasis of certain malignant tumours. The tumours that most commonly spread to bone marrow are carcinomas and the most frequent primary cancers include:

- breast carcinoma
- lung carcinoma (Fig. 16.14C and D)
- carcinoma of the kidney
- carcinoma of the thyroid (particularly the follicular type)
- carcinoma of the prostate (Fig. 16.14A and B).

In most cases, the growth of metastatic carcinoma in the bone marrow leads to destruction of trabecular bone, leading to *osteolytic* deposits which appear as lucent areas on x-ray. Carcinoma of the prostate often stimulates the active formation of new woven bone, producing *osteosclerotic* deposits that appear as increased areas of bone density on X-ray examination. Another tumour which frequently metastasises to bone marrow is neuroblastoma, an aggressive tumour which usually occurs in childhood.

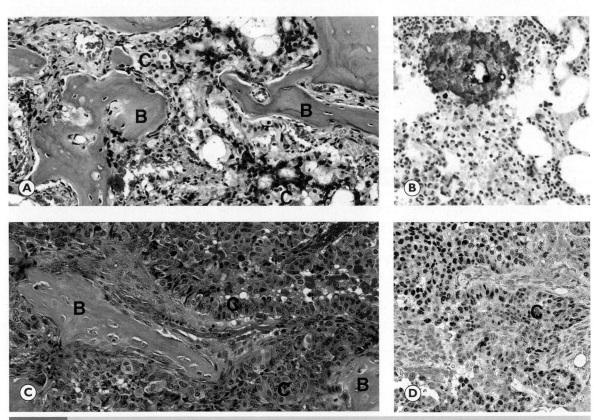

Fig. 16.14 Metastatic tumour in bone marrow. (A) H&E of bone marrow with metastatic prostatic carcinoma (MP); **(B)** immunohistochemical staining for prostate-specific antigen (PSA) (MP); **(C)** H&E of bone marrow with metastatic lung carcinoma (MP); **(D)** immunohistochemical staining for thyroid transcription factor 1 (TTF-1) (MP).

The bone marrow is a frequent site for deposits of metastatic carcinoma, the common primary tumours being from prostate, bronchus, breast, thyroid and kidney. Widespread replacement of bone marrow by metastatic tumour may induce *extramedullary haematopoiesis* (Fig. 16.19) in liver and spleen.

Most metastatic deposits cause bone destruction and, when widespread, can be associated with hypercalcaemia. Metastases from carcinoma of the prostate may, however, be associated with new bone formation and result in *osteosclerosis*. This is shown in Fig. 16.14A, where replacement of marrow by prostatic adenocarcinoma cells **(C)** is associated

with reactive trabecular bone formation **(B)**. In Fig. 16.14B, an immunohistochemical staining method is employed to demonstrate prostate-specific antigen (PSA), a specific marker for prostatic adenocarcinoma in metastatic tumour. The clumps of tumour cells are stained dark brown.

Figs 16.14C and D illustrate metastatic lung carcinoma, again using an immunohistochemical stain (TTF-1), which is useful in identifying bronchogenic carcinoma cells. This antibody targets a nuclear transcription factor that is found almost exclusively in thyroid and lung tissue (see Table 1.3). The site of staining in this case is within the tumour cell nuclei.

KEY TO FIGURES
B bone **C** carcinoma

Multiple myeloma

This group of disorders falls within the WHO category of mature B-cell neoplasms but is considered here because its most frequent presentation is as a disseminated disease, characterised by widespread bone marrow involvement. Myeloma is a neoplastic proliferation of terminally differentiated B cells that have developed the features of plasma cells and so can produce large amounts of immunoglobulin. The features of myeloma are diverse and are a product of various interrelated processes, including displacement of normal haematopoietic elements by the tumour (leading to anaemia, thrombocytopenia and immune dysfunction), bone destruction (E-Fig. 16.9**G**) (causing pain, lytic lesions on X-ray and increased risk of fracture), renal disease and hypercalcaemia, with its associated metabolic consequences. In some patients, the excess immunoglobulin molecules produced may be deposited in the tissues in the form of *amyloid*, an abnormal fibrillar protein with a ß-pleated sheet configuration (see Ch. 15 and E-Fig. 16.10). These insoluble deposits may cause end-organ damage, particularly in the kidney.

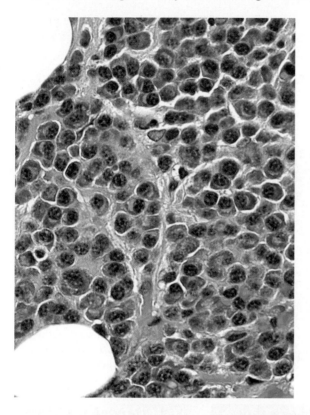

Fig. 16.15 Multiple myeloma (HP).

In Fig. 16.15 from a patient with diffuse marrow involvement, the haematopoietic tissue is replaced by abnormal plasma cells which, in normal marrow, are only a very minor constituent. These have eccentric nuclei, a paranuclear hof (a pale area indicating the site of the prominent Golgi apparatus) and clock-face chromatin. Atypical, binucleate or multinucleate cell forms and more primitive plasmablasts may also be seen.

Molecular or immunohistochemical investigation reveals evidence of **light chain restriction** (i.e. all of the cells produce either κ or λ light chains, indicating monoclonality). This monoclonal immunoglobulin can be identified by **serum electrophoresis** and the light chain component can be excreted in urine, known as **Bence-Jones protein**.

Osteolytic lesions of myeloma lead to bone pain and sometimes fracture, whereas diffuse bone marrow infiltration may lead to destruction of normal haematopoietic cells, resulting in leukoerythroblastic anaemia. Solitary mass lesions in bone are termed **plasmacytomas**.

Leukaemias

Leukaemias are characterised by neoplastic proliferation of white cells within the bone marrow, which then circulate within the peripheral blood. General characteristics of leukaemias include:

■ neoplastic proliferation of marrow derived cells, forming one or more neoplastic cell lines

■ circulation of the neoplastic cells in the peripheral blood

■ suppression of normal haematopoietic activity by the expanding leukaemic cell population.

Because the neoplastic leukaemic cells circulate in the blood, the cells are usually deposited in other tissues and organs, particularly lymph nodes, liver and spleen. Leukaemias are classified according to the cell of origin, but a useful general division is into two main types: chronic leukaemias and acute leukaemias.

■ *Chronic leukaemias* are characterised by neoplastic proliferation of relatively mature white cells. Typically, the clinical course is indolent, with a long natural history. Although the neoplastic cells predominate in the marrow, other haematopoietic cells can survive alongside and adequate numbers of red cells and platelets are produced. Chronic leukaemias are mainly seen in adults over the age of 40 years, but some may eventually transform into a more aggressive acute leukaemia.

■ *Acute leukaemias* are characterised by neoplastic proliferation of very immature white cells (*blast cells*). The course of the disease is very rapid, with destruction of all other haematopoietic cell lines in the marrow. Without treatment, acute leukaemias are rapidly fatal.

■ *Chronic lymphocytic leukaemia (CLL)* is considered in the previous section owing to its overlap with small lymphocytic lymphoma (Fig. 16.5), but its appearance in the bone marrow is illustrated here (Fig. 16.16).

■ *Chronic myeloid leukaemia (CML)* is a neoplastic proliferation of the more mature precursors of neutrophils (for example myelocytes and metamyelocytes) and occurs most commonly in adults.

■ *Acute lymphoblastic leukaemia (ALL)* is a tumour of immature lymphocyte precursors (lymphoblasts), and occurs most commonly in children (see also clinical box 'Clinical features of some T-cell non-Hodgkin lymphomas').

■ *Acute myeloid leukaemia (AML)* is a tumour of immature precursor cells in the myeloid series (mainly myeloblasts) and is most common in adults (Fig. 16.17). It is the most common of a group of acute leukaemias derived from various myeloid precursors, collectively called acute non- lymphoblastic leukaemias.

Some lymphomas that originate in lymph nodes may also eventually spread to involve bone marrow and there may be enough circulating lymphoma cells in the blood to be detected in a blood film, highlighting again that there are areas of overlap between leukaemia and lymphoma.

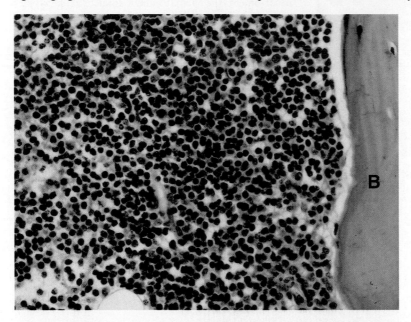

Fig. 16.16 Chronic lymphocytic leukaemia; bone marrow (HP).

In CLL, shown in Fig. 16.16, the marrow between bone trabeculae (**B**) becomes infiltrated by small lymphocytes, similar to those seen in small lymphocytic lymphoma (see Fig. 16.5). Very large numbers of similar cells appear in the peripheral circulation. Although occupation of the marrow is extensive, destruction of the normal haematopoietic marrow elements is not as rapid or severe as in acute lymphoblastic leukaemia and the condition runs an indolent course. This is a disease seen mainly in later life. Lymphadenopathy, splenomegaly and anaemia are commonly encountered.

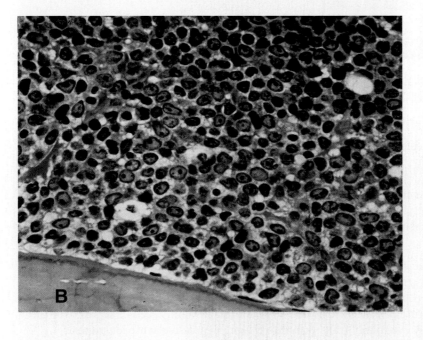

Fig. 16.17 Acute myeloid leukaemia; bone marrow (HP).

AML is characterised by proliferation of primitive myeloid cells in the bone marrow. There are several subgroups, depending on degree of maturation of the neoplastic cells, from primitive *myeloblasts* through types with *promyelocyte* morphology to types with both myeloid and monocytic morphologies. As seen in Fig. 16.17, the marrow is replaced by large atypical myeloid blast cells with few maturing cells (compare with Fig. 16.18). This type of leukaemia predominates in adults under 60 years of age and presents acutely with anaemia and bleeding secondary to thrombocytopenia. Diagnosis is made on blood and marrow examination.

KEY TO FIGURES
B bone

Myeloproliferative neoplasms and myelodysplastic syndromes

This complex group of disorders is also part of the WHO classification. In broad terms, *myeloproliferative neoplasms* are the result of abnormal proliferation of stem cells in the bone marrow, which can differentiate into red cell (erythroid) precursors, white cell (myeloid or granulocytic) precursors, megakaryocytes or fibroblasts. As a result, the peripheral blood usually contains increased numbers of these cells, e.g. excess erythrocytes in *polycythaemia vera* and excess platelets in *essential thrombocythaemia*. *Chronic myeloid leukaemia* is also considered to be one of the myeloproliferative neoplasms. *Myelofibrosis* occurs due to excessive fibroblast proliferation within the marrow, obliterating the marrow cavity due to collagen deposition and so displacing normal haematopoietic progenitors (Fig. 16.19). The myeloproliferative disorders, as well as showing frequent overlap and transition from one form to another, have a tendency to terminate in an acute leukaemic phase.

Myelodysplastic syndromes are also due to proliferation of abnormal stem cells within the marrow, but here, the maturation of cells is abnormal and terminally differentiated blood cells are not produced. They are characterised by various *cytopenias* (reduced numbers of cells in the peripheral blood) and by the presence of some abnormal circulating cells. Morphologically, there is abnormal maturation of bone marrow cells, often involving more than one haematopoietic lineage. This is termed *dysplasia*. Again, there is a spectrum of disorders that overlap, including some which affect only a single cell lineage (e.g. causing only anaemia due to defective red cell maturation, previously referred to as refractory anaemia) and others showing by abnormal cellular maturation affecting multiple different cell lineages. Some variants may have other identifying features such as the presence of ringed sideroblasts (abnormal nucleated red blood cells with granules of iron in the cytoplasm) or the presence of excess blast cells. Cytogenetic abnormalities also play a key role in classification. All of these disorders have a risk of transformation to acute myeloid leukaemia.

Accurate diagnosis of both myeloproliferative neoplasms and myelodysplastic syndromes requires correlation of peripheral blood counts, marrow aspirates and marrow trephine biopsies, usually involving both pathologists and haematologists. There is some overlap between these two groups of diseases and this is recognised within the current WHO classification. In addition, some cases are associated with previous drug therapy with cytotoxic agents and a comprehensive clinical history is always required. Detailed consideration of this group of disorders is outside the scope of this text.

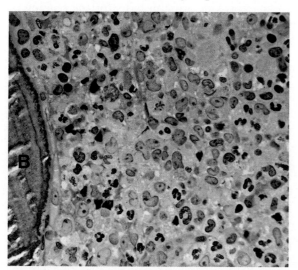

Fig. 16.18 Chronic myelogenous leukaemia; bone marrow (HP) (resin section).

In this disease, there is low-grade neoplastic proliferation of neutrophil precursors. Increased numbers of *myeloblasts* produce greatly increased numbers of *myelocytes*, *metamyelocytes* and mature *neutrophils*, all of which appear in the peripheral blood in greatly increased numbers. The marrow between bone trabeculae **(B)** is packed with neutrophils and late neutrophil precursors, particularly myelocytes and metamyelocytes (Fig. 16.18). Increased numbers of the most primitive precursor, the myeloblast, are also present, but they are a minority population compared with acute myeloid leukaemia (Fig. 16.17). Despite the abnormal myeloid proliferation, normal haematopoietic activity continues, although at a reduced rate. Chronic myeloid leukaemia is characterised by the presence of a t(9;22) translocation known as the *Philadelphia chromosome*.

THE PHILADELPHIA CHROMOSOME

This is a reciprocal translocation involving exchange of genetic material between chromosomes 9 and 22. It is characteristically seen in chronic myeloid leukaemia but also occurs occasionally in acute lymphoblastic leukaemia and acute myeloid leukaemia. It results in the fusion of part of the **breakpoint cluster region (BCR)** gene on chromosome 22 with part of the **Abelson (ABL**, named after a similar viral protein) **gene** on chromosome 9. The **chimaeric protein** formed has tyrosine kinase activity and is constitutively active, altering cell cycle proteins to promote increased proliferation, impaired DNA repair and reduced apoptotic cell death.

Clearly, this translocation is important in tumour progression and our understanding of the molecular basis of this disease has now allowed the development of specifically targeted therapy. In recent years, drugs have been developed to inhibit this abnormal tyrosine kinase activity within the tumour cells. These drugs dramatically reduce proliferation of the malignant cells and reduce the risk of transformation into an acute leukaemic form **(blast crisis)**. Drugs such as **imatinib** and its newer derivatives have also been used with considerable success in the treatment of other tumours such as gastrointestinal stromal tumours (see Fig. 13.14).

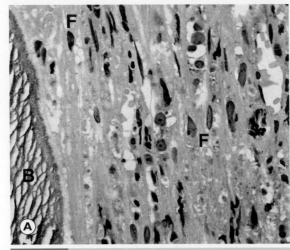

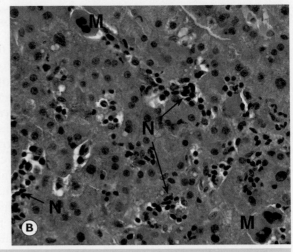

Fig. 16.19 **Myelofibrosis. (A)** Bone marrow, thin resin section (HP); **(B)** liver (HP).

In this disorder, replacement of haematopoietic marrow by progressive *fibrosis* leads to loss of capacity to produce erythrocytes, leukocytes and platelets. In Fig. 16.19A, the marrow space between bone trabeculae **(B)** is infiltrated by spindle-shaped fibroblastic cells **(F)**. This is partly compensated for by *extramedullary haematopoiesis*, when other organs of the lymphoreticular system re-acquire their fetal potential for haematopoiesis. The liver and spleen are the principal organs involved in this compensatory process and the spleen may become greatly enlarged.

Fig. 16.19B shows the liver sinusoids to be distended by a population of immature erythropoietic and granulopoietic elements, as well as occasional megakaryocytes **(M)**. Erythroid islands are recognisable as clusters of small normoblasts **(N)** with densely staining nuclei.

Chapter review.

This table summarises important features of the diseases discussed but is by no means comprehensive. Brief mention is made of typical patterns of immunostaining seen in some lymphomas. It is not expected that these should be memorised, but this *aide-memoire* may provide a useful basis for the reading of more advanced texts by those training in diagnostic pathology.

Table 16.1 **Chapter review.**

Disorder	Main features	Immunostaining	Genetic change	Figure
Reactive lymphadenopathy				
Follicular hyperplasia	Enlarged reactive germinal centres Reflects humoral (B-cell) response			16.1B
Paracortical hyperplasia	Expansion of paracortex, small follicles Reflects cell-mediated (T-cell) response			16.1C
Sinus histiocytosis	Prominence of histiocytes lining sinuses Common in nodes draining carcinoma			16.1D
Non-Hodgkin lymphoma (NHL)				
CLL/SLL	Older adults, often leukaemic Diffuse small B-cell infiltrate Proliferation centres pathognomonic	CD5+ CD23+	Deletion 13q,11q or 17p Trisomy 12	16.5 16.16
Follicular lymphoma	Usually nodular (follicular) architecture Centroblasts and centrocytes but no tingible body macrophages in follicles	CD10+ bcl6+ bcl2+	t(14;18)	16.4
Mantle cell lymphoma	Often GI tract (lymphomatous polyposis) Diffuse or nodular architecture Slightly larger cells	CD5+ CD23– cyclinD1+	t(11;14)	16.6
MALT lymphoma	Extranodal sites with MALT, often gastric Associated with chronic inflammation Lymphoepithelial lesions (cytokeratin+)		t(11;18)	16.7
Diffuse large B-cell lymphoma (DLBCL)	Common, high-grade tumour Sheets of large B cells Brisk proliferation	CD20+ Ki67 high		16.9

| Table 16.1 | Chapter review—cont'd. |

Disorder	Main features	Immunostaining	Genetic change	Figure
Burkitt lymphoma (E-Fig. 16.7**G**)	EBV associated, especially African form Sheets of intermediate-sized cells 'Starry sky' appearance	CD20+ Ki67 100%	t(8;14) c-MYC	16.8
Mycosis fungoides (MF)	Cutaneous disease, mimics psoriasis Atypical T cells infiltrate epidermis Patch, plaque and tumour stages	CD3+ CD4+		16.11
Anaplastic large cell lymphoma	Sheets of large, pleomorphic cells Irregular convoluted nuclei, mitoses ++ Usually children or young adults	ALK1+ CD30+ CD3+	t(2;5)	16.12
Hodgkin lymphoma				
Nodular lymphocyte predominant HL (nLPHL)	Vague nodularity at low power 'L+H' or 'popcorn' variant RS cells Small lymphocytes in background	CD20+ EMA+ CD30–		16.13A
Lymphocyte rich HL	Morphology as for nLPHL Different immunophenotype; need immunohistochemistry to distinguish; both indolent	CD20– CD30+ CD15+		Like 16.13A
Mixed cellularity HL	Classical RS cells Surrounding lymphocytes, histiocytes, neutrophils, eosinophils & plasma cells	CD20– CD30+ CD15+		16.13B
Lymphocyte depleted HL	Many RS cells and variants Few reactive cells Worse prognosis	CD20– CD30+ CD15+		16.13C
Nodular sclerosing HL	Nodules with bands of collagen Classic RS cells and lacunar types Mixed reactive cells, including eosinophils	CD20– CD30+ CD15+		16.13D
Bone marrow disorders				
Myeloma (E-Fig. 16.9**G**, E-Fig. 16.10)	Plasma cell tumour Production of excess immunoglobulin Bence-Jones proteinuria	CD138+ EMA+		16.15
Acute lymphoblastic leukaemia	Primitive lymphoid cell proliferation Usually in children, good prognosis Presents as a result of marrow replacement	TdT+		
Acute myeloid leukaemia	Myeloid precursor cells proliferate Various degrees of differentiation Usually adults, aggressive disease			16.17
Chronic myeloid leukaemia	Part of myeloproliferative spectrum Tumour of more mature neutrophil precursors		t(9;22) Philadelphia chromosome	16.18
Myeloproliferative neoplasms	Bone marrow stem cell producing excess numbers of mature cells of one or more lineage in peripheral blood			16.19A
Myelodysplastic syndromes	Bone marrow stem cell proliferation but failure of normal maturation and so peripheral blood cytopenias			
Other disorders				
Metastatic tumours (E-Fig. 16.6**G**)	Mainly carcinoma and melanoma Common cancers metastatic to bone: lung, breast, prostate, kidney, thyroid			16.2 16.14
Extramedullary haematopoiesis	Response to marrow replacement or need for increased haematopoiesis Primarily spleen and liver			16.19B

KEY TO FIGURES
B bone **F** fibroblast **M** megakaryocyte **N** normoblasts

17 Female reproductive system

Introduction

The female reproductive tract comprises the vulva, vagina, uterus, fallopian tubes and ovaries. As in other systems, a wide range of pathological conditions may occur in these organs. Malignant tumours and their precursor conditions are of major pathological importance. An interesting feature of the female genital tract is that there is a range of epithelial malignancies that can occur at almost any site in the tract. For example, serous adenocarcinoma is most commonly found in the ovary but can also present in the uterus and cervix.

Disorders of the vulva and vagina

The vulva is subject to many of the conditions affecting skin elsewhere in the body, including inflammatory conditions such as *dermatitis* and *lichen planus* (see Ch. 21), but is also an important site for sexually transmitted infections, including the chancre of primary syphilis. Many vulval inflammatory lesions lead to intense itching and the histological features of these conditions are therefore complicated by the effects of trauma from scratching *(lichen simplex chronicus)*. In some post-menopausal women, the vulval mucosa tends to become thickened and white as a result of epithelial atrophy and subepithelial fibrosis, a condition known as *lichen sclerosus et atrophicus* (Fig. 17.1).

Benign tumours of the vulva are relatively uncommon and include Bartholin's gland cysts, fibroepithelial polyps (skin tags), haemangiomas (see Fig. 11.8) and benign naevi. *Hidradenoma papilliferum*, a benign tumour of apocrine sweat gland origin, typically presents as a firm ulcerated nodule in the vulva and has a distinctive histological appearance of uniform apocrine cells arranged in papillary fronds and surrounded by a fibrous stroma (Fig. 17.2).

The majority of malignant tumours arising in the vulva are well differentiated squamous cell carcinomas, similar to those of the skin and mucous membranes (Figs 7.3 and 17.8). Squamous cell carcinoma of the vulva is preceded by epithelial dysplasia, known as *vulval intraepithelial neoplasia (VIN)*. There are now two recognised types of VIN: *'usual type'*, which is associated with HPV infection, and *'differentiated'*, which is associated with lichen sclerosus et atrophicus (Table 17.1 and Fig. 17.3). Clinically, it can be difficult to differentiate these conditions from inflammatory lesions and biopsy is necessary for diagnosis.

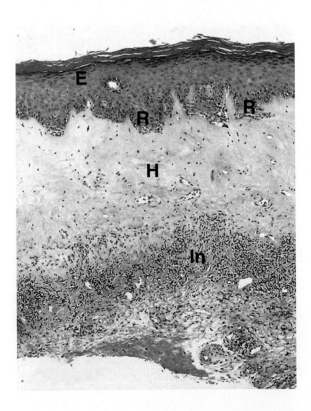

Fig. 17.1 Lichen sclerosus et atrophicus (LP).

This condition of unknown aetiology presents clinically as very itchy, smooth, whitish plaques around the vulva, often with narrowing of the introitus.

Histologically, there may be marked atrophy of the epidermis **(E)** with virtual disappearance of rete pegs **(R)** and skin appendages. Characteristically, the dermis contains a band of inflammatory cells **(In)**, mainly lymphocytes and plasma cells, the inflammatory zone being separated from the epidermis by a layer of acellular hyalinised collagen **(H)** in the superficial dermis.

Although this condition does not exhibit epithelial dysplasia, there is an association with differentiated VIN and the development of subsequent invasive well differentiated squamous cell carcinoma.

Paget's disease of the vulva or *extramammary Paget's disease (EMPD)* is a rare vulval tumour that has an identical histological appearance to Paget's disease of the breast (see Fig 18.13). In most cases, EMPD is confined to the epidermis but there are rare cases of an associated invasive primary vulval adenocarcinoma. EMPD can also arise secondary to adenocarcinomas in the nearby anus, rectum or bladder and this should be excluded clinically. Other rare malignant tumours of the vulva include basal cell carcinoma, malignant melanoma and adenocarcinoma arising in Bartholin's glands.

Disorders of the vagina include infections such as *Candida* (see Fig.5.15) and *Trichomonas* (see Fig 5.20), cysts and endometriosis. Rarely, dysplasia can occur in the vagina, similar to that in the vulva, perianal region and cervix *(vaginal intraepithelial neoplasia, VAIN)*. Primary tumours of the vagina include *squamous cell carcinoma* and *adenocarcinoma*.

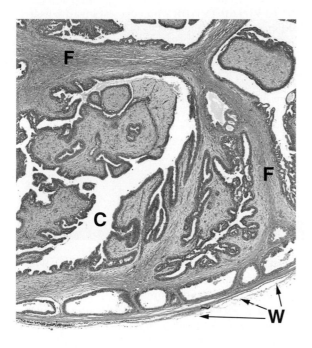

Fig 17.2 Hidradenoma papilliferum (LP).

Hidradenoma papilliferum is a benign tumour of apocrine origin that often presents clinically as a less than 1cm flesh coloured nodule in the vulva. As seen in Fig. 17.2, the tumour is usually well circumscribed **(W)**, with a smooth edge separating the lesion from the surrounding subcutaneous tissue. It is composed of uniform, bland apocrine type cells displaying decapitation secretion (E-Fig. 17.1 **H**) and forming tubules and papillary structures with surrounding cystic spaces **(C)**. The glandular elements typically display an outer layer of myoepithelial cells and an inner layer of cuboidal epithelial cells with eosinophilic cytoplasm, surrounded by a fibrous stroma **(F)**. This 'bilayer' is reassuringly benign and is also seen in other types of benign tumour such as intraductal papilloma of the breast (see Fig 18.8). Malignant transformation is very rare.

Table 17.1 Vulval intraepithelial neoplasia.

	Usual Type VIN	Differentiated VIN
Age	Young women	Older women
Key histological features	Basaloid/warty: conventional dysplasia	Dysmaturation
Grading	Can be low or high grade dysplasia	Always high grade
Associations	High risk HPV	Lichen sclerosus et atrophicus
Immunohistochemical markers	p16	p53

KEY TO FIGURES
C cystic space   **E** epidermis   **F** fibrous stroma   **H** hyalinised collagen   **In** inflammation   **R** rete pegs
W well circumscribed edge

FEMALE REPRODUCTIVE SYSTEM

BASIC SYSTEMS PATHOLOGY

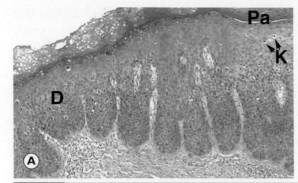

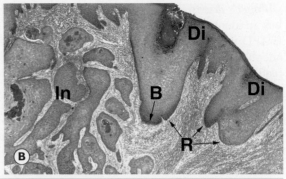

Fig. 17.3 **Vulval dysplasia. (A)** Usual type VIN3/HSIL (HP); **(B)** differentiated VIN (MP).

Vulval dysplasia *(vulval intraepithelial carcinoma VIN)* is a precursor of invasive squamous cell carcinoma. As described in Ch. 7, VIN is graded according to the severity of dysplasia as either high grade squamous intraepithelial lesion (HSIL/VIN2 or 3) or LSIL (VIN1).

Fig. 17.3A shows HSIL/VIN3, characterised by full thickness dysplasia of the epidermis **(D)** with the atypical epithelial cells showing irregular nuclei, mitotic figures extending throughout the full thickness of the epithelium and surface parakeratosis **(Pa)**. There are also superficial koilocytes **(K)** in keeping with HPV infection.

This is in contrast to Fig. 17.3B showing differentiated VIN (dVIN) **(Di)** with adjacent invasive well differentiated squamous cell carcinoma **(In)**. This is often a difficult histological diagnosis as dVIN is characterised by thickened (acanthotic) squamous epithelium with elongated rete ridges **(R)**, which shows features of dysmaturation, including dyskeratosis, eosinophilia ('pinking up') of the epithelial cells and basal nuclear atypia **(B)**. Differentiated VIN is always regarded as a high grade lesion and is associated with lichen sclerosus et atrophicus (Fig. 17.1) or squamous hyperplasia.

Diseases of the uterine cervix

The cervix frequently exhibits chronic inflammatory changes, known as chronic cervicitis (Fig. 17.4), which may also be associated with polypoid hyperplasia of the endocervical mucosa. This can result in the formation of a pedunculated *polyp* containing distended endocervical glands and stroma (Fig. 17.5). Clinically, the most important lesions of the cervix are *epithelial dysplasia* of varying degrees of severity and *squamous cell carcinoma*. These related conditions and their pathogenesis are considered in detail in Figs 17.6 to 17.8. Neoplastic, pre-invasive changes are termed *cervical intraepithelial neoplasia* or *CIN*. The terminology for grading these lesions is evolving and is discussed in Fig. 17.7. Glandular dysplasia also occurs in the cervix and is known as *cervical glandular intraepithelial neoplasia (CGIN)*. CGIN and invasive adenocarcinoma of the cervix are less common than CIN and squamous cell carcinoma.

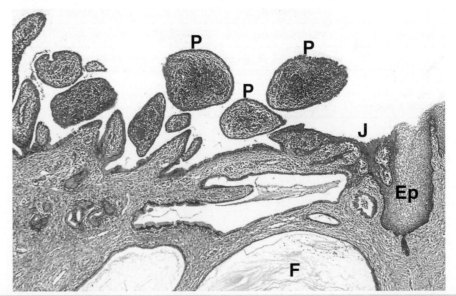

Fig 17.4 **Chronic cervicitis (MP).**

In chronic cervicitis, the ectocervical squamous epithelium **(Ep)** is slightly thickened (acanthosis). There is *micropolyposis* **(P)** in the endocervix (E-Fig. 17.2 **H**) above the squamocolumnar junction **(J)** where there is a heavy chronic inflammatory cell infiltrate composed mainly of lymphocytes and plasma cells. Cervical glands may develop cystic dilatation, often termed Nabothian follicles **(F)**. Long-standing inflammation may lead to *squamous metaplasia* of the endocervical surface epithelium (see Fig. 6.5).

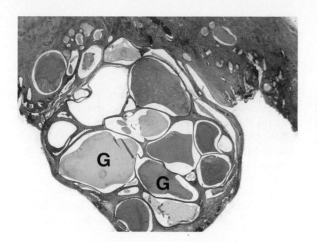

Fig. 17.5 **Endocervical polyp (LP).**

Fig. 17.5 shows a small endocervical polyp arising from the endocervical canal. The polyp is composed of cystically dilated glands **(G)** of varying sizes, each distended by mucin and lined by columnar endocervical mucin secreting epithelium. As the polyp enlarges, it may develop a fibrous stroma between the cystic glands. Extrusion through the cervical os may lead to surface ulceration. Cervical polyps are therefore an important, benign, cause of vaginal bleeding.

Cervical dysplasia and cancer

The understanding that most, if not all, invasive cervical carcinomas are preceded by a long period of pre-invasive neoplastic change in the cervix has led to a revolution in the treatment of cervical carcinomas. These changes are detectable on cytological examination of smears of the cervix, permitting early treatment and prevention of progressive disease. Cytological screening programmes in many countries have reduced the number of deaths from cervical carcinoma. Almost all cervical dysplasia and cancers are caused by persistent infection by oncogenic types of human papillomavirus (HPV), a very common sexually transmitted virus.

In most screening programmes, a positive cytology result is followed up with direct visualisation of the cervix by colposcopy along with a biopsy for definitive diagnosis. HPV testing is increasingly being used to help 'triage' those with positive cytology or to assess cytological smears in women who have had colposcopic treatment (test of cure). More recently, there is a drive to perform primary HPV testing on cervical smears so that only women with a positive HPV test would require cytological examination of their smear. This will potentially have major implications on cytology laboratory infrastructure and staffing.

In the UK, cervical smears taken as part of the national screening programme are reported based on guidelines from the British Association of Cytopathology. Biopsies and large loop excisions of the transformation zone (LLETZ) are reported using the World Health Organization (WHO) system. These classifications are described in further detail in Figs 17.6 and 17.7; however, it should be noted that both systems now also use a simplified two-tier classification (low or high grade) rather than the old three-tier classification (CIN 1/2/3, mild, moderate and severe dyskaryosis), allowing improved reporting consistency. In practice, many pathologists use both the old and new classifications in clinical reports.

The ectocervix is covered by stratified squamous epithelium while the endocervix has a lining of simple columnar mucin-secreting cells. The junction between the two varies during reproductive life with changes in the volume of the cervical stroma. This expands under the influence of hormones during each menstrual cycle, at menarche and during pregnancy and this causes eversion of the vaginal end of the endocervical canal, thus exposing some of the simple columnar epithelium to the vaginal environment. This exposed epithelium appears red in relation to the surrounding stratified squamous epithelium and hence became inaccurately known as a cervical ***erosion;*** more appropriate is the term ***cervical ectropion.*** Under the influence of the vaginal environment, the ectopic columnar epithelium may undergo squamous metaplasia (see Fig. 6.5) to form stratified squamous epithelium. This metaplastic area, known as the ***transformation zone***, appears to be sensitive to the oncogenic effects of HPV. HPV can also infect other squamous cells in the vagina, vulva and perianal region, as well as at more distant sites such as the oesophagus (see clinical box 'Human papillomavirus (HPV) and cancer').

KEY TO FIGURES

B basal atypia **D** dysplastic epidermis **Di** differentiated VIN **Ep** squamous epithelium **F** Nabothian follicle **G** gland **In** Invasive well differentiated squamous cell carcinoma **J** squamocolumnar junction **K** koilocytes **Pa** parakeratosis **P** polyp **R** elongated rete ridges

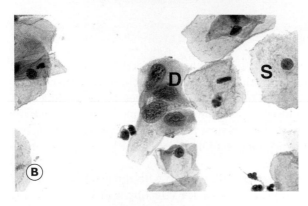

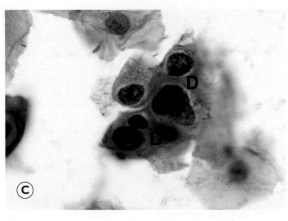

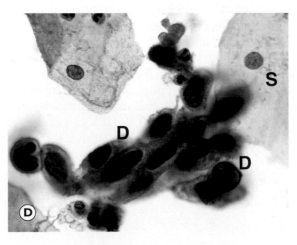

Fig. 17.6 **Cervical cytology (HP). (A)** Koilocytes (low grade dyskaryosis); **(B)** low grade dyskaryosis; **(C)** high grade dyskaryosis (moderate); **(D)** high grade dyskaryosis (severe) (Papanicolaou stain).

Fig. 17.6A–D are from liquid-based cytology (LBC) preparations obtained at cervical smear and stained by the ***Papanicolaou method (Pap)*** (E-Fig. 17.3 **H**). LBC technology has replaced the older method of smearing the cervical cells directly onto a glass slide because of the improved preservation of material and lower false positive and negative rates.

The terminology used in reporting cervical smears has evolved over the last few decades. The current classification has the following categories:

■ Negative

■ Borderline change (in squamous or endocervical cells)

■ Low grade dyskaryosis (including koilocytes with borderline change)

■ High grade dyskaryosis (moderate or severe)

■ High grade ? invasive

■ Glandular abnormality (endocervical or non-cervical)

Fig. 17.6A shows ***koilocytes*** indicative of HPV infection **(K).** Note the clearing of the cytoplasm surrounding the nucleus and compare with the koilocytes in Fig. 17.7. In Fig. 17.6B, again showing ***low grade dyskaryosis***, there are both normal cervical squamous cells **(S)** and clumps of low grade dyskaryotic cells **(D)**, which have large dark-stained nuclei, an irregular nuclear contour and a coarse pattern of nuclear chromatin.

Fig. 17.6C shows ***high grade (moderate) dyskaryosis*** In this smear, the abnormal epithelial cells **(D)** have larger nuclei and a higher nuclear to cytoplasmic ratio than in low grade dyskaryosis, with coarser, more hyperchromatic nuclei.

In ***high grade (severe) dyskaryosis*** as shown in Fig. 17.6D, the nuclear to cytoplasmic ratio is even greater although the cells overall are smaller **(D)**. The abnormal surface cells of dysplastic epithelium are collected when a cervical smear is taken. Most dysplasia occurs at the transformation zone, which is an area of metaplastic squamous epithelium found at the squamocolumnar junction. It is therefore important that the endocervical cells are seen in the cervical smear to ensure that the correct area is sampled.

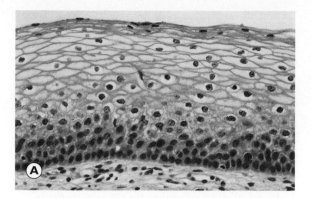

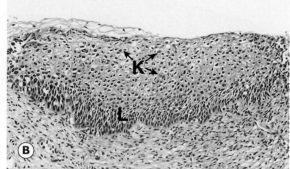

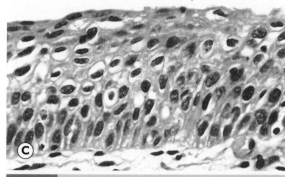

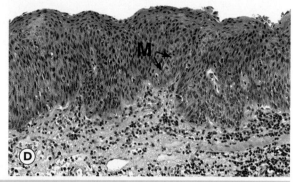

Fig. 17.7 **Cervical intraepithelial neoplasia (CIN).** **(A)** Normal ectocervix (HP); **(B)** LSIL/CIN 1 (HP); **(C)** HSIL/CIN 2 (MP); **(D)** HSIL/CIN 3 (MP).

The consensus from the most recent WHO classification is to use a two-tier classification for CIN, i.e. low grade and high grade squamous intraepithelial lesion (LSIL and HSIL). LSIL is equivalent to HPV change/CIN1 and HSIL is equivalent to CIN 2 and 3. Often both classifications are used in practice to aid understanding for clinicians, therefore both will be described below.

Figs 17.7A–D illustrate the spectrum of cervical epithelial appearances from normal stratified squamous epithelium (E-Fig. 17.4**H**) through to CIN 3 (HSIL).

As seen in Fig. 17.7A, normal ectocervical epithelium is stratified squamous with all cell division being confined to a single basal layer of small, darkly staining cuboidal cells. As the cells undergo maturation, their eosinophilic cytoplasm expands greatly and the cells are pushed upwards towards the epithelial surface.

In CIN 1 (LSIL; Fig. 17.7B), the cells in the lower third of the epithelium **(L)** are enlarged, crowded and hyperchromatic and show increased mitotic activity. There are also *koilocytes* **(K),** in keeping with HPV infection, which are characteristically found in the upper layers of the epithelium and have enlarged irregular nuclei with cleared cytoplasm (compare with Fig. 17.6).

HSIL is characterised by dysplastic cells involving the middle and upper thirds of the epithelium with suprabasal mitotic activity **(M)**. Abnormal mitotic figures may also be seen. The epithelium often appears 'basaloid' or blue as there is lack of cytoplasmic maturation of the dysplastic cells. In the old classification, if the dysplastic cells are mainly in the lower two-thirds of the epithelium then the lesion is termed CIN2 (Fig. 17.7C). Numerous koilocytes are also present. When there are dysplastic cells involving the full thickness of the epithelium, the lesion is termed CIN3 (Fig. 17.7D).

Classification of CIN into LSIL (CIN1) and HSIL (CIN2 and 3) is important as the management is different. Many low grade lesions will regress spontaneously with time and patients are therefore usually monitored with regular smears and colposcopy. High grade lesions, however, are more likely to progress to cancer and are therefore treated by a LLETZ (large loop excision of transformation zone) to remove all the abnormal epithelium.

Note that in all of the above lesions, the basement membrane is intact and well defined. Extension of atypical cells beyond the membrane into the underlying tissues would be termed *invasive carcinoma* (Fig. 17.8).

KEY TO FIGURES
D dyskaryotic cells   **K** koilocytes   **L** lower third of epithelium   **M** mitotic figures   **S** cervical squamous cell

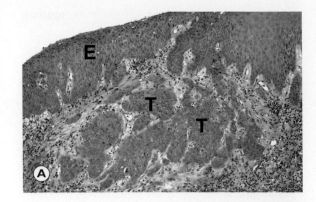

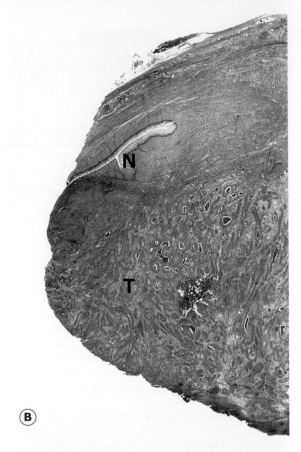

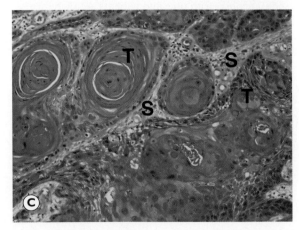

Fig. 17.8 **Invasive squamous cell carcinoma of the cervix. (A)** Superficial invasion (MP); **(B)** invasive carcinoma (LP); **(C)** well differentiated carcinoma (HP).

Squamous carcinomas account for about 90% of cervical malignancies, most of the remainder being adenocarcinomas arising in the endocervix. In most countries, gynaecological cancers are staged according to the *International Federation of Gynaecology and Obstetrics (FIGO) classification*. In cervical cancer, pathological measurement of depth and horizontal extension is important to stage the tumour correctly and for subsequent management.

Invasion may be diagnosed incidentally following LLETZ for CIN and may not be suspected clinically. On histological examination, some of these specimens exhibit the earliest form of invasive carcinoma with only superficial invasion of the cervical stroma. In the UK, if the depth of invasion is less than 3 mm and horizontal extent less than 7 mm, this is staged as *FIGO Stage* IA1 and may be managed more conservatively with a repeat LLETZ procedure, particularly if the patient wishes to preserve her fertility. In some countries, this superficial invasion is termed *microinvasive carcinoma*.

As seen in Fig. 17.8A, the surface epithelium **(E)** shows HSIL/CIN3 (Fig. 17.7D). Small nests of squamous carcinoma **(T)** are seen lying separately within the supporting stroma, the tumour cells having breached the epithelial basement membrane. Typically, the invasive component has a more squamous appearance, the cells having more plentiful eosinophilic cytoplasm than is seen in the overlying CIN 3/HSIL.

If the tumour is clinically visible, it is regarded as at least FIGO stage IB, regardless of its actual size. More extensive carcinoma is treated by surgical removal of the uterus along with the parametrium and a cuff of vaginal tissue *(radical hysterectomy)*. Such an invasive squamous carcinoma of the cervix is illustrated at low magnification in Fig. 17.8B. Note that purple staining tumour **(T)** has replaced most of the cervical stroma, although a portion of normal vaginal mucosa **(N)** remains at the tumour margin. The surface of the tumour is ulcerated and this accounts for the presenting feature of *post-coital bleeding*.

If the patient is young and fertility conservation is a consideration, removal of the cervix and paracervical tissues may be performed *(radical trachelectomy)*. Pelvic lymph nodes are also removed in both procedures. More advanced disease is usually treated with chemoradiotherapy.

At higher magnification (Fig. 17.8C), the tumour consists of sheets of mildly pleomorphic squamous cells **(T)** invading the cervical stroma **(S)**. The cells have plentiful eosinophilic and are separated by a small space where intercellular bridges would be seen at higher magnification. Compare this example with well and poorly differentiated squamous cell carcinoma in Fig. 7.3.

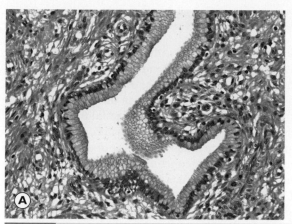
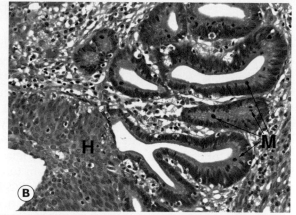

Fig. 17.9 **Cervical glandular intraepithelial neoplasia. (A)** Normal endocervical gland (MP); **(B)** high grade cervical glandular neoplasia (CGIN) (MP).

Adenocarcinoma of the cervix is less common than squamous carcinoma and is often preceded by dysplastic changes in the glandular epithelium. Fig. 17.9B shows *cervical glandular intraepithelial neoplasia (CGIN)* with adjacent HSIL/CIN3 **(H)**. Note the glands show nuclear stratification, hyperchromasia and an increased nuclear to cytoplasmic ratio. Basal apoptotic bodies and mitotic figures **(M)** are also present. Compare these changes to the normal endocervical gland in Fig. 17.9A. CGIN may be detected on cervical smears where a glandular

abnormality is seen. Most adenocarcinomas are associated with high risk HPV types, particularly 16 and 18.

An interesting rare type of cervical cancer is *minimal deviation adenocarcinoma (adenoma malignum)*. This tumour is not associated with HPV and is composed of relatively bland, well differentiated glands, which can make diagnosing this tumour very challenging, especially in superficial biopsies. Other rare types of cervical cancer include clear cell, serous and mesonephric adenocarcinoma.

HUMAN PAPILLOMAVIRUS (HPV) AND CANCER

It is now well established that persistent infection with high risk types of HPV causes a number of cancers, including cervical, anal, vulval, penile and oropharyngeal cancers (OPSCC). HPV is transmitted via skin/mucous membrane contact during sexual activity and is usually asymptomatic. The majority of infections are cleared quickly by the host immune system. A small number remain persistent. There are over 100 types of HPV, which can be broadly divided into two categories:

- **High risk**: There are at least 13 oncogenic types, the commonest being HPV 16 and 18.

- **Low risk**: HPV 6 and 11 are the commonest and cause condyloma acuminata (genital warts) and respiratory papillomatosis.

High risk types of HPV possess viral genes, which can act as **oncogenes** (see Ch. 1). The early E6 and E7 genes are particularly important in carcinogenesis. For example, the E6 gene product is known to bind and inactivate p53 in the host cell. p53 has a key role in **tumour suppression** as it normally inhibits the cell cycle and promotes cell death if DNA damage is present. Its inactivation by the E6 protein can therefore allow unregulated proliferation of genetically abnormal cells, leading to dysplasia and cancer.

There are a number of factors that can increase the risk of persistent infection, development of pre-invasive changes (dysplasia) and subsequent cancer, including smoking, early first sexual contact, multiple sexual partners and immunodeficiency (HIV/AIDS).

PCR-based tests for detection of HPV are used in cervical cancer screening as a primary screening test or to guide further management. In general, HPV positive tumours respond better to chemoradiation and therefore these patients have better outcomes than those with HPV negative tumours. Immunohistochemistry for the HPV surrogate marker p16 can also be used in this setting.

HPV vaccination programmes are now established in many countries. In the UK, girls aged 12–13 years are vaccinated with a quadrivalent vaccine, which protects against HPV6, 11, 16 and 18, with cross protection against some other high risk types. However, it should be remembered that this will not prevent all cases of cervical cancer and attendance at cervical screening tests is still important.

KEY TO FIGURES
E surface epithelium **H** HSIL/CIN3 **M** mitoses **N** normal vaginal mucosa **S** stroma **T** tumour

PART 2

CHAPTER
17

BASIC SYSTEMS PATHOLOGY ■ FEMALE REPRODUCTIVE SYSTEM

241

Disorders of the uterus

The uterine endometrium undergoes monthly cyclical changes under the influence of hormonal stimuli during the reproductive years, except during pregnancy. Before menarche and after the menopause, the endometrial glands and stroma are compact and inactive. At menarche, around the menopause and for the first few cycles after a pregnancy, the endometrium shows a mixture of inactive and normal functional patterns. Iatrogenic factors such as oral contraceptive drugs, other hormonal treatments and intrauterine contraceptive devices may also modify the appearance of the endometrium.

The myometrium is the site of one of the most common benign mesenchymal tumours, the *leiomyoma* (Fig.17.10), often known as a fibroid. Leiomyoma must be differentiated from its much rarer malignant counterpart, *leiomyosarcoma*, as well as from tumours that are difficult to classify, known as *smooth muscle tumours of unknown malignant potential (STUMP)*.

The myometrium may also contain islands of ectopic endometrium known as *adenomyosis* (Fig. 17.11A), which can cause pain and other menstrual disturbances. Such ectopic endometrial tissue may also be found in various other sites throughout the pelvis and sometimes the abdominal cavity, where it is called *endometriosis* (Fig. 17.11B). In this case, it may respond to the normal cyclical hormonal changes resulting in bleeding into the tissues and consequent fibrosis.

Endometrial infection is uncommon but may be associated with retained products of conception after childbirth or miscarriage, pelvic inflammatory disease or with intrauterine contraceptive devices. Endometrial tuberculosis is rare in developed countries, but much more common in countries where TB is common. Localised areas of polypoid hyperplasia forming *endometrial polyps* are common and benign (Fig. 17.12). Excessive or uncoordinated hormonal stimulation of the endometrium may produce *endometrial hyperplasia* (Fig. 17.13B), some variants of which are pre-malignant.

The most common malignant tumour of the endometrium is *endometrioid carcinoma*, an adenocarcinoma derived from endometrial glands (Fig. 17.14A). Other types of adenocarcinoma of the endometrium occur rarely, including tumours typical of the ovary such as *serous* and *clear cell carcinomas* (Figs 17.14B and C). Other rare tumours of the endometrium include *endometrial stromal sarcoma* and carcinosarcoma (previously known as malignant mixed Müllerian tumour, MMMT). *Carcinosarcoma* is a highly aggressive tumour showing a biphasic appearance with malignant epithelial elements in a sarcomatous stroma.

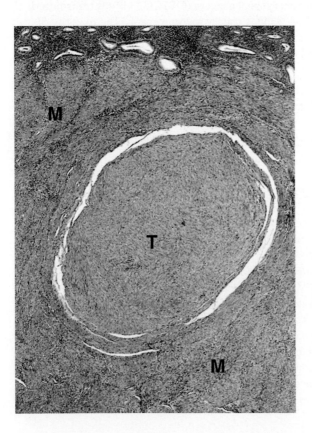

Fig. 17.10 Leiomyoma (fibroid) of myometrium (LP).

This benign tumour of myometrial smooth muscle (E-Fig. 17.5 **H**) is a common cause of abnormal or excessive uterine bleeding and pelvic discomfort (E-Fig. 17.6 **G**). The tumour **(T)** is composed of fascicles (bundles) of smooth muscle cells with blunt ended nuclei and eosinophilic cytoplasm. Gradual expansion of the tumour compresses the surrounding myometrium **(M)**.

In this example, the tumour lies in the myometrium *(intramural)* but some tumours may protrude into the endometrial cavity to produce a polypoid *submucosal* fibroid or protrude onto the serosal surface *(subserosal)*. Secondary changes may also occur, including extensive collagenisation, calcification (especially with increasing age) and cystic degeneration. Growth of these tumours is usually hormone-dependent, as they almost always shrink and partially regress after the menopause.

These tumours are differentiated from *smooth muscle tumours of unknown malignant potential* and *leiomyosarcomas* of the myometrium on the basis of the degree of mitotic activity, cellular pleomorphism and presence of coagulative necrosis.

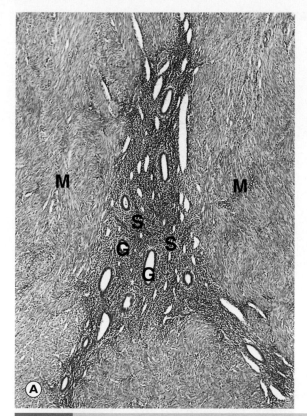
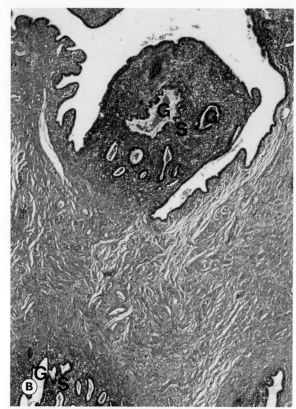

Fig. 17.11 **Adenomyosis and endometriosis. (A)** Adenomyosis; **(B)** endometriosis of Fallopian tube (MP).

Endometrial glands **(G)** and stroma **(S)** may be found outside the endometrium (Fig. 17.11A). If the ectopic endometrium is found embedded deep within the myometrium **(M)**, the condition is known as *adenomyosis*; similar deposits at other sites are known as *endometriosis*. Adenomyosis is often associated with a symmetrical increase in myometrial volume resulting in enlargement of the uterus; occasionally, there is a localised increase in smooth muscle to produce a leiomyoma-like mass containing endometrial islands, a lesion called an *adenomyoma*.

This ectopic endometrium represents an outgrowth of the basal endometrial layer and in most cases is not responsive to ovarian hormones. It is not usually shed during menstruation and therefore, in contrast to endometriosis, no evidence of bleeding is seen in the tissue.

Fig. 17.11B shows endometrial glands **(G)** and stroma **(S)** embedded within the wall of the Fallopian tube. Deposits are seen within the mucosa at the top of the micrograph and in the muscular wall in the bottom corners. Unlike adenomyosis, this endometrium is hormone-responsive and bleeds during menstruation, causing pain. Evidence of bleeding may be seen as haemosiderin-laden macrophages in the tissue and in the lumen of the glands. The presence of free blood within the tissue often causes a marked fibrotic reaction that may cause adhesions between loops of bowel.

Fibrosis of the Fallopian tubes owing to endometriosis is a common cause of infertility and can result in tubal ectopic pregnancy.

Endometriosis of the ovary may give rise to a cyst filled with altered blood, known as a *chocolate cyst* (E-Fig. 17.7**G**). The most common sites for endometriosis include the fallopian tubes, paratubal connective tissues and ovaries. It is, however, not uncommon in the abdomen and is occasionally seen in the thorax. Longstanding endometriosis is associated with clear cell and endometrioid adenocarcinomas of the ovary.

KEY TO FIGURES

G endometrial gland   **M** myometrium   **S** endometrial stroma   **T** tumour

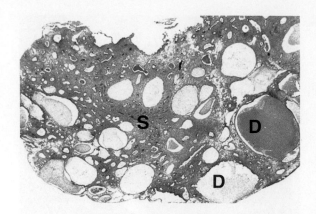

Fig. 17.12 Endometrial polyp (LP).

Endometrial polyps are an important but innocuous cause of abnormal uterine bleeding and often present around the menopause. They may have a stalk or pedicle and are often multiple. Most are composed of cystically dilated glands **(D)** in a fibrotic endometrial stroma **(S)** and covered by a layer of flattened endometrial surface cells. Thick walled blood vessels are a useful diagnostic feature. The glands and stroma in some polyps are responsive to hormonal stimulation and may thus resemble proliferative, secretory (rarely) or hyperplastic endometrium. Polyps are more common in women taking drugs such as tamoxifen. Occasionally, endometrial carcinomas may arise in a polyp.

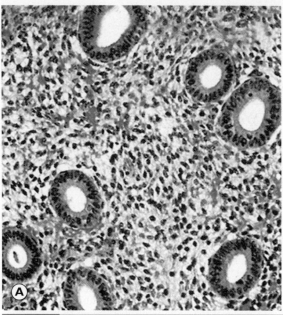

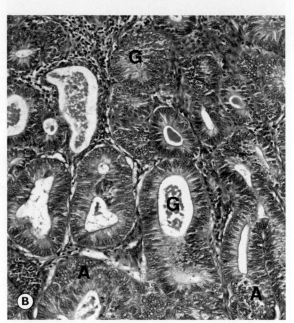

Fig. 17.13 Endometrial hyperplasia. (A) Normal proliferative endometrium (HP); (B) hyperplasia with atypia (atypical hyperplasia) (HP).

Endometrioid endometrial carcinoma (EC) usually arises from pre-existing *endometrial hyperplasia (EH)*. EH occurs as a result of prolonged or unopposed oestrogenic stimulation, examples of which include anovulatory cycles, ovarian lesions such as granulosa cell tumours, ovarian stromal hyperplasia and obesity. The classification of EH was recently updated by the WHO, moving to a two-tier classification in 2014. EH can be classified as (1) *hyperplasia without atypia* or (2) *atypical hyperplasia* (synonyms: hyperplasia with atypia/ endometrial intraepithelial neoplasia or EIN). In the former, there is an increased gland to stroma ratio but no cytological atypia. There is a low rate of progression to EC (1%–3%) and changes may resolve on removal of the oestrogenic stimulus In the latter, cytological atypia is present and these lesions

often harbour the same genetic mutations as EC. Up to a third of patients with atypical hyperplasia will have co-existing invasive cancer or will be at high risk of developing it in the year following diagnosis. Therefore, these patients are often treated with a total hysterectomy. Patients who are not fit enough for surgery are usually managed with progestogens and close follow-up with repeat biopsies.

Note in Fig. 17.13B the glands **(G)** are irregular and crowded together with little intervening stroma. Compare this with the normally spaced glands in Fig. 17.13A. In addition, there is marked cytological atypia **(A)** with 'rounding up' of the nuclei, nucleoli, nuclear stratification and pleomorphism and an increased nuclear to cytoplasmic ratio. Squamous morules and stromal 'foamy' macrophages are also common features (Fig. 17.14).

KEY TO FIGURES

A cytological atypia   **C** cytoplasmic clearing   **D** dilated gland   **E** crowded malignant glands
G endometrial gland   **F** cell budding   **M** myometrium   **P** papillary architecture
S endometrial stroma   **SM** squamous morule   **SL** slit-like spaces

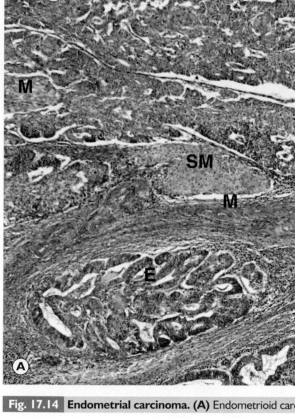

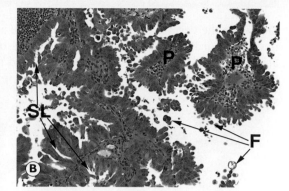

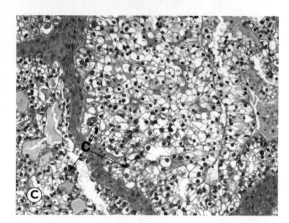

Fig. 17.14 **Endometrial carcinoma.** **(A)** Endometrioid carcinoma; **(B)** serous carcinoma; **(C)** clear cell carcinoma (HP).

The most common type is *endometrioid adenocarcinoma* (Fig. 17.14A) (E-Fig. 17.8 **G**), which resembles endometrioid glands and can have a variety of architectural appearances such as crowded, infiltrating glands lacking intervening stroma **(E)** (pictured) or papillary, cribriform and solid forms. Tumours are graded according to the **FIGO** system, based on the percentage solid component of the tumour (Grade 1<5%, Grade 2=5%–50%, Grade 3=>50%). If there is nuclear atypia disproportionate to the architectural grade then the overall grade can be increased by one. Note in Fig. 17.14A malignant glands infiltrate the myometrium **(M)**. There are also associated squamous morules **(SM)**.

Serous carcinoma is an uncommon type but is highly aggressive and often presents with advanced disease (Fig. 17.14B). Note the tumour displays a papillary architecture **(P)** with cells budding off the papillae

(F) and lying 'free'. Note also, some of the glands have slit-like spaces **(SL)** rather than the rounded glandular spaces of endometrioid carcinoma. Serous carcinomas in the endometrium are always high grade. *Psammomatous calcification* may also be seen (not illustrated) and is further discussed in Fig. 17.22. It is important to exclude a uterine metastasis from a primary ovarian serous carcinoma, as this would show identical histology.

Clear cell carcinoma (Fig. 17.14C) is another uncommon type. The classic pattern shows nests and glands of cells with cleared cytoplasm **(C)** along with occasional eosinophilic granules due to glycogen accumulation, although there are other histological variants. Nuclei are atypical and irregular with prominent nucleoli. Both clear cell and serous carcinomas are regarded as high grade tumours and have a worse prognosis than endometrioid adenocarcinoma.

MOLECULAR ASPECTS OF ENDOMETRIAL CANCER (EC)

There have been significant recent advances in the molecular understanding of EC. Current risk stratification is based on the histological subtype of EC, FIGO grade and stage. More recently, the *Cancer Genome Atlas Classification* has shown that at a genomic level, there are four main subtypes of EC that can predict outcome and potentially help guide clinical management, particularly in high grade tumours. Further studies have shown that immunohistochemical markers can also be used to demonstrate the same stratification. This could potentially be used in routine histopathology departments. The subgroups are listed below in order of outcome (best at the top). In the future, these molecular tests are likely to be part of the routine pathological assessment of ECs.

■ **Ultramutation of POLE**: This is a gene involved in DNA repair, and ultramutation is associated with an excellent outcome, regardless of stage or grade.

■ **Microsatellite instability (MSI) high**: This can occur in Lynch syndrome, somatic mutations and epigenetic alterations such as MLH1 hypermethylation (see Ch. 1).

■ **Copy number low:** This group of tumours lacks specific molecular signatures and typically show on endometrioid morphology.

■ **Copy number high**: Serous type carcinomas. *TP53* mutation testing or immunohistochemistry can be used as a surrogate marker. These typically have a very poor prognosis.

Placental disorders

Details of the various structural and functional abnormalities of the placenta, decidua, membranes and umbilical cord are generally outside the scope of this book; however, hydatidiform mole (Fig. 17.15) and choriocarcinoma (Fig. 17.16) are included as examples of disorders of placental growth. Ectopic pregnancy is discussed in Fig. 17.18.

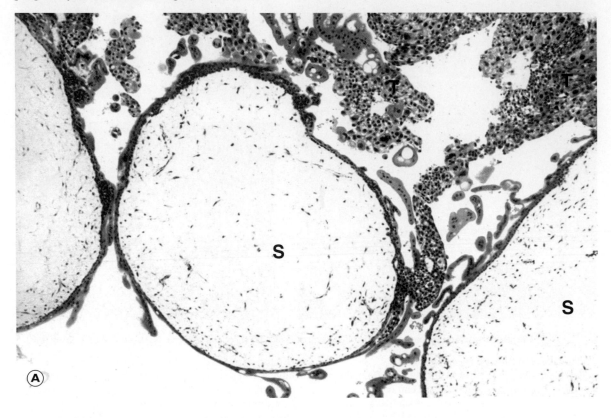

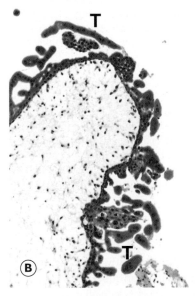

Fig. 17.15 **Hydatidiform mole: complete. (A)** MP; **(B)** HP.

This condition known as *hydatidiform mole* arises in a small proportion of pregnancies after miscarriage, termination of pregnancy or even years after a normal pregnancy (E-Fig. 17.9 **H**). Moles may be *partial or complete*. In a complete mole, as seen in Fig. 17.15A, the chorionic villi become oedematous with central cystic spaces *(cisterns)* **(S)**. The cisterns are invested by a layer of hyperplastic cytotrophoblast and syncytiotrophoblast (Fig. 17.15B). In addition to hyperplasia and proliferation of the trophoblast, there are disconnected masses of trophoblast cells **(T)** lying apparently free of the villi and showing mild cellular pleomorphism. Hydatidiform moles exhibit a wide spectrum of behaviours: some are eradicated by simple curettage, others persist despite repeated curettage and a small number develop into undoubtedly malignant *choriocarcinoma* (Fig. 17.16).

Complete hydatidiform mole almost always has a 46,XX karyotype, but all the chromosomes are derived from the spermatozoa with none from the ovum. Partial moles have similar, but less prominent, histological abnormalities that rarely develop into choriocarcinoma and have a triploid karyotype such as 69,XXY.

KEY TO FIGURES

C cytotrophoblast   **H** haemorrhage   **M** tubal mucosa   **P** purulent exudate   **S** cistern   **Sy** syncytiotrophoblast   **T** trophoblast

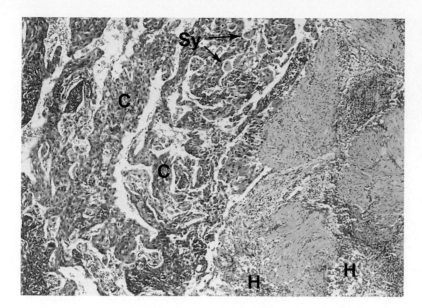

Fig. 17.16 Choriocarcinoma (HP).

Choriocarcinoma (Fig. 17.16) is a malignant tumour derived from trophoblast cells, usually from abnormal gestations. The tumour consists of malignant cells resembling either cytotrophoblast cells **(C)** or multinucleate syncytiotrophoblast cells **(Sy)**. The two cell types are arranged in alternating layers, mimicking the structure of chorionic villi. No true chorionic villi are found. The tumour is typically haemorrhagic **(H)** because of the propensity of trophoblast cells to invade blood vessel walls. Areas of necrosis in the tumour are common. Choriocarcinoma is remarkably invasive, metastasising widely via lymphatics and the bloodstream, particularly to the lungs. Fortunately, this tumour responds well to chemotherapy. Choriocarcinoma may also rarely occur in the ovary and in the testis, in the latter case, usually as part of a mixed germ cell tumour.

Diseases of the fallopian tubes

The fallopian tubes may become infected by pyogenic bacteria, particularly Gonococcus and chlamydia species, resulting in acute inflammation known as *acute salpingitis* (Fig. 17.17). This may be complicated by obstruction of the tubal lumen, leading to chronic suppurative inflammation and abscess formation. Along with tuberculosis of the fallopian tube, these conditions constitute an important cause of female infertility worldwide owing to obliteration of the tubal lumen. In developed countries, endometriosis (Fig 17.11) is a common cause of infertility. Scarring of the tube and other disorders may prevent the free passage of a fertilised ovum into the endometrial cavity and implantation may occur in the tube leading to *tubal ectopic pregnancy* (Fig. 17.18); this usually culminates in massive intraperitoneal haemorrhage caused by the placenta eroding through the tubal wall.

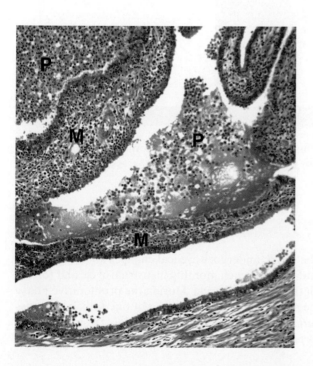

Fig. 17.17 Acute salpingitis (MP).

In *acute salpingitis*, the tubal mucosa **(M)** becomes hyperaemic, oedematous and infiltrated with neutrophils and the lumen becomes filled with a purulent exudate **(P)**. Blockage of the tubal lumen often follows, preventing drainage and leading to distension of the tube by pus *(pyosalpinx)* or fluid *(hydrosalpinx)*. Sometimes the inflammation produces a *tubo-ovarian abscess* as a result of adhesions between tube, fimbriae and ovary, and extension of suppuration to these areas may produce multiple locules of pus. Without the intervention of antibiotics, the combination of adhesions and suppuration rarely permits total resolution of the acute inflammation and a state of chronic inflammation generally ensues. This state, known as *chronic salpingitis*, may persist for many years, resulting in fibrosis and tubal obstruction and is an important cause of female infertility. Chronic salpingitis may be a component of more widespread chronic inflammation involving ovaries, clinically termed *pelvic inflammatory disease (PID)*.

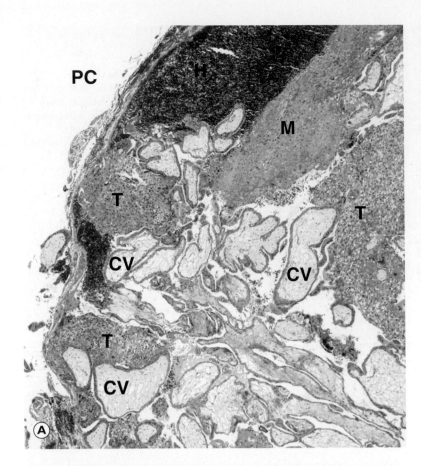

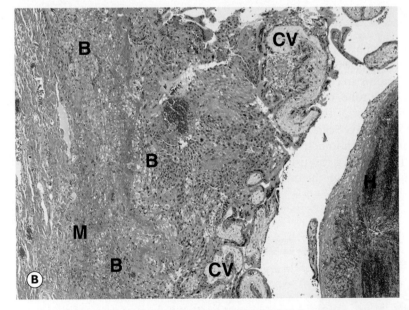

Fig. 17. 18 Tubal ectopic pregnancy. **(A)** MP; **(B)** MP.

The fallopian tube is the most frequent location for ectopic implantation of the fertilised ovum, resulting in *ectopic pregnancy*. Other much rarer sites include the abdominal cavity and the ovary. The tubal lumen becomes filled and expanded by the developing embryo (not seen in Fig. 17.18) and the placenta.

In Fig. 17.18A, the fallopian tube has already ruptured and chorionic villi **(CV)** and sheets of trophoblast **(T)** can be seen spilling into the peritoneal cavity **(PC)**. The muscular wall of the fallopian tube **(M)** has been breached by trophoblast burrowing into it **(B)** (shown in Fig. 17.18B). Haemorrhage **(H)** is also seen within the peritoneal cavity. Haemorrhage into the lumen of the tube **(H)** causes *haematosalpinx.*

Ectopic pregnancies usually become dramatically apparent by severe haemorrhage into the lumen, often followed by tracking of blood into the peritoneal cavity. Thus, tubal ectopics most often present as acute abdominal emergencies; only very rarely does the pregnancy continue to near normal term. The most common cause of tubal ectopic pregnancy is obstruction of the lumen, usually caused by infection, endometriosis and intra-abdominal adhesions; however, 50% occur in normal fallopian tubes.

Disorders of the ovary

The ovary may be affected by a variety of non-neoplastic disorders including endometriosis (Fig. 17.11), as well as being involved by chronic inflammation in the form of tubo-ovarian abscesses caused by primary infection of the fallopian tube (Fig. 17.17)

Non-neoplastic cysts

Under the influence of pituitary gonadotrophins, the ovary undergoes cyclical changes allowing for the development and release of a mature ovum at the mid-point of each monthly menstrual cycle and for the production of the ovarian hormones, which control the menstrual cycle. During the proliferative phase of the menstrual cycle, a number of *follicles* enlarge culminating in maturation of one follicle that discharges its single *ovum* into the fallopian tube *(ovulation)*. The follicle, until this time also responsible for production of oestrogens, now develops into the *corpus luteum*, responsible for producing progesterone until the beginning of the next menstrual cycle when the follicle atrophies to form the redundant, collagenous *corpus albicans*. This regular sequence of changes is normally only interrupted by pregnancy, in which case the corpus luteum persists until the end of the first trimester. On occasion, however, the sequence is arrested at some stage and small *follicular* or *luteal cysts* may form. Some small cysts may also form by inclusion of islands of surface 'germinal' epithelium of the ovary; these are known as *epithelial inclusion cysts*. These three types of cyst are shown in Fig. 17.19.

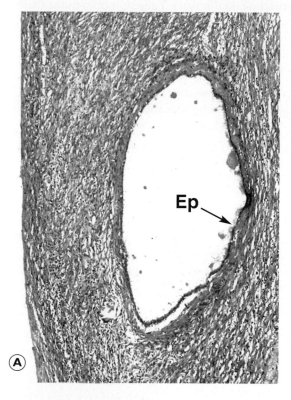

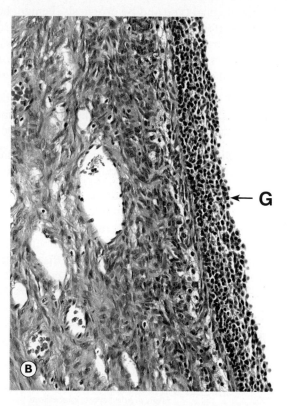

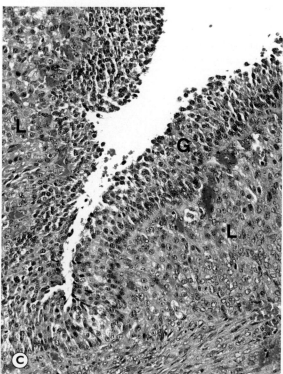

Fig. 17.19 Non-neoplastic ovarian cysts. (A) Epithelial inclusion cyst (LP); **(B)** follicular cyst (MP); **(C)** luteal cyst (MP).

The most common type of ovarian cyst is the *epithelial inclusion cyst* as illustrated in Fig. 17.19A. These cysts are commonly multiple, small and lined by a simple cuboidal epithelium **(Ep)**. They are thought to be derived from entrapped portions of the ovarian surface epithelium, which is erroneously but traditionally referred to as germinal epithelium. *Follicular cysts*, as seen in Fig. 17.19B, are lined internally by granulosa cells **(G)**, which usually form a thicker layer than the flattened cells lining the germinal inclusion cyst. Continuing enlargement of the follicular cyst leads to atrophy of the lining cells so that distinction between a large follicular cyst and a germinal inclusion cyst may be difficult. Multiple follicular cysts are found in the ovaries of patients with polycystic ovarian syndrome, frequently associated with obesity, anovulation and hirsutism.

The *luteal cyst* is probably derived from a corpus luteum that has not undergone the normal transition to a corpus albicans. The cyst is usually ovoid with a slightly irregular outline. Microscopically, it contains clear or brownish fluid, and there are luteinised cells in its wall **(L)**.

KEY TO FIGURES
B placental site reaction   **CV** chorionic villi   **Ep** epithelium   **G** granulosa cells   **H** haemorrhage
L luteal cells   **M** muscular wall of fallopian tube   **PC** peritoneal cavity   **T** trophoblast

Tumours of the ovary

Tumours may arise from each of the specialised elements that make up the ovary and may be classified into four broad groups based on the current WHO classification. These groups of tumours and their major subtypes are listed in Table 17.2 below.

■ **Epithelial tumours**: Tumours of the surface ovarian epithelium are the commonest and are defined by histological type and by prognosis (benign, borderline, malignant). These tumours range from benign (often cystic) to frankly malignant. Intermediate between these two ends of the spectrum are tumours with low malignant potential. This group is called *borderline* or *atypical proliferating tumours*. Classification of serous carcinoma into two distinct tumours (high and low grade) is important and is described in detail in Figs 17.20 and 17.21 and Table 17.3.

■ **Sex cord stromal tumours**: These tumours may develop from *granulosa cells* and *theca cells* (Fig. 17.27), as well as from spindle cells of the ovarian stroma forming *fibromas*. These may produce oestrogenic hormones and cause endocrine effects such as endometrial hyperplasia (Fig. 17.13).

■ **Germ cell tumours**: The classification and morphology of ovarian germ cell tumours is quite similar to those for testicular germ cell tumours (see Fig. 19.1).

■ **Metastatic tumours**: The ovary is a common site for metastatic carcinoma, which is frequently bilateral. A well-known example is the *Krukenberg tumour* in which there is infiltration of the ovary by mucin secreting adenocarcinoma of signet ring type (see Fig. 17.25); such tumours are usually derived from stomach or colon and probably reach the ovary by either transcoelomic or lymphatic spread. Tumours from other parts of the genital tract, including uterus and cervix, commonly involve the ovaries. Breast and pancreaticobiliary carcinomas also frequently metastasise to this site. The ovaries may also be involved by lymphoma.

Table 17.2 Overview of ovarian tumours.

Tumour type	Subtype
Epithelial tumours ~70%	**Low grade serous:** serous cystadenoma, serous borderline tumour (SBT), low grade serous carcinoma **High grade serous carcinoma** **Mucinous:** mucinous cystadenoma, borderline mucinous tumour, invasive mucinous carcinoma **Endometrioid:** resembles endometrioid carcinoma of the uterus and may arise from endometriosis **Seromucinous:** a new category, associated with endometriosis. **Brenner (transitional cell) tumour:** almost all benign, rarely malignant **Clear cell:** almost all malignant and high grade – may arise from endometriosis **Undifferentiated:** too poorly differentiated to categorise **Neuroendocrine:** large cell and small cell types
Sex-cord-stromal tumours ~20%	**Fibroma** **Thecoma** **Fibrothecoma** **Granulosa cell tumour** – adult type, juvenile type **Sertoli-Leydig cell tumour**
Germ cell tumours ~5%	**Mature teratoma** (dermoid cyst): very common and benign **Immature teratoma:** immature tissues, usually neuroepithelial elements **Dysgerminoma** (testicular equivalent is seminoma) **Yolk sac tumour** **Choriocarcinoma**
Metastatic tumours ~5%	From stomach, colon, breast, uterus, cervix May also be involved by lymphoma

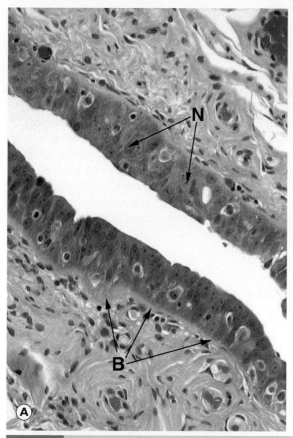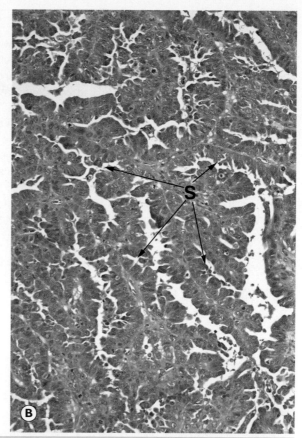

Fig. 17.20 **Serous carcinoma. (A)** Serous tubal intraepithelial carcinoma (STIC HP); **(B)** high grade serous carcinoma (MP).

Until recently, *high grade serous carcinomas (HGSC)* were thought to arise from the epithelial surface of the ovary. Now, most are thought to arise from carcinoma in situ at the distal end of the fallopian tube, known as *serous tubal intraepithelial carcinoma* or *STIC*. Compare Fig. 17.20A with normal fallopian tubal epithelium (E-Fig. 17.10**H**). Note the atypical cells show nuclear irregularity and stratification **(N)** with prominent nucleoli. Mitotic figures are often seen. The atypical cells are confined to the epithelium and the basement membrane is intact **(B)**. STIC lesions also harbour TP53 mutations similar to HGSC and this can be detected with immunohistochemistry for p53 (Fig. 17.21).

HGSC is a distinct disease from *low grade serous carcinoma* (LGSC, Fig. 17.22) and is the commonest

malignant epithelial tumour of ovary. HGSC is often diagnosed at a late stage with extra-ovarian spread and follows a rapid, aggressive clinical course. HGSC can display a variety of architectural patterns histologically, including papillary, glandular, solid, transitional cell-like and endometrioid-like appearances. Fig. 17.20B shows the typical branching papillary glandular pattern with 'slit-like' spaces **(S)**. The tumour cells show marked nuclear atypia with nuclear pleomorphism and nucleoli and there are frequent mitoses. Necrosis is often a feature. Treatment usually consists of a combination of debulking surgery and chemotherapy, depending on the stage of the disease.

Table 17.3 **Serous carcinoma.**

Serous carcinoma	High grade serous carcinoma	Low grade serous carcinoma
Frequency	Commonest malignant tumour of ovary	Uncommon
Genetics	Genetically unstable (high copy number alterations)	Genetically stable
Molecular	Majority *TP53* mutations	RAS pathway mutations (*KRAS/BRAF/ErbB2*)
Origin	Fallopian tube (STIC)	Serous cystadenoma via serous border-line tumour
Clinical course	Aggressive, fast	Indolent, slow

KEY TO FIGURE
B basement membrane   **N** nuclear atypia   **S** slit-like spaces

P53 AND SEROUS CARCINOMA

Classification of ovarian serous carcinomas into low and high grade reflects recent evidence showing that these two tumours are biologically and molecularly distinct diseases that develop two different pathways. As described in Fig. 17.22, low grade serous carcinoma develops from the serous cystadenoma/serous borderline tumour pathway, whereas high grade serous carcinoma is thought to develop from STIC lesions in the distal fallopian tube (Fig. 17.20).

TP53, a **tumour suppressor gene**, is mutated in almost all high grade serous carcinomas. Mutations can result in different types of protein expression in the nucleus, which can be detected by immunohistochemical stains. **Overexpression** is the commonest pattern, giving strong and diffusely positive staining. **Null expression** results in completely negative staining, which can be misinterpreted as 'normal'. As low grade serous carcinomas do not harbour TP53 mutations, they show a **'wild type'** or phenotypically normal expression pattern with variable staining of the nuclei. Rarely, high grade serous carcinomas can show cytoplasmic or wild type pattern of staining. These patterns are illustrated in Fig. 17.21.

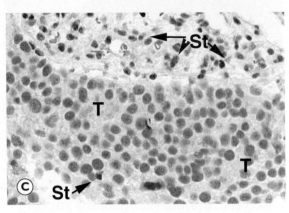

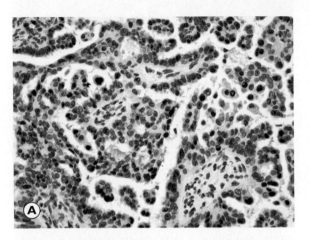

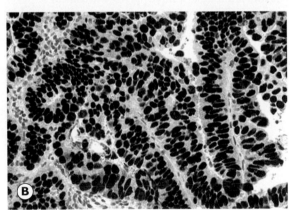

Fig. 17.21 P53 Immunohistochemistry. (A) Wild type; **(B)** over expression; **(C)** absent/null.

The commonest expression patterns of p53 are illustrated in Fig. 17.21. Note wild type staining is variable with some strongly positive nuclei, some weakly positive and some negative. This is in contrast to Fig. 17.21B where there is strong and diffuse positive staining of almost all the tumour nuclei. In Fig. 17.21C, the tumour nuclei show absent staining (T) but note there are stromal cells (St) showing 'wild type' (variable) staining. This serves as a useful internal positive control to confirm that the antibody has worked correctly.

KEY TO FIGURES
H hierarchical branches   **P** psammoma bodies   **S** stroma   **St** stromal cell nuclei   **T** tumour cells

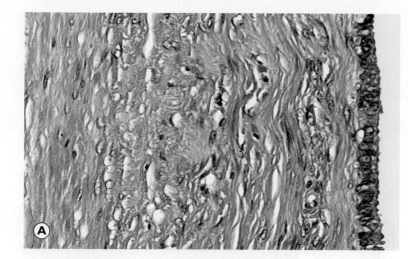

Fig 17.22 **Serous tumours. (A)** Serous cystadenoma (HP); **(B)** serous borderline tumour (LP); **(C)** low grade serous carcinoma (HP).

Benign serous cystadenomas, which range from tiny to huge (watermelon sized), are often unilocular and are filled with a clear, watery (serous) fluid. The benign cysts are lined by columnar epithelium, resembling that which lines the fallopian tube (Fig. 17.22A). *Cystadenofibromas* have a similar epithelial lining but contain a collagenised stromal component.

Serous borderline tumours (SBT) are usually cystic lesions containing complex, branching papillary structures (Fig. 17.22B). Histologically, these display 'hierarchical branching' from large papillary excrescences to single cells lying apparently 'free' in the cyst **(H)**. The lining cells show atypia with nuclear stratification, pleomorphism and nucleoli. SBTs can be associated with invasive or non-invasive *implants* in the peritoneum. *micropapillary variant* of SBT, composed of long slender papillae without hierarchical branching, is associated with a poorer prognosis than conventional SBT.

As described earlier, *low grade serous carcinomas* (Fig. 17.22C) develop in a 'step-wise' fashion from pre-existing cystadenomas or SBTs and are a distinct disease from high grade serous carcinoma. Note the prominent papillary architecture and low grade cytological atypia. Stroma is also highlighted **(S)**. Spherical, concentrically laminated calcified bodies known as *psammoma bodies* **(P)** are common in serous tumours of all grades as a result of dystrophic calcification. Note that they are not unique to the ovary and are also seen in high grade serous tumours in the uterus and papillary tumours at other sites such as thyroid (see Fig. 20.7) and meningiomas (see Fig. 23.14).

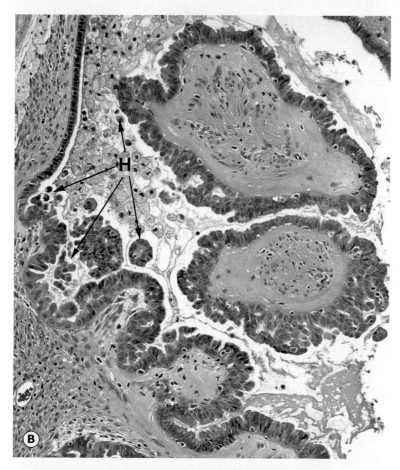

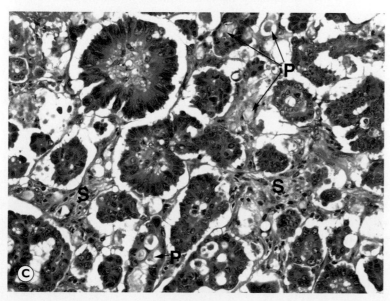

BASIC SYSTEMS PATHOLOGY ■ FEMALE REPRODUCTIVE SYSTEM

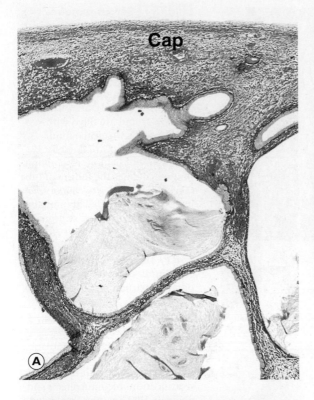

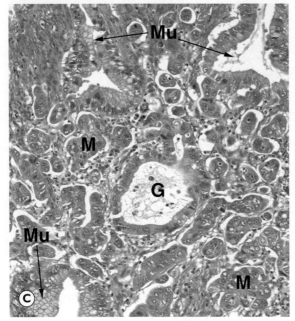

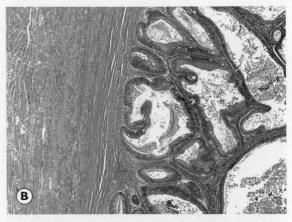

Fig 17.23 **Mucinous ovarian tumours. (A)** Mucinous cystadenoma (LP); **(B)** borderline mucinous tumour (LP); **(C)** invasive mucinous adenocarcinoma (MP).

Benign mucinous cystadenoma, (E-Fig. 17.11 **G**) as shown in Fig. 17.23A, has a characteristically smooth outer surface composed of the ovarian capsule **(Cap)**. The cystic locules are filled with mucin and lined by tall columnar epithelium with uniform basal nuclei and copious mucin-containing cytoplasm at the luminal aspect.

The epithelium of mucinous tumours can be of intestinal type (majority), resembling the epithelium of the GI tract with goblet cells, or endocervical in type. *Borderline mucinous tumours (BMT)* (Fig. 17.23B) show proliferation of the epithelial lining with cytological atypia. Often the epithelium is arranged into complex glandular and papillary forms with a lobular pattern at low power. The cytological atypia often resembles that of adenomas in the colon. These tumours require meticulous sampling for histological examination to exclude areas of frank invasion. BMTs can contain areas of high grade dysplasia/ intraepithelial carcinoma or microinvasion but stage 1 intact tumours usually have a good prognosis regardless of these features.

Invasive mucinous carcinoma (Fig. 17.23C) is less common than serous carcinoma. As the majority of mucinous carcinomas are of intestinal type, these tumours often have similar histological and immunohistochemical features to metastatic adenocarcinomas of the gastrointestinal tract and diagnosis of a primary ovarian tumour can only be made after clinical exclusion of a gastrointestinal primary. Bilateral ovarian involvement, extra ovarian disease and lymphovascular invasion favour metastatic disease over a primary tumour. Note there are infiltrating micropapillary elements **(M)** and glands **(G)** in which the cells contain mucin **(Mu)**.

KEY TO FIGURES
B Call-Exner body   **C** cystic spaces   **Cap** capsule   **CS** collagenous stroma   **G** malignant glands
L luteinised cells   **M** micropapillary tumour   **Mu** mucin   **N** nests of transitional cells   **Sp** spindle
cells   **SR** signet ring cells   **T** tumour

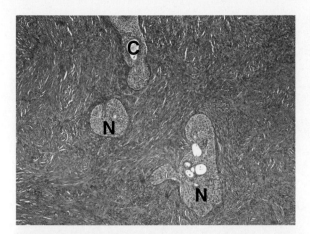

Fig. 17.24 Brenner tumour (LP).

Brenner tumours are almost always benign and are often incidental findings in ovaries removed for another reason. Brenner tumours consist of nests **(N)** of epithelial cells resembling the transitional cells of the normal bladder epithelium. The epithelial cell nests may contain small cystic spaces **(C)** and are set in a fibrous stroma consisting of spindle cells, which may occasionally contain lipid. Most Brenner tumours are small but they may be 20 cm or more in diameter. Rare borderline and frankly malignant variants occur. They sometimes occur in association with mucinous cystadenomas.

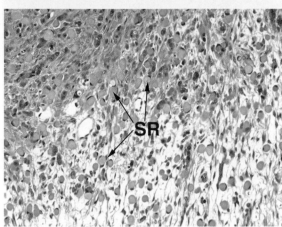

Fig. 17.25 Krukenberg tumour (HP).

Krukenberg tumours are malignant ovarian tumours as a result of metastasis. Classically, this is from a signet ring type gastric adenocarcinoma though it can arise from other primary sites in the GI tract (e.g. appendix, colon) and the breast (e.g. lobular carcinoma). Macroscopically, metastatic ovarian tumours often involve both ovaries, which show nodular surfaces. Often, there are deposits elsewhere in the body (extra-ovarian disease). Note the numerous signet ring cells **(SR)** with abundant cytoplasm and eccentric nuclei situated in an oedematous stroma.

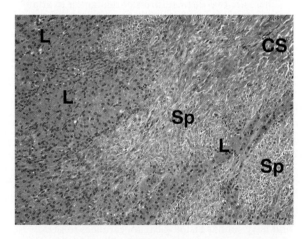

Fig. 17.26 Fibrothecoma (MP).

Fibrothecoma is an uncommon sex cord stromal tumour. However, it is useful as it illustrates the features of both a *fibroma* and a *thecoma*, which are more common. *Fibromas* are the commonest sex cord stromal tumour, presenting as a unilateral or bilateral solid ovarian mass with a whorled white cut surface. Histologically there are spindle cells **(Sp)** in a collagenous stroma **(CS)**. *Thecomas* are composed of luteinised cells **(L)** with abundant cytoplasm, which contains steroids, responsible for the classic gross appearance of a solid yellow mass. *Thecomas* can present with the effects of excess oestrogens (e.g. endometrial hyperplasia) or excess androgens (virilisation).

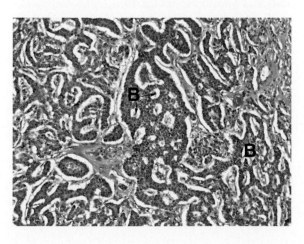

Fig. 17.27 Granulosa cell tumour (MP).

Most adult *granulosa cell tumours* occur in middle-aged to older women and are unilateral. They are composed of uniform ovoid to spindle cells resembling normal granulosa cells. The cells typically have a longitudinal nuclear groove. These may be arranged in a variety of patterns, including one mimicking follicle formation, the *Call-Exner body* **(B)**, which is shown here. Less well differentiated forms may be arranged in a variety of other patterns such as the 'watered-silk' pattern. Most early stage tumours have a good prognosis, but the tumour has a tendency to recur locally after many years. The juvenile type, which is much rarer, has a distinctive histological appearance and occurs mainly, but not always, in a younger age group.

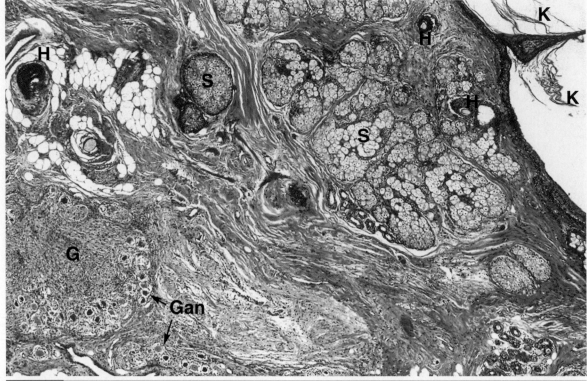

Fig. 17.28 **Benign (mature) cystic teratoma (MP).**

Mature cystic teratoma (E-Fig. 17.12 **G**) is composed of mature components of the three germ cell layers. Ectodermal elements usually predominate (skin and skin appendages) and therefore these tumours are commonly referred to as *dermoid cysts*. Mesodermal (e.g. cartilage and smooth muscle) and endodermal (e.g. respiratory and intestinal epithelium) elements can also occur. Uncommonly, monodermal teratomas can occur with differentiation of one mature tissue type, e.g. struma ovarii, which is composed mostly of thyroid tissue.

Mature cystic teratoma takes the form of a unilocular cyst filled with a thick, yellowish, pasty material composed of masses of degenerating keratin (**K**), often containing hair. This is produced by keratinising stratified squamous epithelium resembling skin. At one end of the cyst wall, there is often a raised area within which are other teratomatous components including hair follicles (**H**), sebaceous glands (**S**) and, occasionally, teeth. Neuroectodermal tissues may also be found; in this example, note the area of glial tissue

(**G**) and a ganglion (**Gan**) alongside. Cystic teratomas are most common in young women and are almost always benign.

There are two distinct forms of malignant ovarian teratoma. *Malignant transformation* can occur within the differentiated elements of an otherwise mature teratoma (e.g. squamous cell carcinoma, melanoma) or teratomas may be immature, composed of primitive embryonal tissues.

Immature teratoma is an uncommon tumour that presents most commonly in childhood/adolescence. Histologically, there are fetal or embryonic tissues present that are usually neuroepithelial in nature. Grading is based on the proportion of neuroepithelium present in the cyst, therefore thorough sampling is important. Prognosis depends on the grade and stage of disease. Other germ cell tumours of the ovary such as dysgerminoma, choriocarcinoma and yolk sac tumour are very rare and have similar histological appearances to their testicular equivalents (see Ch. 19).

KEY TO FIGURES
G glial tissue   **Gan** ganglion   **H** hair follicles   **K** keratin   **S** sebaceous glands.

Table 17.4 Chapter review.

Site	Pathological condition	Main pathological features	Figure
Vulva	Lichen sclerosus et atrophicus	Thin/thick epithelium, band of hyalinised collagen under epithelium with underlying band of chronic inflammation	17.1
	Dysplasia (VIN)	Neoplastic epithelial cells confined to the epithelium. VIN usual type and differentiated	17.3
	Hidradenoma papilliferum	Apocrine benign tumour with papillary architecture.	17.2
	Invasive SCC	Similar to SCC at other sites	Like 17.8
Cervix and vagina	Chronic cervicitis	Chronic inflammation with papillary hyperplasia of the mucosa	17.4
	Endocervical polyp	Dilated endocervical glands in an inflamed fibrous stroma	17.5
	CIN	Atypical epithelial cells confined to the epithelium, either 3 grades, (CIN 1, 2 and 3) or 2 (LGSIL and HGSIL)	17.6 and 17.7
	SCC	Similar to SCC at other sites	17.8
	Adenocarcinoma in situ	Dysplastic cells lining pre-existing cervical glands	17.9
	Adenocarcinoma	Adenocarcinoma - usually mucin-producing but rarely endometrioid or clear cell types	
Uterus	Adenomyosis/endometriosis	Endometrial glands in the myometrium/at other sites	17.11
	Endometrial polyp	Disorganised endometrial glands in fibrotic stroma	17.12
	Endometrial hyperplasia: with/without atypia	Proliferative endometrial glands with varying degrees of crowding and cytological atypia	17.13
	Endometrial carcinoma • most endometrioid • less common serous/clear cell	Adenocarcinoma invading the endometrium or myometrium	17.14
	Leiomyoma (fibroid)	Well defined nodule of smooth muscle cells in the myometrium	17.10
Placenta	Hydatidiform mole	Abnormal chorionic villi, often with cystic spaces and atypical proliferating trophoblast	17.15
	Choriocarcinoma	Frankly malignant tumour consisting of layers of syncytiotrophoblast and cytotrophoblast	17.16
Fallopian tube	Acute salpingitis	Typical acute inflammation with plentiful neutrophils	17.17
Ovary	Benign, non-neoplastic cysts: epithelial inclusion cyst, follicular cyst, luteal cyst	Bland cysts lined by flattened epithelium, granulosa cells or luteinised granulosa cells	17.19
	Epithelial tumours • Serous • Endometrioid • Clear cell • Mucinous • Brenner tumour	Various types • Fallopian tube differentiation • Like uterine endometrioid carcinoma • Atypical cells with clear cytoplasm • Like cervical adenocarcinoma • Resembles urothelial tumours	17.20–17.23 Like 17.14 Like 17.14 17.23 17.24
	Sex-cord stromal tumours • Thecomas • Granulosa cell tumours – adult/juvenile	 • Spindled cells, may be luteinised • Ovoid cells forming follicular structures (Call-Exner bodies)	17.26 17.27
	Germ cell tumours • Teratoma – most are mature • Dysgerminoma • Yolk sac tumour • Choriocarcinoma	 • Mixture of mature (adult) tissues • Resembles seminoma	17.28 Like 19.4 Like 19.7 17.16
	Metastatic tumours: primaries from gastric, colon, pancreas, kidney, others	Resembles primary tumour morphology	17.25

18 Breast

Introduction

The female breast (E-Fig. 18.1**H**) is dependent for its normal activity on oestrogen and progestogens and thus exhibits considerable structural and functional variation throughout life. Apart from the overt changes occurring during puberty, pregnancy, lactation (E-Fig. 18.2**H**) and menopause, subtler changes also occur within the normal menstrual cycle. As a corollary, hormonal disturbances probably underlie various benign breast disorders and probably also play some part in the pathogenesis of more serious conditions such as **breast cancer**. Likewise, the male breast normally remains rudimentary unless breast enlargement, **gynaecomastia** (Fig. 18.5), is induced by exogenous or endogenous hormone imbalance; it may also result from the use of certain drugs, for example spironolactone.

Most clinically significant breast disorders present as a lump and the major imperative is to identify those that are malignant tumours so that the patient may be treated promptly. Breast cancer screening programmes use radiological techniques (**mammography** and/or **ultrasound**) to identify clinically unde-tectable, suspicious breast lesions, including abnormal calcifications. A tissue diagnosis is then made by **fine needle aspiration (FNA)** and/or **core biopsy** before definitive treatment is undertaken. It is expected that early removal of very small tumours will be curative.

Inflammatory disorders of the breast

Infections of the breast are uncommon and mainly occur during lactation; bacteria (usually *Staphylococcus aureus*) gain access through cracks and fissures in the nipple and areola. Without early antibiotic therapy, the resulting **bacterial mastitis** may be followed by the development of a **breast abscess** that may require surgical drainage. More commonly, localised areas of inflammation of the breast follow trauma, which may be of sufficient severity to produce a condition known as **fat necrosis** (Fig. 18.1).

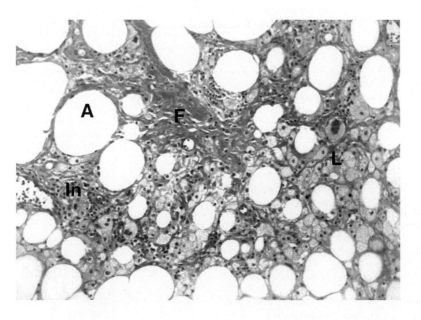

Fig. 18.1 Fat necrosis (MP).

Trauma to the breast, sometimes quite trivial, may result in necrosis of mammary adipose tissue (E-Fig. 18.3**G**). The presence of necrotic adipose tissue (**A**) excites a chronic inflammatory cell infiltrate (**In**), in which lipophages (**L**) (macrophages containing lipid, giving their cytoplasm a foamy appearance) and plasma cells may be present in large numbers. Fibrosis (**F**) of the damaged area produces a hard, often irregular, breast lump, which may resemble a breast carcinoma on palpation. Similar, more localised, changes may be seen in the breast following FNA, core biopsy or other surgical procedures.

KEY TO FIGURES
A adipose tissue   **Ap** apocrine metaplasia   **C** cyst   **F** fibrosis   **In** inflammatory infiltrate   **L** lipophages

Non-neoplastic breast disease

Non-neoplastic breast disease includes a number of disorders that may give rise to a palpable mass or a mammographic abnormality. These conditions may include alterations to the stroma, to the glandular architecture or to the glandular epithelium; usually more than one element is involved. Calcification is not uncommon in these benign lesions and must be differentiated from calcification seen in malignant breast disease. This is not always possible using imaging techniques and biopsy may be required to determine the nature of the lesion.

Simple *fibrocystic change* (E-Fig. 18.4**G**) involves cystic dilatation of ducts, apocrine metaplasia of the epithelium and fibrosis of stroma (Fig. 18.2). *Adenosis* refers to a benign proliferation of glands that may be combined with fibrosis (sclerosis) of the stroma to give rise to *sclerosing adenosis* (Fig. 18.3), which can be difficult to differentiate from invasive carcinoma both clinically and pathologically. Similar changes with proliferation and distortion of benign breast ducts and lobules along with fibrosis of the stroma may be seen in *radial scars* and *complex sclerosing lesions*. A third type of benign lesion is *usual ductal hyperplasia (UDH)* where there is an increase in the number of layers of cells lining the ducts, i.e. more than the normal two layers. This is generally graded as mild, moderate or florid ductal hyperplasia. *Atypical ductal hyperplasia (ADH)* (Fig. 18.4) is a condition intermediate between hyperplasia and *carcinoma in situ* and carries with it a small, but significantly increased, risk of developing carcinoma. *Columnar cell change* or *hyperplasia* is another benign lesion often associated with micro-calcifications and, when there is associated epithelial atypia, it may confer a slight increase in the risk of developing cancer.

With the exception of ADH, sclerosing adenosis and atypical columnar cell lesions, the above conditions carry little or no increased risk of malignancy. Benign breast disorders may be difficult to differentiate clinically from carcinoma. Furthermore, these conditions are common and thus may occur concurrently with, but independently of, invasive carcinoma.

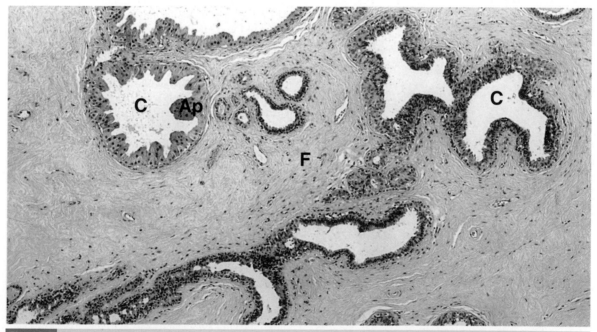

Fig. 18.2 Fibrocystic change (MP).

This breast lesion is so common that it is considered a normal physiological variant. It is nevertheless of great clinical importance since it may give rise to firm palpable masses and/or large cysts that require biopsy to exclude carcinoma. Calcification may also be seen in these lesions.

Typically, as in this micrograph, there is dilatation of acinar structures to form cysts (**C**), accompanied by *apocrine metaplasia* (**Ap**) of epithelial cells. In apocrine metaplasia, the epithelial cells have strongly eosinophilic cytoplasm, often with apical buds and enlarged nuclei, mimicking the apocrine secretory pattern of lactation. In addition, there is variable fibrosis (**F**) of the stroma, which may give the mass an irregular outline.

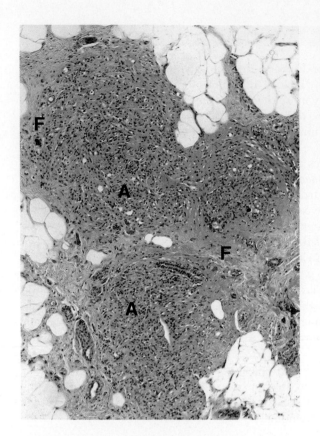

Fig. 18.3 Sclerosing adenosis (LP).

In this condition, there is fibrosis of the intralobular stroma in association with **adenosis**, i.e. proliferation of benign terminal duct–lobular units. This common lesion may give rise to a poorly defined, palpable mass in the breast or to a mammographic abnormality, including calcification. The lesion is centred on the lobules and the overall lobular pattern can still be discerned, in contrast to carcinoma in which it is usually lost. The condition is associated with a slight increase in risk of carcinoma.

As seen in Fig. 18.3, there is a proliferation of small acinar structures (**A**), which are distorted by the surrounding fibrosis (**F**).

Radial scars (<10 mm) and **complex sclerosing lesions** (>10 mm) are related benign lesions that share some characteristics with sclerosing adenosis. As the name suggests, these lesions radiate out from a central fibrous scar.

It is most important not to mistake these benign lesions for invasive breast carcinoma. Diagnosis can be difficult on routine H&E stains, especially on a core biopsy, but immunostaining for smooth muscle actin or other muscle specific antigens will highlight the myoepithelial cells that are prominent in these lesions and absent in invasive carcinomas.

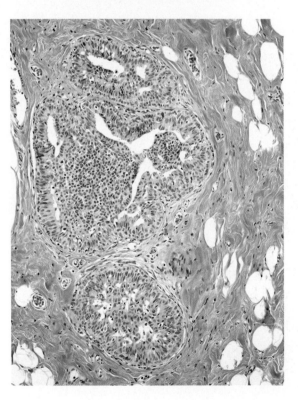

Fig. 18.4 Ductal hyperplasia (MP).

Ductal hyperplasia is another common form of benign breast disease. In **usual ductal hyperplasia (UDH)**, shown in Fig. 18.4, the thickness of the epithelial layer lining the ducts is increased from the normal two cells thick to three, four or many more, depending upon the severity of the hyperplasia. In severe forms, as illustrated here, the ducts are distended by a marked proliferation of epithelial cells, forming a swirling, streaming pattern. There are often tufts of cells and irregular bridges of cells extending across the ductal lumina, forming cleft-like spaces. Myoepithelial cells are also present within the proliferation. This hyperplastic process is associated with a small increase in subsequent cancer risk.

In contrast, **atypical ductal hyperplasia (ADH)** is associated with a significantly greater risk of carcinoma. ADH displays many of the features of low grade **ductal carcinoma in situ (DCIS)** (see next section and Fig. 18.9) but is more limited in extent, by definition being less than 2 mm in size and/or involving not more than two membrane-bound spaces.

ADH is commonly seen in breast specimens in association with both invasive and in situ carcinoma. When it is identified in isolation in small biopsies, this should prompt further surgical sampling to exclude adjacent areas of DCIS or invasive carcinoma.

KEY TO FIGURES

A acinar structures   **D** duct   **F** fibrosis

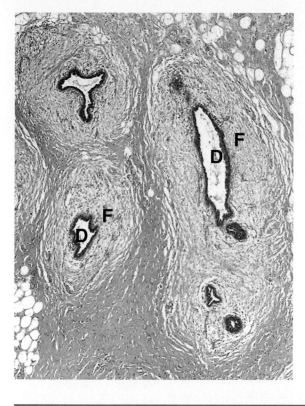

Fig. 18.5 Gynaecomastia of male breast (MP).

The male breast is normally rudimentary and inactive, consisting of fibroadipose tissue containing atrophic mammary ducts. Oestrogenic changes may result in breast hyperplasia *(gynaecomastia)*. The simple mammary ducts **(D)** become enlarged, often with thickening of the epithelial layer and an increase in periductal fibrous tissue **(F)**, shown in Fig. 18.5.

Gynaecomastia may develop at puberty because of a rise in circulating oestrogens or by administration of exogenous oestrogens, for example sex change or drugs used in treatment of prostatic carcinoma. Various other drugs such as spironolactone, heroin and marijuana also cause gynaecomastia in some individuals. It may also result from alcohol abuse and, in particular, cirrhosis of the liver, which results in abnormal metabolism of androgens into oestrogens.

Neoplasms of the breast

The most common benign neoplasm of the breast is the *fibroadenoma* (Fig. 18.6), a localised proliferation of breast ducts and stroma. Such lesions occur most frequently in isolated form in women aged 25–35 years. The *phyllodes tumour* (Fig. 18.7) is related to the fibroadenoma except that it has a tendency to recur and some are frankly malignant. The only other benign tumour of much clinical significance is the *benign intraductal papilloma* (Fig. 18.8), usually occurring as a solitary lesion in one of the larger mammary ducts. Histologically similar papillary lesions may also be multifocal, a condition known as *intraductal papillomatosis*. These lesions tend to occur in the smaller ducts and are associated with a small but definite increase in the risk of carcinoma.

Malignant tumours of the female breast are extremely common, with a peak incidence in the decade before the menopause. Most are adenocarcinomas arising from the epithelium of the terminal duct–lobular unit. Traditionally, these tumours were thought to resemble ductal or lobular breast structures and were named accordingly. The most recent edition of the World Health Organization (WHO) Classification of breast tumours recommends the term *invasive carcinoma of no special type* for those tumours that would previously have been called ductal carcinomas, recognising that this is essentially a default diagnostic group, used only after excluding all of the other 'special' types of breast carcinoma, including *lobular carcinoma*. These 'special' subtypes of invasive carcinoma are associated with distinct clinical and pathological features, often with a good prognosis; examples are *tubular carcinoma* and *mucinous carcinoma* of the breast (Fig. 18.10). *Medullary carcinoma* (not illustrated) is a rare variant characterised by high grade histological features and a prominent inflammatory infiltrate. A range of histological appearances of breast carcinoma is illustrated in Figs 18.9 to 18.12.

In many cases, the development of invasive breast cancer is preceded by carcinoma in situ, in which the malignant cells proliferate within the mammary ducts or lobules but do not breach the basement membrane (*ductal* or *lobular carcinoma in situ* (*DCIS* or *LCIS*)). Risk factors for breast carcinoma include younger age at menarche, later first live birth, family history of breast cancer and previous biopsy with ADH.

In some cases of breast carcinoma, both in situ and invasive, malignant cells may spread along mammary and lactiferous ducts onto the surface of the nipple resulting in *Paget's disease of the nipple* (Fig. 18.13).

Sarcomas also occur in the breast, the most common being *angiosarcoma* (see Fig. 11.12). This may follow previous radiotherapy for treatment of breast carcinoma. Carcinoma of the breast does occur in males but is extremely uncommon.

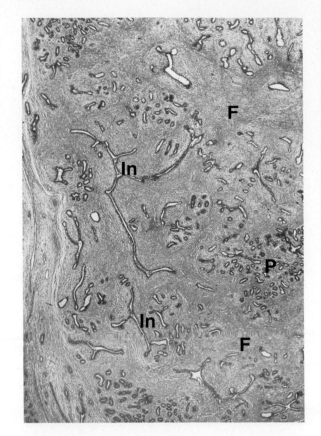

Fig. 18.6 Fibroadenoma (LP).

Fibroadenoma is a common, benign, solitary lesion found in the breasts of women of all ages, but most often in women less than 30 years old. It is usually considered to be a tumour but may well represent a nodular form of benign mammary hyperplasia. The mass is well circumscribed (E-Fig. 18.5**G**) with a pseudo-capsule of connective tissue and is composed of both epithelial and stromal components. The epithelial components form glandular structures lined by mammary duct-type epithelium, whilst the stromal component is a loose, cellular form of fibrous tissue (**F**). In some cases, the stroma may be myxoid.

Two patterns of growth are seen, often in the same lesion. In the *peri-canalicular pattern* (**P**), the epithelial component takes the form of rounded ducts that remain small and undistorted, with the stroma arranged round them in a roughly symmetrical and regular manner. By contrast, in the *intra-canalicular pattern* (**In**), the ducts appear elongated, but actually represent sections cut through flattened spaces compressed by nodular proliferation of the stromal component; in general, this latter pattern is more prominent in larger fibroadenomas. In both patterns of fibroadenoma, hormonal changes, such as occur in pregnancy and lactation, may induce hyperplasia of the epithelial component.

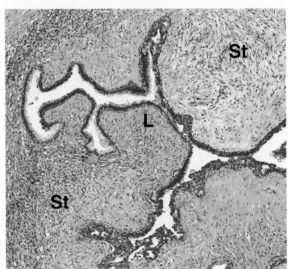

Fig. 18.7 Phyllodes tumour (MP).

The *phyllodes tumour* is related to the fibroadenoma, consisting of a mixture of epithelial and stromal elements. The stroma (**St**) is, however, more prominent in the phyllodes tumour, consisting of crowded atypical spindle cells. The stroma thus bulges into the lumen of the duct to give the characteristic leaf-like pattern (**L**), seen in Fig. 18.7, and there may be occasional mitotic figures.

These tumours have a tendency to recur locally but are usually cured by wide excision. A small proportion behave in a frankly malignant fashion with distant metastases and are thus called *malignant phyllodes tumours* (previously *cystosarcoma phyllodes*). These tumours generally have more crowded, pleomorphic stromal cells with more mitoses, stromal overgrowth and an infiltrative margin. A borderline category has also been described with features intermediate between benign and malignant phyllodes tumour.

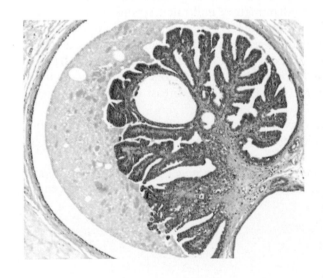

Fig. 18.8 Intraductal papilloma (MP).

Papillomas of mammary duct epithelium may arise as solitary or multiple lesions. Solitary lesions, as shown here, are usually located in the larger lactiferous ducts near the nipple and present with a blood-stained discharge from the nipple. The lesions are usually small, consisting of a delicate, pink-staining supporting stroma covered by a single or double layer of cuboidal or low columnar epithelial cells, resembling the normal lining of the mammary duct; with larger lesions, the duct is often dilated. Multiple duct papillomas *(florid duct papillomatosis)* are rare but may occur in smaller ducts in younger patients.

Epithelial hyperplasia and carcinoma in situ may also arise in a breast papilloma. Malignant change is rare but carcinomas with a papillary architecture are sometimes seen.

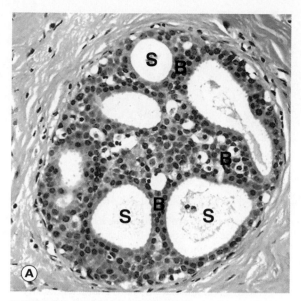

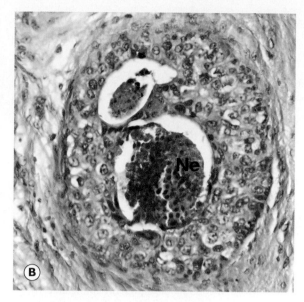

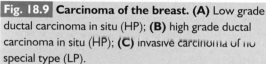

Fig. 18.9 **Carcinoma of the breast. (A)** Low grade ductal carcinoma in situ (HP); **(B)** high grade ductal carcinoma in situ (HP); **(C)** invasive carcinoma of no special type (LP).

Breast carcinoma (E-Fig. 18.6**G**) is divided into invasive and in situ types depending on whether the malignant cells have breached the basement membrane of the duct and invaded the stroma. Both invasive and in situ carcinomas may be associated with abnormal calcifications that may provide the only mammographic clue to the presence of small tumours.

Ductal carcinoma in situ (DCIS) is graded according to the cytological and architectural features of the lesion, with low grade lesions conferring a moderate increase in the likelihood of invasive carcinoma while high grade lesions are associated with a marked increase in the likelihood of invasive carcinoma. Fig. 18.9A shows an example of low grade DCIS. The epithelial cells fill and expand the ducts, forming sharply defined glandular spaces **(S)** separated by 'rigid' bridges **(B)** of cells; low grade DCIS may form a *cribriform pattern* (as shown here), a *micropapillary* or a *solid pattern*. The cells are uniform in size and regularly placed in relation to each other.

In contrast, in high grade DCIS, the duct is expanded by a proliferation of large, highly pleomorphic cells. As seen in Fig. 18.9B, there is often central necrosis **(Ne)** (often called *comedo necrosis*), which may be calcified.

Invasive carcinoma of no special type (previously called *ductal carcinoma, NOS*, i.e. *Not Otherwise Specified* or *ductal carcinoma, NST*, i.e. *No Special Type*) is the most common form of invasive carcinoma and has the worst prognosis. As seen in Fig. 18.9C, the invading malignant epithelial cells form small duct-like structures **(D)**, solid nests **(N)** and even solid sheets of cells. The stroma **(St)**, as in this example, is frequently very fibrotic, which gives the characteristic firm texture on palpation (see Fig. 7.13).

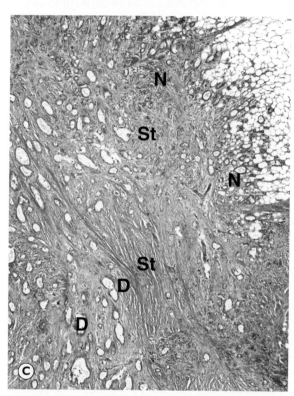

Tumours are graded in an attempt to predict likely clinical behaviour and to inform the need for treatment. The most commonly used scheme assigns a numerical grade to each of three features of the tumour; namely, the degree of gland formation, the nuclear features of the tumour cells and the frequency of mitotic figures. The sum of these grades is then converted to a numerical grade 1, 2 or 3, with grade 1 being a low grade lesion with a better prognosis and grade 3 a high grade lesion.

KEY TO FIGURES

B rigid cell bridges   **D** ductal structures   **F** fibrous tissue   **In** intra-canalicular pattern   **L** leaf-like pattern   **P** peri-canalicular pattern   **N** solid cell nests   **Ne** necrosis   **S** glandular space   **St** stroma

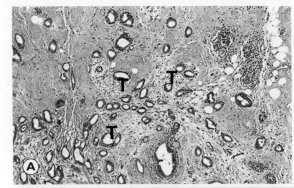

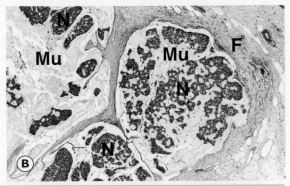

Fig. 18.10 **Variants of invasive breast carcinoma. (A)** Tubular carcinoma (MP); **(B)** mucinous carcinoma (MP).

Certain variants of invasive breast carcinoma have a much better prognosis than invasive carcinoma, NST. These are much less common, but two of the commoner types are invasive *tubular carcinoma* and *mucinous carcinoma*. Tubular carcinoma, as shown in Fig. 18.10A, consists of malignant epithelial cells, which form well-defined tubular or ductal structures **(T)**, with no solid nests of cells or single cell invasion. The tubules are lined by a single layer of mildly pleomorphic cells and invade into the surrounding fat with no evidence of an overall lobular architecture;

this is in contrast to *sclerosing adenosis* (Fig. 18.3), which may be confused with tubular carcinoma.

Mucinous carcinoma (E-Fig. 18.7**G**), as seen in Fig. 18.10B, is characterised by pools of mucin **(Mu)** in which nests of malignant cells **(N)** are suspended. Mucinous carcinoma is characteristically soft to palpation and has a well-defined margin of fibrous tissue **(F)**. Other breast carcinoma variants with a good prognosis that are not illustrated here include invasive *cribriform carcinoma* and *medullary carcinoma*.

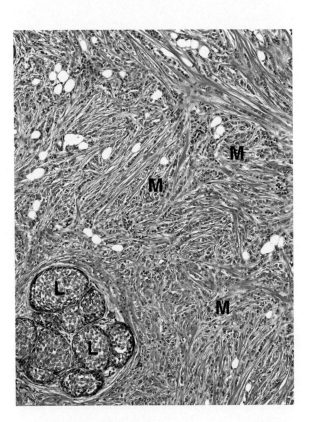

Fig. 18.11 **Lobular carcinoma of the breast (MP).**

Lobular carcinomas are also divided into in situ and invasive forms; both are often present in the same lesion. Fig. 18.11 shows *lobular carcinoma in situ (LCIS)* at the lower left, adjacent to an area of invasive carcinoma.

In LCIS, the lobules **(L)** are expanded and filled by small, evenly spaced epithelial cells that do not form ducts. In the rest of the micrograph, *invasive lobular carcinoma* consists of similar malignant cells **(M)** infiltrating the stroma in rows of cells (often described as *Indian files*) and as single cells that do not form ducts.

Lobular carcinoma in situ is often found incidentally in biopsies taken for another purpose as it usually does not give rise to a mammographic or palpable lesion. LCIS is often multifocal and is considered as a marker lesion for invasive carcinoma, rather than a premalignant lesion. Invasive lobular carcinoma is thought to imply a better prognosis than invasive carcinoma, NST, but is more likely to be bilateral and multifocal.

KEY TO FIGURES
F fibrous tissue   **L** lobular carcinoma in situ   **M** malignant cells   **Mu** mucin   **N** malignant cell nests   **T** tubular structures

PREDICTIVE FACTORS IN BREAST CANCER

The ideal aim is to give each patient exactly the right type and amount of treatment for their particular cancer. Breast cancer is not a single disease, but a group of conditions that progress at different rates and respond differently to treatments. The difficulty is to identify those cancers that need extra treatment (in addition to surgery and radiotherapy) and those that will respond to hormonal therapies.

Treatment is primarily dependent on the type, grade and clinical and pathological stage of the tumour. Patient factors such as age, other health problems and patient preferences are also important. However, in addition, the presence of oestrogen and progestogen receptors (ER and PR) in breast cancer cells has been shown to confer an improved prognosis and to render the cancer susceptible to hormonal treatment. Testing cancers for ER and PR has been standard practice for many years. More recently, the presence of **human epidermal growth factor 2** (**HER-2** or **erbB2**) has been shown to confer a worse prognosis. *HER-2* is a normal component of normal cells but it is overexpressed in about 20% of breast cancers, usually high grade, high stage, poor prognosis tumours. Tumours that overexpress her-2 (usually because of gene amplification) are likely to respond to treatment with drugs such as **trastuzumab**. These are monoclonal antibodies, specifically targeting the her-2 protein and able to switch it off.

More recently, **genomic testing** has offered the hope of even better risk stratification, determining which patients are at highest risk of disease recurrence and which will benefit most from chemotherapy and radiotherapy. Tumour gene expression is analysed and a score is assigned to estimate likely patient risk and benefit from therapy.

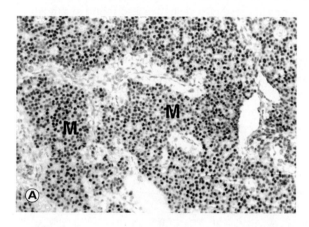

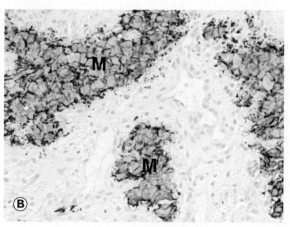

Fig. 18.12 **Predictive tests in breast carcinoma.**
(A) Oestrogen receptors immunohistochemistry (MP);
(B) her-2 immunohistochemistry (HP).

Testing for oestrogen and progestogen receptors (ER and PR) has been standard practice in pathology laboratories for many years. The usual method used is immunohistochemistry, using specific monoclonal antibodies to detect the receptors. These methods and the scoring systems used must be carefully standardised to ensure accuracy. One commonly used scoring system is the **Allred** method, which gives a value of 0 to 3 for the intensity of nuclear staining and value of 0 to 5 for the proportion of cells showing a positive reaction. These two components are summed, giving possible scores of 0 or 2 to 8.

Fig. 18.12A shows a section of a low grade invasive breast carcinoma of no special type that has been stained by the immunohistochemistry method (IHC) using a monoclonal antibody specific for oestrogen receptors. Most of the malignant tumour cells **(M)** show strong brown staining of the nuclei, indicating oestrogen receptor positivity and thus a relatively improved prognosis. Both ER and PR are normal proteins found in the nucleus and are present in normal breast epithelial cells.

Fig. 18.12B at high magnification shows a positive IHC test for her-2. This protein is found on the cell surface and therefore strong membrane staining is required for a positive result, as seen here. Note that the cell nucleus is not stained, in contrast to the ER test in Fig. 18.12A. The test is typically validated or, in borderline cases, confirmed by in situ hybridisation to confirm gene amplification by demonstrating multiple copies of the *HER-2* gene in the nucleus.

CHEMORADIOTHERAPY IN BREAST CANCER

Combinations of surgery, hormonal therapy, chemotherapy and radiotherapy are typically used in managing breast carcinoma, depending upon patient fitness, tumour stage at presentation and other features such as tumour hormone receptor status and *HER-2* status. Where feasible, most tumours are treated by initial surgical excision, often with sampling of axillary lymph nodes to look for nodal metastases (see box 'Sentinel node biopsy' in Ch. 7). If the resected tumour demonstrates high risk features, the patient is then more likely to be offered additional or **adjuvant chemoradiotherapy** post-operatively.

In some patients, primary surgical excision of the tumour may not be feasible. This may be due to the tumour being locally advanced or even known to be metastatic at the time of diagnosis. Some of these patients with advanced disease may benefit from **neoadjuvant chemoradiotherapy**, which aims to reduce the extent of disease, and may facilitate subsequent surgical removal. Use of neoadjuvant treatment in breast cancer has increased greatly in recent years. From a pathological perspective, this often necessitates more detailed assessment of diagnostic biopsies than would traditionally have been required. For example, small biopsy specimens of tumour should be provisionally graded and also tested for hormone receptors and *HER-2*. These features may guide selection of patients for neoadjuvant therapy.

HEREDITARY BREAST CARCINOMA

Familial breast cancer constitutes about 5%–10% of all breast cancers and up to 40% in women less than 35 years of age. Of familial breast cancers, up to 20% occur in women with mutations in the breast cancer susceptibility genes **BRCA1 and 2**. Mutations in these two genes are also found in almost all women with hereditary ovarian carcinomas. These discoveries offer the hope of genetic testing for members of affected families and the possibility of prophylactic treatment. In addition, although the histopathological appearances of these tumours are somewhat different from non-hereditary types of breast cancer, the discovery of these genes offers new insights into the mechanisms of carcinogenesis.

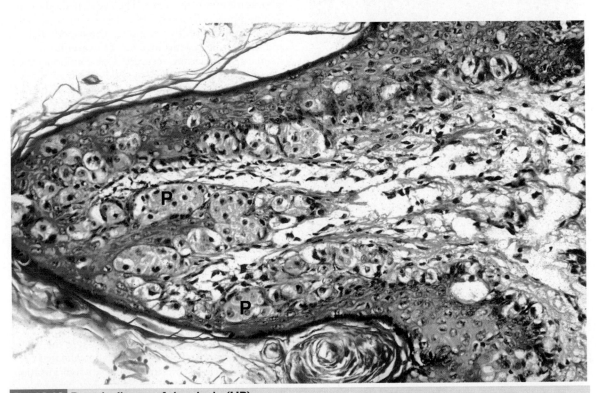

Fig. 18.13 **Paget's disease of the nipple (HP).**

Some patients with carcinoma of the breast develop reddening and thickening of the skin of the nipple (E-Fig. 18.8**H**) and areola (E-Fig. 18.9**G**), occasionally followed by ulceration. The epidermis of the nipple and areola becomes infiltrated by malignant epithelial cells with hyperchromatic nuclei and pale cytoplasm.

These cells, known as **Paget's cells** (**P**), are breast carcinoma cells that have spread along the epithelium of the mammary and nipple ducts to the epidermis from an underlying in situ or invasive carcinoma.

KEY TO FIGURES
P Paget's cells

Table 18.1 Chapter review.

Disorder	Main features	Figure
Fat necrosis (E-Fig. 18.3**G**)	Fat cells with loss of nuclei, inflammatory infiltrate rich in foamy histiocytes	18.1
Fibrocystic change (E-Fig. 18.4**G**)	Dilated ducts with apocrine metaplasia of the epithelium, fibrosis of the stroma	18.2
Sclerosing adenosis	Proliferation and distortion of small benign ducts in a fibrotic stroma	18.3
Ductal hyperplasia	Increase in thickness of epithelial cell layers lining ducts	18.4
Atypical ductal hyperplasia (ADH)	Increased epithelial cells within a duct with many of the features of low grade ductal carcinoma in situ but more limited in extent	
Gynaecomastia	Enlargement of ducts, increased thickness of epithelial layers, increased peri-ductal fibrous tissue in the male breast	18.5
Fibroadenoma (E-Fig. 18.5**G**)	Mixture of benign epithelial and stromal components forming a discrete, usually mobile mass	18.6
Phyllodes tumour	Mixture of epithelial and stromal elements with overgrowth of the stromal component giving a 'leaf-like' pattern, increased cellularity and cytological atypia of the stroma: a few are malignant	18.7
Intraductal papilloma	Branching stromal structures covered by cuboidal or low columnar epithelial cells	18.8
Ductal carcinoma in situ (DCIS)	Atypical cells filling and expanding breast ducts (various patterns) may be high or low grade	18.9A and B
Invasive breast carcinoma (NST) (E-Fig. 18.6**G**)	Invasive atypical cells forming duct-like structures or solid nests – graded as 1–3 depending on architecture, cytological atypia and mitotic activity	18.9C
Tubular carcinoma	Invasive carcinoma consisting of well-formed small ductal structures	18.10A
Mucinous carcinoma (E-Fig. 18.7**G**)	Invasive carcinoma with plentiful mucin production, often with nests of malignant cells floating in pools of mucin	18.10B
Lobular carcinoma in situ (LCIS)	Expanded lobular structures filled with small atypical cells showing no gland formation	18.11
Invasive lobular carcinoma	Invasive carcinoma consisting of small cells, resembling lobular cells, invades as single cells or as lines of cells known as 'Indian files'	18.11
Paget's disease of the nipple (E-Fig. 18.9**G**)	Invasion of malignant cells into the epidermis of the nipple, usually an underlying invasive carcinoma or DCIS	18.13

19 Male reproductive system

Introduction

The male reproductive system includes the testes with their related duct systems, the prostate and the penis. These organs are responsible for the production, storage and periodic emission of the male gametes, spermatozoa, as well as the production of male sex hormones, principally testosterone. The organs of this system are prone to the full range of pathological conditions seen in other organ systems. However, clinically, the most important pathological conditions are inflammation (mainly caused by infection) and tumours.

Disorders of the testis and epididymis

Inflammation of the testis *(orchitis)* may result from viral infections, for example mumps; the testis may also be the site of a gumma in the tertiary stage of syphilis (see Fig. 5.11). Other bacterial infections usually arise as a complication of infection of the lower urinary tract or following surgical instrumentation. A non-infective cause of testicular inflammation is ***granulomatous orchitis***, which may follow an episode of trauma to the testis. Focal granulomatous inflammation, known as ***sperm granulomas***, may also occur because of sperm retention, for example after vasectomy. Venous infarction of the testis owing to ***torsion*** is an important cause of testicular pain in childhood and young adulthood and is illustrated in Fig. 19.1.

The most important pathological lesions of the testes are tumours, most of which are derived from germ cells; a system of classification is shown in Table 19.1 and examples are illustrated in Figs 19.3 to 19.7.

Like the testis, the epididymis may become infected by pyogenic bacteria, associated with lower urinary tract infection and/or surgical instrumentation. When infection occurs, usually both the testis and epididymis are involved, a condition known as ***acute epididymo-orchitis***. The epididymis is occasionally the site of disseminated tuberculous infection, ***tuberculous epididymitis***, usually secondary to active pulmonary or renal tuberculosis.

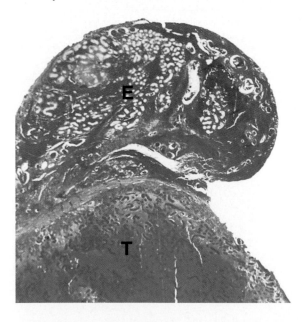

Fig. 19.1 Torsion of the testis (LP).

The arterial supply and venous drainage of the testis (E-Fig. 19.1 **H**) pass in the long course of the spermatic cord from and to the major vessels in the abdomen and pelvis. The spermatic cord is liable to twist, leading to compression of the thin-walled veins and obstruction of venous drainage from the testis. If this state persists for several hours or more without correction, the testis **(T)** and epididymis **(E)** may become deeply congested and subsequently undergo venous infarction, in which necrosis is associated with severe congestion and extravasation of blood. Two small embryological remnants, the appendix testis and the appendix epididymis, are also liable to torsion. The histological changes are similar to those seen in venous infarction of the bowel following volvulus or strangulation (see Fig. 10.5).

Testicular tumours

Testicular tumours may arise in any of the normal components of the testis, but by far the most common are the ***germ cell tumours***, thought to be derived from multipotential germ cells of the seminiferous tubules. Most testicular germ cell tumours are thought to arise from a pre-malignant change in the cells lining the seminiferous tubules known by the term ***germ cell neoplasia in situ (GCNIS)***. Foci of GCNIS are commonly found in the testis adjacent to tumours. These (with the exception of the rare spermatocytic tumour) are highly malignant tumours in young men, which may be cured by a combination of surgery and modern chemotherapy regimens. Most countries now use the current World

Health Organization (WHO) classification to subtype tumours. Approximately two-thirds of testicular tumours contain elements of two or more different tumour types, for example *seminoma* plus *embryonal carcinoma*. There are some similarities between testicular and ovarian germ cell tumours, but it should be remembered that most ovarian germ cell tumours are mature teratomas (dermoid cysts) and behave in a benign fashion, whereas most germ cell tumours in males are malignant.

Testicular germ cell tumours can be broadly divided into two main groups and this is an important distinction as the two groups are treated differently:

■ **Seminoma:** This tumour type consists of malignant cells resembling the normal cells lining the seminiferous tubules (Fig. 19.3).

■ **Non-seminomatous germ cell tumours:** This group includes a variety of tumours that exhibit differentiation towards embryonal or extra-embryonal structures (Figs 19.4 to 19.6)

In the current WHO classification, tumours are divided into those derived from GCNIS and those not derived from GCNIS. Only the main subtypes are shown in Table 19.1. A small proportion of testicular tumours arise from the other cells in the testes, for example Leydig cell tumours and Sertoli cell tumours; the majority of these tumours are benign but they may secrete inappropriate sex hormones. In older men, the most common tumour of the testis is *lymphoma*, usually in association with lymphoma at other sites in the body. Rarely, a testicular mass may be the first indication of lymphoma. Testicular lymphomas are almost always non-Hodgkin diffuse large B cell lymphomas (see Ch. 16).

Table 19.1 Classification of germ cell tumours of the testis.

Tumour type	WHO (2016) classification
Germ cell tumours derived from GCNIS	Seminoma Teratoma (post pubertal type) Embryonal carcinoma Yolk sac tumour (endodermal sinus tumour) Choriocarcinoma
Germ cell tumours not derived from GCNIS	Spermatocytic tumour Pre pubertal teratomas, e.g. epidermoid cyst
Combination of two or more of any type	Mixed germ cell tumour

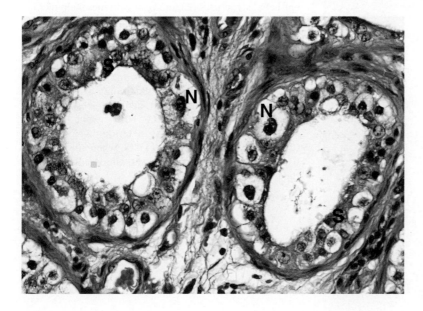

Fig. 19.2 Germ cell neoplasia in situ (HP).

Germ cell neoplasia in situ (GCNIS) is commonly found in testicular tissue adjacent to germ cell tumours. It is thought to be the precursor lesion of most germ cell tumours and is found also in cases of cryptorchidism and in individuals with a contralateral germ cell tumour or a strong family history.

The most common pattern, as shown here, consists of undifferentiated neoplastic cells (**N**), arranged circumferentially around the basement membrane of the seminiferous tubule (E-Fig. 19.2 **H**). The Sertoli cells (**S**) are pushed towards the centre to the tubule. There is no evidence of normal spermatogenesis.

KEY TO FIGURES
E epididymis **N** neoplastic germ cells **S** Sertoli cells **T** testis

MALE REPRODUCTIVE SYSTEM

BASIC PATHOLOGICAL PROCESSES

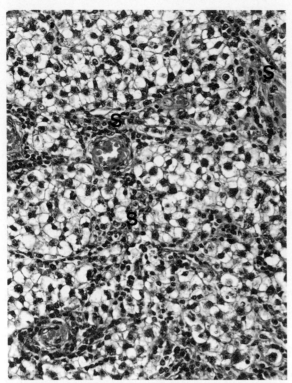

Fig. 19.3 Classical seminoma (HP).

Seminoma is the most common tumour of the testis, with a peak incidence between 30 and 45 years. Macroscopically, the tumour is well circumscribed, pale, creamy-white and homogeneous, with a faint lobular pattern (E-Fig. 19.3 **G**); necrosis and haemorrhage are rare unless the tumour is very large. Seminoma is a malignant tumour and tends to spread via lymphatics, initially to iliac and para-aortic lymph nodes.

Histologically, most seminomas show the classical appearance illustrated in Fig. 19.3. The tumour consists of sheets of uniform polygonal cells with clear cytoplasm and a round central nucleus with a prominent nucleolus. The cells are divided into clusters by fine fibrous septa **(S),** which are usually infiltrated by small lymphocytes. Sometimes, the inflammation is very marked and even granulomatous and it may in these cases be difficult to identify the tumour. The precursor lesion of seminoma is GCNIS (Fig. 19.2) and this can often be seen in the seminiferous tubules adjacent to the tumour.

Spermatocytic tumour, previously known as spermatocytic seminoma, typically presents in older men and has an excellent prognosis with orchidectomy usually being sufficient for treatment. It is now known that this tumour is unrelated to seminoma as it is not associated with GCNIS.

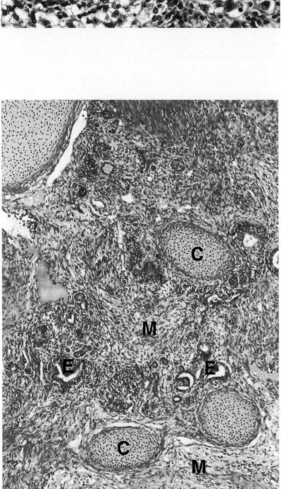

Fig. 19.4 Teratoma (MP).

In adults, testicular teratomas are usually composed of a mixture of mature and immature tissues. The immature components often consist of fetal-type tissues such as cartilage **(C)**, poorly differentiated epithelial structures **(E)** and primitive mesenchyme **(M)**, as shown in Fig. 19.4. Despite having both mature and immature elements, these tumours usually behave in a malignant fashion, in contrast to ovarian teratomas, which are almost always benign. Some teratomas in adults show frank malignant transformation with areas of carcinoma or sarcoma. Teratoma is a common component of mixed germ cell tumours and is preceded by GCNIS.

Compare this with the mature teratoma of the ovary (dermoid cyst) shown in Fig. 17.28, where all the tissues are fully differentiated and almost identical to the normal adult equivalents.

KEY TO FIGURES
C cartilage   **D** Schiller–Duval body   **E** epithelial structure   **G** glandular structures   **M** primitive mesenchyme   **R** reticular pattern   **S** septum   **T** tubular structures

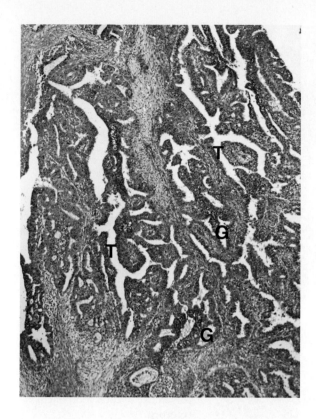

Fig. 19.5 Embryonal carcinoma (MP).

These tumours most often occur in men aged 20–30 years and tend to be more aggressive than seminomas. Embryonal carcinoma can present in a pure form, but most commonly occurs as a component of a mixed germ cell tumour.

Grossly, the tumour is often poorly circumscribed with areas of haemorrhage and necrosis.

The tumour at low power resembles a carcinoma and is composed of primitive epithelial tumour cells with high grade cytological features. The large anaplastic tumour cells may form gland-like structures (**G**) and tubular structures (**T**) as seen in Fig. 19.5 or solid sheets of cells or papillary structures. Mitotic figures are frequent. Vascular and lymphatic invasion are common in this tumour, along with infiltration beyond the testis into adjacent structures such as the epididymis.

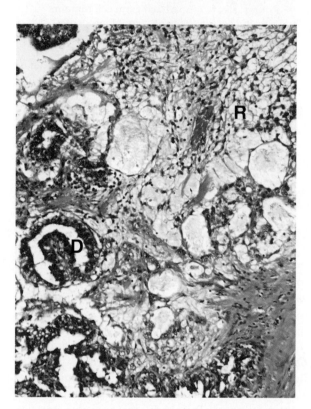

Fig. 19.6 Yolk sac tumour (MP).

Pure **yolk sac tumour** (or **endodermal sinus tumour**) is rare in adult men but is the most common malignant germ cell tumour in male infants and young boys. Yolk sac tumour resembles the yolk sac of the developing embryo. In practice, there is a wide range of histological patterns, the most common being a lace-like (**microcystic** or **reticular**) pattern (**R**) of large poorly differentiated cells, as seen in Fig. 19.6. A characteristic, but not common, feature is the **Schiller–Duval body** (**D**), which resembles a fetal glomerulus. Other features include intracytoplasmic hyaline globules and extracellular deposits of basement membrane material. Often, more than one pattern will be found in an area of yolk sac tumour.

Yolk sac tumour is frequently an element of mixed germ cell tumours in adults. Yolk sac tumour secretes **alpha-fetoprotein (αFP)**, which is easily measured in blood to monitor tumour progression.

BASIC PATHOLOGICAL PROCESSES ■ MALE REPRODUCTIVE SYSTEM

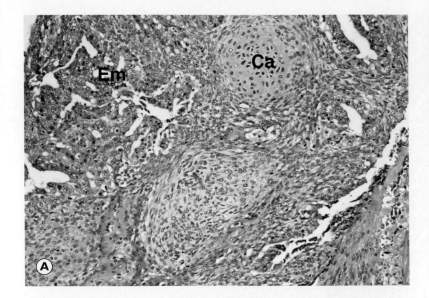

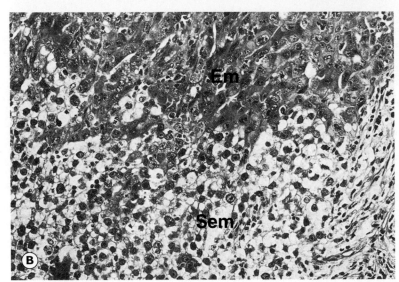

Fig. 19.7 Mixed testicular germ cell tumours. (A) Embryonal carcinoma and teratoma (MP); **(B)** embryonal carcinoma and seminoma (HP).

Certain germ cell tumours are composed of a mixture of elements. Fig. 19.7A shows a germ cell tumour consisting of immature teratoma and embryonal carcinoma. In the top left corner, the embryonal carcinoma **(Em)** shows glandular forms as well as solid areas. In the teratoma component, there is some immature cartilage **(Ca)** E-Fig. 19.4**G**).

In Fig. 19.7B, pale-staining cells of the seminoma component **(Sem)** contrast with darker-staining cells of an embryonal carcinoma **(Em)**. In the WHO system, this tumour is classified as *embryonal carcinoma with seminoma* and usually the percentage of each component is recorded.

Mixed germ cell tumours may also contain foci of *choriocarcinoma* or *yolk sac tumour*. *β-hCG* is produced by trophoblastic elements and can be used as a biochemical marker for the presence of choriocarcinoma, as well as to detect tumour recurrence.

Disorders of the prostate

The prostate gland (E-Fig. 19.5**H**) undergoes *benign nodular hyperplasia (hypertrophy)* in almost all men from middle age onwards, probably because of an alteration in hormone balance. This important lesion, shown in Fig. 19.8, produces obstruction to bladder outflow as a result of pressure on the prostatic urethra; in turn, the obstruction may produce pressure effects on the proximal conducting system of the urinary tract, leading to *hydroureter* and *hydronephrosis* with pressure atrophy of the renal parenchyma. Prostatic hyperplasia also predisposes to infection and stone formation.

Invasive carcinoma of the prostate is a common and important malignant tumour in men and is illustrated in Fig. 19.10. Carcinoma of the prostate may be associated with dysplasia of the glandular epithelium. This has been named *prostatic intraepithelial neoplasia (PIN)* and is shown in Fig. 19.9. The prognosis of carcinoma of the prostate can be predicted by careful grading and staging. Staging takes into consideration the size (volume) of the tumour, the degree of spread within the prostate, extension beyond the prostate and lymph node and distant metastases. Perineural and vascular invasion also contributes to assessment of prognosis. Some of these features may only be determined in radical prostatectomy specimens whereas others can be assessed on core biopsies. Imaging is also important for the detection of distant metastases, for example to bone. Small foci of low-grade tumour that are not palpable may be found in prostates removed for benign hyperplasia. Most of these tumours progress too slowly for them to cause clinically significant disease in elderly patients and, for this reason, are often called *latent carcinomas*.

KEY TO FIGURES

A acinus   **C** corpora amylacea   **Ca** immature cartilage   **D** high-grade PIN   **E** normal epithelium   **Em** embryonal carcinoma   **H** hyperplastic prostate nodule   **M** fibromuscular connective tissue   **N** compressed peripheral glands   **P** papillary fold   **Sem** seminoma

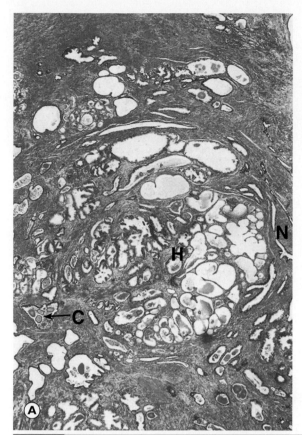

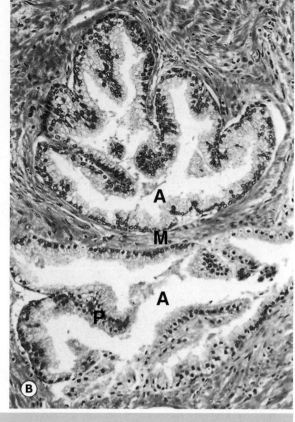

Fig. 19.8 Benign prostatic hyperplasia. (A) LP; (B) MP.

Benign prostatic hyperplasia is a common condition affecting middle-aged to elderly men in which the transitional and para-urethral components of the prostate gland undergo glandular hyperplasia accompanied by hypertrophy of the intervening fibromuscular stroma of the gland. The peripheral zone of the prostate is not involved in the hyperplastic process and becomes compressed and atrophic at the outer margin (E-Fig. 19.6 **G**).

At low magnification in Fig. 19.9A, note the rounded nodules of hyperplastic prostatic tissue (**H**) in the transitional/para-urethral part of the gland and the compressed peripheral zone (**N**) at the periphery. Since the para-urethral component of the prostate gland is involved, compression of the urethral lumen is a frequent occurrence and is responsible for typical clinical features such as hesitancy, poor urinary stream and urinary retention. Macroscopically, the typical hyperplastic prostate has a nodular microcystic appearance, the tiny cysts representing enormously dilated hyperplastic prostatic glandular acini, which often contain small, laminated concretions known as *corpora amylacea* (**C**).

At high magnification as in Fig. 19.9B, the acini (**A**) are lined by tall columnar prostatic epithelial cells with small basal nuclei. The cells have a regular arrangement but are sometimes thrown up into papillary folds (**P**). Adjacent acini are separated by a variable amount of fibromuscular connective tissue (**M**) in which the muscular component may be hypertrophied; muscular hypertrophy is often particularly prominent in the region of the bladder neck.

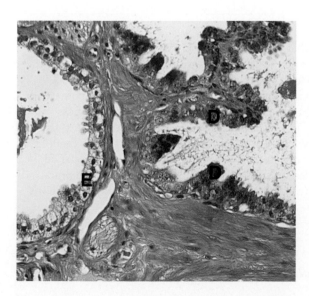

Fig. 19.9 Prostatic intraepithelial neoplasia (HP).

Prostatic intraepithelial neoplasia (PIN) represents dysplasia of the tall columnar epithelium. PIN may be subclassified as high or low grade. In clinical practice, as the significance of low-grade PIN is uncertain, it is usually ignored. High-grade PIN, however, tends to occur in prostates with invasive carcinoma and therefore the finding of high-grade PIN should prompt an intensified search for invasive carcinoma.

The gland on the right in Fig. 19.9, consisting of highly atypical epithelial cells (**D**), is a good example of high-grade PIN. These cells, in contrast to the normal prostatic epithelium (**E**) (left), have enlarged pleomorphic nuclei and prominent nucleoli. The cytoplasm is more basophilic than normal. These cells are very similar to those of invasive carcinomas, but there is no evidence of stromal invasion. A layer of basal cells can be detected around the periphery of the gland, although sometimes immunohistochemical staining is required to demonstrate this.

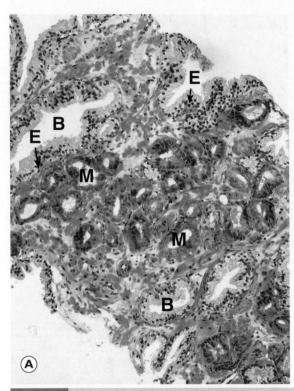
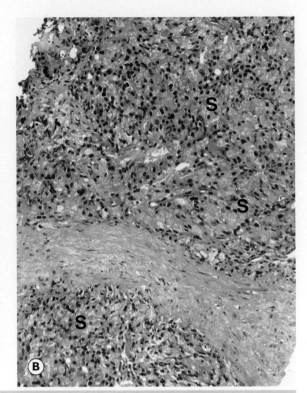

Fig. 19.10 **Adenocarcinoma of the prostate. (A)** Well differentiated (MP); **(B)** poorly differentiated (MP).

This common tumour usually arises in the peripheral zone of the prostate gland, as opposed to benign prostatic hyperplasia, which characteristically develops in the peri-urethral and transitional zones of the gland (Fig. 19.8). Almost all prostatic primary malignant tumours are adenocarcinomas.

Prostatic adenocarcinomas are traditionally graded by the **_Gleason grading system_** according to their architectural features. Gleason grade 1 lesions consist of nodules of small, well-defined glands with limited infiltration of the surrounding tissue. In contrast, grade 5 lesions consist of sheets of malignant cells with no discernible glandular differentiation and which infiltrate widely. Grades 2, 3 and 4 are intermediate. Most prostatic tumours include components of two or more of these patterns and therefore current practice gives the grade of the two most prominent components and their sum. This is known as the combined Gleason grade or score, for example combined Gleason score 3+5=8, with the first number representing the most common component. As

mentioned above, accurate grading along with staging is important to estimate the prognosis of prostatic adenocarcinoma and to guide treatment. More recently, a new simplified 5 grade group system was introduced, acknowledging that both the predominant pattern of adenocarcinoma and the total Gleason score are important in predicting outcome.

Fig. 19.10A shows an area of Gleason grade 3 carcinoma. Small, round, malignant glands **(M)** lined by enlarged atypical epithelial cells are seen infiltrating between benign glands **(B)**. The contrast between the benign and malignant cells is particularly well demonstrated, the malignant cells being larger with prominent nucleoli and less cytoplasm. A very important feature is that the malignant glands lack the basal cell layer **(E)**, which is prominent in the benign glands.

Fig. 19.10B shows an area of Gleason grade 5 prostatic adenocarcinoma where the malignant cells form sheets **(S)** of pleomorphic cells invading the stroma. No glandular structures are seen.

SCREENING FOR PROSTATE CANCER

Screening for disease is dependent on the principle that early detection increases cure rate and reduces morbidity and/or mortality. Screening is, by definition, applied to large numbers of healthy individuals. Blood testing for **_prostate-specific antigen (PSA)_** has been available for several years, but, as yet, there is no national government-funded screening programme as there is for breast carcinoma. Although the test is cheap and has minimal side effects, the benefits of applying it to large numbers of asymptomatic men have yet to be demonstrated. The test has a significant false positive rate, thus triggering prostatic biopsies, a more expensive test with more potential side effects, in healthy men. It is also likely that the test would detect many cases of indolent, low-grade carcinoma that would be unlikely to cause appreciable problems during the lifespan of the individual. However, in clinical practice, many men are screened for prostate cancer on an individual basis, usually because they themselves have requested the test.

KEY TO FIGURES
B benign glands   **E** basal epithelial cell   **M** small malignant glands   **S** sheets of malignant cells
T islands of squamous cell carcinoma

Disorders of the penis

The most important pathological lesion of the penis is *squamous cell carcinoma* (Fig. 19.11), which is usually preceded by squamous dysplasia similar to that in the vulva (see Fig. 17.3) known as *penile intraepithelial neoplasia PeIN* (human papillomavirus (HPV) associated lesions) or *differentiated PeIN* (non–HPV associated lesions). Genital wart or *condyloma acuminatum* also occurs on the penis and is caused by infection with certain types of HPV, as in the lower genital tract in the female. Phimosis is a common clinical condition that can be caused by an inflammatory and fibrosing condition of the fore-skin termed *balanitis xerotica obliterans*, similar to lichen sclerosus in women (see Fig. 17.1).

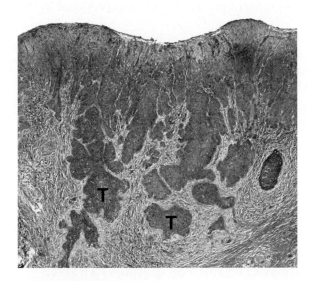

Fig. 19.11 **Squamous carcinoma of penis (LP).**

Fig. 19.11 shows a well-differentiated keratinising squamous cell carcinoma of the glans penis, with islands of tumour **(T)** extending deeply into the stroma. Metastatic spread is by lymphatics to superficial inguinal nodes.

Squamous cell carcinoma (SCC) of the penis is now classified as HPV related or non-HPV related, similar to tumours of the vulva and perianal region (see Ch. 17). HPV-related SCCs are typically basaloid or warty in appearance and show strong positivity for the surrogate HPV marker p16. Non-HPV related tumours can be subdivided into various histological subtypes, including veruccous carcinoma and sarcomatoid or spindle cell SCC.

Table 19.2 **Chapter review.**

Organ	Disorder	Main features	Figure
Testis	Torsion	Necrosis of tissue with extensive congestion and haemorrhage due to venous infarction	19.1
	Epididymo-orchitis	Acute inflammation, similar to acute inflammation in other tissues	Like 3.4
	Germ cell neoplasia in situ	Malignant germ cells within seminiferous tubules, usually as a single layer around the basement membrane with the Sertoli cells pushed inwards	19.2
	Seminoma	Sheets of large, undifferentiated cells separated by delicate fibrous septa usually with a lymphocytic infiltrate in the septa	19.3
	Teratoma	Tumour consists of mixtures of fetal tissues, e.g. cartilage, primitive mesenchyme, epithelial structures, bone, etc.	19.4
	Embryonal carcinoma	Large malignant cells forming gland-like structures, solid sheets, tubular structures and papillary structures Often large necrotic areas	19.5
	Yolk sac tumour	Primitive germ cells resembling yolk sac structures Various patterns including reticular (microcystic), Schiller–Duval bodies, hyaline cytoplasmic globules	19.6
	Choriocarcinoma	Alternating layers of syncytiotrophoblast and cytotrophoblast with haemorrhage	17.16
	Mixed germ cell tumour	Consists of a mixture of one or more different germ cell tumours	19.7
Prostate	Benign hyperplasia	Nodular enlargement of glandular and stromal elements of the prostate gland; usually affects the transitional and para-urethral components	19.8
	High grade prostatic intraepithelial neoplasia	Highly atypical cells similar to those seen in invasive carcinoma but confined within prostatic acini	19.9
	Adenocarcinoma	Malignant cells invading the prostate as glands, cribriform structures or sheets	19.10
Penis	Balanitis xerotica obliterans	Hyalinisation of the subepithelial collagen of the foreskin with an underlying band of inflammation	Like 17.1
	Squamous cell carcinoma (SCC)	Similar to SCC of vulva: invasion of underlying tissue by nests of atypical squamous cells, often with formation of keratin pearls. HPV related and non-related types.	19.11

20 Endocrine system

Pituitary gland disorders

Structural defects of the pituitary gland are few, although functional abnormalities are potentially numerous, leading to under- or overproduction of one or more of the many hormones produced by the pituitary gland and its target endocrine glands.

The most important histopathological lesions of the pituitary gland are benign *adenomas* derived from the anterior pituitary (adenohypophysis). These commonly secrete anterior pituitary hormones and result in the development of endocrine syndromes. Adenomas may be derived from any of the normal anterior pituitary cell types and can be classified by the hormones they secrete:

■ **Prolactinomas:** secrete prolactin and may lead to infertility and, occasionally, inappropriate breast milk production.

■ **Corticotroph adenomas:** secrete adrenocorticotrophic hormone (ACTH) and result in *Cushing's disease* (Fig. 20.1).

■ **Somatotroph adenomas:** secrete excess growth hormone and lead to *acromegaly* or rarely *gigantism* (Fig. 20.2) (E-Fig. 20.1**G**).

■ **Thyrotroph** and **gonadotroph adenomas:** both types are rare.

■ **Non-secretory adenomas:** a large number of pituitary adenomas have no demonstrable hormone secretion; such tumours only become manifest by impinging on vital local structures such as the optic chiasm, causing visual disturbance, or by expanding to a size large enough to destroy the surrounding normal functioning tissue, resulting in clinical *hypopituitarism.*

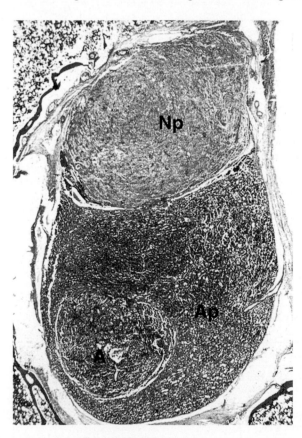

Fig. 20.1 Pituitary adenoma (LP).

Fig. 20.1 shows a pituitary gland in situ in the pituitary fossa and cut in sagittal section, showing the anterior pituitary (adenohypophysis, **Ap**) (E-Fig. 20.7 **H**) and the posterior pituitary (neurohypophysis, **Np**). Within the substance of the anterior pituitary lies a small *pituitary adenoma* (**A**) composed of cells of uniform type. The tumour is benign, as evidenced by its well-circumscribed, non-invasive, spherical appearance, and is small enough to have caused no distortion of the pituitary outline or undue compression of adjacent normal pituitary cells.

In this particular case, the tumour cells secreted ACTH in gross excess and the patient died as a result of the metabolic and cardiac complications of *Cushing's disease*. In all, the illness lasted no more than 7 or 8 weeks despite its benign pathogenesis.

Cushing's syndrome can also be caused by an *adrenal cortical adenoma* or *carcinoma*. Clinically, a pituitary cause for Cushing's disease can be differentiated from an adrenal cause by examining the plasma ACTH concentration. If plasma ACTH concentration is low, it suggests a primary adrenal cause and if the plasma ACTH is normal or high, a pituitary cause is most likely. This can be explained by the normal *feedback mechanism* controlling ACTH production. A high level of *glucocorticoid* within the blood inhibits the production of ACTH from the anterior pituitary. This normal feedback loop is lost in Cushing's disease resulting in uncontrolled production of glucocorticoids and the resulting clinical manifestations of this disease.

KEY TO FIGURES
A pituitary adenoma **Ap** adenohypophysis **Np** neurohypophysis

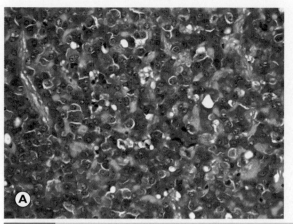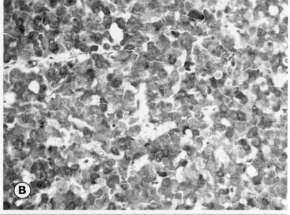

Fig. 20.2 **Pituitary adenoma. (A)** HP; **(B)** immunohistochemistry for growth hormone (HP).

As noted above, symptoms of pituitary tumours often reflect activity of the hormones they secrete. In addition, their location in the pituitary fossa can lead to compression of the optic chiasm with symptoms/signs of visual disturbance, specifically bitemporal hemianopia.

As shown in Fig. 20.2A, the typical histological appearance of a pituitary adenoma is of fields of somewhat monotonous, small to medium-sized tumour cells with moderate amounts of cytoplasm. In this case, immunocytochemistry for growth hormone is positive, shown in Fig. 20.2B.

This patient presented with endocrine symptoms related to excess growth hormone secretion. In adults, this manifests as *acromegaly*, with abnormal growth of the viscera (including the heart), skin, soft tissues and skeleton. This last feature is particularly evident in the bones of the face, with protrusion of the jaw *(prognathism)*, and in the bones of the hands and feet. In children, before the epiphyseal plates have fused, excess growth hormone secretion leads to *gigantism*, often also with features of acromegaly.

Disorders of the thyroid gland

A variety of pathological processes may affect the thyroid gland (E-Fig. 20.8 **H**), leading to either diminished or excessive output of the thyroid hormone thyroxine. *Hypothyroidism* may result from dysfunction at any level of the hypothalamo-pituitary-thyroid axis and, as such, may be regarded as either primary (arising from a disorder within the thyroid gland) or secondary (as a consequence of pituitary disease).

There are a number of causes of primary hypothyroidism, some of which have an autoimmune basis, for example *Hashimoto's thyroiditis* (Fig. 20.3) (E-Fig. 20.2 **G**). Hypothyroidism can be treated with thyroid hormone supplementation in the form of *thyroxine* tablets.

As with hypothyroidism, *hyperthyroidism (thyrotoxicosis)* may be considered as primary (abnormality within the gland) or secondary (abnormality outside of gland). Most cases of hyperthyroidism arise as a result of diffuse hyperplasia of the thyroid acinar cells, most commonly in the condition known as *Graves' disease* (Fig. 20.4). Sometimes the hyperplasia is confined to a single *benign thyroid adenoma* (E-Fig. 20.3**G**) , a so-called *toxic nodule*. Nevertheless, most thyroid adenomas (Fig. 20.6) are non-functional and do not lead to disturbances of thyroid hormone output.

Multinodular goitre is one of the most common types of thyroid tissue in which the thyroid becomes enlarged due to the presence of numerous hyperplastic thyroid nodules (Fig. 20.5) (E-Fig. 20.4**G**).

Four main forms of *thyroid carcinoma* occur, namely *papillary*, *follicular*, *medullary* and *anaplastic* (in order of frequency). Papillary, follicular and anaplastic carcinomas arise from cuboidal follicular lining cells. Medullary carcinoma of the thyroid is an uncommon malignant tumour of calcitonin-producing (parafollicular or C) cells and is particularly notable for its production of amyloid. Examples of papillary, follicular and medullary carcinomas are illustrated in Fig. 20.7. *Anaplastic carcinomas* usually occur in the very elderly and are composed of sheets of poorly differentiated cells with little cytoplasm. These tumours grow very rapidly and extensively invade local tissues, often presenting as a bulky mass in the neck associated with symptoms of tracheal compression. *Lymphoma* may also arise in the thyroid gland, usually following longstanding Hashimoto's thyroiditis.

NON-INVASIVE FOLLICULAR PATTERNED NEOPLASM WITH PAPILLARY-LIKE NUCLEAR FEATURES (NIFTP)

Through the molecular sequencing of a subtype of papillary thyroid carcinoma, known as an encapsulated follicular variant of papillary thyroid carcinoma, it has been possible to reclassify some of these cases. A proportion of these lesions have been shown to have a similar molecular profile to follicular adenomas and are now classified as *non-invasive follicular patterned neoplasm with papillary-like nuclear features (NIFTP).* These lesions are thought to have benign/indolent behaviour, similar to a follicular adenoma. This is an example of how new technologies can be a useful adjunct to the more traditional histopathology and allied techniques (see Ch. 1).

BASIC SYSTEMS PATHOLOGY ■ ENDOCRINE SYSTEM

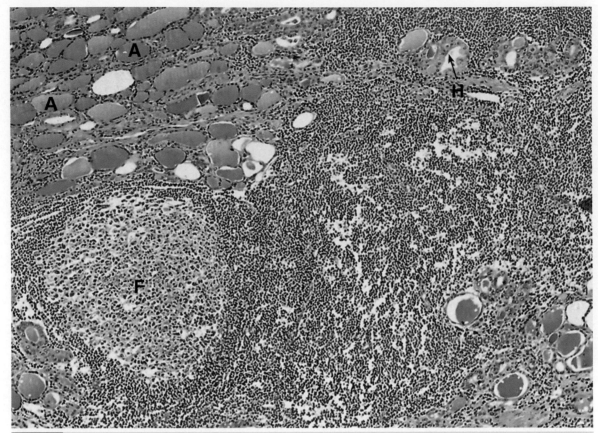

Fig. 20.3 **Hashimoto's thyroiditis (MP).**

This disease is an autoimmune thyroiditis in which thyroid acini **(A)** are progressively destroyed by immunological processes and the gland becomes diffusely infiltrated by lymphocytes and plasma cells. In some areas, the small darkly staining lymphocytes aggregate to form typical lymphoid follicles **(F)**, often with germinal centres. In the early stages of the disease, the extensive lymphoid infiltrate produces a diffusely enlarged, firm thyroid gland with a pale cut surface, resembling a lymph node. Thyroid epithelial cells in this condition commonly show *oncocytic* or

Hürthle cell transformation, the Hürthle cells **(H)** having strongly eosinophilic granular cytoplasm and slightly enlarged nuclei.

As thyroid follicles are progressively destroyed, the patient, who at the outset is euthyroid or even mildly hyperthyroid, becomes increasingly hypothyroid *(myxoedematous)*. When almost all thyroid acini are destroyed, the lymphoid infiltrate becomes less obvious and fibrosis supervenes, with progressive reduction in size of the gland.

INVESTIGATION OF A SOLITARY THYROID NODULE

Solitary thyroid nodules (defined as palpable, discrete nodules in an otherwise unremarkable thyroid) are detectable in approximately 5% of the population, the figure increasing with age and higher in women than in men. The differential diagnosis of these solitary nodules is wide and ranges from benign disease (such as thyroiditis or adenoma) to malignant disease (metastatic or primary), though the overwhelming majority are benign. Indications of a more concerning diagnosis may be revealed through careful history taking and/or clinical examination. However, as in many fields of medicine, the clinical clues to differentiate benign from malignant disease are not foolproof and further investigations are often required.

Ultrasound guided *fine needle aspiration (FNA)* is the most commonly used procedure in investigating solitary thyroid nodules. This is a relatively simple procedure that can be undertaken in the out-patient department. In the majority of cases, the results can provide insight into the nature of the nodule to allow planning of further management. Thus, if the lesion is small and benign, no further action may be indicated. Alternatively, if the lesion is malignant, surgical excision can be planned, with the extent of surgery guided by the nature of the malignancy.

A proportion of lesions will be reported as follicular lesions of uncertain significance. In this setting, molecular profiling tests can be performed on cytology aspirate material to look for high risk molecular signals that would prompt surgical management. If these high risk molecular signals are absent, then the patient can be reassured that the lesion is likely to be benign and no further treatment is required.

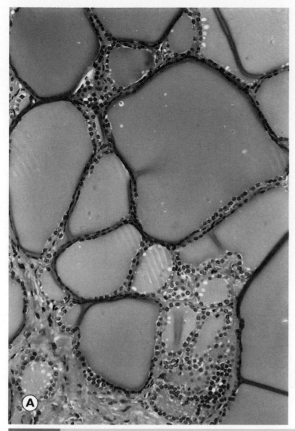
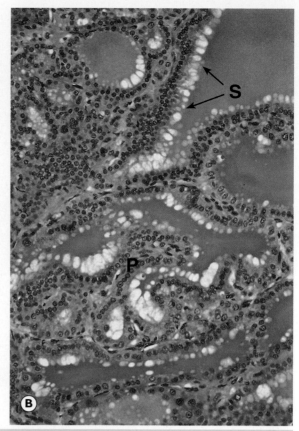

Fig. 20.4 **Graves' disease. (A)** Normal thyroid (HP); **(B)** hyperplastic thyroid (HP).

Thyroid function is normally under the control of the hypothalamic–pituitary axis via the release of thyroid-stimulating hormone (TSH) from the pituitary, which stimulates thyroid acinar cells to liberate thyroxine. The resulting level of circulating thyroxine then regulates TSH production by a negative feedback mechanism.

Under certain circumstances this balance may be disrupted leading to hyperplasia and hypertrophy of thyroid acinar cells through prolonged, unchecked stimulation; this gives rise to the histological appearance known as *thyroid hyperplasia*.

Graves' disease is by far the commonest cause of pathological thyroid hyperplasia. This autoimmune disease is characterised by a triad of clinical features, namely hyperthyroidism, *exophthalmos* (protruding eyes) and non-pitting oedema of the lower limbs *(pre-tibial myxoedema)*. In the majority of cases, circulating antibodies to the TSH receptor are produced, such as a circulating immunoglobulin called

thyroid-stimulating immunoglobulin. This binds to TSH receptors on thyroid acinar cells, mimicking the effects of TSH and resulting in excess secretion of thyroxine. The resulting glandular appearance is described as *thyrotoxic hyperplasia* and is illustrated in Fig. 20.4B.

Compared with the normal thyroid in Fig. 20.4A, the hyperplastic acinar cells are taller and have larger nuclei, reflecting a greater degree of metabolic activity. The acini themselves are smaller than normal because of the reduced amount of colloid resulting from increased thyroxine secretion. The hyperplastic acinar cells may crowd up on one side of the acini, projecting into the lumen as papillary structures **(P)**. The colloid in hyperplastic follicles shows peripheral scalloping **(S)**, reflecting the increased utilisation of stored thyroid colloid to produce thyroxine by the hyperactive thyroid acinar cells. In addition to these features, the thyroid may sometimes contain prominent lymphocytic aggregates (not shown in this figure).

KEY TO FIGURES
A thyroid acini   **F** lymphoid follicle   **H** Hürthle cells   **P** papillary structure   **S** scalloping

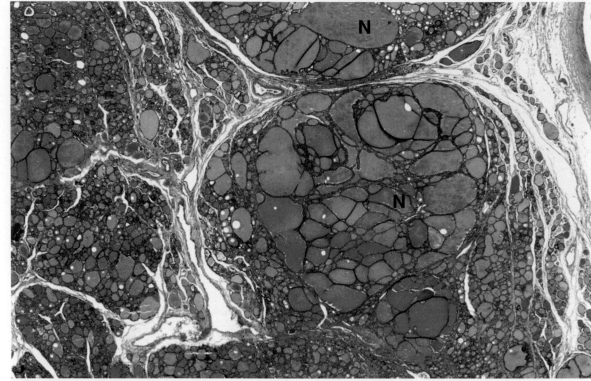

Fig. 20.5 Multinodular goitre (MP).

Goitres may be either *diffuse* or *multi-nodular* (E-Fig. 20.4**G**), depending on the pattern of involvement of the gland. In most instances, deficiency of dietary iodine leads to impaired thyroid hormone synthesis. Thus, to maintain the euthyroid state, the gland becomes enlarged, driven by a compensatory rise in TSH. Initially, this is achieved through formation of larger than normal follicles, known as a *diffuse (colloid) goitre*. This may progress to *multinodular goitre*, as illustrated in Fig. 20.5, in which the gland consists of multiple nodules (**N**) composed of follicles of varying size.

Fibrosis, haemorrhage and calcification (not illustrated) are common. Some cases of multinodular goitre have a *dominant nodule*, a single very large nodule that may be difficult to distinguish clinically from an adenoma. However, histologically, the nodular appearance of the rest of the gland will usually identify the lesion as part of multinodular goitre.

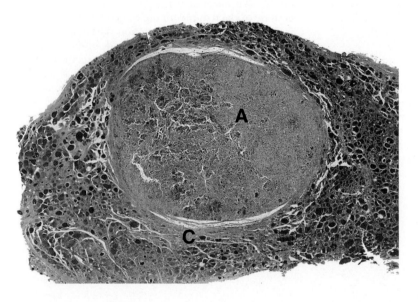

Fig. 20.6 Thyroid adenoma (LP).

Thyroid adenomas are benign tumours of follicular epithelium forming solitary, encapsulated, round nodules. In the majority of instances they are non-functional, with relatively few producing thyroid hormones.

Fig. 20.6 illustrates the typical low-power appearance of a thyroid adenoma (**A**), forming a readily identifiable, discrete lesion with a well-formed surrounding capsule (**C**).

Occasionally, an adenoma may be difficult to differentiate from a well-differentiated *follicular carcinoma* (Fig. 20.7C). In such cases, thorough sampling and careful attention to the surrounding capsule is required to identify evidence of capsular or vascular invasion, both features of follicular carcinoma.

KEY TO FIGURES
A adenoma   **C** capsule   **F** follicular carcinoma   **N** nodule   **OA** Orphan Annie eye nuclei
S stromal core   **Sp** spindle cells   **T** surrounding thyroid gland

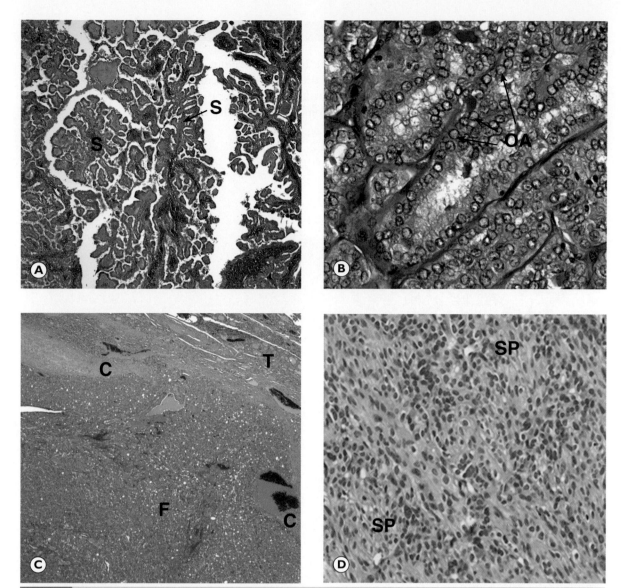

Fig. 20.7 **Thyroid carcinoma. (A)** Papillary carcinoma (MP); **(B)** papillary carcinoma (HP); **(C)** follicular carcinoma (LP); **(D)** medullary carcinoma (LP).

Papillary carcinomas are the most common of the thyroid malignancies. As illustrated in Fig. 20.7A, the tumours form complex papillary structures, each composed of a narrow stromal core **(S)** covered with a layer of glandular epithelium. The stromal cores sometimes contain small, calcified, laminated bodies known as *psammoma bodies* (not shown here). At higher magnification in Fig. 20.7B, the dispersed chromatin typical of papillary carcinoma cells can be appreciated. This imparts a characteristic, *optically clear* appearance to the nuclei, sometimes referred to as *Orphan Annie eye* nuclei **(OA)**. This slow-growing tumour tends to spread via lymphatics to regional nodes but has the best prognosis of all thyroid cancers.

Follicular carcinomas are the second most common of the thyroid carcinomas. Typically, they appear as solitary lesions that may be *encapsulated* or *widely invasive*.

Microscopically, they can be difficult to distinguish from a benign follicular adenoma (Fig. 20.6). In such cases, extensive sampling of the tumour is required, in particular the capsule, looking for capsular and/or vascular invasion. Fig. 20.7C shows a *minimally invasive* follicular carcinoma **(F)** that has breached the capsule **(C)** to invade the surrounding gland **(T)**. Bloodstream spread is the major mode of metastasis, with lung and bone as common sites of secondary tumour deposits.

Medullary carcinomas are rare (Fig. 20.7D). These develop from the parafollicular or C cells of the thyroid. They may be solitary or multifocal. The constituent cells vary in appearance from spindled **(Sp)** to plasmacytoid in shape. The chromatin pattern as seen within the nuclei appears granular and the cells have abundant eosinophilic cytoplasm. These tumours can be associated with the production of amyloid (not seen here).

THE ROLE OF MOLECULAR PATHOLOGY IN TREATMENT OF THYROID CANCER
Molecular pathology is becoming increasingly important in the diagnosis and treatment of thyroid cancer. Up to 80% of papillary thyroid carcinomas show an activating mutation in the ***BRAF V600E*** gene, which can be demonstrated by appropriate molecular tests, for example using sequencing.
Other pathways important in thyroid cancer are being investigated including ***TERT promotor mutations***. Drugs that specifically target these mutations are being developed to provide a personalised treatment pathway for thyroid cancer patients.

BASIC SYSTEMS PATHOLOGY ■ ENDOCRINE SYSTEM

Disorders of the parathyroid glands

The overproduction of parathyroid hormone due to an underlying abnormality of the parathyroid gland may result in **hyperparathyroidism** leading to altered calcium metabolism, bone disease and hypercalcaemia. This may be primary, secondary or tertiary, depending on the underlying cause. Primary abnormalities of parathyroid hormone and carcinoma of the parathyroid are very rare (see Fig. 20.8).

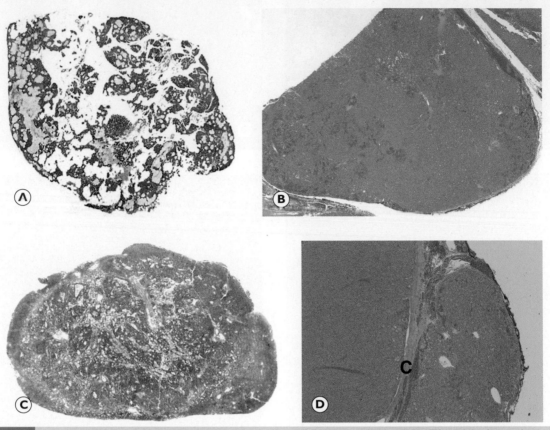

Fig. 20.8 **Parathyroid hyperplasia, adenoma and carcinoma. (A)** Normal gland (LP); **(B)** nodular hyperplasia (LP); **(C)** adenoma (LP); **(D)** carcinoma (MP).

The normal adult parathyroid gland contains small endocrine (known as **chief** and **oxyphil**) cells arranged in nests or cords intermixed with adipose tissue. Should the need arise for a greater output of parathyroid hormone, for example in cases of excessive urinary calcium loss in chronic renal failure, the endocrine cells undergo **hyperplasia** with loss of the adipose tissue.

Compare the hyperplastic gland in Fig. 20.8B with the normal parathyroid gland in Fig. 20.8A. The hyperplastic gland is not only larger than the normal gland, but the hormonally active endocrine component has also increased replacing some of the adipose tissue component. If demand for excessive parathyroid hormone persists, the gland may become markedly enlarged. These hyperplastic changes usually affect all four glands uniformly and can be **nodular** or **diffuse**. However, involvement can occasionally be asymmetrical, leading to difficulty in distinguishing hyperplasia from an adenoma. This is known as **asymmetrical hyperplasia**.

Autonomous benign tumours of the parathyroid gland, **parathyroid adenomas**, usually affect only one of the four glands, although occasionally they may be multiple. In Fig. 20.8C, a parathyroid adenoma replaces the normal gland. A compressed rim of normal parathyroid gland can sometimes be seen, a useful clue in differentiating from hyperplasia.

When there is an adenoma, the remaining normal glands may show a suppressed parathyroid pattern, making them more difficult to find at the time of surgical exploration. A nuclear medicine scan such as a **technetium (99mTc) sestamibi scan** can be used to demonstrate the position of the abnormal glands prior to surgery.

Parathyroid carcinoma is rare (Fig. 20.8D). Patients often present with a very high serum calcium and parathyroid hormone level. The malignant gland can be large and difficult to remove at the time of operation. Histological assessment reveals parathyroid tissue separated by fibrous bands. There is capsular **(C)** and vascular invasion, the ubiquitous features of malignancy within endocrine organs.

KEY TO FIGURES
C capsular invasion

Disorders of the adrenal glands

The adrenal gland (Fig. 20.9A) has two distinct morphological and functional components:

- The **cortex**: This secretes three groups of steroid hormones, namely glucocorticoids (e.g. cortisol), mineralocorticoids (e.g. aldosterone) and small quantities of sex hormones. With the naked eye, the adrenal cortex appears yellow because of its high content of lipid (mainly cholesterol), which is the substrate for synthesis of steroid hormones.

- The **medulla**: This forms part of the neuroendocrine system and is responsible for the production of the catecholamines adrenaline (epinephrine) and noradrenaline (norepinephrine).

Disorders of the adrenal cortex

In response to acute stress, *atrophy of the adrenal cortex* (Fig. 20.9B) may arise as the normally lipid-rich cortical cells breakdown lipid for the production of steroid hormones, thus becoming *lipid depleted*. This is commonly seen in adrenal glands at post-mortem, particularly when a patient has died with features of shock. It is manifest by atrophy of the gland with loss of the normal lipid vacuolation of cells of the cortex seen on microscopy. Adrenocortical atrophy may also result from steroid therapy (iatrogenic) or, occasionally, through primary autoimmune disease *(Addison's disease)*. Other important, though less common, causes of adrenocortical insufficiency are tumour metastases and Waterhouse–Friderichsen syndrome in which there is haemorrhage of both adrenal glands caused by coagulation abnormality in the setting of bacterial meningitis.

In contrast to the picture with acute stress, with more prolonged stress the adrenal glands may become enlarged through hypertrophy and hyperplasia of cortical cells. Alternatively, *hyperplasia of the adrenal cortex* (Figs 20.9C and 20.9D) may arise as a consequence of prolonged stimulation of the adrenal cortex by pituitary-derived adrenocorticotrophic hormone (ACTH; *Cushing's disease*) or secretion of ectopic ACTH by non-pituitary tumours *(Cushing's syndrome)*.

The adrenal cortex may be the site of benign *adrenocortical adenomas* (Fig. 20.10) or, rarely, malignant *adrenocortical carcinomas*. These tumours of the adrenal cortex may be functional, resulting in the following endocrine syndromes:

- **Cushing's syndrome:** caused by cortisol secreting tumours

- **Conn's syndrome:** resulting from aldosterone secreting tumours

- **Adrenogenital syndrome:** owing to excess production of androgens.

Often, cortical hyperplasia is nodular rather than diffuse and it may be difficult to distinguish between a benign cortical adenoma and a large nodule forming part of nodular cortical hyperplasia.

Disorders of the adrenal medulla

Developmentally, the adrenal medulla arises from embryonal neural crest cells and is part of the *paraganglion system* along with a number of clusters of cells known as the *extra-adrenal paraganglia*, of which the carotid body is perhaps the best known. This paraganglion system is closely associated with the functioning of the autonomic nervous system.

The most important lesions of the adrenal medulla are tumours of the catecholamine-producing *(chromaffin)* cells, known as *phaeochromocytoma*, or neuronal tumours *(neuroblastomas, ganglion cell tumours)*.

Phaeochromocytomas (Fig. 20.11) (E-Fig. 20.5**G**) produce excessive adrenaline and noradrenaline and are usually benign. When these originate outwith the adrenal gland, they are referred to as *extra-adrenal paragangliomas* (Fig. 20.12). In some cases, these are associated with familial syndromes such as *von Hippel–Lindau syndrome (VHL)*. Some familial syndromes such as *succinic dehydrogenase B (SDH-B) deficiency* are associated with a greater chance of malignancy; thus, most patients with adrenal tumours will undergo routine genetic testing during their investigations.

Neuroblastomas (Fig. 20.13) (E-Fig. 20.6**G**) are highly malignant embryonal tumours of neuroblasts, typically arising in childhood.

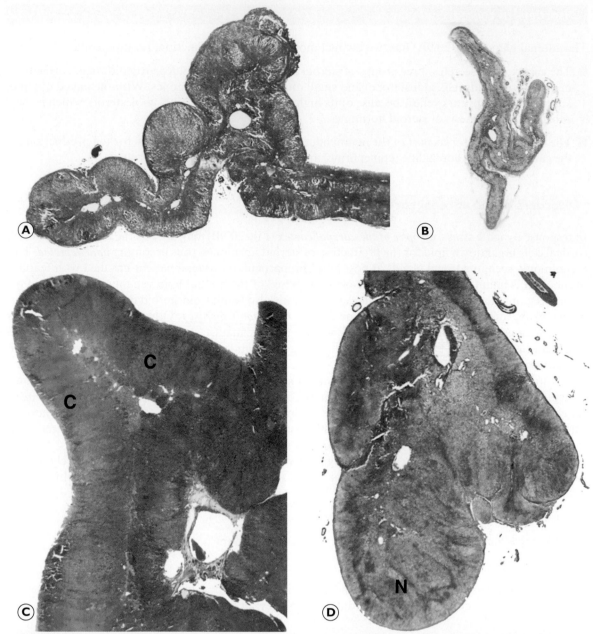

Fig. 20.9 **Adrenal cortical atrophy and hyperplasia. (A)** Normal gland (LP); **(B)** atrophic gland (LP); **(C)** diffuse hyperplasia (LP); **(D)** nodular hyperplasia (LP).

Figs 20.9A–D, all at the same magnification, compare the normal gland (Fig. 20.9A) with adrenal atrophy and hyperplasia.

In *adrenal atrophy*, as shown in Fig. 20.9B, marked reduction in the size of the gland is due to atrophy of the cortex. In this example, the atrophy was caused by long-term administration of corticosteroids, resulting in suppression of pituitary ACTH.

Adrenocortical hyperplasia occurs in either *diffuse* or *nodular* forms, as illustrated in Figs 20.9C and Fig. 20.9D, respectively. In the diffuse form, the cortex

(C) is uniformly and regularly thickened, often by cells of one type. In the much more common nodular form, the cortex contains adenoma-like nodules **(N)** of hyperplastic cortical cells, usually of zona fasciculata type. Diffuse adrenal cortical hyperplasia is usually caused by excess stimulation by ACTH from the pituitary *(Cushing's disease)* or by ectopic ACTH secreted by a non-pituitary tumour, for example from a small cell carcinoma of lung *(Cushing's syndrome)*. Nodular hyperplasia is commonly idiopathic and non-functional.

KEY TO FIGURES
A adenoma   **C** cortex   **N** hyperplastic nodule

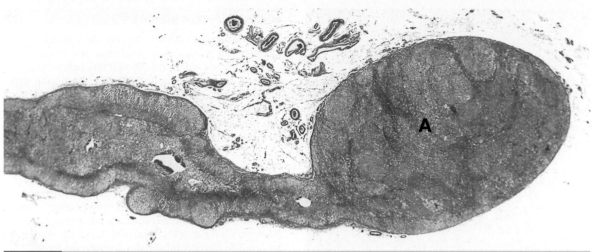

Fig. 20.10 Adrenal cortical adenoma (LP).

Hyperadrenal syndromes may result from excess secretion of hormones by a solitary benign *adrenal cortical adenoma*, the activity of which is independent of regulation by pituitary ACTH. As shown in Fig. 20.10, these tumours form a circumscribed, spherical mass **(A)** within the cortex and may be composed of a single cell type (e.g. zona glomerulosa cells in *Conn's syndrome*), but more often contain a mixture of cortical cell types.

Note how similar the adenoma is to the nodules in nodular cortical hyperplasia in Fig. 20.9D.

Cortical adenomas are a fairly frequent incidental finding at autopsy, a fact that leads to the belief that most are non-functioning and asymptomatic. Almost all cortical adenomas have a yellow cut surface, thereby distinguishing them from phaeochromocytomas, which typically appear brown.

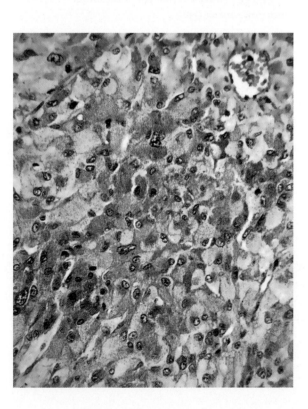

Fig. 20.11 Phaeochromocytoma (HP).

Phaeochromocytomas arise from the catecholamine-producing chromaffin cells of the adrenal medulla. Most tumours are benign in their growth characteristics but produce symptoms related to excess catecholamine secretion such as palpitations and sweating and, on occasion, may lead to potentially lethal hypertension. These tumours have a convenient association with 10%: approximately 10% are extra-adrenal (termed *paragangliomas*; Fig. 20.12), 10% are bilateral and 10% are malignant.

Macroscopically, the cut surface of the tumour is pale brown. Histologically, the tumour is composed of nests or *zellballen* (not seen here) of plump, irregular cells, often with pink granular cytoplasm, reflecting a high content of catecholamine-containing granules. Diagnosis of malignancy is based on evidence of invasion and spread, since purely cytological criteria are unreliable.

These tumours commonly secrete catecholamines. A diagnostic marker is *vanillylmandelic acid (VMA)*, a metabolite that can be measured in the urine.

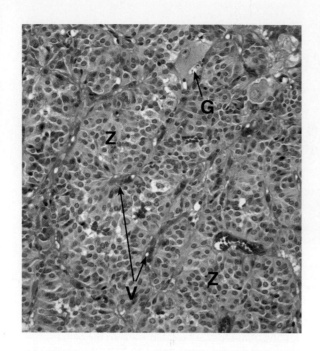

Fig. 20.12 Paraganglioma (HP).

The *paraganglion system* comprises the adrenal medulla and groups of extra-adrenal neuroendocrine cells, which are widely distributed throughout the body (in or near the midline) in close association with the autonomic nervous system. Perhaps the most recognisable of these are the *carotid bodies* in the neck and the *organs of Zuckerkandl* at the bifurcation of the abdominal aorta.

Tumours may arise in these extra-adrenal paraganglia, which, in all but name, are equivalent to phaeochromocytomas of the adrenal medulla (Fig. 20.11). These tumours, known as *paragangliomas*, most commonly arise in relation to the paraganglia of the abdomen and thorax, with a small number arising from paraganglia of the head and neck. Those arising adjacent to the carotid arteries are referred to as *carotid body tumours*.

In Fig. 20.12, the histological similarities to adrenal phaeochromocytoma are evident, with nests (*zellballen*) (**Z**) of plump tumour cells with a granular cytoplasm intersected by fine vascular channels (**V**). Close inspection may reveal ganglion cells (**G**) in some examples, as in this case.

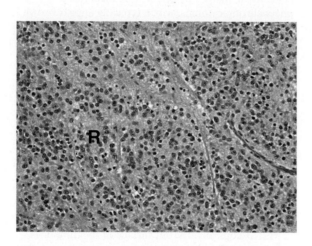

Fig. 20.13 Adrenal embryonal tumours: neuroblastoma (HP).

Neuroblastoma is an example of a 'small round blue cell tumour' believed to be derived from primitive neuroblasts in the adrenal medulla. It is highly malignant and represents the most common extra-cranial solid tumour of infancy.

The typical appearance of neuroblastoma is shown in Fig. 20.13. There is usually extensive haemorrhage and necrosis, but the viable areas are composed of small, undifferentiated tumour cells in a pink-staining fibrillary stroma; the cells have a densely stained nucleus with scanty cytoplasm. A characteristic feature is occasional clumps of cells arranged in the form of a *Homer Wright rosette* (**R**) surrounding a central zone of neurofibrils.

MULTIPLE ENDOCRINE NEOPLASIA SYNDROMES

The *multiple endocrine neoplasia (MEN)* syndromes are a group of inherited conditions characterised by tumours (benign and malignant) of multiple endocrine glands. Whilst the tumours involved may not be unique to MEN, they are distinguished from sporadic lesions by:

■ a younger age at onset

■ tumours preceded by hyperplasia in the gland

■ presentation with multiple organs involved

■ several tumours arising in one organ

■ a more aggressive clinical course.

The main syndromes are MEN-1 and MEN-2 (further subdivided to MEN-2A, MEN-2B and familial medullary thyroid cancer), both of which are inherited in an autosomal dominant manner. In MEN-1 (Werner syndrome), abnormalities of the parathyroid, pancreas and pituitary predominate, whereas in MEN-2A and -2B, phaeochromocytomas and thyroid (medullary carcinoma) tumours are typical, with mucocutaneous neuromas distinguishing MEN-2B.

KEY TO FIGURES
G ganglion cell   **R** Homer Wright rosette   **V** vascular channels   **Z** zellballen

Table 20.1 Chapter review.

Disorder	Main features	Figure
Pituitary gland		
Pituitary adenoma	Derived from cells of anterior pituitary. May present with endocrine symptoms if hormone secreting. Typically, expanded nests of monotonous cells with moderate amounts of cytoplasm. Immunohistochemistry to identify secreted hormones.	20.1 20.2
Thyroid gland		
Hashimoto's thyroiditis	Autoimmune thyroiditis with destruction of thyroid acini. Inflammatory cell infiltrate in gland with formation of lymphoid follicles.	20.3
Graves' disease	Autoimmune disease. Commonest cause of pathological thyroid hyperplasia. Triad of hyperthyroidism, exophthalmos, pre-tibial myxoedema. Thyrotoxic hyperplasia with small acini and scalloping of colloid.	20.4
Multinodular goitre	Majority as result of iodine deficiency. Nodules of varying sizes	20.5
Thyroid adenoma	Benign tumours of follicular epithelium. Encapsulated. Solitary. Majority non-functioning.	20.6
Non-invasive follicular patterned neoplasm with papillary-like nuclear features	These are newly described, thyroid lesions that are well circumscribed or encapsulated. They are composed exclusively of thyroid follicles lined by cells that show the typical nuclear features of papillary carcinoma. Molecular profiling of these lesions has shown that they have a similar molecular profile to follicular adenomas and are regarded as indolent.	
Papillary carcinoma	Most common thyroid malignancy. Papillary architecture with tumour cells lining stromal cores. Optically clear nuclei (Orphan Annie eye).	20.7A and B
Follicular carcinoma	Solitary, encapsulated or invasive lesions. May be difficult to differentiate from adenoma. Extensive sampling for capsular and/or vascular invasion indicated.	20.7C
Medullary carcinoma	Uncommon tumour of parafollicular cells. Notable for amyloid production.	20.7D
Anaplastic carcinoma	Aggressive, undifferentiated tumour arising in elderly.	
Parathyroid glands		
Hyperplasia	Increased demand for parathyroid hormone results in expansion of endocrine component. Normally all four glands involved.	20.8B
Adenoma	Benign. Usually only in one of four glands. Adenoma cells replace normal gland architecture. May be surviving rim of normal gland.	20.8C
Carcinoma	Rare. Presents with very high serum calcium. Invasion of the tumour beyond the capsule together with vascular invasion.	20.8D
Adrenal glands		
Cortical atrophy	Response to stress or long-term corticosteroid administration.	20.9B
Cortical hyperplasia	May be diffuse or, more commonly, nodular. Diffuse hyperplasia may be response to pituitary or ectopic ACTH. Nodular commonly idiopathic.	20.9C and D
Cortical adenoma	Independent of ACTH secretion. Solitary nodule in cortex, often of multiple cell types. Common incidental finding at autopsy.	20.10
Phaeochromocytoma	Arise from medullary chromaffin cells. Symptoms of catecholamine secretion. Nests (zellballen) of plump cells with granular cytoplasm.	20.11
Paraganglioma	Tumour of extra-adrenal paraganglion system. Equivalent of adrenal phaeochromocytoma. Carotid body tumour is one example.	20.12
Neuroblastoma	Adrenal embryonal tumour. Highly malignant. Most common childhood extracranial solid malignancy.	20.13

21 Skin

Introduction

The skin is commonly affected by a wide range of pathologies. Some of these are cutaneous manifestations of systemic disease processes whilst others are primary disorders of the skin. Common systemic viral illnesses such as measles and chickenpox are associated with characteristic skin rashes and many autoimmune and vasculitic disorders, such as systemic lupus erythematosus, dermatomyositis, scleroderma and Henoch–Schönlein purpura, present with skin manifestations. Primary disorders of the skin are extremely common and the vast majority of these are inflammatory or neoplastic in type.

Inflammatory disorders

Skin has a limited repertoire of responses to injury. The most common of these are illustrated in Figs 21.1 to 21.4. Most stimuli result in a combination of these changes, each with varying degrees of severity. As a result, definitive diagnosis of inflammatory dermatological conditions requires careful correlation of clinical and histological findings. Few skin conditions have pathognomonic histological appearances.

Dermatitis is a common clinical term used to describe a wide variety of inflammatory skin conditions with diverse causes. Histologically, there are changes of acute or chronic inflammation (Figs 21.5 and 21.6). Some disorders have additional histological features that may indicate a more specific diagnosis or aetiology. Two relatively common inflammatory dermatoses with characteristic clinical and microscopic features are *lichen planus* (Fig. 21.7) and *psoriasis* (Fig. 21.8).

Systemic viral infections frequently cause skin rashes, some of which have typical histological features, e.g. herpes simplex virus (HSV) infection (see Fig. 5.12), chickenpox and shingles. The latter two disorders are different clinical manifestations of infection by the herpes zoster virus and the histological changes closely resemble those of HSV infection. Other viruses give rise to apparently localised skin lesions by causing proliferation of the cells of the epidermis. Common examples include *viral warts* (Fig. 21.9), which are caused by human papillomavirus infection (see also Ch. 17), and *molluscum contagiosum* (Fig. 21.10), which is due to infection by a poxvirus.

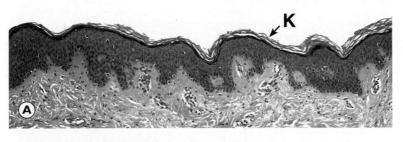

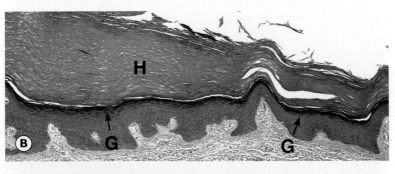

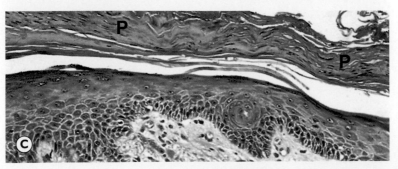

Fig. 21.1 Abnormalities of surface keratin (MP); (A) normal keratin; **(B)** hyperkeratosis; **(C)** parakeratosis.

Figs 21.1A to C compare the appearance of normal keratin **(K)** of thin skin (Fig. 21.1A) with two common abnormalities of keratin (E-Fig. 21.1 **H**). Fig. 21.1B illustrates *hyperkeratosis* **(H)**. Here, the keratin layer is thickened, but otherwise histologically normal *(orthokeratosis)*. This change is usually associated with thickening of the underlying granular layer **(G)** (stratum granulosum), termed *hypergranulosis*. Orthokeratosis is commonly seen in skin that has been chronically traumatised by scratching and, in this setting, it is usually associated with thickening of the epidermis *(acanthosis*, Fig. 21.2).

Fig. 21.1C shows *parakeratosis* **(P)**. In this case, the keratin is histologically abnormal in that it contains spindly nuclear remnants. Parakeratosis is usually associated with loss or severe thinning of the underlying granular layer. It can occur in a range of conditions but may be associated with *dysplasia* affecting the underlying epidermis (Fig. 21.14).

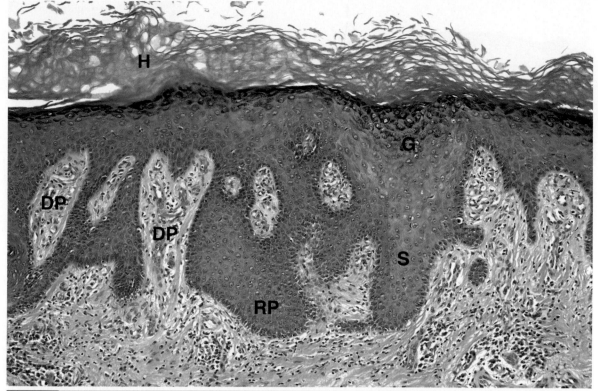

Fig. 21.2 Abnormal epidermal thickening: acanthosis (MP).

Acanthosis is the term given to thickening of the epidermis, usually due to an increase in the depth of the stratum spinosum **(S)** (prickle cell layer). It is a common feature of many skin conditions, particularly chronic inflammatory conditions (Figs 21.6 and 21.7). The thickening of the epidermal layer is particularly marked in the rete pegs **(RP)**, which are expanded and elongated with prominent interdigitating dermal papillae **(DP)**. Note that there is associated thickening of the granular layer **(G)** (hypergranulosis) and overlying orthokeratotic hyperkeratosis **(H)**.

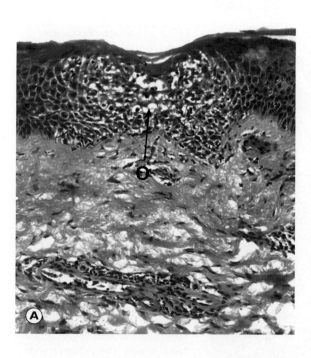

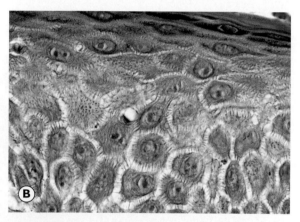

Fig. 21.3 Intra-epidermal oedema: spongiosis. **(A)** MP; **(B)** HP.

Oedema of the epidermis causes separation of epithelial cells, particularly in the prickle cell layer (E-Fig. 21.2 **H**), a condition known as *spongiosis*.

Accumulation of oedema fluid **(O)** between epidermal cells causes gaps to appear. This accentuates the intercellular junctions as illustrated in Fig. 21.3B. This oedema fluid may coalesce to form intra-epidermal vesicles.

Spongiosis with vesicle formation is a feature of acute dermatitis (Fig. 21.5).

KEY TO FIGURES

DP dermal papillae   **G** granular layer   **H** hyperkeratosis   **K** keratin   **O** oedema   **P** parakeratosis
RP rete peg   **S** stratum spinosum

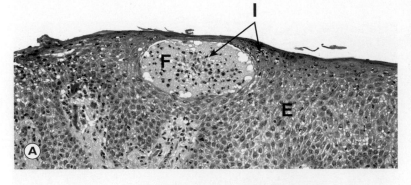

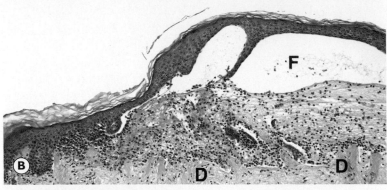

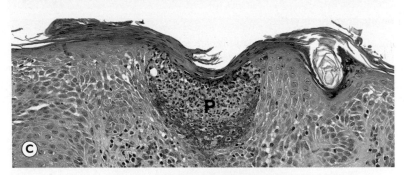

Fig. 21.4 Other epidermal inflammatory reactions. (A) Vesicle (MP); (B) bulla (LP); (C) pustule (MP).

Accumulations of fluid beneath or within the epidermis may cause small raised blebs on the skin.

Most are due to inflammation in the epidermis. When small, such lesions are termed *vesicles*. In Fig. 21.4A, note the small area of fluid accumulation **(F)**, forming a vesicle within the epidermis **(E)**. Some inflammatory cells **(I)** are present within the fluid and in the adjacent epidermis.

Larger collections of fluid are termed *bullae*. A bulla is shown in Fig. 21.4B. The collection of fluid **(F)** here is larger and includes inflammatory cells and fibrin. In this case, the roof of the bulla consists of the full thickness of the epidermis and its base is the upper dermis **(D)**.

The term *pustule* is used to describe a collection consisting of neutrophils with some fluid, lying within or beneath the epidermis. Fig. 21.4C shows a pustule **(P)** beneath the corneal layer of the epidermis.

Bullae and pustules are further categorised by their location, which may be *subepidermal*, *intra-epidermal* or *subcorneal*.

Fig. 21.5 Acute dermatitis (MP).

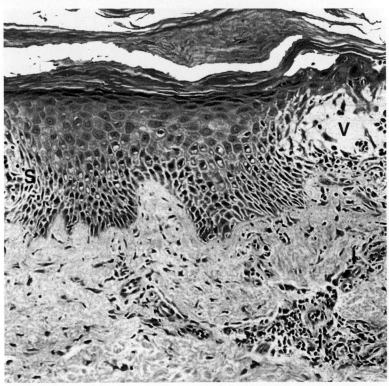

In early acute dermatitis (Fig. 21.5), the major changes involve the epidermis, with fluid accumulating between the prickle cells causing spongiosis **(S)**. As the lesion progresses, the spongiotic areas may become converted into fluid-filled vesicles **(V)** containing a few inflammatory cells, mainly lymphocytes and neutrophils, with variable infiltration of the epidermis by these cells. If the vesicles rupture onto the surface, crusts or scabs composed of fibrin and polymorph nuclei form. In the earlier stages, the upper dermis shows only oedema, but later there may be a mixed acute and chronic inflammatory cell infiltrate **(I)**, particularly around upper dermal blood vessels. This pattern is seen in the acute phase of the common inflammatory skin disease *eczema*, which is thought to have an allergic aetiology (E-Fig. 21.3**G**).

KEY TO FIGURES

A acanthosis **C** chronic inflammation **CB** Civatte bodies **D** upper dermis **DC** dilated capillary
DP dermal papilla **E** epidermis **F** fluid **G** granular layer **H** hyperkeratosis **I** inflammatory cells
M microabscess **P** pustule **PK** parakeratosis **R** rete peg **S** spongiosis **V** vesicle

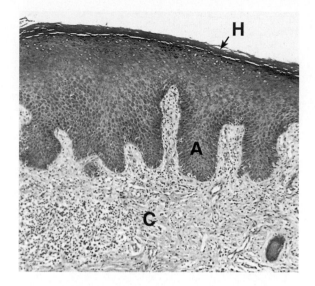

Fig. 21.6 Chronic dermatitis (MP).

The histological features of chronic dermatitis are seen in many skin rashes with a variety of causes. The characteristic features shown in Fig. 21.6 are epidermal thickening, i.e. acanthosis **(A)**, and a variable degree of hyperkeratosis **(H)**. There is no infiltration of the epidermis by inflammatory cells, but the upper and mid dermis show a moderate to heavy infiltrate of chronic inflammatory cells **(C)**, mainly lymphocytes and plasma cells, particularly around blood vessels.

The acanthosis and hyperkeratosis may produce the clinical appearance of *lichenification*, a leather-like thickening of the skin due to chronic scratching or irritation (E-Fig. 21.4**G**). This feature is recognised in the term *lichen simplex chronicus*, used to describe a form of chronic, non-specific dermatitis that occurs mainly in response to scratching of skin affected by acute dermatitis.

When the dermatitis is still active, the thickened epidermis will contain the same sort of spongiotic vesicles seen in Fig. 21.5, for example in long-standing eczema.

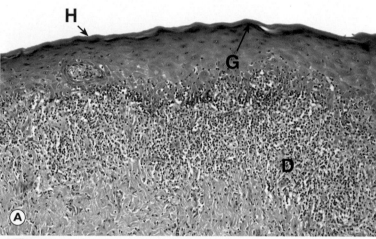
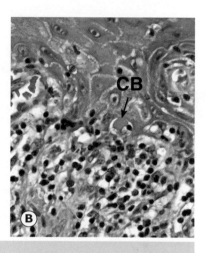

Fig. 21.7 Lichen planus. **(A)** MP; **(B)** HP.

Lichen planus is a clinically and histologically distinct type of dermatitis. In the epidermis, as seen in Fig. 21.7A, there is hyperkeratosis **(H)** and thickening of the granular layer **(G)** (hypergranulosis). A characteristic feature is the disruption of the normally regular basal layer by vacuolar degeneration and destruction of basal cells. As seen in Fig. 21.7B, this leaves a ragged and irregular dermo-epidermal

junction in which *colloid* or *Civatte bodies* **(CB)** (apoptotic keratinocytes) may be seen. The dermis **(D)** shows a dense chronic inflammatory cell infiltrate, mainly confined to the upper third. Lichen planus may affect the mucosal surfaces of the mouth and vulva where basal cell layer damage may lead to blistering and erosion.

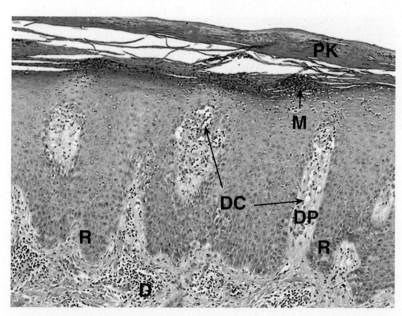

Fig. 21.8 Psoriasis (MP).

Psoriasis is a chronic skin disease characterised by well-demarcated, erythematous, scaly lesions (E-Fig. 21.5**G**).

As shown in Fig. 21.8, the major feature is acanthosis with greatly elongated, narrow rete pegs **R**. Between the rete pegs, the epidermis is thinned over oedematous and expanded dermal papillae **(DP)** in which dilated capillaries **(DC)** are prominent. The alternately thick and thin epidermis is covered by a parakeratotic layer **(PK)** of keratin, which contains small aggregations of the nuclear debris of inflammatory cells, forming *Munro micro-abscesses* **(M)**. There is a variable chronic inflammatory infiltrate in the upper dermis **(D)**.

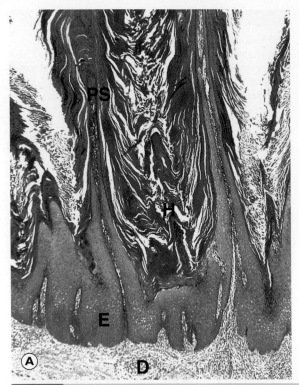

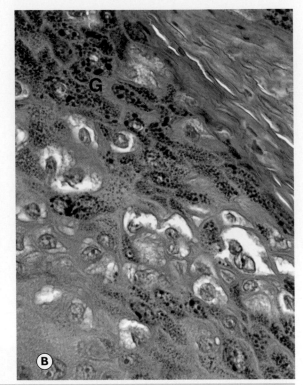

Fig. 21.9 Viral wart. **(A)** LP; **(B)** HP.

A *viral wart*, or *verruca vulgaris*, which occurs on non-traumatised skin, has an exophytic papillary form as illustrated in Fig. 21.9A. Histologically, the epidermis **(E)** is irregularly thickened and covered by a thick layer of hyperkeratosis **(H)** in which there are *parakeratotic spires* **(PS)** over the tips of the more prominent papillary epidermal outgrowths.

The epidermal cells in an active viral wart usually show focal prominence of the granular layer **G** as illustrated in Fig. 21.9B, with occasional areas of large,

pale vacuolated cells in the upper stratum spinosum. The dermis **(D)** shows a chronic inflammatory cell infiltrate.

In skin areas prone to trauma, warts have a much less papillary form and may be dome-shaped (e.g. in *juvenile warts* of the hands) or inverted (e.g. *plantar warts* of the sole of the foot).

These lesions are caused by the human papillomavirus.

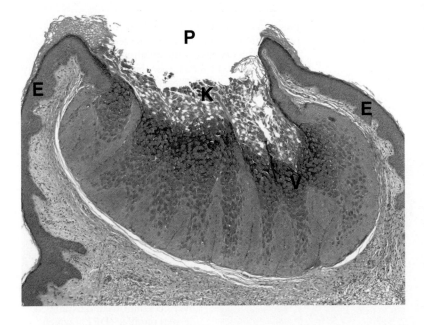

Fig. 21.10 Molluscum contagiosum (LP).

Molluscum contagiosum (Fig. 21.10) is a localised nodular thickening of the epidermis. This condition occurs more commonly in children and is due to infection by a poxvirus. There are lobules of epithelial proliferation with an inverted, endophytic architecture. Viral inclusion bodies **(V)** are easily visible, both in the proliferating epidermis, where they stain a reddish colour, and in the overlying keratin plug **(K)**, where they appear more darkly stained. The keratinous plug extrudes through a central pit **(P)** at the apex of the dome-shaped nodule, which is surrounded by normal epidermis. Lesions usually resolve spontaneously.

KEY TO FIGURES
D dermis **E** epidermis **G** granular layer **H** hyperkeratosis **K** keratin plug **N** keratin nest **P** pit
PS parakeratotic spires **V** viral inclusion bodies

Neoplastic disorders

Common primary skin tumours may be divided broadly into those arising from epithelial cells, those arising from melanocytes and those arising within dermal and subcutaneous tissues. Much less commonly, skin can be involved by metastatic tumour from other sites (e.g. lung or renal cancer) or by direct invasion from an underlying neoplasm (most commonly breast cancer). Lymphoma may also affect the skin either primarily (e.g. *mycosis fungoides*, see Fig. 16.11) or in cases of systemic lymphoma.

Epithelial neoplasms

Seborrhoeic keratosis and *basal cell papilloma* are terms used interchangeably to describe a very common benign skin lesion seen predominantly in elderly patients. *Basal cell carcinoma* is a low-grade malignant tumour that resembles the basal cells of the epidermis; *squamous cell carcinoma* is a more aggressive tumour that resembles the cells of the prickle cell layer (stratum spinosum) of the epidermis. Both of these malignant tumours are strongly associated with chronic sun exposure. Chronic sun damage is also associated with premalignant change in the skin in the form of epidermal *dysplasia*, with disordered maturation of keratinocytes. Severe dysplasia, the skin equivalent of CIN 3 (see Fig. 17.7), can be described as *carcinoma in situ*, *intra-epidermal carcinoma* or using the eponymous term *Bowen's disease*. Lesser degrees of epidermal dysplasia are termed *actinic* or *solar keratosis*.

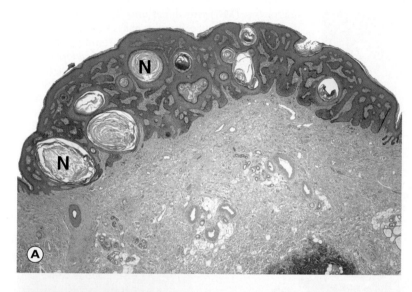

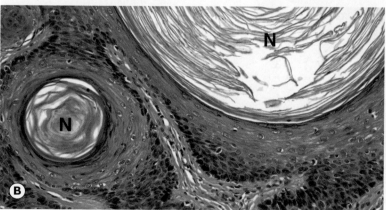

Fig. 21.11 **Seborrhoeic keratosis. (A)** LP; **(B)** HP.

Seborrhoeic keratosis (sometimes called *basal cell papilloma* or *seborrhoeic wart*) is a common lesion of the elderly. This is characterised by a localised proliferation of cells that resemble the normal basal cells of the epidermis, usually forming a raised warty lesion as illustrated in Fig. 21.11A (E-Fig. 21.6 **G**).

Such outgrowths are vulnerable to chronic trauma, leading to overlying hyperkeratosis and formation of keratin nests **(N)** in the lesion. These whorls of keratin (sometimes referred to as 'horn cysts') are characteristic and this is illustrated at higher magnification in Fig. 21.11B. There is often prominent melanin pigment within the cells of the basal layer and, as a result, these lesions often appear dark brown or black in colour.

Examination of the cells at high magnification shows that the nuclei are bland and uniform and there is no evidence of significant mitotic activity. These features may be compared with those of a malignant skin tumour, basal cell carcinoma, illustrated in Fig. 21.12. The aetiology of this lesion is unknown, but it is usually regarded as a benign skin tumour.

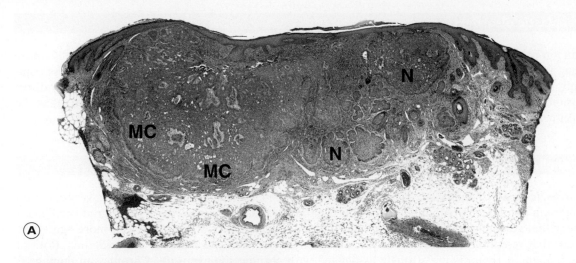

(A)

Fig. 21. 12 Basal cell carcinoma. (A) LP; (B) HP.

Basal cell carcinoma is a common tumour, composed of cells with dark-staining nuclei and sparse, poorly defined cytoplasm. Fig. 21.12A shows the typical appearances of the common nodular form (E-Fig. 21.7 **G**), with a mixture of solid nodular **(N)** and microcystic **(MC)** growth patterns. In addition to this nodular form, basal cell carcinomas show a wide range of growth patterns. The *morphoeic* variant presents as a flat, hard area of skin and the *superficial* form as a reddish, scaly lesion (E-Fig.21.8 **G**). As seen in Fig. 21.12B, the cells at the periphery of the tumour are characteristically arranged in a palisaded pattern **(P)**, whereas the central cells are more randomly arranged. Basal cell carcinoma arises from the basal cells of the epidermis or epidermal appendages. It behaves as a malignant tumour in that it invades dermis and any deeper underlying structures, but it almost never metastasises. Basal cell carcinomas occur most frequently on the light-exposed areas of skin, particularly the face, and usually present as nodular lesions, which may undergo ragged ulceration, giving rise to the colloquial term *rodent ulcer*.

(B)

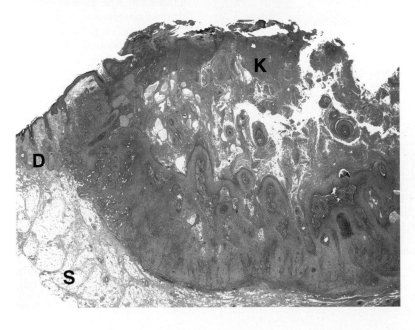

Fig. 21.13 Squamous cell carcinoma (LP).

Squamous cell carcinoma of the skin (E-Fig. 21.9 **G**) histologically resembles squamous cell carcinomas in many other sites (see Fig. 7.3). The skin tumours are usually well differentiated and highly keratinising. In Fig. 21.13, there is a large central plug of keratin **(K)** with surrounding infiltrating carcinoma.

The tumour invades through the dermis **(D)** and into underlying subcutaneous fat **(S)**. It may spread via the lymphatic channels to regional lymph nodes. Invasive squamous cell carcinoma of the skin can develop from *intra-epidermal carcinoma* (*squamous cell carcinoma in situ*, Fig. 21.14).

KEY TO FIGURES
BM basement membrane **D** dermis **K** keratin **MC** microcystic pattern **N** nodular pattern
P palisading cells **TM** tripolar mitosis **S** subcutaneous fat

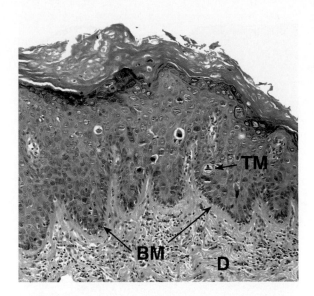

Fig. 21.14 **Intra-epidermal carcinoma (HP).**

Invasive squamous carcinoma (Fig. 21.13) may be preceded by epidermal dysplasia. When the dysplasia is severe and involves the full thickness of the epidermis, it is termed *intra-epidermal carcinoma*, *carcinoma in situ* or *Bowen's disease*. This eponymous term is reserved for lesions with a plaque-like clinical appearance.

In Fig. 21.14, there is severe dysplasia extending through the full thickness of the epidermis, with loss of the normal organisation and stratification. The basement membrane **(BM)** is intact and there is no invasion of the dermis **(D)**. Numerous mitotic figures are seen and some of these appear atypical, with occasional tripolar forms **(TM)**. When the epidermal dysplasia is restricted to lower levels of the epidermis, the condition is known as *actinic (solar) keratosis*.

Melanocytic lesions

In normal skin, melanocytes are scattered in the basal layers of the epidermis, their fine cytoplasmic processes ramifying between the keratinocytes towards the skin surface (E-Fig. 21.10 **H**). Melanocytes are responsible for the synthesis of the brown pigment melanin, which is then transferred to adjacent keratinocytes. There are significant racial and genetic differences in the melanin synthetic activity of melanocytes, resulting in the varying degrees of normal pigmentation seen in the skin. Exposure to sunlight enhances melanin synthesis and transfer into keratinocytes.

Benign pigmented skin lesions are very common and are known colloquially as 'moles'. This term encompasses a large group of benign lesions called *naevi*, which are characterised histologically by aggregates of melanocytic cells at various sites within the skin. The three main subtypes, *junctional*, *compound* and *intradermal naevi*, are shown in Fig. 21.15.

Malignant melanoma is an important and highly malignant tumour of melanocytic cells. Its main features and histological variants are illustrated in Figs 21.16 to 21.19. There are also melanocytic lesions with features intermediate between a benign naevus and a malignant melanoma. These are described as *atypical* or *dysplastic naevi* and may progress to melanoma in some cases.

Benign melanocytic naevi

These are of three main types, defined according to the location of the melanocytic nests:

- **Junctional melanocytic naevus:** Nests of melanocytes are confined to the lower epidermis.

- **Compound melanocytic naevus:** Nests are located in both the lower epidermis and upper dermis.

- **Intradermal melanocytic naevus:** Nests of melanocytes are present in the dermis only.

Benign naevi (E-Fig. 21.11 **G**) have a predictable natural history and are illustrated in Fig. 21.15. Most begin as flat, pigmented *junctional naevi*, with nests of pigmented melanocytes confined to the lower levels of the epidermis, sitting on the epidermal basement membrane. Purely junctional naevi are most commonly found in children. As the child grows older, some of these junctional melanocytes migrate across the basement membrane into the upper dermis where they lose most of their pigment and the cells become smaller and tightly packed together. There are some remaining pigmented junctional nests in the epidermis and smaller non-pigmented naevus cells in the dermis. At this stage, the naevus is called a *compound naevus* and the intradermal nests produce a lesion that is raised above the level of skin to form a brown, raised nodule. In early adulthood, most of the junctional nests of melanocytes migrate into the dermis until no more are present in the epidermis. At this stage, the naevus is a completely *intradermal naevus*. All of these lesions are completely benign but, rarely, a previously benign naevus will transform into a malignant melanoma. This usually occurs by a well recognised route: the junctional nests do not completely migrate into the dermis but proliferate abnormally and show features of cytological and architectural atypia, producing a *dysplastic* or *atypical naevus*. If untreated, a proportion of these eventually become superficial spreading malignant melanoma (Figs 21.16 and 21.17)

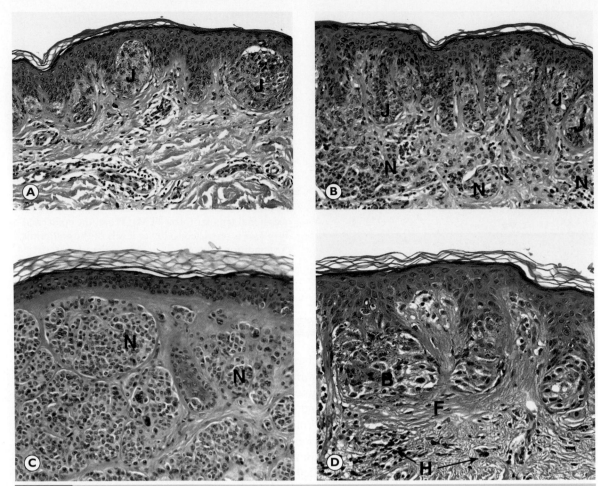

Fig. 21.15 **Melanocytic naevi. (A)** Junctional naevus (MP); **(B)** compound naevus (MP); **(C)** intradermal naevus (MP); **(D)** dysplastic junctional naevus (HP).

In a junctional naevus (Fig. 21.15A), the melanocytes aggregate in junctional nests **(J)** in the lower layers of the epidermis but do not encroach into the underlying dermis. The nests are round to oval and well circumscribed and the melanocytes are pigmented.

A compound naevus (Fig. 21.15B) contains both intra-epidermal junctional nests **(J)** and nests of naevus cells in the upper dermis **(N)**. The cells in the dermis become small and densely packed and are said to be *'maturing'*. As time passes, more and more naevus cells occupy the dermis and there are fewer junctional nests in the epidermis.
Eventually, all the naevus cells that formed the junctional nests have migrated into the upper dermis to form an intradermal naevus, as shown in Fig. 21.15C.

Sometimes, the junctional melanocyte nests do not migrate completely into the dermis but develop features of both cytological and architectural atypia, forming a dysplastic naevus (Fig. 21.15D). Nuclear pleomorphism is seen. Architectural atypia often takes the form of elongated nests composed of spindle-shaped melanocytes running transversely, bridging adjacent epidermal rete pegs **(B)**. There is usually associated fibrosis within the superficial dermis, termed *fibroplasia* **(F)**, and prominent *melanophages* **(H)** (histiocytes containing melanin pigment) may be seen.

Some pathologists use the term *atypical naevus* for lesions of this type and may then describe the degree of cytological and architectural atypia as mild, moderate or severe. This information may be helpful for clinicians when planning further patient follow-up.

Malignant melanocytic lesions (malignant melanoma)

Malignant melanoma (E-Fig. 21.12**G**) is a malignant tumour of melanocytes, the incidence of which is increasing dramatically in white-skinned people around the world. Excessive sun exposure, particularly sunburning, is believed to be the principal cause. Neglected malignant melanomas have frequently metastasised at the time of presentation, but public awareness is leading to patients presenting earlier, such that many malignant melanomas may now be completely cured by primary excision of the lesion. Malignant melanoma spreads initially via lymphatics to regional lymph nodes and subsequently via the blood-stream, by which time control of the disease is extremely difficult.

KEY TO FIGURES
AM atypical melanocyte nests   **B** bridging melanocyte nests   **F** fibroplasia   **H** melanophages
J junctional nest   **N** intradermal nest   **SM** single melanocytes

---

The risk of metastasis, and therefore the prognosis, depends mainly on the following factors:

■ **Depth of tumour invasion**

- *Melanoma in situ* indicates that tumour cells have not breached the basement membrane. This indicates that the lesion lacks any metastatic potential and so excision is curative.

- *Breslow depth* is one of the main prognostic indicators in melanoma. This is measured perpendicularly from the granular cell layer of the epidermis down to the deepest invasive tumour cell. Lesions with a Breslow depth of less than 1 mm have an excellent prognosis.

- *Clark level* is an alternative means of assessing the extent of tumour invasion and is most valuable in lesions less than 1 mm in depth. This system identifies the deepest anatomical layer of the skin that is involved, e.g. Clark level 2 indicates that the tumour is limited to the papillary dermis, whilst Clark level 5 describes invasion of subcutaneous tissues.

■ **Growth phase**

- *Radial growth phase* describes a lesion with predominantly horizontal (lateral) growth and without evidence of deep dermal infiltration. This pattern of growth is associated with a relatively favourable prognosis and is typically seen early in the development of the superficial spreading form of malignant melanoma. This is one of the common subtypes encountered in clinical practice (Figs 21.16 and 21.17).

- *Vertical growth phase*, in contrast, indicates that the malignant cells show predominantly vertical growth, invading deeper into the dermis. This is typical of nodular malignant melanoma and is associated with an adverse prognosis (Fig. 21.18).

■ **Lymphatic, vascular or perineural invasion**

- When present, these histological features indicate an adverse prognosis and are associated with a high risk of lymph node and distant metastases.

Other subtypes of melanoma include *lentigo maligna* (a pre-invasive form of the disease that occurs in sun-damaged skin of older patients, illustrated in Fig. 21.19), *invasive lentigo maligna melanoma* (the invasive form of the same disorder) and *acral lentiginous malignant melanoma,* which, as the name suggests, occurs at acral sites (sites with thick skin such as the palms and soles). This lesion is uncommon in white-skinned populations, but occurs with relatively greater frequency in black populations owing to the presence of lesser quantities of protective melanin pigment at these sites.

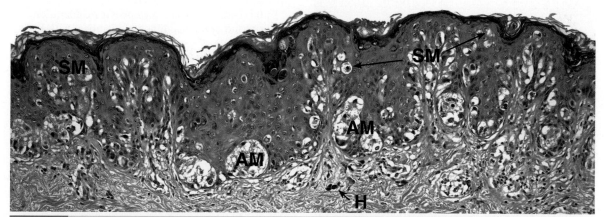

Fig. 21.16 Superficial spreading malignant melanoma in situ (HP).

In Fig. 21.16, the epidermis contains irregular nests of atypical melanocytes (**AM**). Unlike in junctional naevi (Fig. 21.15) where these are confined to the tips of rete pegs, here the nests are more randomly distributed and some extend into upper layers of the epidermis. The nests are variable in size and shape and the melanocytes they contain are atypical and pleomorphic. Numerous single melanocytes (**SM**) are scattered through the upper layers of the epidermis. This is termed *Pagetoid spread* due to the resemblance to Paget's disease of the nipple (see Fig. 18.13). Some *melanophages* (**H**) (histiocytes containing melanin pigment) are present in the papillary dermis, but here there is no invasion of the dermis by the malignant cells (compare with Fig. 21.17).

CLINICAL ASPECTS OF MALIGNANT MELANOMA

Malignant melanoma usually presents as a new or changing pigmented lesion. On examination, the edge of the lesion is often irregular and rather ill-defined, whilst benign naevi tend to be round and uniform with a sharply defined border. Naevi also tend to be evenly pigmented whereas melanomas typically exhibit variable pigmentation, often with several different shades of black and brown. More advanced tumours can have nodular areas and sometimes show surface ulceration because the expanding mass of tumour cells destroys the overlying epidermis. Occasional lesions are not pigmented and these are termed *amelanotic melanomas*. These tumours are more difficult to recognise and may be confused with other lesions such as intradermal naevi and basal cell carcinomas. Complete excision is the initial treatment of choice in cases of melanoma.

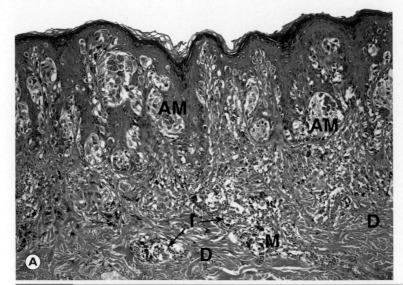

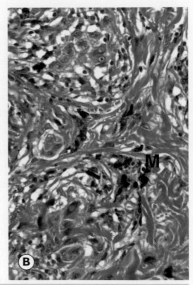

Fig. 21.17 **Superficial spreading malignant melanoma: dermal invasion. (A)** LP; **(B)** HP.

As in the superficial spreading malignant melanoma in situ shown in Fig. 21.16, there are nests of atypical melanocytes in all layers of the epidermis **(AM)**, but in this example malignant cells have broken through the epidermal basement membrane to invade the dermis **(D)** in a radial/horizontal growth pattern. Again, there are prominent melanophages **(M)**, and some

lymphocytic inflammatory cells **(I)** are also present in the surrounding dermis.

In Fig. 21.17B, the infiltrating cells show obvious nuclear pleomorphism and are seen to have prominent nucleoli. In contrast to Fig. 21.16, the malignant cells lie between dermal collagen fibres and there is no basement membrane around them.

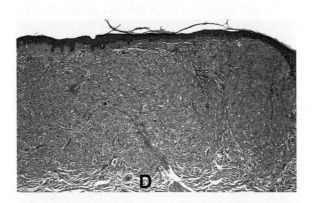

Fig. 21.18 **Malignant melanoma: nodular (LP).**

The low-power image in Fig. 21.18 shows the architectural pattern of a malignant melanoma with a nodular (vertical) growth phase component, which invades into the deep dermis **(D)**.

In this case, there is no melanocyte proliferation at the dermo-epidermal junction (compare with Fig. 21.17).

The Breslow thickness of this lesion is much greater than 1 mm and the prognosis is poor, with a high chance of metastatic spread.

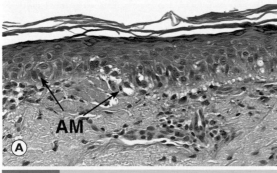

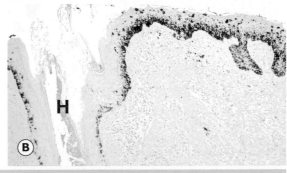

Fig. 21.19 **Lentigo maligna. (A)** H&E (HP); **(B)** immunohistochemical staining for MelanA (MP).

Lentigo maligna is a form of in situ melanoma that usually presents as an enlarging, flat, pigmented patch on the faces of elderly people. Fig. 21.19A shows an almost continuous line of single, atypical melanocytes **(AM)** in the basal layer. The cells show pleomorphism with enlarged, hyperchromatic nuclei. Typically, these abnormal melanocytes extend down the basal layer of skin appendages such as hair follicles **(H).** This is illustrated in Fig. 21.19B,

using an immunohistochemical method to highlight melanocytes (stained brown). Eventually, invasion of the dermis may occur *(lentigo maligna melanoma)*.

In general, lentigo maligna has a prolonged period of in situ growth and invasive disease is relatively uncommon. When this occurs, it is usually manifest by the development of a nodule within the previously flat, pigmented lesion.

MOLECULAR MEDICINE AND TARGETED TREATEMENT OF MALIGNANT MELANOMA
Management of malignant melanoma is challenging as the disease often responds quite poorly to conventional chemotherapy. Newer drug treatments have been developed that are designed to target specific drivers of tumour growth whilst avoiding effects on normal tissues. An important example is testing for *BRAF v600e* and *v600k* mutations as these predict disease response to BRAF inhibitor drugs. In many centres, all cases of locally advanced or metastatic melanoma are tested for these mutations at the point of diagnosis in order to guide patient treatment.

Immunotherapy is also evolving, based upon developments in our understanding of immune tolerance and the key role of PD-1/PD-L1 in a range of tumour types, including non–small cell lung cancer (see Ch. 12) and melanoma. PD-L1 has a role in allowing some tumour cells to avoid immune surveillance (so-called **immune escape**). New drug treatments are available that can block this pathway and therefore allow the patient's own immune system to target tumour cells.

Some melanomas harbour mutations in *c-KIT* (see Fig.13.14) and treatment with tyrosine kinase inhibitor drugs such as imatinib may have a role. Pathologists have a key role in determining which patients will benefit from these new treatment options.

Cysts and other skin lesions

Some common skin lesions are difficult to classify because their aetiologies are incompletely understood. Examples include the various cysts commonly referred to as 'sebaceous cysts' by clinicians. Common skin cysts fall into two main categories histologically, *epidermoid cysts* (Fig. 21.20) and *pilar cysts* (Fig. 21.21). Other lesions such as the *pyogenic granuloma* (Fig. 21.22) and *dermatofibroma* (Fig. 21.23) share some features with benign neoplasms, but are considered by others to be reactive proliferations, often occurring after minor injury. *Dermatofibrosarcoma protuberans* (Fig. 21.24) shows some histological similarities to dermatofibroma, but as the name suggests, this is a malignant soft tissue neoplasm (a sarcoma). Other soft tissue lesions are considered in Ch. 22.

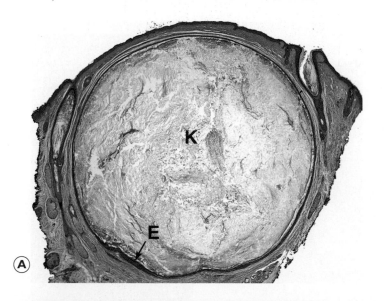

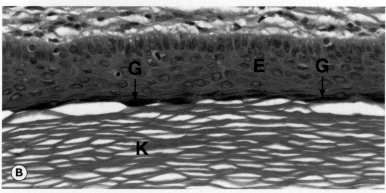

Fig. 21.20 Epidermoid cyst. (A) LP; **(B)** HP.

Epidermoid cysts (sometimes called *epidermal cysts*) are intradermal lesions that may open onto the skin surface through a punctum. The cyst contains lamellated keratin **(K)** and is lined by a thin, flattened squamous epithelium **(E)**, which, like the epidermis, has a granular layer **(G)**. This is illustrated at higher magnification in Fig. 21.20B.

Trauma to the cyst may lead to rupture, associated with escape of keratin into the surrounding dermis where its presence excites a granulomatous foreign body giant cell reaction (see Fig. 4.9), with swelling, tenderness and redness around the cyst.

Clinically, these lesions are often (inaccurately) called sebaceous cysts and traumatised, ruptured cysts are said to be infected sebaceous cysts, again inaccurately. The features of inflammation around ruptured cysts are due to the reaction to leaked keratin.

BASIC SYSTEMS PATHOLOGY ■ SKIN

KEY TO FIGURES
AM atypical melanocytes **D** dermis **E** epithelium **G** granular layer **H** hair follicle **I** inflammatory cells **K** keratin **M** melanophages

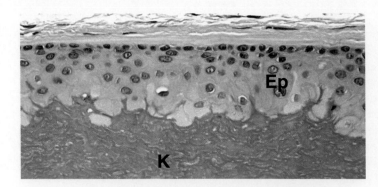

Fig. 21.21 Pilar cyst (HP).

Pilar cysts (sometimes called *tricholemmal cysts*) are similar to epidermoid cysts, but occur almost entirely on the scalp. They differ from epidermal cysts in the nature of the keratin **(K)**, which is compact and cohesive, and in the lining squamous epithelium **(Ep)**, which resembles hair follicles, lacking a granular layer (Fig. 21.21).

These lesions are also mistakenly called sebaceous cysts.

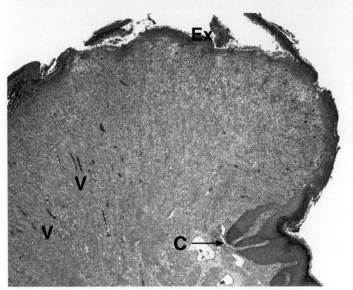

Fig. 21.22 Pyogenic granuloma (LP).

Pyogenic granuloma (sometimes called *lobular capillary haemangioma*) is a common lesion, which may occur following a minor penetrating injury, for example by a rose thorn. It consists of a raised nodule composed of lobules of capillary-sized vessels **(V)**, somewhat resembling a capillary haemangioma (Fig. 21.22). It may represent an abnormal overgrowth of the vascular element of normal granulation tissue. The surface of the lesion is frequently ulcerated and, in this example, there is an overlying inflammatory exudate **(Ex)**. A characteristic histological feature is a collarette **(C)** of proliferating epidermis at the base of the lesion.

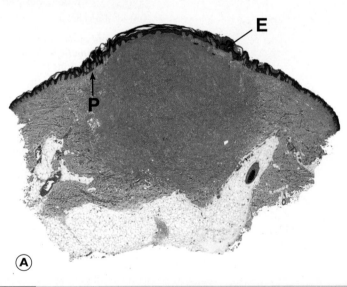

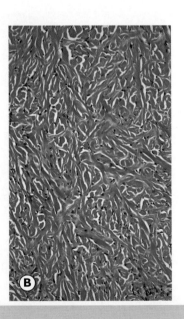

Fig. 21.23 Dermatofibroma. (A) LP; (B) HP.

Dermatofibroma (sometimes called *benign fibrous histiocytoma*) is a common skin lesion, usually occurring on the limbs of young and middle-aged people in the form of a single, firm, raised nodule, ranging in colour from white to brown (E-Fig. 21.13**G**).

As seen in Fig. 21.23A, the lesion lies in the dermis and has ill-defined margins, being composed of irregularly arranged spindle cells resembling fibroblasts with intervening collagen fibres. The degree of cellularity seen in these lesions is variable and some forms contain abundant collagen with fewer fibroblastic cells. Scattered foamy or haemosiderin-laden histiocytes are present in some lesions, probably due to degeneration within the lesion. The overlying epidermis **(E)** tends to show prominent basal layer pigmentation **(P)** and is often irregularly thickened, a feature described as *pseudoepitheliomatous hyperplasia*. When this change is very marked, the appearance may mimic invasive carcinoma.

Although the dermatofibroma resembles a group of soft tissue tumours described as *'fibrohistiocytic'* (owing to the presence of cells similar to fibroblasts and histiocytes), dermatofibromas are generally considered to be reactive lesions rather than true benign tumours. The lesion is shown at higher magnification in Fig. 21.23B.

Sometimes, there is a clinical history of previous minor injury at the site of the lesion.

KEY TO FIGURES
C collarette of proliferating epidermis **E** epidermis **Ep** lining epithelium **Ex** inflammatory exudate
K keratin **P** basal layer pigmentation **V** vascular tissue

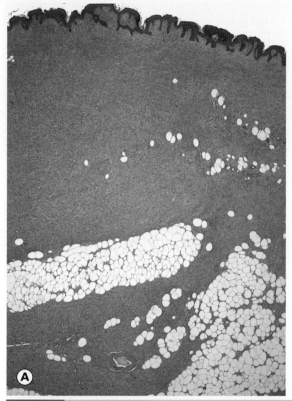
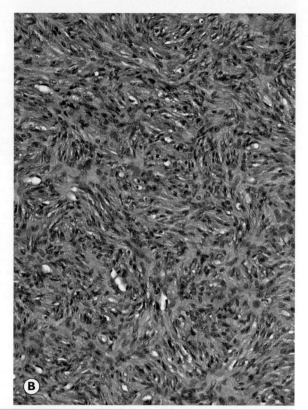

Fig. 21.24 **Dermatofibrosarcoma protuberans.** **(A)** LP; **(B)** HP.

This is a low-grade sarcoma that usually occurs in young adults. It arises in the skin, most commonly affecting the trunk, and presents as a hard and gradually enlarging plaque. Over time, it may become raised and nodular, hence the designation 'protuberans'.

Histologically, the tumour is composed of spindle cells that show variable but usually mild pleomorphism (Fig. 21.24B). There are occasional mitotic figures. Although originating in the dermis, it enlarges by infiltrating laterally into adjacent dermis and deeply into subcutaneous adipose tissue, as in Fig. 21.24A. It often infiltrates much more extensively than is apparent clinically and complete excision at

first attempt can be difficult. Incomplete excision is invariably followed by recurrence and continued local spread.

Metastasis does occur rarely and, in common with other sarcomas, this is usually blood-borne in type (rather than the pattern of lymphatic spread to local lymph nodes typically seen in carcinomas) and results in lung metastases.

Over time, some tumours may develop areas of higher-grade malignancy, resembling *fibrosarcoma*, a soft tissue tumour that can also occur at other sites. This transformation is manifest clinically by a rapid increase in the size of the tumour.

Table 21.1 **Chapter review.**

Disorder	Main features	Figure
Responses of skin to injury		
Orthokeratosis	Thickened layer of normal keratin. No nuclear fragments. Often associated prominence of granular layer (hypergranulosis).	21.1B
Parakeratosis	Abnormal surface keratin with residual flecks of nuclear material. Often associated with loss or diminution of granular layer.	21.1C
Acanthosis	Thickening of epidermis, usually associated with increased depth of the rete pegs.	21.2
Spongiosis	Intra-epidermal oedema due to acute inflammation, resulting in gaps between keratinocytes and highlighting intercellular junctions.	21.3
Vesicle	Small accumulation of oedema fluid within epidermis due to acute inflammation, sometimes containing a few inflammatory cells.	21.4A
Bulla	Large collection of fluid within or beneath epidermis, sometimes containing inflammatory cells and fibrin.	21.4B
Pustule	Collection of neutrophil polymorphs and some fluid within or beneath the epidermis. May be subcorneal, intra-epidermal or subepidermal.	21.4C

BASIC SYSTEMS PATHOLOGY ■ SKIN

Table 21.1	Chapter review—cont'd.	

Disorder	Main features	Figure
Inflammatory disorders		
Acute dermatitis (E-Fig. 21.3 **G**)	Intra-epidermal oedema resulting in spongiosis and vesiculation. Some inflammatory cells in epidermis. Later, chronic inflammation in dermis.	21.5
Chronic dermatitis (E-Fig. 21.4 **G**)	Acanthosis and hyperkeratosis with chronic inflammation around vessels in superficial dermis.	21.6
Lichen planus	Irregular acanthosis with chronic inflammation blurring dermo-epidermal junction. Basal cell vacuolar damage and apoptotic keratinocytes.	21.7
Psoriasis (E-Fig. 21.5 **G**)	Regular acanthosis with thinning of suprapapillary epidermis and dilated capillaries in oedematous papillary dermis. Munro micro-abscesses.	21.8
Viral lesions		
Viral wart (verruca vulgaris)	Exophytic papillary lesion of epidermis with parakeratotic spires, hyper-granulosis and occasional koilocytic cells. HPV infection.	21.9
Molluscum contagiosum	Inverted lobules of proliferating epithelium with viral inclusions (molluscum bodies) and a central plug of keratin. Poxvirus infection.	21.10
Epithelial neoplasms		
Seborrhoeic keratosis (basal cell papilloma) (E-Fig. 21.6 **G**)	Benign proliferation of bland cells resembling basal cells of epidermis. Hy-perkeratosis and nests of keratin. Usually exophytic.	21.11
Basal cell carcinoma (E-Figs 21.7 **G** and 21.8 **G**)	Low grade malignant tumour. Small, hyperchromatic cells resembling basal cells of epidermis. Peripheral palisading. Mitotic. Various patterns.	21.12
Squamous cell carcinoma (E-Fig. 21.9 **G**)	More aggressive than BCC. Larger cells with eosinophilic cytoplasm. Kerati-nisation. May arise from carcinoma in situ (Bowen's disease).	21.13
Intra-epidermal carcinoma (carci-noma in situ, Bowen's)	Full thickness dysplasia of epidermis. Disordered architecture and cytologi-cal atypia. Basement membrane intact.	21.14
Actinic keratosis (solar keratosis)	Mild to moderate epidermal dysplasia. Associated with chronic sun damage.	
Melanocytic lesions		
Junctional naevus	Nests of uniform and bland pigmented melanocytic cells at dermo-epidermal junction. No naevus cells in dermis.	21.15A
Compound naevus (E-Fig. 21.11 **G**)	Nests of naevus cells at dermo-epidermal junction and in dermis. Dermal nests smaller, less pigmented and showing maturation.	21.15B
Intradermal naevus	No remaining junctional melanocyte nests. Mature naevus cells only within dermis.	21.15C
Atypical naevus (dysplastic naevus)	Cytological and architectural atypia of melanocyte nests. Often more spin-dle-shaped cells and superficial desmoplasia.	21.15D
Superficial spreading malignant melanoma in situ	Nests of severely atypical melanocytes with Pagetoid spread of single cells within epidermis. Basement membrane remains intact.	21.16
Invasive superficial spreading malig-nant melanoma (E-Fig. 21.12 **G**)	Atypical melanocytes in epidermis and also invading into dermis. Breslow depth and Clark level important for prognosis.	21.17
Nodular malignant melanoma	Tumour in vertical growth phase with nodule of tumour cells in dermis and minimal junctional activity. Adverse prognosis due to lesional depth.	21.18
Lentigo maligna	Form of melanoma in situ found on face of elderly patients. Linear prolifera-tion of atypical melanocytes at dermo-epidermal junction.	21.19
Lentigo maligna melanoma	Invasive malignant melanoma arising from long-standing lentigo maligna. Often nodule forms within flat, pigmented patch.	
Other lesions		
Epidermoid cyst (epidermal cyst)	Clinical term sebaceous cyst. Cyst filled with lamellated keratin. Lined by stratified squamous epithelium. Granular layer present.	21.20
Pilar cyst (tricholemmal cyst)	Clinical term sebaceous cyst. Usually scalp. Firm, amorphous keratin. Squamous lining without granular layer.	21.21
Pyogenic granuloma (lobular capil-lary haemangioma)	Often after minor penetrating injury. Lobules of capillary size vessels. Collarette of epidermis at base.	21.22
Dermatofibroma (benign fibrous histiocytoma) (E-Fig. 21.13 **G**)	Probably reactive lesion. Fibroblasts and collagen, ill-defined edge. Scattered histiocytes. Overlying epidermal hyperplasia.	21.23
Dermatofibrosarcoma protuberans	Low-grade sarcoma of skin. Resembles dermatofibroma but deeply invasive and locally aggressive. May rarely metastasise.	21.24

22 Bone and soft tissues

Bone

Bone is a highly specialised tissue (E-Fig. 22.1**H**), composed of a particular type of collagen embedded in a ground substance matrix, *osteoid*. Osteoid becomes mineralised by the deposition of calcium salts in the form of **hydroxyapatite**. The osteoid is synthesised by **osteoblasts,** which, in their resting state, are inactive, spindle-shaped cells lying unobtrusively on bone surfaces. When there is a need to synthesise more osteoid, osteoblasts become cuboidal and actively synthesise protein (E-Fig. 22.2**H**). Bone is constantly being remodelled through the removal of old bone by resorptive cells called *osteoclasts* (E-Fig. 22.3**H**) and deposition of new osteoid by osteoblasts. Thus, the bulk and architectural arrangement of bone can be modified in response to changing functional demands and stresses. As well as its structural role, the calcified bone also provides a large calcium pool from which calcium can be withdrawn (by resorptive activity of osteoclasts) to maintain serum calcium homeostasis.

Bone fracture

Bone fracture is a common and important result of trauma. Where there is an underlying bone abnormality, for example osteoporosis, osteomalacia, Paget's disease or metastatic tumour, the trauma or extra stress required to produce bone fracture may be minimal. This is called **pathological fracture**. The healing of a bone fracture is briefly outlined in Fig. 3.11 as an example of a specialised form of tissue repair.

Bone infection

Infections of the bone are now comparatively uncommon, although bacterial osteomyelitis, both pyogenic and tuberculous, were formerly important crippling diseases. Acute osteomyelitis (E-Fig. 22.4**G**) is caused by pyogenic bacteria such as *Staphylococcus aureus* (Fig. 22.1). This usually occurs in infants and young children, the bacteria gaining access to the marrow cavity via the bloodstream. It may also follow penetrating trauma in people of any age, for example after compound (open) fracture. Pathologically, acute osteomyelitis represents abscess formation in the medullary space of the bone, but the course of the disease in bone is complicated by two factors. First, increased pressure in the confined space causes infarction of further large areas of bone. Second, masses of dead bone *(sequestra)* behave as foreign bodies, inhibiting normal repair processes and providing a haven for bacteria that is inaccessible to body defence mechanisms. Chronic osteomyelitis (E-Fig. 22.5**G**) may follow if treatment is delayed or inadequate. Tuberculous osteomyelitis is illustrated in Fig. 5.7.

Metabolic bone disease

Osteoporosis (osteopenia) is a condition in which total bone mass is decreased due to reduction in the number or size of bone trabeculae (usually both) and thinning of cortical bone. Despite this, the bone otherwise appears structurally normal. In contrast, *osteomalacia* is a disease in which osteoid fails to undergo normal mineralisation, usually because of deficiency of vitamin D, although other causes of total body calcium depletion may also be responsible. *Rickets* is the childhood equivalent of osteomalacia. The appearances of normal bone, osteoporosis and osteomalacia are compared in Fig. 22.2.

Paget's disease of bone (Fig. 22.3) is a condition of unknown aetiology that occurs in the elderly. It is characterised by haphazard and inappropriate osteoclastic erosion of formed bone and concurrent, haphazard osteoblastic deposition of new bone. *Hyperparathyroidism*, due to excessive secretion of parathyroid hormone by a parathyroid adenoma or parathyroid hyperplasia, may cause rather similar haphazard osteoclastic erosion of bone.

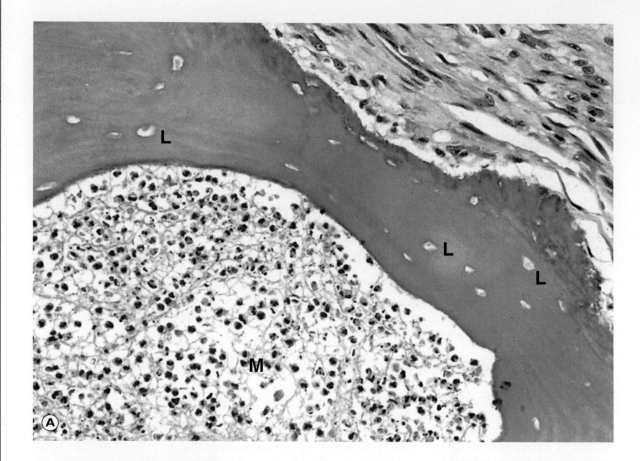

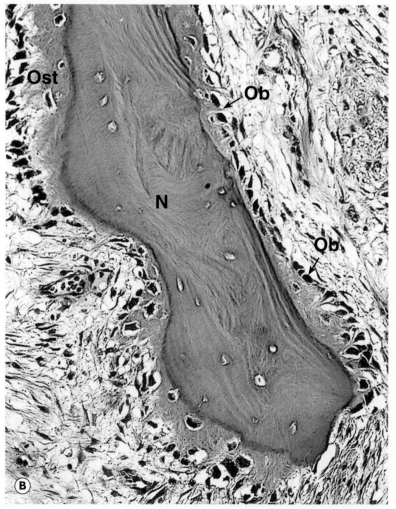

Fig. 22.1 Osteomyelitis. **(A)** (HP); **(B)** necrotic bone (HP).

Fig. 22.1A shows a high power view of acute purulent osteomyelitis in the amputated toe of a diabetic patient. There is an acute inflammatory reaction in the marrow space (**M**) at the lower left of the field, which is infiltrated by plentiful neutrophils within a fibrin meshwork. The bony trabecula is necrotic, with no viable osteocytes in the lacunae (**L**). In the upper right, the marrow is fibrotic, indicating ongoing repair.

In Fig. 22.1B, the process has progressed to a chronic phase with necrotic bone undergoing *remodelling*. The trabecula of necrotic bone (**N**) in the centre is surrounded by active osteoblasts (**Ob**), which are laying down new matrix or osteoid (**Ost**) on the outer surface of the dead bone. This newly formed, immature bone is termed *woven bone*, because of the haphazard arrangement of its collagen fibres. This is in contrast to the highly ordered arrangement of collagen in mature, lamellar bone. This difference can be demonstrated by viewing the specimen using polarised light.

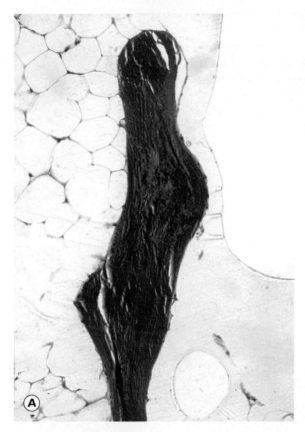

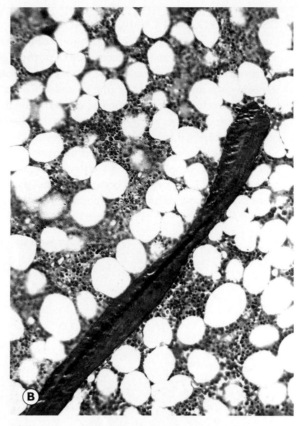

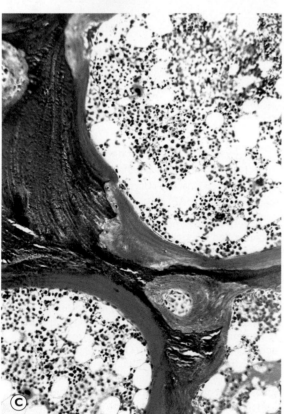

Fig. 22.2 **Osteoporosis and osteomalacia (undecalcified resin sections, Goldner's trichrome) (MP).** **(A)** Normal bone; **(B)** osteoporosis; **(C)** osteomalacia.

In the normal trabecular bone, shown in Fig. 22.2A, the entire trabecula is fully calcified (stained green by the Goldner's trichrome method).

Fig. 22.2B illustrates *osteoporosis*, in which the bone appears qualitatively normal but its mass is diminished, with the trabeculae being reduced in both number and size. Osteoporosis is extremely common in the elderly, especially in post-menopausal women, and is exacerbated by immobility (E-Fig. 22.6**G**). It may also occur in an isolated limb if it is immobilised for any reason. This is a form of *disuse atrophy*. Osteoporosis is also caused by some endocrine disorders and is particularly common with corticosteroid excess (see clinical box, 'Osteoporosis in clinical practice').

Fig. 22.2C shows *osteomalacia*. Here, the trabeculae are of normal or increased thickness, but there is deficient mineralisation so that each trabecula has a central core of calcified bone (stained green) coated by an outer shell of unmineralised osteoid (stained orange-red). Osteomalacia is usually the result of vitamin D deficiency. Vitamin D deficiency in the growing child (rickets) is pathologically identical to osteomalacia. It results in gross skeletal deformity by disruption of bone mineralisation at growth plates.

KEY TO FIGURE
L lacunae **M** marrow space **N** necrotic bone **Ob** osteoblasts **Ost** osteoid

OSTEOPOROSIS IN CLINICAL PRACTICE

Loss of bone mineral density is a common clinical problem that gives rise to considerable morbidity and mortality owing to the occurrence of *pathological fractures* through the weakened bones. Such fractures occur most often in post-menopausal women and typical sites of fracture include vertebrae, femoral neck and distal radius (the so-called *Colles' type fracture*). Such injuries can result in prolonged periods of reduced mobility, exacerbating the underlying problem of reduced bone mass.

Interventions focus on trying to reduce the risk of such fractures, as well as aiming to avoid subsequent immobility if fractures do occur. Prevention of osteoporosis requires a range of interventions, aimed at maximising bone mass by promoting weight-bearing exercise and good nutrition. In higher-risk patient groups, supplementation with calcium and vitamin D may be encouraged. Drugs such as *bisphosphonates* act by preventing bone resorption by osteoclasts, and are widely used in clinical management of osteoporosis and other metabolic bone disorders.

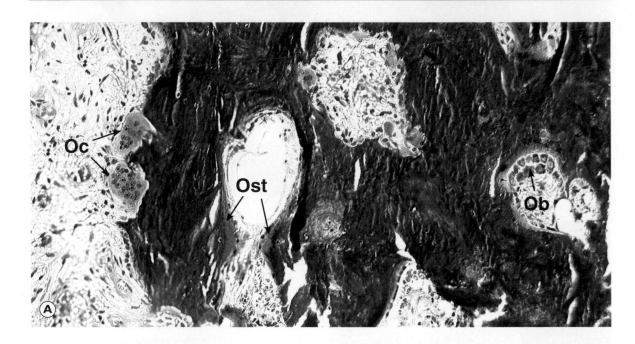

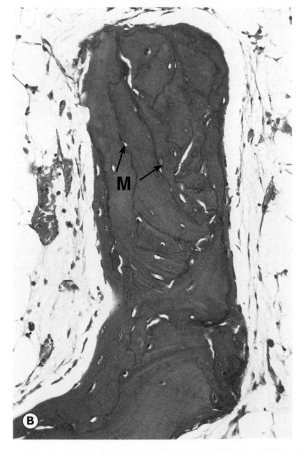

Fig. 22.3 **Paget's disease of bone (MP). (A)** Active osteolytic lesion (undecalcified resin section, Goldner's trichrome); **(B)** inactive sclerotic lesion (decalcified paraffin section, H&E).

In *Paget's disease of bone*, there is indiscriminate and uncontrolled osteoclastic erosion of bone followed by excessive osteoblastic activity, producing excess osteoid, which subsequently becomes mineralised, leading to irregular trabecular thickening. Fig. 22.3A shows abnormally large multinucleate osteoclasts **(Oc)** actively eroding a bone surface. Another trabecular surface shows a layer of newly deposited red-staining osteoid **(Ost)**, underlying rows of large active cuboidal osteoblasts **(Ob)**. This progressive, haphazard remodelling results in gross distortion of bone, often with marked thickening. The condition tends to be confined to a relatively small number of long bones, vertebrae or cranial bones, which may become inadequate to withstand functional stresses, leading to severe skeletal deformity, e.g. bowing of long bones (E-Fig. 22.7**G**), or pathological fracture.

With time, disease activity slowly diminishes. The initially highly cellular bone becomes progressively sclerotic. Usually, the bone is left thicker than before, but paradoxically weaker because much of the former strong lamellar bone is replaced by weaker woven bone. The disruption of the optimum lamellar pattern can be readily viewed by polarising microscopy, and, in old lesions as in Fig. 22.3B, the limits of separate episodes of previous bone destruction and irregular new bone formation are marked by thin, dark mosaic lines **(M)**.

Bone is a frequent and important site of *haematogenous metastatic spread* of malignant epithelial tumours, particularly carcinomas of bronchus, breast, kidney, thyroid and prostate (see Fig. 16.14). Metastatic tumour deposits usually destroy bone trabeculae, although carcinoma of the prostate (see Fig. 19.10) sometimes stimulates excessive new bone formation, resulting in *osteosclerotic* rather than the more usual *osteolytic* deposits.

Primary tumours of bone are much less common. These may arise from any of the cell types found in bone. The essential features of the more important of these tumours are given in Table 22.1.

■ **Osteoid osteoma** is a benign but painful tumour of bone, which is illustrated in Fig. 22.4.

■ **Osteogenic sarcoma** or **osteosarcoma** is the most common malignant primary tumour of bone (Fig. 22.5). This occurs mainly in children and adolescents.

■ **Chondromas** (Fig. 22.6) are benign tumours of hyaline cartilage, which may arise either on the surface of bone or within the medullary cavity where they are known as *enchondromas.* These may rarely undergo malignant transformation.

■ **Chondrosarcomas** (Fig. 22.7) are malignant cartilage tumours that mainly arise in middle-aged and elderly individuals.

As discussed in Ch. 16, malignant tumours may also arise from the haematolymphoid cells of the bone marrow, for example myeloma, lymphoma, leukaemia, etc.

In addition to true bony neoplasms, there is a miscellaneous group of tumour-like lesions that are also found in bone. The main features of these lesions are presented in Table 22.2. The cartilage-capped *exostosis* or *osteochondroma* is the most common of these and is illustrated in Fig. 22.8.

Table 22.1 **Important primary tumours of bone.**

Name of tumour	Main pattern of cellular differentiation	Age and sex incidence	Common sites	Behaviour
Osteoid osteoma (Fig. 22.4)	Osteoblast	Adolescents, M>F	Long bones, lower limb	Benign, painful, osteosclerotic
Osteosarcoma (Osteogenic sarcoma) (Fig. 22.5)	Primitive osteoblast	Mainly adolescent Elderly, M>F	Around knee Sites of Paget's	Highly malignant, metastasis to lungs
Chondroma (Enchondroma) (Fig. 22.6)	Chondrocyte	Common, any age	Hands and feet, long bones	Benign, very rare malignant change
Chondrosarcoma (Fig. 22.7)	Chondrocyte	Middle aged/elderly, M>F	Pelvis, ribs, vertebrae	Malignant, local spread and metastasis
Non-ossifying fibroma	Fibroblast	Mainly children and young adults	Long bones of lower limbs	Benign, osteolytic, may be multiple
Chondromyxoid fibroma	Uncertain	Young adults	Long bones, mainly tibia	Benign, osteolytic, may be painful
Giant cell tumour	Osteoclast	20–40 years, M>F	Long bones, mainly around knee	Benign, may recur locally
Chordoma	Notochord tissue	Middle aged/elderly, M>F	Sacrum, skull base	Locally aggressive bone destruction
Ewing's tumour (Fig. 7.6B)	Uncertain	Children/adolescents, M>F	Shaft of long bones	Highly malignant, early metastases

KEY TO FIGURE
M mosaic lines   **Ob** osteoblast   **Oc** osteoclast   **Ost** osteoid

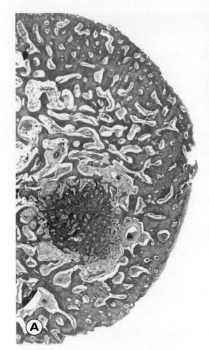

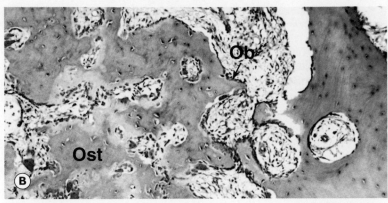

Fig. 22.4 **Osteoid osteoma. (B)** Osteoid osteoma in medullary cavity (LP); **(B)** histology of edge of lesion (MP).

Osteoid osteoma (E-Fig. 22.8**G**) is a benign tumour of osteoblasts that usually arises in the medullary cavity of the shaft of long bones, commonly the tibia or femur. Fig. 22.4A shows the typical low-power appearance of this benign tumour. Fig. 22.4B shows the edge of the lesion. There is a central *nidus* composed of partially mineralised osteoid **(Ost)** in irregular masses, surrounded by a rim of actively proliferating osteoblasts **(Ob)**.

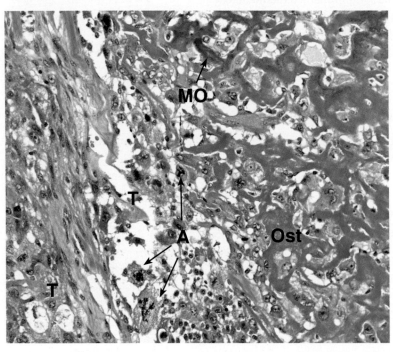

Fig. 22.5 **Osteogenic sarcoma (osteosarcoma) (HP).**

This relatively uncommon tumour is, nevertheless, the most frequently occurring primary malignant tumour of bone (E-Fig. 22.9**G**). Most cases occur in children and adolescents (usually around the knee), but it may occasionally occur in elderly patients with long-standing Paget's disease.

Histologically, there are highly pleomorphic tumour cells **(T)** and, towards the right of Fig. 22.5, these cells are producing irregular seams of delicate, pink-stained osteoid **(Ost)**. This osteoid is partly mineralised **(MO)**, producing a granular, purple appearance. There are several atypical mitotic figures **(A)** within this field.

These tumours are generally highly vascular and early bloodstream metastasis to the lungs is common.

SOME CLINICAL ASPECTS OF BONE TUMOURS

Primary malignant bone tumours occur mainly in children and adolescents and, traditionally, the prognosis has been extremely poor. In the past, surgical excision of the primary tumour mass was the mainstay of treatment and this normally required amputation of the affected part. With the development of newer chemotherapeutic agents, treatment and outcome in these cases has altered considerably.

Following initial biopsy for diagnosis and classification of the tumour, most patients are now treated with chemotherapy in the first instance and the tumour response is monitored closely by regular radiological imaging. After this, complete surgical excision of the residual tumour is undertaken. Amputation of limbs is avoided whenever possible by the use of new bone and/or joint prostheses, which can be surgically inserted to replace the affected parts of the skeleton, leaving surrounding tissues intact. This strategy of initial treatment with systemic chemotherapy has dramatically improved the outlook for children with malignant bone tumours.

KEY TO FIGURES
A atypical mitosis   **B** binucleate tumour cells   **C** chondrocytes   **H** hyaline matrix   **MO** mineralised osteoid   **Ob** osteoblast   **Ost** osteoid   **T** tumour

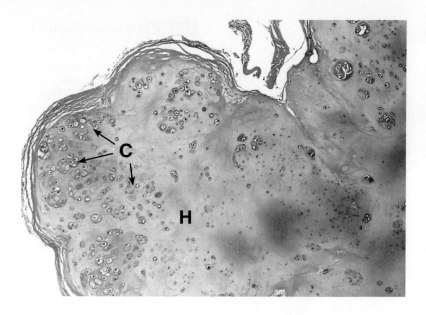

Fig. 22.6 Chondroma (LP).

Chondromas are composed of well circumscribed nodules of benign hyaline cartilage (E-Fig. 22.10**H**). The gross appearance is characteristic (E-Fig. 22.11**G**) with a semi-translucent, grey-blue appearance that is due to the hyaline matrix (**H**). The neoplastic chondrocytes (**C**) seen within the lacunae are benign, with no dysplastic features, and are embedded in a well-formed cartilage matrix. *Enchondromas* appear identical histologically, but occur within the medullary cavity of the bone. Multiple benign cartilaginous tumours occur in rare syndromes such as *multiple enchondromatosis* or *Ollier's disease*.

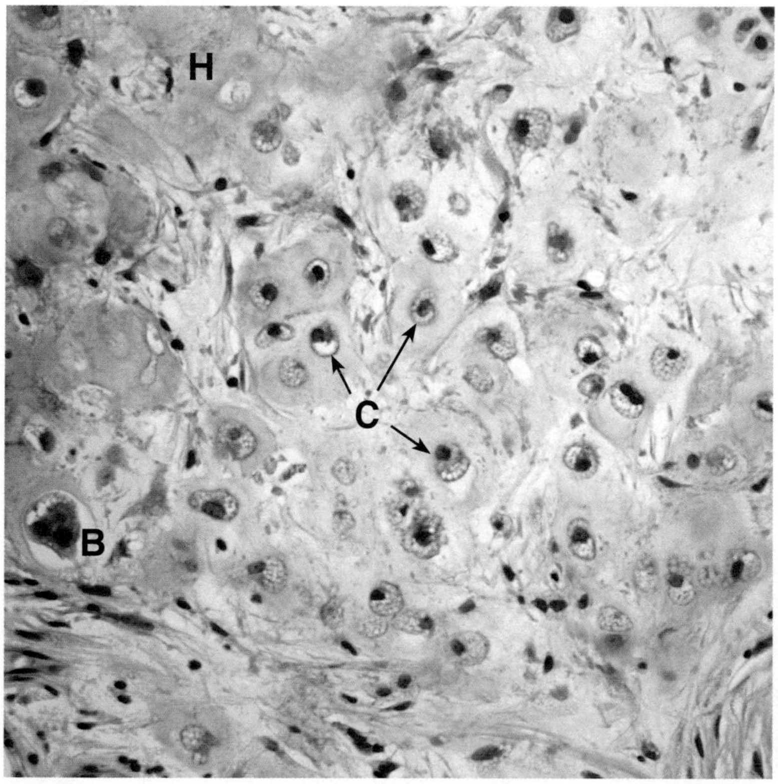

Fig. 22.7 Chondrosarcoma (HP).

Chondrosarcoma is a malignant cartilaginous tumour that usually arises in the axial skeleton in middle age and later (E-Fig. 22.12 **G**.) The tumours vary in their behaviour from indolent low-grade malignancy to very poorly differentiated and aggressive neoplasms with little obvious cartilage formation.

The tumour shown in Fig. 22.7 consists of nodules of pale hyaline matrix (**H**). Malignant chondrocytes (**C**) lie embedded within lacunae in the matrix. These cells differ from normal chondrocytes in that they are enlarged, atypical cells that may be binucleate (**B**) or show crowding of two or more cells in a single lacuna. Mitotic figures may be seen in higher-grade tumours. Well-differentiated chondrosarcoma may be difficult to differentiate from benign chondroma. Careful correlation with clinical and radiological findings is essential for diagnosis.

BASIC SYSTEMS PATHOLOGY ■ BONE AND SOFT TISSUES

Table 22.2 Tumour-like lesions of bone.

Name of lesion	Age and sex	Common sites	Behaviour
Osteochondroma (exostosis)	Children/adolescents, M>F	Upper tibia, lower fibula	Non-neoplastic outgrowth of bone and cartilage, possibly derived from growth plate.
Aneurysmal bone cyst	Children/adolescents, M>F	Long bones, spine	Reactive, cause unknown. Osteolytic, risk of fracture at site.
Fibrous dysplasia	Children/adolescents, M>F	Long bones, facial bones	Developmental abnormality, 20% involve multiple bones. Osteolytic, risk of fracture.
'Brown tumour' of hyperparathyroidism	Adults, M>F	Anywhere	Osteolytic, often multiple. Resemble giant cell tumour. Treat hyperparathyroidism.

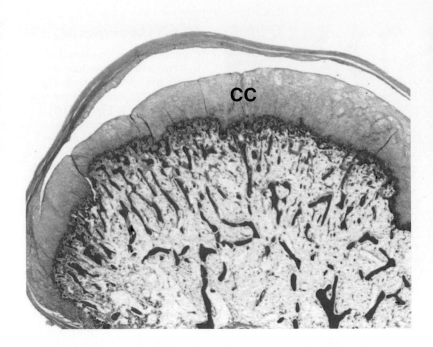

Fig. 22.8 **Osteochondroma (LP).**

Osteochondromas or *exostoses* are mushroom-shaped bony protuberances, with a cartilage cap **(CC)**, arising in the region of the epiphysis (E-Fig. 22.13**G**). It is thought that these may be derived from displacement of part of the growth plate.

Endochondral ossification takes place at the deep surface of the cartilage to form cortical bone **(B)**. The stalk of medullary bone is continuous with the medulla of the underlying bone, without intervening cortex.

Rarely, chondrosarcoma may arise in an osteochondroma. This is much more common in individuals with the syndrome *multiple hereditary exostoses*.

In Fig. 22.8, there has been artefactual separation of the perichondrium.

Diseases of the joints

The three most important disorders of joints are *osteoarthritis, gout* and *rheumatoid arthritis*. Osteoarthritis (Fig. 22.9) is the name given to the wear and tear degenerative changes that occur in some joints with increasing age. Gout is an inflammatory arthropathy caused by the deposition of urate crystals within the joints and soft tissues (illustrated in Fig. 22.10). Rheumatoid arthritis is a systemic chronic inflammatory disorder of autoimmune origin characterised by synovitis and arthritis (Fig. 22.11).

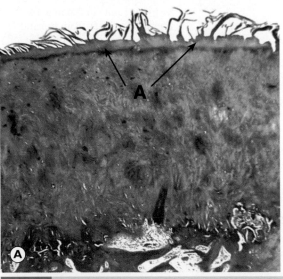
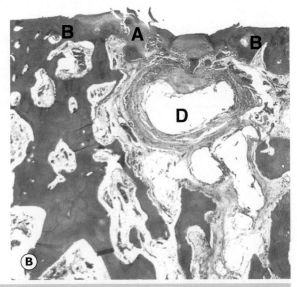

Fig. 22.9 **Osteoarthritis. (A)** Early changes (MP); **(B)** established lesion (LP).

Osteoarthritis is a degenerative disorder of articular cartilage as a result of excessive wear and tear. Secondary inflammatory changes occur in the soft tissue components of the joint.

In the earliest stages, the articular cartilage **(A)** loses its smooth appearance and develops surface fibrillations and flaking as shown in Fig. 22.9A. The damaged cartilage is progressively eroded until the underlying cortical bone **(B)** is exposed. After prolonged articulation of naked bone with the opposing surface, the bone becomes slightly thickened, hard, dense and highly polished, a process known

as *eburnation*. At the same time, there is irregular outgrowth of new bone *(osteophytes)* at the articular margins.

In the established case shown in Fig. 22.9B, only a small amount of articular cartilage **(A)** remains and the exposed bone **(B)** has undergone eburnation. The bone underlying the traumatised eburnated surface may undergo cystic degeneration **(D)**.

All of these changes lead to joint pain and progressive limitation of movement at the joint. The hips, knees and finger joints are most commonly and severely affected.

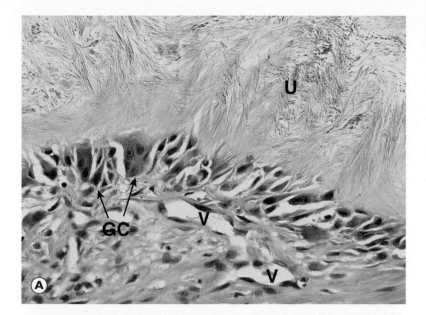

Fig. 22.10 **Gout. (A)** H&E (MP); **(B)** as above, viewed using plane polarised light.

Gout is an acute relapsing form of arthritis seen in individuals with *hyperuricaemia*. Gout is most often primary, i.e. of unknown cause; however, a small proportion of cases arise due to increased nucleic acid turnover, as in leukaemia or in patients with chronic renal disease who cannot excrete urate effectively.

Acute attacks of gout are precipitated by crystallisation of urate within joints, causing an acute inflammatory reaction. Over time, chronic arthritis may develop. The synovium becomes inflamed and fibrotic and this inflammatory mass or pannus may erode the underlying cartilage. *Gouty tophi* are deposits of crystalline material within the soft tissues. These have a similar histological appearance.

Fig. 22.10A shows a chronic granulomatous reaction to urate crystals. The needle-shaped crystals **(U)** occupy the upper part of the image and there is a surrounding band of reactive histiocytes, giant cells **(GC)** and organising granulation tissue with numerous small vessels **(V)**.

The optical properties of the crystals are useful in allowing easy microscopic identification. Urate crystals exhibit strong *negative birefringence* when viewed using plane polarised light, as illustrated in Fig. 22.10B. This concept is considered further below.

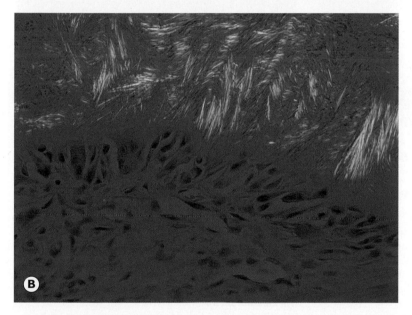

EXAMINATION OF SYNOVIAL FLUID

Joint pain is a fairly common symptom, but one that requires careful assessment. In particular, the rapid onset of severe pain in a single joint should be investigated immediately.

Gout can present in this way, as can another crystal arthritis called *pseudogout*, but acute pyogenic joint infection *(septic arthritis)* is a very important differential diagnosis since this requires urgent antibiotic treatment to prevent destruction of the joint. Other forms of arthritis, such as rheumatoid disease, tend to affect multiple joints *(polyarthropathy)*, but the initial presentation is sometimes with involvement of a single joint.

Clinical examination and initial investigations such as a full blood count should be followed by aspiration of synovial fluid from the joint. Immediate examination of this specimen can be helpful in guiding treatment. Fluid can also be submitted for microbiological culture in cases of suspected joint sepsis.

Normal synovial fluid is virtually acellular but, in acute pyogenic infection, it may be transformed into pus, consisting of numerous neutrophil polymorphs. Some neutrophils are also seen in cases of acute crystal arthropathy but here, polarisation reveals the presence of crystals. As illustrated above, uric acid forms fine, needle-shaped crystals that show strong *negative birefringence*. This term refers to the physical property of rotating polarised light in a particular direction as it passes through the specimen.

In contrast, *pseudogout* is caused by precipitation of calcium pyrophosphate crystals that are rhomboid in shape and show positive birefringence. This disorder tends to affect large joints such as the knees, often in elderly patients who are being treated with diuretic drugs.

KEY TO FIGURES
A articular surface **B** bone **CC** cartilage cap **D** cystic degeneration **GC** giant cell **U** urate crystals
V vessels

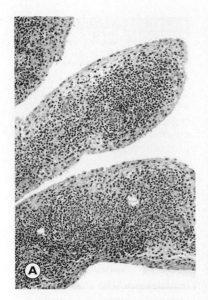

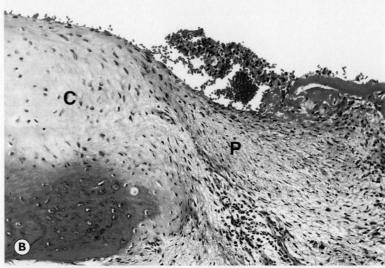

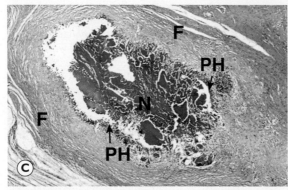

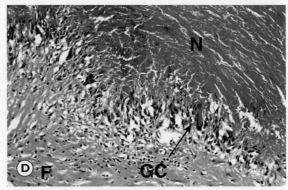

Fig. 22.11 **Rheumatoid arthritis. (A)** Synovium (MP); **(B)** articular cartilage (MP); **(C)** rheumatoid skin nodule (LP); **(D)** rheumatoid skin nodule (HP).

Rheumatoid arthritis is a systemic disorder, the predominant feature of which is chronic relapsing inflammation of articular joints, particularly the small joints of the hands. The disease affects both the synovium lining the joint capsule and the cartilage on the articular surfaces.

The earliest changes occur in the synovium, which becomes thickened, excessively vascular and thrown up into papillary folds as a result of oedema and infiltration by numerous lymphocytes and plasma cells. This is illustrated in Fig. 22.11A. This is accompanied by exudation of excess fluid into the joint space with precipitation of fibrin on the synovial surface.

The articular cartilage changes shown in Fig. 22.11B follow later and involve localised destruction of cartilage C and its replacement by fibrovascular granulation tissue known as *pannus* (P).

Initially, joint mobility is limited by pain and swelling, then later by gross cartilage and bone destruction and fibrous ankylosis across the joint space owing to fusion of granulation tissue pannus.

Rheumatoid nodules are found in the subcutaneous tissues, most commonly in individuals with seropositive rheumatoid arthritis, i.e. those who have *rheumatoid factor* in their serum. The nodules are usually found on the extensor surfaces of the limbs and, clinically, these are firm, non-tender and mobile. Rheumatoid nodules may also occur in almost any other tissue, for example lung and spleen.

The rheumatoid nodule shown at low power in Fig. 22.11C consists of a central core of necrosis (**N**), rimmed by a palisade of histiocytes and fibroblasts (**PH**), which is in turn surrounded by fibrous tissue (**F**) containing lymphocytes and plasma cells.

This *palisading* or lining up of histiocytes and fibroblasts is better appreciated at high magnification in Fig. 22.11D. An occasional giant cell (**GC**) can be identified. The rheumatoid nodule in fact represents a large granuloma with central necrosis.

KEY TO FIGURES
C cartilage   **F** fibrous tissue   **GC** giant cell   **N** necrosis   **NB** nerve branches   **P** pannus   **PH** palisading histiocytes

Soft tissue lesions

Many benign tumours and reactive tumour-like lesions commonly occur in soft tissue. Malignant soft tissue tumours *(sarcomas)* are rare and their diagnosis and classification form a highly specialist area of pathology. Here, we will illustrate some of the reactive lesions and benign tumours frequently encountered in clinical practice and also review the broad concepts of sarcoma pathology by consideration of a few specific tumour types.

Reactive processes and tumour-like lesions

Some soft tissue masses do not satisfy the usual criteria to be classified as true benign neoplasms and are considered to be *reactive* rather than *neoplastic*. These lesions may arise following a minor injury or in areas exposed to repetitive trauma, but such a history is not always obtained. The line between benign soft tissue tumours and reactive tumour-like lesions is not always clear and, in recent times, molecular evidence of clonality has begun to emerge for some of the entities conventionally considered to be reactive.

It is of great importance to note that some reactive soft tissue lesions may be very rapidly growing, causing clinical suspicion of malignancy. Such lesions may also appear alarming histologically, showing active proliferation with numerous mitotic figures. This possibility must always be considered before suggesting a diagnosis of soft tissue sarcoma.

A large number of soft tissue masses fall into this broad group, but the majority are encountered only rarely in clinical practice. A few of the more common lesions are considered here. The *traumatic* or *amputation neuroma* is a reactive mass that may form following damage to a peripheral nerve (Fig. 22.12). A *ganglion* is a fairly common lesion that is probably related to repeated minor damage around sites of excessive tendon and joint use, e.g. around the wrists and hands of pianists and typists (Fig. 22.13). *Giant cell tumour of tendon sheath* (also known as *nodular tenosynovitis*) also tends to occur around the hands and wrists (Fig. 22.14). As the name suggests, the nature of this lesion has been the subject of considerable debate and there is increasing evidence that it may be a true benign neoplasm.

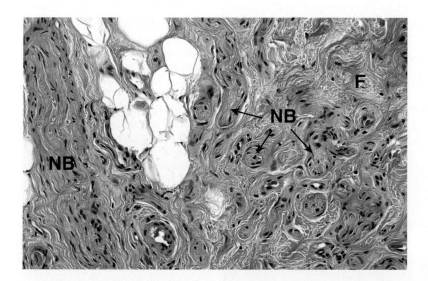

Fig. 22.12 **Traumatic neuroma.**

Traumatic neuroma typically arises following transection of a peripheral nerve, often at the time of amputation of a limb or digit. Histologically, there is a proliferation of tiny nerve branches **(NB)** within the fibrous connective tissue **(F)** of the scar.

The eponymously named *Morton's neuroma* is a similar lesion that arises on the foot from the plantar digital nerve, usually between the third and fourth toes. It is thought to be due to chronic, pressure-related nerve injury and may be exquisitely painful.

PSEUDOSARCOMA

Some reactive processes in soft tissue appear extremely alarming, both clinically and histologically, and may be described as *pseudosarcomas*. One example is *nodular fasciitis*. This typically presents as a very rapidly growing soft tissue swelling, appearing over the course of a few weeks. On close questioning, there may be a history of preceding trauma. The mass tends to be situated in the superficial fascia and usually has ill-defined margins (unlike most benign tumours, which tend to be encapsulated). Histologically, this is a proliferation of spindle cells, often with very numerous mitotic figures. There is a high risk of over-diagnosing malignancy in this setting and great care is required to recognise that this is a reactive process, rather than a sarcoma.

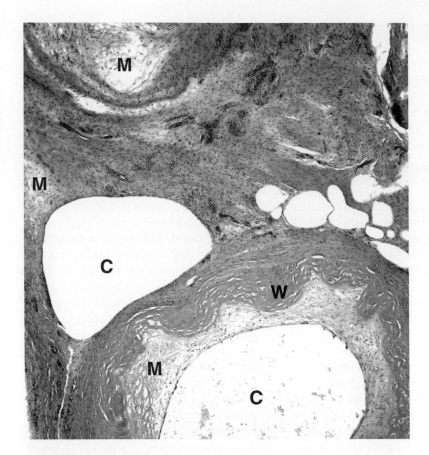

Fig. 22.13 Ganglion (LP).

Ganglia most commonly affect the hands and wrists, presenting as a firm and mobile mass in the vicinity of tendons and synovial joints (E-Fig. 22.14 **G**). The size of these lesions may fluctuate and, historically, treatment involved striking the affected part with a heavy book! This simple intervention often causes the lump to disappear by dispersing fluid contents, but most lesions recur over time and surgical excision provides a more definitive solution.

Histologically, there is usually a cystic space (**C**) with a fibrous wall (**W**) and no discernible lining (Fig. 22.13). Foci of myxoid change (**M**) are present in the surrounding connective tissue. Sometimes, the cystic spaces may be lined by histiocytic cells resembling synovial lining cells.

Most lesions appear to arise from the sheath of synovium, which invests the tendons, although some can be shown to connect with an adjacent synovial joint.

Fig. 22.14 Giant cell tumour of tendon sheath (nodular teno-synovitis). (A) LP; (C) HP.

Giant cell tumour of tendon sheath is a common lesion that typically occurs around the fingers. It is usually a firm nodule with a lobulated surface (E-Fig. 22.15**G**).

At low power in Fig. 22.14A, there is a proliferation of bland polygonal cells with eosinophilic cytoplasm, as well as a scattering of multinucleate, osteoclast-like giant cells (**GC**) (Fig. 22.14B). Some lesions show areas of haemosiderin (**H**) deposition within macrophages and collections of foamy macrophages (**FM**) containing lipid may also be prominent.

It is closely related to another soft tissue lesion with the highly descriptive name *pigmented villonodular synovitis*. This disorder usually affects the synovium of the knee joint and typically presents with swelling, joint pain and reduced joint mobility. Although the histological features are extremely similar, this process diffusely affects the joint and frequently recurs following treatment.

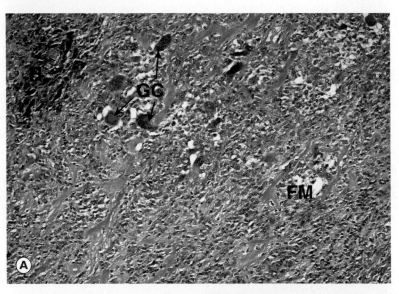
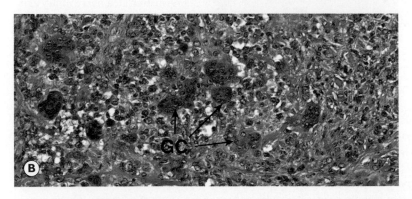

KEY TO FIGURES
C cystic space   **FM** foamy macrophages   **GC** giant cells   **H** haemosiderin   **M** myxoid change   **T** fibrin thrombus   **W** fibrous wall

One of the commonest of all soft tissue lesions is the *lipoma*, a benign tumour that resembles normal adipose tissue (Fig. 22.15). Other benign soft tissue tumours may show patterns of differentiation resembling smooth muscle (*leiomyoma*, see Figs 17.10 and 7.12), blood vessels (*haemangioma*, see Fig. 11.8, peripheral nerves (*Schwannoma*, see Fig. 23.15 and *neurofibroma,* see Fig. 23.16), striated muscle (*rhabdomyoma*) or fibrous tissue (*fibroma*).

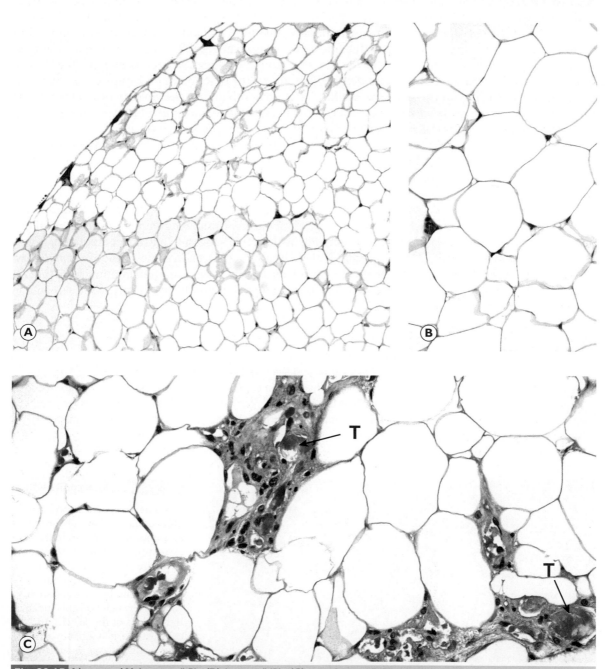

Fig. 22.15 **Lipoma.** **(A)** Lipoma (LP); **(B)** lipoma (HP); **(C)** angiolipoma (HP).

The lipoma is a very common tumour that usually occurs within the subcutaneous fatty tissue (E-Fig. 22.16**H**) of the trunk or limbs. They are soft, fairly well-defined lesions that are usually painless (E-Fig. 22.17**G**). Fig. 22.15A shows a low power view of a benign lipoma with a well-defined edge. The lesion is composed of sheets of uniform adipocytes. These cells have a very small nucleus, which is displaced to the periphery of the cell by a large globule of lipid, illustrated at higher magnification in Fig. 22.15B. In some patients, multiple tender lesions occur and, histologically, these differ from usual lipomas in that they contain multiple small blood vessels, some of which contain fibrin thrombi (**T**). These lesions are called *angiolipomas* and an example is shown in Fig. 22.15C.

Malignant tumours

Primary malignant tumours of soft tissue or *sarcomas* are rare and form a highly specialist area of practice. The approach to diagnosis is rather similar to that used in haematolymphoid pathology and typically requires careful correlation of the clinical and radiological findings with the histological appearance and pattern of immunohistochemical staining. Molecular studies may also be of value because many soft tissue tumours have characteristic non-random chromosomal rearrangements.

Classification of soft tissue tumours is complex and is currently based upon the *World Health Organization (WHO)* system. This uses a combination of clinical, histological, immunohistochemical and molecular features. In the past, sarcomas were often considered to arise from the tissue type that they resembled, e.g. *liposarcomas* were thought to develop due to malignant transformation of normal or benign adipose tissue. It is now accepted that most sarcomas do not arise from benign precursor lesions. Classification is therefore based upon the concept that tumour cells may *differentiate* so that they resemble normal tissues to a lesser or greater degree. This allows the description of groups of tumours that resemble tissues such as fat (*liposarcoma*, see Fig. 22.16), smooth muscle (*leiomyosarcoma*, illustrated in Fig. 7.6), striated muscle *(rhabdomyosarcoma)*, blood vessels (*angiosarcoma*, illustrated in Fig. 11.12), nerves *(malignant peripheral nerve sheath tumour)*, fibrous tissue *(fibrosarcoma)*, etc.

Some sarcomas lack any resemblance to normal tissues or structures but have sufficiently distinctive clinical, histological, immunohistochemical and molecular features to allow reliable identification. These are described within the WHO classification as *tumours of uncertain histogenesis*. The entity *synovial sarcoma*, despite its rather misleading name, is included within this group.

The term *undifferentiated sarcoma* is used for very aggressive and highly malignant tumours that do not resemble any normal tissues. By definition, these sarcomas show no immunohistochemical evidence of a particular pattern of differentiation and, as the name suggests, they are composed of highly pleomorphic malignant cells. An older term for these tumours still seen in some textbooks is *malignant fibrous histiocytoma*, based upon the supposed resemblance of the large and often multinucleate tumour cells to histiocytes. Pleomorphic sarcoma is one of the more common forms of soft tissue sarcoma in adults. An example is shown in Fig. 22.17.

SOME FEATURES OF SOFT TISSUE SARCOMAS
Soft tissue sarcomas occur over a wide age range and are one of the most common forms of malignancy in childhood. Benign soft tissue tumours usually occur in superficial sites whereas sarcomas are more likely to form deep-seated masses. Sarcomas are typically larger than benign tumours and, unlike carcinomas (which tend to spread through lymphatic channels to regional lymph nodes in the first instance), sarcomas typically metastasise via the bloodstream, giving rise to lung and bony metastases

---

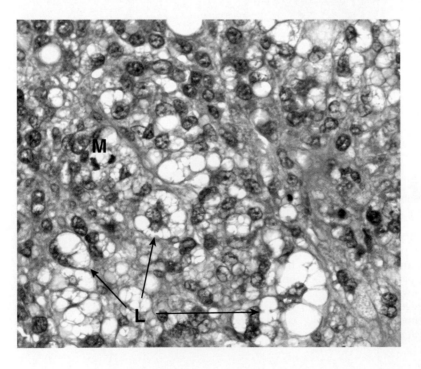

Fig. 22.16 Liposarcoma (HP).

Liposarcomas tend to occur in older adults and usually arise at deep soft tissue sites in the extremities or retroperitoneum. Most are characterised by the presence of *lipoblasts*, tumour cells with multiple cytoplasmic vacuoles, which typically indent the nucleus of the cell (**L**). In contrast, normal adipocytes have a single, large vacuole in the cytoplasm that displaces the nucleus to the periphery of the cell. This example is a pleomorphic tumour that includes many lipoblasts. There is evidence of mitotic activity (**M**). There are several different morphological subtypes of liposarcoma, including myxoid, well differentiated and dedifferentiated variants. In common with many other sarcomas, molecular methods are useful in diagnosis (see below).

MOLECULAR METHODS IN SARCOMA PATHOLOGY

Most malignant tumours, such as the common carcinomas, exhibit a wide range of genetic abnormalities, but these are rarely helpful in clinical diagnosis. In contrast, many soft tissue tumours exhibit highly characteristic non-random chromosomal rearrangements.

These are diagnostically useful in many cases and their recognition has also brought about advances in the understanding of tumour classification and in the development of some targeted drug therapies for the management of malignant disease (e.g. use of imatinib in treatment of gastrointestinal stromal tumours as discussed in Ch. 13).

Liposarcomas are interesting because molecular biology has contributed to the understanding of tumour classification. Myxoid liposarcomas typically exhibit a t(12;16) translocation, whilst well-differentiated and de-differentiated variants usually show evidence of a supernumerary giant ring or marker chromosome (formed of amplified genetic material from chromosome 12). If fresh tumour tissue is available, classical cytogenetic techniques can be used to demonstrate these abnormalities. Molecular methods have revealed that the area amplified on chromosome 12 typically includes the gene *MDM2* (important in regulation of cell cycle). This *MDM2* amplification can be detected using FISH techniques and the overexpressed protein can also be detected using immunohistochemical staining methods, which is helpful in routine diagnostic practice.

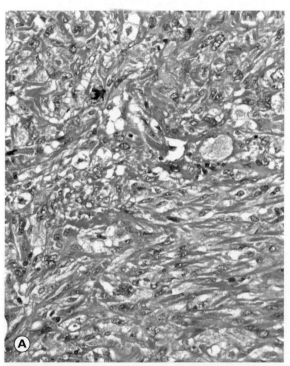

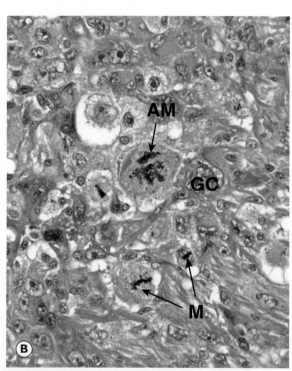

Fig. 22.17 **Undifferentiated pleomorphic sarcoma. (A)** MP; **(B)** HP.

Fig. 22.17A shows a highly pleomorphic tumour composed of plump, spindle-shaped cells and very large, histiocyte-like cells. There is no resemblance to any normal tissue.

At high magnification in Fig. 22.17B, the nuclei are large, irregular and have prominent nucleoli. Some giant cell forms are present **(GC)** and there are several mitotic figures **(M)**, including an atypical form **(AM)**.

In the past, the term 'malignant fibrous histiocytoma' was used to describe a large number of sarcomas with pleomorphic morphology and with no clear evidence of any specific pattern of differentiation. With increasing application of immunohistochemical and molecular techniques, many of these tumours can now be assigned to more specific diagnostic categories.

KEY TO FIGURES
AM atypical mitosis   **GC** tumour giant cells   **L** lipoblast   **M** mitotic figures

Table 22.3 Chapter review.

Disorder	Main features	Figure
Non-neoplastic bone disorders		
Fracture	Common following trauma. Specialised form of repair with callus. Pathological fracture occurs through bone weakened by disease.	3.11
Osteomyelitis	Pyogenic organisms such as *Staphylococcus aureus*, TB now rare. Haematogenous spread or after penetrating injury, e.g. open fracture. Sequestrum of dead bone inhibits resolution.	22.1
Osteoporosis	Reduction in bone mass. Qualitatively normal bone mineralisation. Common cause of pathological fracture in postmenopausal women.	22.2B
Osteomalacia/rickets	Incomplete mineralisation of normal sized trabeculae. Due to vitamin D deficiency. Called rickets in children and associated with deformity.	22.2C
Paget's disease of bone	Uncontrolled osteoblastic and osteoclastic activity. Thickened but weakened bone. Mosaic cement lines. Risk secondary osteosarcoma.	22.3
Benign and tumour-like lesions of bone		
Osteochondroma (exostosis)	Non-neoplastic outgrowth of bone with cartilage cap at epiphysis. Hereditary form with multiple lesions. Small risk of chondrosarcoma.	22.8
Osteoid osteoma	Benign bone-forming tumour in medullary cavity of long bones. Central nidus. Typically painful and relieved by aspirin.	22.4
Chondroma (enchondroma)	Benign cartilage-forming tumour. Enchondroma in medullary cavity. Rare syndromes with multiple lesions, e.g. Ollier's disease.	22.6
Malignant bone tumours		
Metastatic carcinoma	Commonest form of malignant tumour in bone. Typically from lung, breast, prostatic, renal and thyroid carcinomas. Usually lytic on X-ray examination.	16.14
Osteosarcoma	Malignant bone-forming tumour. Children/adolescents or secondary to Paget's in elderly. Long bones, early haematogenous spread.	22.5
Chondrosarcoma	Malignant cartilage-forming tumour. Axial skeleton, usually older adults.	22.7
Ewing's sarcoma	Small round blue cell tumour. Usually children, typically shaft of long bones. Highly aggressive behaviour.	7.6B
Joint disease		
Osteoarthritis	Common degenerative disease. Fibrillation of hyaline cartilage, eburnation, subchondral cysts and osteophyte formation.	22.9
Gout	Crystal arthropathy. Deposition of uric acid crystals in synovial fluid and/or forming tophi. Needle-shaped, strong negative birefringence.	22.10
Pseudogout	Crystal arthropathy. Deposition of calcium pyrophosphate crystals in large joints. Rhomboid crystals, weak positive birefringence.	
Septic arthritis	Pyogenic and tuberculous types. Usually single acutely painful joint. Needs urgent antibiotic treatment to limit joint damage.	
Rheumatoid arthritis	Systemic inflammatory disease with symmetrical small joint polyarthropathy. Inflamed synovium, sometimes rheumatoid nodules.	22.11
Benign and reactive soft tissue lesions		
Traumatic neuroma (amputation neuroma)	Reactive proliferation of small nerve branches in scar following transaction of peripheral nerve. Morton's neuroma on foot similar.	22.12
Ganglion	Reactive cystic lesion, usually hands or wrists. Myxoid degeneration and cysts associated with tendon sheath or near joint.	22.13
Giant cell tumour of tendon sheath (nodular tenosynovitis)	Common, typically fingers. Localised firm nodule. Mixture of giant cells and mononuclear cells with haemosiderin and foamy histiocytes.	22.14
Pigmented villonodular synovitis	Similar to giant cell tumour but diffusely affects single joint. Commonly knee, often locally recurrent after treatment.	Like 22.14
Lipoma	Common benign tumour of fat. Soft swelling, usually in subcutaneous tissues. Mature adipose tissue.	22.15A
Angiolipoma	Similar to lipoma but often painful due to small, capillary vessels with fibrin thrombi. Often multiple.	22.15B
Leiomyoma	Benign smooth muscle tumour. In skin, well-defined and derived from vessels (angioleiomyoma) or with irregular edge (from pilar muscle).	7.12 17.10

Table 22.3	Chapter review—cont'd.	
Disorder	**Main features**	**Figure**
Haemangioma	Benign proliferation of blood vessels. Common in skin. In liver, association with hormonal contraceptives. Capillary or cavernous sized channels.	11.8
Schwannoma	Benign tumour of Schwann cells. Encapsulated. Spindle-shaped cells with cellular Antoni A (nuclear palisading) and myxoid Antoni B areas.	23.15
Neurofibroma	Benign tumour of peripheral nerves. Ill-defined edges. Spindle cells. Multiple in von Recklinghausen's disease (neurofibromatosis).	23.16
Rhabdomyoma	Rare benign tumour of striated muscle. Cardiac rhabdomyomas typically occur in young children.	
Malignant soft tissue tumours		
Liposarcoma	Malignant fatty tumour. Adults, deep soft tissue sites. Lipoblasts typical. Various types. Molecular methods helpful.	22.16
Leiomyosarcoma	Malignant tumour of smooth muscle. Pleomorphic spindle-shaped cells with eosinophilic cytoplasm.	7.6
Angiosarcoma	Malignant tumour forming vessels. Aggressive behaviour. May complicate chronic lymphoedema or follow irradiation.	11.12
Malignant peripheral nerve sheath tumour	Malignant tumour derived from peripheral nerves. Association with neurofibromatosis.	
Fibrosarcoma	Malignant proliferation of fibroblasts. Typically, fascicles of spindle cells with 'herringbone' architecture.	
Synovial sarcoma	Sarcoma of uncertain histogenesis. Typical combination of spindle cells and epithelioid areas (biphasic). Cytogenetics shows t(X;18).	
Undifferentiated pleomorphic sarcoma	Pleomorphic, high grade tumour with no clear evidence of differentiation. Older adults, aggressive behaviour.	22.17

23 Nervous system

Introduction

Although, in common with any other organ system, the central nervous system (CNS) is susceptible to infection, trauma and the processes of infarction, inflammation and neoplasia, the anatomy and metabolic requirements of the CNS modify its response to common injurious agents and render it prone to unique pathological processes.

Tissues of the CNS

Neurones are the functional units of the nervous system (E-Fig. 23.1**H**). A typical neurone is composed of a cell body *(soma)* rich in rough endoplasmic reticulum *(Nissl substance)*, short afferent cell processes *(dendrites)* and a main efferent cell process (the *axon*). Except in development, neurones are not capable of replication and hence, once a neuronal cell body dies, regeneration is not possible. Damage to the axon with preservation of the soma can, however, be repaired by regeneration of the axon.

Specialised support cells (glial cells) are of four types: astrocytes, oligodendrocytes, microglia and ependymal cells. *Astrocytes*, (E-Fig. 23.2**H**) with their delicate cytoplasmic processes, form a 'fibrillary' supporting framework for neurons and other cells of the CNS, participate in maintenance of the blood–brain barrier and proliferate following damage. *Oligodendrocytes* form myelin sheaths around axons in the CNS (E-Fig. 23.3**H**). Their counterparts in the peripheral nervous system are the *Schwann cells*. *Microglia* (E-Fig. 23.4**H**) are cells with short processes and are the CNS equivalent of quiescent macrophages. *Ependymal cells* (E-Fig. 23.5**H**) provide a lining to the ventricles and central canal of the spinal cord.

Blood vessels in the brain have a specialised structure for maintenance of the *blood–brain barrier*. This limits transport and diffusion from the vascular compartment into the CNS. Connective tissues in the CNS are limited to the meninges (E-Fig. 23.6**H**), choroid plexuses and around blood vessels. The relative paucity of fibroblastic cells means that healing in the CNS is generally not marked by fibrous scarring. In the peripheral nervous system, connective tissue and associated blood vessels are found in association with individual axons *(endoneurium)*, bundles of axons *(perineurium)* and peripheral nerves *(epineurium)*.

Response of CNS tissues to injury

Neurones have a limited ability to survive significant changes in their metabolic or physical environment and are said to be *selectively vulnerable* compared to the more robust astrocytes or microglial cells. Neurones may undergo reversible cell damage, which is recognisable histologically by swelling of the cell body associated with loss of Nissl substance, a process termed *chromatolysis*. This process is particularly seen in the cell body of a neurone after damage to the axonal process. As discussed in Ch. 2, necrosis of brain tissue usually results in liquefaction, leaving a fluid-filled space.

Following injury or necrosis, healing through granulation tissue and fibrous scarring is an uncommon event in the CNS, a result of a relative lack of fibroblasts. Initially, there is an exudative response with activation of local microglia and recruitment of phagocytic monocytes to phagocytose dead tissue. This is followed by proliferation of astrocytes to form an *astrocytic scar*. This process is generally termed *gliosis* and is a common end product of damage to the specialised structures of the CNS. If there is extensive tissue necrosis, for example following infarction, the gliotic response is insufficient to repair the whole defect and a fluid-filled space lined by gliosis *(glia limitans)* remains.

Where healing through granulation tissue and collagenous fibrosis occurs, it is in relation to healing of inflammatory processes such as around a cerebral abscess. It also occurs in disease involving the meninges, such as acute bacterial meningitis and tuberculous meningitis (see Fig. 5.7) (E-Fig. 23.7**G**).

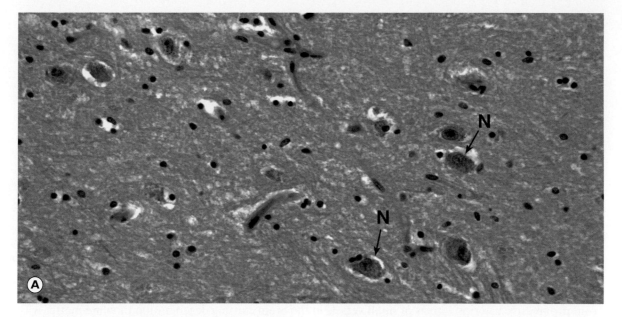

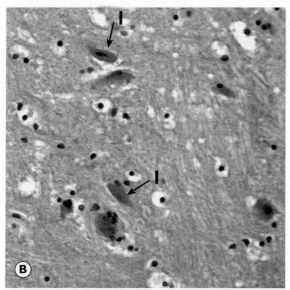

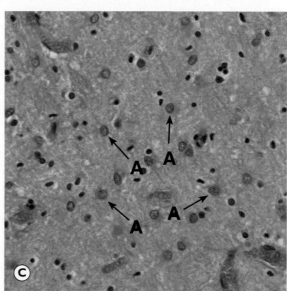

Fig. 23.1 **Neuronal death and astrocytic response. (A)** Normal (HP); **(B)** early hypoxic/ischaemic response (HP); **(C)** later response (HP).

Neurones are especially vulnerable to hypoxia such as may occur following cardiac or respiratory arrest. At an early stage, dead neurones become shrunken and eosinophilic with pyknosis of the nuclei. This change particularly affects large neurones and is shown in Fig. 23.1B where recently dead neurones **(I)** in the thalamus are present. Compare the neurones in this field with the normal neurones **(N)** in Fig. 23.1A of a normal thalamus. Note that surrounding cells such as oligodendrocytes and astrocytes are unaffected.

Following such damage, dead neurones will be removed by phagocytic cells and there is associated proliferation of astrocytes in the damaged area. This is seen in Fig. 23.1C, which is a similar area of the thalamus to that shown in Figs 23.1A and B, but subject to an episode of hypoxia several weeks earlier. No neurones are seen in this field where a large number of pink-stained astrocytes **(A)** are noted. This process, termed *gliosis*, is a common end result of damage to the central nervous system.

KEY TO FIGURES
A astrocyte   **I** ischaemic neurone   **N** normal neurone

Vascular disorders of the CNS

The brain is responsible for approximately 20% of total body oxygen consumption at rest. Under normal circumstances, cerebral blood flow is maintained through the process of *cerebral autoregulation* such that delivery of oxygen to the brain is not compromised. Where this process fails, the consequence is the *ischaemic cell process*, with decreasing vulnerability from neurones through glia to microglia and blood vessels. Hence, brief interruptions in blood flow are reflected in *selective neuronal necrosis*, whilst longer interruptions or cessation of flow result in *cerebral infarction* or *stroke*, a term used to describe the sudden onset of a persistent focal neurological deficit such as paralysis, disturbance of speech, coordination or sensation. The majority of strokes arise as a consequence of atheroma, thrombosis or embolism (Fig. 23.2). *Cerebral haemorrhage* is also an important cause of stroke and may arise following reperfusion of a vessel occluded by thrombus or through rupture of small intracerebral vessels.

Cerebral infarction may follow thrombosis of a cerebral artery, often superimposed on atheroma of cerebral vessels. This is commonly seen in the vertebrobasilar territory, resulting in brainstem infarction. Cerebral infarction may also result from occlusion of a vessel by embolus. Such emboli most commonly arise from complicated atheroma of the carotid arteries (usually at the bifurcation), from the left side of the heart (frequently from mural thrombus after myocardial infarction), from atrial thrombosis in atrial fibrillation or from thrombotic vegetations on the aortic or mitral valves. More insidious disease results from progressive arteriosclerosis of small vessels in the brain causing degeneration of white matter with small areas of micro-infarction in the cerebral cortex. This is a common cause of dementia (progressive intellectual deterioration) in the elderly and is termed *multi-infarct dementia*.

Primary intracerebral haemorrhage is most often a complication of hypertension (E-Fig. 23.8**G**). The muscular walls of small vessels in the brain are replaced by collagenous tissue, which leaves the vessels prone to rupture. Typically, hypertension related intracerebral haemorrhages occur in or around the basal ganglia. Where intracerebral haemorrhage arises elsewhere in the brain (lobar haematomas), other aetiologies should be considered. Accumulation of β-amyloid in the walls of small vessels in the superficial cerebral cortex and adjacent meninges, *cerebral amyloid angiopathy*, represents a further important pathology, which may predispose to intracerebral haemorrhage. Less common causes of primary intracerebral haemorrhage include congenital abnormalities of cerebral vessels forming *arteriovenous malformations*, saccular aneurysms, vasculitis and haemorrhage into primary or secondary brain tumours.

Intracranial haemorrhage may also occur from vessels outside the brain. *Subarachnoid haemorrhage* arises as a result of rupture of vessels in the subarachnoid space. The most common reason is rupture of a small aneurysm arising on one of the main cerebral arteries, descriptively termed a *saccular (berry) aneurysm* (see Fig. 11.4). *Subdural haemorrhage* results from bleeding from fragile veins, which traverse the subdural space. This most commonly occurs in the elderly as a result of trauma, which may be relatively trivial. *Extradural haemorrhage* (E-Fig. 23.9**G**) is a result of bleeding from arterial vessels outside the dura, a common complication of trauma to the head, especially with skull fracture. The middle meningeal vessels are most vulnerable.

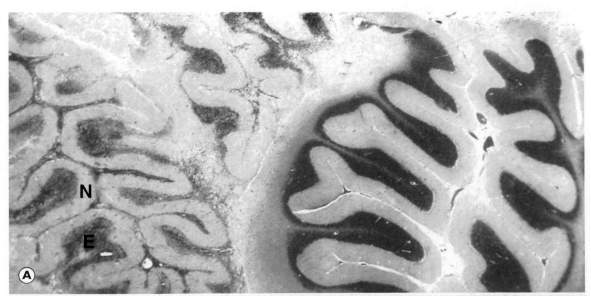

Fig. 23.2 Infarction. *(Caption opposite)*

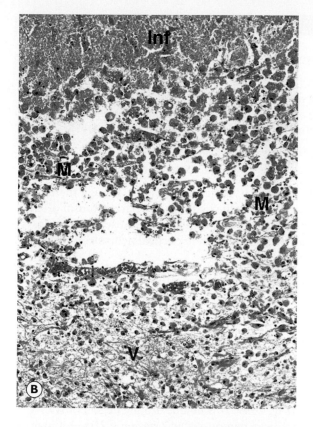

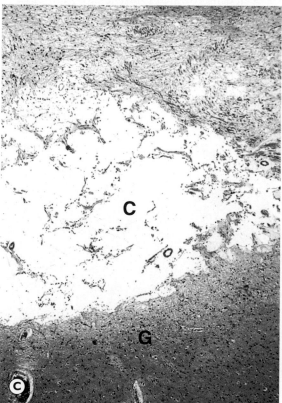

Fig. 23.2 **Infarction. (A)** Early infarct (LP); **(B)** later infarct (MP); **(C)** old (cystic) infarct (LP). (*Illustration* **(A)** *opposite*).

Fig. 23.2A–C illustrate histological features of cerebral infarction at a variety of stages in evolution.

The earliest histological manifestations involve neurones, which become shrunken, eosinophilic and exhibit nuclear pyknosis. These changes are detectable within hours of infarction and established by 6 to 12 hours. Typically, microscopic disruption of small capillary vessels with extravasation of red cells is also present at this stage. Unlike other tissues, in cerebral infarction a neutrophilic response is only transient and macrophage infiltration dominates the cellular reaction from about 2 days post-infarction. This is accompanied by proliferation of small vessels at the margin of the infarcted territory.

Macroscopically, cerebral infarcts can be either haemorrhagic or anaemic (pale) (E-Fig. 23.10**G**). The haemorrhagic pattern is thought to be a result of reperfusion of capillaries damaged by the initial ischaemic episode.

Fig. 23.2A illustrates an area of infarction in the cerebellum of a patient who died 2 days after infarction. The infarcted area on the left exhibits loss of basophilia because of necrosis (**N**) of the small neurones of the granular layer and extravasation of erythrocytes (**E**).

Following infarction, organisation and repair take place. The dead tissue becomes infiltrated by macrophages recruited from blood monocytes, which phagocytose lipid-rich myelin and take on a foamy appearance. By about 7 to 10 days post-infarction, the infarct has become liquefied and partly cystic.

Fig. 23.2B shows this phase in a cerebral infarct. The infarcted area (**Inf**) consists of a homogeneous mass of necrotic tissue with remnants of karyorrhectic nuclei. Surrounding this area is a zone of lipid-containing macrophages (**M**) and beyond this is a peripheral zone of proliferating astrocytes and blood vessels (**V**). Glial proliferation (*gliosis*) is the equivalent of granulation tissue in infarcts elsewhere in the body and is intended to fill the infarcted territory. The resulting glial scar is formed not of fibrous tissue but of the cell bodies and processes of astrocytes. This phase lasts up to 2 months post-infarction.

When an infarct is large, the process of gliosis does not completely fill the defect and a cyst-like cavity remains, lined by dense astrocytic tissue. Fig. 23.2C shows an old cystic infarct in the internal capsule with the central cavity (**C**) surrounded by glial tissue (**G**). There is no neuronal regeneration following a cerebral infarct. Some of the early clinical manifestations of cerebral infarction may be due to oedema occurring in relatively undamaged tissue at the margins of the infarcted territory. This oedema resolves and explains some of the clinical improvement that a patient may experience with time.

BASIC SYSTEMS PATHOLOGY ■ NERVOUS SYSTEM

KEY TO FIGURES
C cystic cavity   **E** erythrocytes   **G** glial tissue   **Inf** infarcted area   **M** macrophages   **N** necrosis
V proliferating astrocytes and blood vessels

Degenerative diseases of the CNS

Certain diseases of the CNS are characterised by progressive degeneration of neurones and/or white matter:

■ **Alzheimer's disease** is a common cause of irreversible cognitive impairment (dementia), mainly in the elderly. The aetiology is unknown, but there are distinct histological abnormalities (Fig. 23.3) that distinguish the condition from dementia with Lewy bodies and vascular dementia.

■ **Parkinson's disease** (Fig. 23.4) causes clinical features of tremor, slow movement and rigidity as a result of degeneration of nerve cells in the substantia nigra. The cause is unknown.

■ **Dementia with Lewy bodies** (Fig. 23.5) is clinically similar to Alzheimer's disease, though there are some key differences with fluctuating cognition, visual hallucinations and parkinsonism often encountered in this type of dementia. It has brainstem pathology identical to that seen in Parkinson's disease but, in addition, similar neuronal pathology is present in cortical neurones and serves as the substrate for cognitive impairment.

■ **Vascular dementia** typically manifests clinically with a stepwise deterioration in cognitive function and focal neurological signs. A number of possible pathologies may be encountered in association with vascular dementias, reflecting whether the disease involves small or large vessels.

■ **Motor neurone disease** is the result of specific degeneration of motor neurones in the cerebral cortex, brainstem and spinal cord. Cells degenerate over a period of a few years resulting in progressive denervation of muscle with insidious paralysis and death. The cause of this disease is unknown.

■ **Creutzfeldt-Jakob disease (CJD)** is a cause of rapid onset, progressive dementia resulting from extensive death of neurones in the cerebral cortex (Fig. 23.6). It is unique among degenerative diseases of the CNS in that a transmissible cause has been demonstrated *(variant CJD)* although poorly characterised. The infective agent, known as *prion protein*, is closely related to that which causes scrapie in sheep and bovine spongiform encephalopathy (BSE) in cattle.

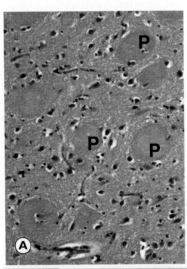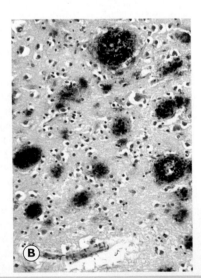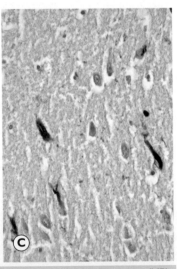

Fig. 23.3 **Alzheimer's disease. (A)** LP; **(B)** amyloid immunohistochemistry (LP); **(C)** tau immunohistochemistry (HP).

Alzheimer's disease (AD) is the commonest neurodegenerative disease, with an incidence that increases with age. The typical presentation is in the seventh decade with symptoms of memory failure, progressing steadily to involve motor skills, speech and sensation. The cause is unknown, although in a small proportion of cases a genetic association has been identified.

Macroscopically there may be striking thinning of gyri, particularly those of the frontal and temporal lobes. Histologically, plaques, neurofibrillary tangles and neuronal loss are identified. *Plaques* **(P)** are accumulations of a peptide *(amyloid)* and appear as amorphous, pink masses in the cortex (Fig. 23.3A) which may be revealed with immunohistochemistry (Fig. 23.3B). *Neurofibrillary tangles* appear as flame-shaped skeins formed by the abnormal accumulation of cytoskeletal filaments, in particular the microtubule associated protein tau, which can be demonstrated using immunohistochemical techniques, as in Fig. 23.3C.

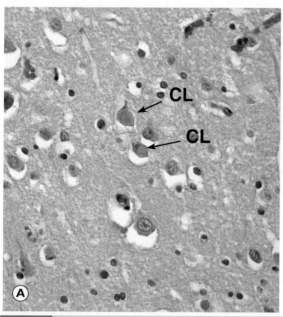

Fig. 23.4 **Parkinson's disease (HP).**

Parkinson's disease is caused by idiopathic destruction of neurones in the substantia nigra, resulting in loss of the neurotransmitter dopamine. Histologically, distinctive inclusions are seen in the remaining neurones.

The specimen from the substantia nigra of a patient with Parkinson's disease (Fig. 23.4) shows a typical neuromelanin-containing neurone within which is a *classical Lewy body* (**L**). These are rounded, pink-staining inclusions, often with a surrounding pale halo. These inclusions are composed of aggregates of the protein *alpha-synuclein* together with a number of other proteins.

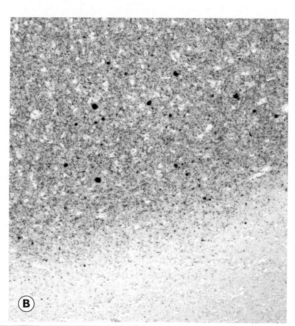

Fig. 23.5 **Dementia with Lewy bodies. (A)** HP; **(B)** alpha-synuclein immunohistochemistry (MP).

Dementia with Lewy bodies (DLB) is the second commonest neurodegenerative disease and shares clinical similarities with AD. However, in contrast to AD, patients with DLB often present with visual hallucinations, prominent fluctuations in cognition and parkinsonian motor symptoms, in particular rigidity and slowness of movement *(bradykinesia)*. Patients may also be highly sensitive to certain antipsychotic medications.

Macroscopically, there may be thinning of the gyri of the frontal and temporal lobes, perhaps not as marked as in AD. Pallor of the substantia nigra is typically present.

In contrast to the classical Lewy bodies of the substantia nigra, *cortical Lewy bodies* (**CL**) appear as ill-defined, pink, cytoplasmic inclusions, most readily identified in the neurones of the deeper layers of the temporal and frontal cortex (Fig. 23.5A). They are perhaps best demonstrated by immunohistochemistry for alpha-synuclein, as in Fig. 23.5B.

KEY TO FIGURES
CL cortical Lewy body   **L** classical Lewy body   **P** senile plaque

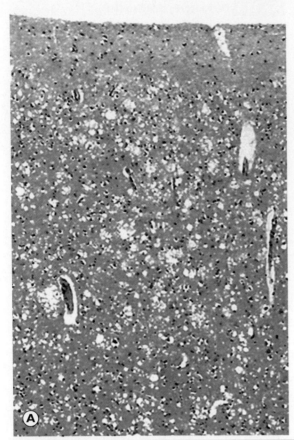

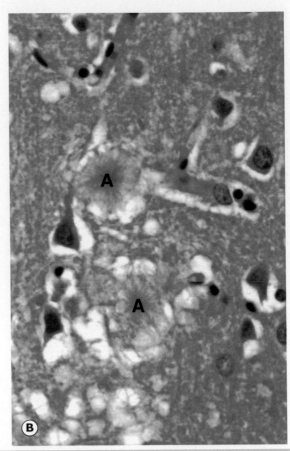

Fig. 23.6 **Prion diseases. (A)** Spongiform change in cerebral cortex (LP); **(B)** amyloid plaque in variant Creutzfeldt-Jakob disease (HP).

The prion diseases are also known as the *spongiform encephalopathies* and have a common molecular pathological basis. Prion diseases occur in several species in addition to man, the most notable being scrapie in sheep and BSE in cattle.

These diseases are biologically unique as they can be transmitted by a protein-only agent. Prion protein is a normal cellular protein associated with the cell membrane. In disease, the three-dimensional configuration of the protein becomes altered such that it aggregates in cells and is resistant to degradation. Importantly, it is believed that the abnormal configuration of the protein is able to bring about conversion of normal prion protein to a pathological form, such that disease can be transmitted.

Most human prion diseases occur sporadically *(sporadic Creutzfeldt-Jakob disease)*. They can, however, be transmitted by inoculation, both to other species and also from person to person iatrogenically by corneal transplantation, use of cadaveric dural grafts, neurosurgery with contaminated instruments and treatment with human growth hormone or gonadotrophins obtained from cadavers *(iatrogenic Creutzfeldt-Jakob disease)*. *Variant Creutzfeldt-Jakob disease (vCJD)* is believed to have been transmitted to humans from BSE-infected cattle through

consumption of contaminated beef. In addition, several human prion diseases can be inherited in an autosomal dominant fashion if there are mutations in the prion gene that give rise to an abnormal protein configuration *(Gerstmann-Sträussler-Scheinker syndrome* and *fatal familial insomnia)*. Importantly, protein derived from a genetic cause can transmit disease by inoculation.

In a healthcare setting, prion diseases represent a potential biological hazard, mainly from inoculation, and so autopsy and histological procedures have to be carried out to appropriate health and safety standards.

The main pathological changes seen in the nervous system are neuronal loss, vacuolation (termed *spongiform change)* and astrocytic gliosis. These features can be seen in Fig. 23.6A where the cerebral cortex shows loss of neurones and is largely replaced by rounded vacuoles. Astrocytic gliosis is best seen if special stains are used to detect astrocyte proliferation. In some cases, accumulated prion protein forms plaques of amyloid. This is particularly seen in vCJD as shown in Fig. 23.6B, where plaques of amyloid **(A)** are surrounded by spongiform change. In vCJD, but not other forms, prion protein accumulates in lymphoid tissues, such as tonsil, where it can be demonstrated using immunohistochemical techniques.

KEY TO FIGURES
A amyloid plaque

Infections of the CNS

Infections in the CNS may arise as a consequence of bacterial, viral or fungal agents and result in inflammatory processes, which may be divided into those involving the meninges *(meningitis)* or the CNS parenchyma *(encephalitis* in the brain; *myelitis* in the spinal cord). *Encephalomyelitis* and *meningo-encephalitis* describe conditions where a mixed pattern of involvement occurs.

Bacterial pathogens

Bacterial meningitis may be a severe life-threatening disease. Survivors are commonly left with brain damage. The common infective agents are the meningococcus (*Neisseria meningitidis*), the pneumococcus (*Streptococcus pneumoniae*) and *Haemophilus influenzae*.

Histologically, there is an acute, purulent, neutrophilic response in the meninges with secondary thrombosis of many of the blood vessels supplying the CNS. Treatment with antibiotics may allow recovery. However, healing may be complicated by fibrosis in the meninges.

In the majority of cases, CNS infections arise as a consequence of haematogenous spread. In the remaining, small proportion of cases, infection may arise as a complication of a surgical procedure (including lumbar puncture) or as a consequence of local spread such as from an infected air sinus.

Where there is impairment in cell-mediated immunity, such as encountered in AIDS, organ transplantation, chemotherapy or haematolymphoid malignancy, there is an increased incidence of tuberculous meningitis. Typically, this takes the form of *granulomatous meningitis* (see Fig. 5.7), though the cellular response may be minimal in situations of severe immunological compromise.

Viral pathogens

Viral meningitis is commonly due to an enterovirus and is rarely fatal. Typically, it results in a transient lymphocytic response in the meninges.

Encephalitis and myelitis are usually caused by viral infections, some having a particular propensity to affect specific types of neurone. In viral encephalitis or myelitis, there are three main histological features:

■ Focal neuronal loss and phagocytosis as a direct result of viral infection.

■ Lymphocytic 'cuffing' of vessels with increase in microglial cells; this is because of a local immune response.

■ Astrocytic reaction with increase in number and size of astrocytes in response to loss of neurones.

The commonest acute necrotising encephalitis is herpes simplex type 1 (HSV-1) infection. Typically, the history is one of fever, confusion, headache and frontotemporal localising signs. This latter feature reflects the preferential involvement of the frontal and temporal lobes, which can be detected as an asymmetrical imaging abnormality on CT scanning. HSV-1 causes a severe form of generalised encephalitis with extensive necrosis of brain tissue (Fig. 23.7).

In contrast, the polio virus tends to attack motor cells of the anterior horn of the spinal cord causing *poliomyelitis* and, for this reason, is termed a *neurotropic virus*. Rabies virus is also neurotropic and results in a meningo-encephalitis with virus inclusions visible in neuronal cells. Papovavirus infection of the CNS occurs in immunosuppressed patients and particularly affects oligodendroglial cells resulting in loss of myelin in white matter. The disease is termed *progressive multifocal leukoencephalopathy*. The human immunodeficiency virus (HIV-1), which causes AIDS, also affects the CNS and can result in *HIV encephalitis* (Fig. 23.8). Persistent viral infection of the brain occurs in some cases of measles virus and results in a chronic degeneration of nerve cells in a disease termed *subacute sclerosing panencephalitis*.

Fungal/protozoal pathogens

Fungal infections of the CNS are rare and mainly confined to immunosuppressed patients. The most common causative organisms are *Aspergillus*, *Rhizopus* (causes mucormycosis) and *Cryptococcus* species (see Fig. 5.18). Lesions usually take the form of abscesses.

BASIC SYSTEMS PATHOLOGY ■ NERVOUS SYSTEM

Brain abscesses

Typical cerebral abscesses may develop as a consequence of meningitis or may be the result of direct spread of infection from the skull (such as complicating middle ear infection) or of blood-borne spread from an infection elsewhere in the body, such as the lung. There is commonly a mixed infection including anaerobic organisms. Histologically, there is a pus-filled cavity walled off by fibrosis generated through granulation tissue derived from local blood vessels. Around this fibrous cavity wall, there is a reactive astrocytic response.

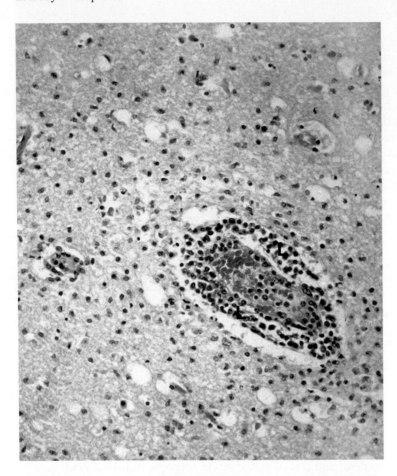

Fig. 23.7 Herpes simplex encephalitis (MP).

Viral encephalitis may be caused by *herpes simplex type 1*, the same virus that causes 'cold sores'. The virus spreads to involve the frontal lobes, limbic system and temporal lobes of the brain. The typical histological features of an encephalitis are seen, namely neuronal death, lymphocytic cuffing of vessels and astrocyte proliferation. There is, however, severe necrosis of the affected areas of brain, which become semi-liquid as macrophages phagocytose dead tissue.

Fig. 23.7 shows an area of cortex replaced by a mixture of macrophages and astrocytes with a small vessel cuffed by lymphocytes (**L**). Careful examination of tissue may reveal eosinophilic viral inclusion bodies in nuclei of remaining neurones. Immunohistochemistry tests can detect herpes viral antigen and are used diagnostically. Electron microscopy is another method used to detect the virus. Prompt treatment with antiviral drugs may halt progression of the disease. However, late presentation commonly results in death or severe neurological deficit.

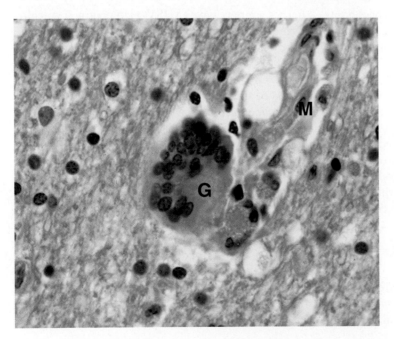

Fig. 23.8 HIV encephalitis (HP).

Neurological dysfunction is common in AIDS, including opportunistic infections, primary central nervous system lymphoma and direct or indirect effects of the HIV virus itself.

One such condition, *HIV encephalitis*, is shown in Fig. 23.8. The characteristic feature is inflammation of white matter with aggregates of mononuclear cells (**M**) and associated multinucleate giant cells (**G**). These are found throughout the central nervous system, usually close to a small blood vessel, and may be associated with foci of necrosis and reactive gliosis. Virus can be detected within cells in these areas. The clinical features are of insidious dementia, mood disorders and motor abnormalities.

KEY TO FIGURES
D demyelinated area   **G** multinucleate giant cell   **L** lymphocytes   **M** mononuclear cells   **W** white matter

Primary demyelinating diseases

Primary demyelinating diseases result in selective loss of myelin sheaths with (relative) preservation of axons. The commonest of these is ***multiple sclerosis (MS)***, where episodes of demyelination occur in multiple different sites in the CNS and at different times (i.e. separated in place and time). The typical lesions of MS are well-defined foci of demyelination, ***plaques***, distributed throughout the cerebral hemispheres, brainstem and spinal cord. It is postulated there is an abnormal immunological reaction, possibly triggered by a viral infection, resulting in focal myelin destruction.

There are three histological stages in the demyelinating process. First, during an acute episode, myelin breakdown occurs associated with lymphocyte and macrophage infiltration of the affected area, termed a plaque. At this stage there is clinical evidence of focal neurological dysfunction. Although the primary damage is against myelin, secondary damage to axons also occurs. In the second phase, astrocytes proliferate and gradually infiltrate the demyelinated area, which exhibits a continued lymphocytic infiltration. In the final phase of evolution of the plaque, cellularity is reduced, astrocytes shrink in size and the process becomes 'burnt out'. This is illustrated in Fig. 23.9.

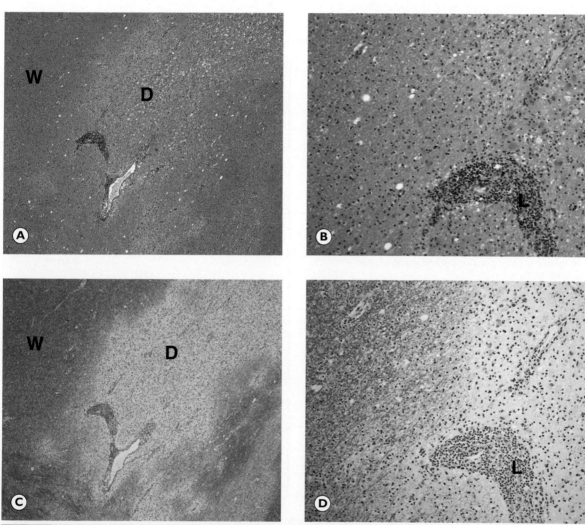

Fig. 23.9 **Multiple sclerosis. (A)** H&E (LP); **(B)** H&E (MP); **(C)** myelin stain (LP); **(D)** myelin stain (MP).

Figs 23.9A and B show the typical H&E appearance of demyelination. The pale-staining demyelinated area **(D)** is easily distinguished from the normal-staining white matter **(W)**. In the medium power image (Fig. 23.9B), the increase in cellularity in these regions is a result of macrophages and reactive astrocytes. Another typical feature is cuffing of small blood vessels by lymphocytes **(L)**. Figs 23.9C and D illustrate the same fields stained by a method to demonstrate myelin. Normal myelin stains dark blue, with areas of demyelination **(D)** appearing pale-stained. Note the well-defined boundary between demyelinated plaque and normal white matter.

Tumours of the CNS

Primary tumours of the CNS are uncommon, accounting for approximately 2% of cancer deaths in adults and 10% in children, although metastases to the brain from extracranial malignancies are, by contrast, relatively common. Despite their rarity, there are numerous different types of tumours arising from the CNS or its coverings with origins in *neuroepithelial tissue* (glia, neurones, embryonal tissues), meninges and lymphoid cells.

A unique system of classification and grading of tumours of the CNS exists that is regularly revised and updated (currently World Health Organization (WHO) 2016). The most recent update reflects the recent explosion in molecular knowledge of CNS tumours and integrates histological features (phenotype) with the results of specific molecular tests (genotype). Tumours are still graded on purely histological grounds from slow growing (*WHO grade I*), to rapidly growing and highly aggressive (*WHO grade IV*). However, molecular subtype is very important in some tumour types for prognostic information. The updated WHO classification contains a large number of entities but only some are considered in this chapter and an abridged classification is given in Table 23.1.

Over and above growth rate and tumour grade, any CNS tumour may exert harmful effects by growing into vital structures or by causing swelling of the brain around the tumour. Hence a small, WHO grade 1 (low grade) tumour may have serious consequences if it is located in or adjacent to the cardiorespiratory control centres of the brainstem.

Table 23.1 **Common examples of tumours of the CNS and its coverings.**

Tumour type	WHO grade	Tumour type	WHO grade
Diffuse astrocytic and oligodendroglial tumours (including molecular subtype)		**Embryonal tumours (including molecular subtype)**	
Diffuse astrocytoma: IDH1 mutant/wild type/NOS	II	Medulloblastoma (abbreviated genomic classification)	IV
Anaplastic astrocytoma: IDH1 mutant/wild type/NOS	III	• WNT activated (good prognosis) • SHH activated • Group 3 (poor prognosis) • Group 4	
Oligodendroglioma (IDH1 mutant and 1p 19q co-deleted / NOS)	II	**Neuronal and mixed glioneuronal tumours**	
Anaplastic oligodendroglioma (IDH1 mutant and 1p19q co-deleted/NOS)	III	Ganglioglioma	I or III
Glioblastoma (IDH1 mutant/wild type/NOS)	IV	Central neurocytoma	II
Oligoastrocytoma NOS	II	**Nerve sheath tumours**	
Anaplastic oligoastrocytoma NOS	III	Neurofibroma	I
Other astrocytic tumours		Schwannoma	I
Pilocytic astrocytoma	I	Malignant peripheral nerve sheath tumour	II, III or IV
Pilomyxoid astrocytoma	II	**Meningeal tumours**	
Ependymal tumours		Meningioma (various subtypes)	I
Ependymoma	II	Atypical meningioma	II
Anaplastic ependymoma	III	Anaplastic meningioma	III

MOLECULAR NEUROPATHOLOGY

CNS tumours are first assessed for histological features and graded accordingly. Following this, a number of specific molecular tests are employed depending on the histological type of tumour. Tests for diffuse gliomas are discussed in their relevant figures. In the new WHO classification, some molecular markers are an essential feature to diagnose a particular tumour type and essentially 'trump' histological features, e.g. a diagnosis of oligodendroglioma requires demonstration of both mutation of IDH1 (immunohistochemistry or sequencing) and co-deletion of chromosomal arms 1p and 19q (FISH). IDH1 also confers a better outcome in diffuse gliomas.

Particular molecular subtypes also give important prognostic information to better inform patients and provide options for more targeted therapies. For example, medulloblastoma is the commonest brain tumour in children, most often arising in the cerebellar vermis, and can show a variety of histological appearances. Recent genomic classification has shown four distinct molecular subtypes of medulloblastoma (Table 23.1) that allow stratification of tumours into prognostic categories and allow for more aggressive treatment of poor prognostic tumours. In the future, histological diagnosis of 'diffuse glioma' may be all that is required at light microscopy and molecular tests will provide the basis of further classification and treatment.

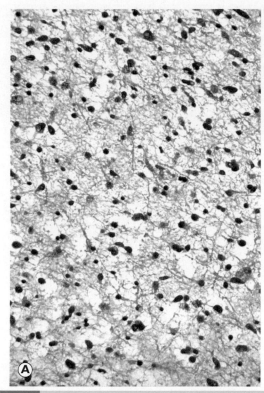
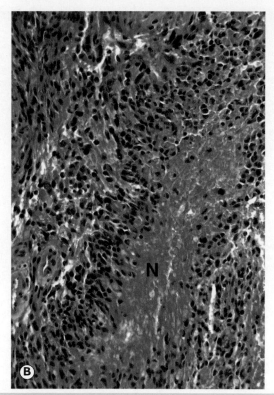

Fig. 23.10 **Tumours of glial origin. (A)** Diffuse astrocytoma (HP); **(B)** glioblastoma (MP).

Recent major revisions to the WHO classification has resulted in astrocytic and oligodendroglial tumours being grouped together, thus acknowledging their similarities as diffusely infiltrating gliomas with shared molecular characteristics, namely isocitrate dehydrogenase (IDH) mutations.

Astrocytomas may arise anywhere in the cerebral hemispheres, brainstem, cerebellum or spinal cord and can present in all age groups from young children to the elderly. They range from the low grade, slow growing and infiltrative *diffuse astrocytoma (WHO grade II)* to the high grade, aggressive, widely infiltrative *glioblastoma (WHO grade IV)*.

A *diffuse astrocytoma (WHO grade II)* is illustrated in Fig. 23.10A. Tumour cells have pink cytoplasm and fine cellular processes imparting a 'fibrillary' appearance to the background. Low-grade astrocytomas may show a degree of pleomorphism but do not contain vascular proliferation or necrosis.

Glioblastoma (WHO grade IV) is a tumour composed of highly atypical glial cells of varying sizes. As seen in Fig. 23.10B, these vary from small cells which exhibit little tendency to differentiation, to cells exhibiting astrocytic morphology to large, bizarre, giant tumour cells. Necrosis **(N)** is a typical feature of this type of tumour, together with high cellularity and vascular proliferation. These tumours have a very poor prognosis. Intermediate between diffuse astrocytomas and glioblastomas are astrocytomas, which exhibit cytological pleomorphism and readily identified mitotic activity. These are termed *anaplastic astrocytomas (WHO grade III)*.

Molecular subtyping of astrocytic tumours is largely based on the presence or absence of IDH mutations with intact chromosomal arms 1p and 19q. IDH mutations can be detected by sequencing or by immunohistochemical staining which detects the commonest IDH 1 mutation (R132H). IDH1 mutation occurs in the majority of diffuse astrocytomas such that, if it is absent, the diagnosis should be questioned. In glioblastoma, around 10% of tumours show IDH mutations, typically in a younger age group, and this is associated with better overall survival. It is thought that these tumours have arisen as a result of progression from lower grade gliomas.

The molecular subcategory 'Not Otherwise Specified' (NOS) is reserved for cases where molecular tests have not been performed or the results do not fit with the histological and clinical picture.

Management of astrocytomas is based on a balance of need for intervention, likely growth rate and risk of surgery. Surgical intervention in low grade gliomas is often delayed until symptoms are such that decompression of the tumour is indicated. Where possible, in the higher grade tumours, surgery to excise as much tumour as possible while preserving brain function is performed. This may then be followed by radiotherapy and, increasingly, chemotherapy.

The diagnosis of mixed tumours known as oligoastrocytomas is now discouraged as the majority of these can usually be placed in the astrocytoma or oligodendroglioma categories with the aid of molecular testing.

BASIC SYSTEMS PATHOLOGY ■ NERVOUS SYSTEM

KEY TO FIGURES
N Necrosis

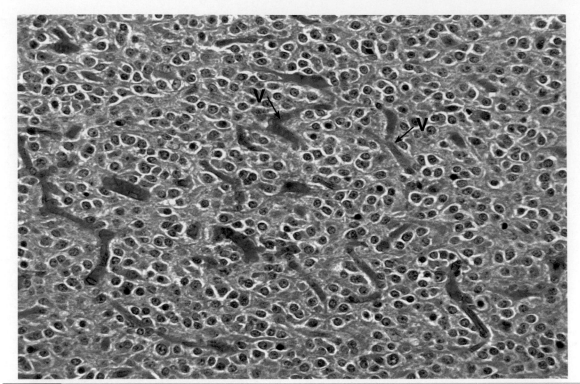

Fig. 23.11 Tumours of glial origin: oligodendroglioma (HP).

Oligodendrogliomas most commonly arise in the cerebral hemispheres, often in the frontal lobes, and are composed of cells resembling oligodendrocytes. The typical *oligodendroglioma (WHO grade II)* (Fig. 23.11) is composed of homogeneous sheets of cells with uniform rounded nuclei, clear cytoplasm forming a 'halo' around the nucleus sometimes referred to as a 'fried egg' appearance with a network of finely branching small blood vessels **(V)**. Microscopic foci of calcification are frequently seen. The presence of a high mitotic count, nuclear pleomorphism, necrosis and vascular proliferation may be associated with more aggressive behaviour. Tumours exhibiting such features are termed *anaplastic oligodendrogliomas (WHO grade III)*.

At a molecular level, oligodendrogliomas must harbour both IDH mutation and co-deletion of complete chromosome arms 1p and 19q to confirm the diagnosis. The latter can be detected by FISH testing.

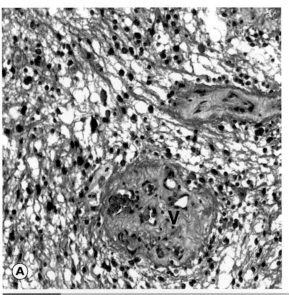

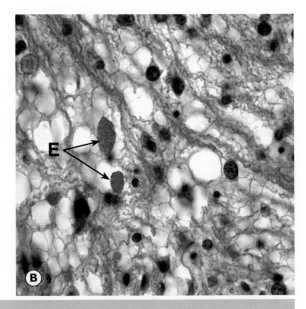

Fig. 23.12 Pilocytic astrocytoma. **(A)** MP; **(B)** HP.

Fig. 23.12A shows an example of a *pilocytic astrocytoma (WHO grade I)*. composed of mildly pleomorphic cells with round to spindle-shaped nuclei, fine, 'hair-like' cellular processes and typically thick-walled blood vessels **(V)**. At higher magnification in Fig. 23.12B another distinctive feature is readily appreciated, the *eosinophilic granular body* **(E)**.

Pilocytic astrocytomas most commonly present in children and young adults as cerebellar tumours, though they can occur at other sites, including the optic nerves where they are known as optic gliomas. They are associated with an excellent outcome and harbour a different molecular profile to the other diffuse glial tumours described above.

KEY TO FIGURES

E eosinophilic granular body   **P** perivascular pseudorosette   **Ps** psammoma body   **T** tubule
W cellular whorl   **V** blood vessel   **VP** vascular proliferation

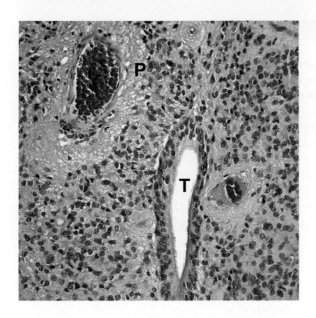

Fig. 23.13 Ependymoma (MP).

These tumours are derived from the ependymal cells that normally line the ventricular system. Histologically, the tumour cells are uniform and arranged around blood vessels, leaving a perivascular 'nuclear free zone' known as a *pseudorosette* (P). In addition, areas of tumour form epithelial tubules (T) that recapitulate the structure of the central canal of the spinal cord (Fig. 23.13).

Ependymomas are most commonly seen in the region of the fourth ventricle and are also the commonest intrinsic tumour of the spinal cord in childhood. Tumours range from low-grade lesions (WHO grade II) to high-grade, anaplastic ependymomas (WHO grade III). There is a propensity for the tumour to spread via CSF pathways, seeding the leptomeninges.

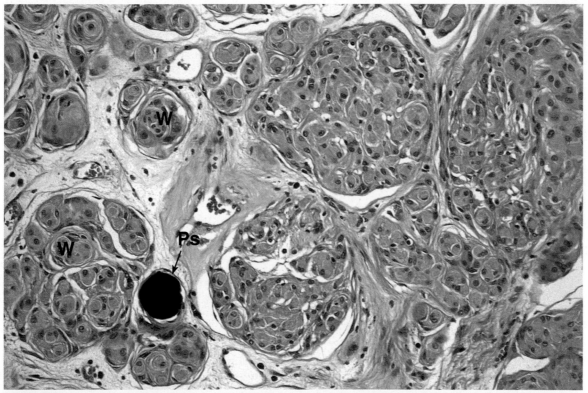

Fig. 23.14 Meningioma (MP).

Meningiomas (E-Fig. 23.11**G**) are thought to arise from arachnoidal cells of the meninges and are common tumours in adults. The tumours are nearly always low grade and produce symptoms by slow compression of underlying brain or spinal cord. There are several histological patterns of meningioma, varying from epithelioid cell lesions to spindle-cell lesions.

Fig. 23.14 illustrates a meningioma composed of epithelioid cells arranged in whorls (W).

At the centre of the whorls there may be circumscribed areas of laminated calcification termed *psammoma bodies* (Ps).

In general, mitotic figures are not common in meningiomas. However, occasional meningiomas show increased mitotic activity or brain invasion and are then termed *atypical meningiomas (WHO grade II)*. Such tumours are prone to local recurrence. Tumours with very high mitotic activity are rare and termed *anaplastic meningiomas (WHO grade III)*.

Disorders of peripheral nerves

Diseases of the peripheral nerves *(peripheral neuropathies)* result in abnormal motor or sensory function in the territory of the affected nerve. There are two main patterns of disease. *Axonal neuropathies* are due to primary damage to axons, while *demyelinating neuropathies* are a result of primary damage to Schwann cells and the myelin sheaths they form.

Generalised peripheral neuropathies may be found in association with a variety of diseases, such as diabetes mellitus, lead poisoning, alcoholism, uraemia and some malignancies. Several specific peripheral neuropathy syndromes are associated with segmental loss of myelin. These include *post-infectious polyneuropathy (Guillain–Barré syndrome)* and a large group of *hereditary sensorimotor neuropathies*. Axonal degeneration underlies other causes of peripheral neuropathy, for example those due to toxins, trauma or ischaemia. As a worldwide problem, an important cause of peripheral nerve disease is leprosy (see Fig. 5.9) in which nerve trunks are infiltrated by large numbers of macrophages filled with *Mycobacterium leprae,* with resulting loss of nerve fibres.

Tumours of peripheral nerve are common and are derived from Schwann cells (the cells forming peripheral myelin sheaths), fibroblasts and perineural cells. Examples are shown in Figs 23.15 and 23.16.

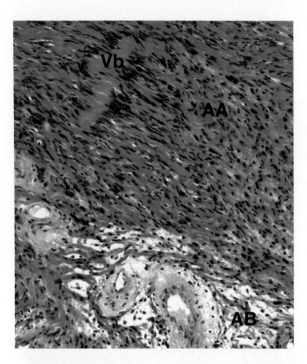

Fig. 23.15 Schwannoma (MP).

These tumours, derived from Schwann cells, typically arise in peripheral nerves and are usually solitary, rounded tumours found in relation to nerve trunks. They are benign and usually slow growing.

Schwannomas arising from the eighth cranial nerve (occasionally referred to as *acoustic neuromas*) can be part of the syndrome of neurofibromatosis type 2 or may arise as solitary tumours.

Two patterns of growth are seen histologically (Fig. 23.15). Compact or *Antoni A* **(AA)** areas are composed of spindle cells with pink cytoplasm forming characteristic palisades, *Verocay bodies* **(Vb)**, while degeneration in the tumour results in loosely arranged vacuolated tumour areas termed *Antoni B* areas **(AB)**.

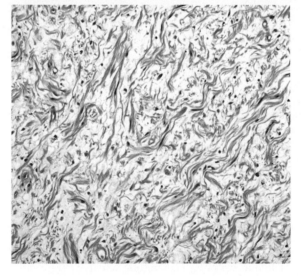

Fig. 23.16 Neurofibroma (HP).

Neurofibromas are tumours of peripheral nerves consisting of a mixture of cell types including Schwann cells, fibroblasts and perineural cells. They may be solitary but are frequently multiple, especially in the genetically determined disease *neurofibromatosis type 1* (NF1; von Recklinghausen's disease).

Histologically, the tumour is composed of loosely arranged spindle cells with varying amounts of intervening collagen (Fig. 23.16). A frequent feature is accumulation of connective tissue mucopolysaccharides resulting in a gelatinous or myxoid tumour. In contrast to Schwannomas, neurofibromas expand the nerve trunks in a diffuse manner. Neurofibromas are benign tumours.

However, malignant tumours arising from peripheral nerve or showing nerve sheath differentiation termed *malignant peripheral nerve sheath tumours (MPNST)* may be encountered, particularly in association with NF1.

KEY TO FIGURES
A atrophic fibres   **AA** Antoni A area   **AB** Antoni B area   **L** lymphoid infiltrate   **N** normal sized fibres   **P** phagocytosis   **Vb** Verocay body

Diseases of skeletal muscle present with weakness, wasting of muscle and/or pain, typically made worse by exercise. These symptoms and signs can be due to either primary disease of muscle *(myopathy)* or secondary to degeneration of or damage to the nerve supplying the muscle *(neurogenic)*. For this reason, muscle diseases are commonly considered together with diseases of the nervous system. Histology often provides the only satisfactory method of distinguishing between myopathic and neurogenic muscle diseases (Fig. 23.17). Myopathies can be acquired *(inflammatory* or *toxic)* or genetically determined *(dystrophies)*.

Inflammatory diseases of muscle are typified by muscle fibre inflammation and destruction. They may be subdivided according to whether the cause is unknown *(idiopathic)* or an infectious agent. A number of idiopathic inflammatory myopathies are thought to be associated with immunologically associated muscle damage. The commonest amongst these are *dermatomyositis*, *inclusion body myositis* and *polymyositis* (Fig. 23.18).

The dystrophies are characterised by degeneration and regeneration of muscle fibres resulting in progressive muscle wasting and weakness. There are several syndromes differing in age and sex incidence, time of onset and clinical course. Many are due to mutations in genes coding for structural proteins in muscle, such as the dystrophin protein producing either *Duchenne* or *Becker muscular dystrophy* (Fig. 23.19).

Mutations in either mitochondrial DNA or the nuclear DNA encoding mitochondrial proteins, whether inherited or acquired, can result in a number of heterogeneous syndromes with particular predilection for the heart, central nervous system and skeletal muscle *(mitochondrial myopathy*; Fig. 23.20).

A number of systemic disease processes may also be associated with muscle weakness and wasting, such as Cushing's disease, thyrotoxicosis and carcinomatosis.

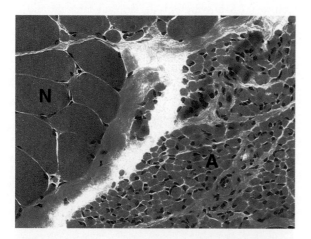

Fig. 23.17 Neurogenic muscular atrophy (HP).

Weakness and wasting of skeletal muscle may occur as a result of lower motor neurone damage rather than primary muscle disease. Histologically, neurogenic muscle atrophy affects groups of muscle fibres supplied by damaged motor neurones, in contrast to the haphazard pattern of atrophy seen in the muscular dystrophies.

In Fig. 23.17, normal-sized fibres (**N**) contrast sharply with a large group of atrophic fibres (**A**) from a denervated motor unit. This is an example of *spinal muscular atrophy* in which there is loss of spinal anterior horn cells. Similar changes are seen in a variety of peripheral nerve diseases.

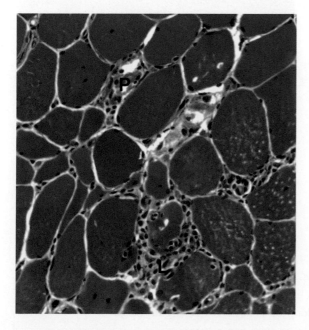

Fig. 23.18 Polymyositis (HP).

Patients with polymyositis present clinically with proximal muscle weakness and have an elevated serum creatine kinase level, reflecting ongoing muscle necrosis. As seen in this biopsy, the characteristic appearance is of necrosis of individual muscle fibres, a lymphoid infiltrate (**L**) and phagocytosis (**P**) of muscle fibre debris. The disease is believed to be autoimmune in origin and is usually treated by immunosuppression.

Dermatomyositis is another form of inflammatory myopathy with characteristic skin rashes and a strong association with systemic malignancy. The histology is similar to that of polymyositis, though with a preferential involvement of perifascicular fibres *(perifascicular atrophy)*.

Inclusion body myositis most commonly presents in the elderly with a steroid resistant, asymmetrical, often distal muscle weakness. The distinguishing feature on microscopy is the presence of cytoplasmic vacuoles, which may stain for Alzheimer associated proteins (e.g. amyloid β).

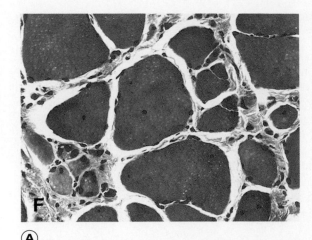

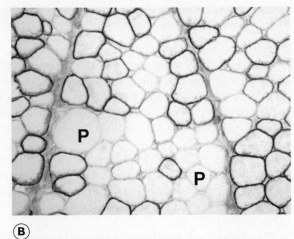

Fig. 23.19 **Muscular dystrophy. (A)** HP; **(B)** immunohistochemistry for dystrophin protein (LP).

Dystrophin protein has a role in connecting the cytoskeleton of muscle to the extracellular matrix. Mutations in the dystrophin gene, located in the Xp21 region, are responsible for the two most common forms of muscular dystrophy, *Duchenne (DMD)* and *Becker (BMD) muscular dystrophies*.

Histologically, there is destruction of muscle fibres with replacement of muscle by fibrous tissue **(F)**. Residual fibres exhibit a markedly abnormal variation in fibre size, with atrophy of some fibres and hypertrophy of others.

As the disease progresses, the muscle becomes virtually replaced by fibrosis and, later, adipose tissue.

This gives rise to apparent swelling of the affected muscles and accounts for the *pseudohypertrophy* of calf muscles seen in DMD affected children.

Immunohistochemistry can be used to reveal the pattern of staining with antibodies to dystrophin, which is normally ubiquitous on muscle fibres. As shown in Fig. 23.19B, in this case there is abnormal patchy and pale staining of many fibres **(P)**.

DMD manifests in early childhood, has a relentless course and results in death in early adult life. In contrast, BMD symptoms develop at a later age and the disease has a less aggressive course.

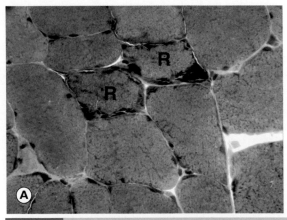

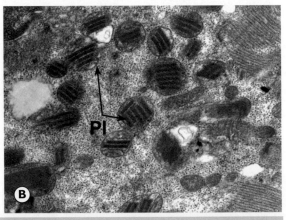

Fig. 23.20 **Mitochondrial myopathy. (A)** Gomori trichrome (HP); **(B)** electron microscopy of mitochondrial inclusions.

Mitochondrial myopathies may present in early adulthood with symptoms of muscle weakness, often involving proximal limb muscles and with prominent involvement of extra-ocular muscles. The muscle symptoms may form part of a complex of symptoms/signs including neurological symptoms and cardiomyopathy.

Morphologically, the most characteristic abnormality is aggregates of abnormal mitochondria, often in a subsarcolemmal location. These are

best appreciated using specialist muscle staining techniques. One such technique is illustrated in Fig. 23.19A where a section of skeletal muscle is stained with the Gomori trichrome stain. Here, abnormal accumulations of mitochondria appear as red-staining, subsarcolemmal deposits, with the affected fibres referred to as *ragged red fibres* **(R)**. Electron microscopy reveals mitochondria with abnormal crystalline inclusions often termed '*parking lot*' *inclusions* **(PI)**.

KEY TO FIGURES
F fibrous tissue   **P** patchy and pale fibres   **PI** 'parking lot' inclusions   **R** ragged red fibre

Table 23.2 **Chapter review.**

Disorder	Main features	Figure
Vascular disorders		
Selective vulnerability	Neurones more vulnerable to hypoxic/ischaemic injury than glial cells. Shrunken, eosinophilic neurones in early stages, followed by phagocytosis of dead neurones and astrocytic proliferation.	23.1
Infarction	Most a result of atheroma, thrombosis or embolism. Haemorrhagic or anaemic. Large infarcts heal with cavitation and gliosis.	23.2
Haemorrhage	Primary intracerebral haemorrhage most often a complication of hypertension. Other causes: cerebral amyloid angiopathy, vascular malformations, aneurysms, tumours. Other intracranial haemorrhages: extradural, subdural, subarachnoid.	
Degenerative diseases		
Alzheimer's disease	Most common cause of dementia. Unknown aetiology. Typically in elderly. Amyloid plaques and neurofibrillary tangles on microscopy.	23.3
Parkinson's disease	Idiopathic destruction of neurones in substantia nigra. Motor symptoms/signs. Inclusions (Lewy bodies) in surviving substantia nigra neurones.	23.4
Dementia with Lewy bodies	Common cause of dementia. May be history of visual hallucinations, fluctuating cognition and parkinsonian symptoms. Inclusions in cortical and nigral neurones.	23.5
Prion diseases	Transmissible via abnormal prion protein. Most common – sporadic Creutzfeldt-Jakob disease. Also iatrogenic, variant and familial forms. Neuronal loss, spongiform change and gliosis.	23.6
Infections		
Bacterial meningitis	Acute, purulent exudates in meninges. Most common organisms – meningococcus, pneumococcus, *Haemophilus influenzae*.	
Herpes simplex encephalitis	Most common acute necrotising encephalitis. Neuronal death, astrocyte proliferation, lymphocytes round blood vessels and necrosis.	23.7
HIV encephalitis	Inflammation of white matter with clusters of mononuclear cells and occasional multinucleated cells.	23.8
Demyelinating diseases		
Multiple sclerosis	Well-defined plaques of demyelination with relative preservation of neuronal elements and inflammatory cell response.	23.9
Tumours of CNS		
Astrocytoma	Graded on histological features from grade I (lowest grade) to grade IV (highest grade, most aggressive; glioblastoma). IDH1 mutation, 1p and 19q intact.	23.10
Oligodendroglioma	Typically sheets of cells with round nuclei and cleared cytoplasm, fine vessels and foci of calcification. IDH1 mutation, 1p19q co-deletion.	23.11
Ependymoma	From ependymal cells lining ventricles. Perivascular pseudorosette arrangements of tumour cells and epithelial tubules.	23.13
Meningioma	From arachnoidal cells of meninges. Cells arranged in whorls with some containing psammoma bodies.	23.14
Peripheral nerves		
Leprosy	Nerve trunks infiltrated by macrophages filled with *Mycobacterium leprae*, with resulting loss of nerve fibres.	5.9
Schwannoma	Derived from Schwann cells. Biphasic appearance with Antoni A (with occasional Verocay bodies) and Antoni B areas.	23.15
Neurofibroma	May be solitary or multiple in association with NF1. Loosely arranged spindle cells with intervening connective tissue.	23.16
Skeletal muscle		
Neurogenic atrophy	Result of damage to nerve innervating muscle. Clusters of atrophic fibres.	23.17
Polymyositis	Inflammatory infiltrate with necrosis and phagocytosis of muscle fibres.	23.18
Duchenne/Becker muscular dystrophy	Mutation of dystrophin gene on X chromosome. Muscle fibre destruction with replacement by fibrous tissue and wide variation in fibre size.	23.19
Mitochondrial myopathy	Aggregates of abnormal mitochondria with trichrome stain (ragged red fibres) and mitochondrial inclusions in electron microscopy preparations.	23.20

Appendix I – Notes on commonly used staining methods

Haematoxylin and Eosin (H&E)
This is the most commonly used stain in routine histopathology. Haematoxylin is a dye that stains acidic structures a purplish-blue and eosin is a dye that stains basic structures pinkish-red. In the mammalian cell, most of the acidic structures reside in the nucleus due to the presence of nuclear DNA, whereas most of the cytoplasmic structures are basic. Thus, nuclei stain purplish-blue and the cytoplasm stain a pinkish-red. If a cell's cytoplasm contains abundant RNA, the cytoplasm may have a purplish tint, e.g. in plasma cells.

The intensity of the staining by H&E depends upon many factors including the thickness of the tissue section and the formulation of the stain. The thickness of the section has the most impact upon the staining intensity as can be seen in some thicker, low power images throughout this text.

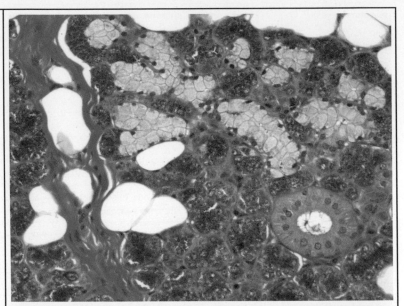

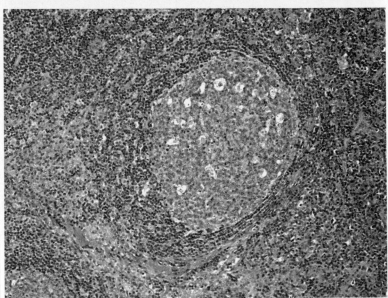

Periodic Acid-Schiff (PAS)
The periodic acid-Schiff (PAS) reaction demonstrates the presence of complex carbohydrates by staining them a deep magenta. PAS will stain pure complex carbohydrates such as glycogen but will also stain carbohydrates when they are bound to lipids and proteins.

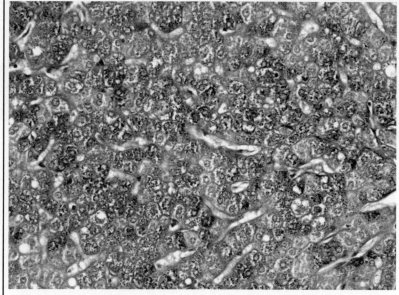

Diastase Periodic Acid-Schiff (D-PAS, PASD, PASF)
Many of these complex carbohydrate, lipid or protein compounds are present in basement membranes, fungal cell walls and some neutral mucin. In order to differentiate between the pure glycogen and these other compounds, glycogen can be eradicated in the tissue section by pre-treatment with the enzyme diastase (amylase).

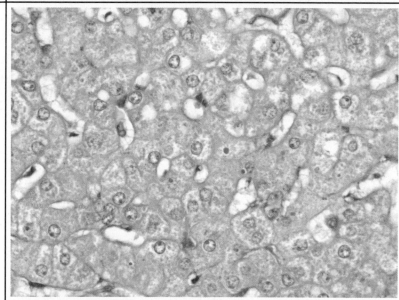

Alcian Blue (Acid Mucin)
Epithelial mucins are secreted by epithelial cells and may be acidic or neutral. Acidic mucins are present in goblet cells and oesophageal submucosal glands. Most adenocarcinomas elaborate acidic mucin. Alcian blue stains acidic mucin a vivid blue. On the other hand, neutral mucins, e.g. those present in gastric foveolar cells and prostate glands, are PAS positive.

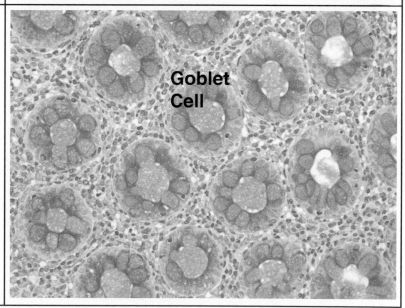

Goblet Cell

Masson Trichrome
This method uses a three-colour method to stain nuclei black, collagen blue and muscle red. It is used routinely in liver and kidney biopsies. It can also be used to demonstrate Reinke crystals in Leydig cell tumours.

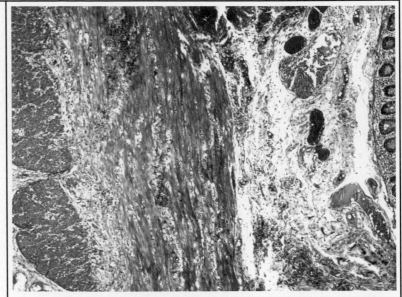

Martius Scarlet Blue (MSB)
This is another three-colour method that stains fibrin red, erythrocytes yellow and collagen blue. It is useful for the examination of thrombi in histological sections, particularly at autopsy.

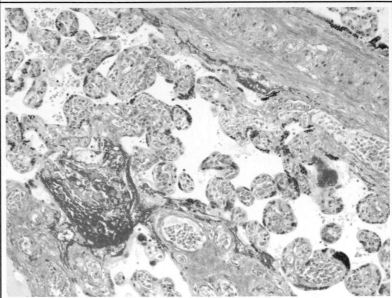

Miller's Elastic van Gieson (EVG)
This stains collagen red and elastic fibres black. It is particularly useful in staining the elastic laminae of arteries (black), the smooth muscle of the media (yellow) and collagenous tissue (red). It can also be used to assess for a breach in the visceral pleural elastic tissue in lung cancers.

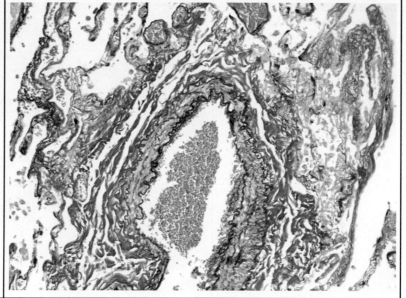

Miller's Elastic H&E (EHE)
This is another elastic stain where the elastic fibres stain dark blue. It is used for the assessment of venous invasion in colorectal cancers, an important factor in staging.

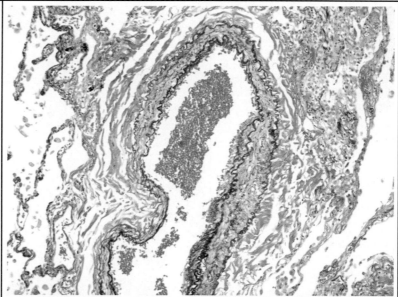

Phosphotungstic Acid Haematoxylin
This stain demonstrates muscle cross-striations. It may also be used to demonstrate the presence of mitochondria in oncocytic neoplasms.

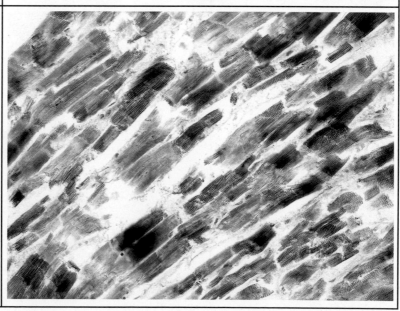

Gordon and Sweet's Reticulin
This is a silver-based stain that demonstrates reticulin fibres. It is particularly useful in the interpretation of liver architecture.

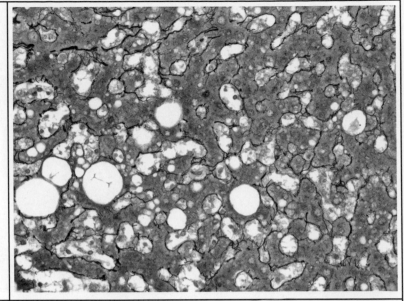

Congo Red and Sirius Red
These two dyes have a special affinity for proteins with a beta pleated sheet pattern, for example, amyloid. Amyloid stains red with both methods and shows apple-green birefringence on polarised light microscopy.

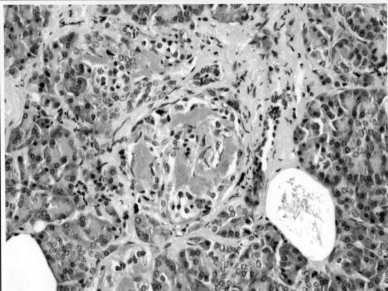

Gram Stain
This method is mainly used in smears of bacteria in diagnostic microbiology but can also be used in histological sections to show whether any bacteria are present and, if so, whether they are Gram-positive or Gram-negative.

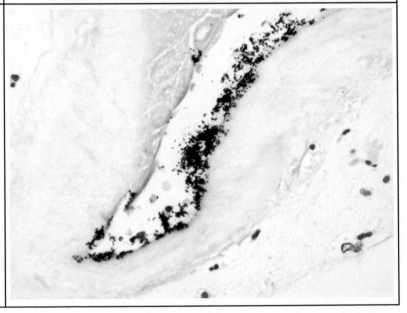

Perl's Stain

This is used to demonstrate the presence of ferric iron in tissues, usually at the site of old bleeding where the iron-containing pigment, haemosiderin (derived from local haemoglobin breakdown), accumulates. It can also be used to demonstrate accumulation of iron in various tissues in the primary iron storage disease haemochromatosis and can be used for the identification of asbestos bodies in tissue sections.

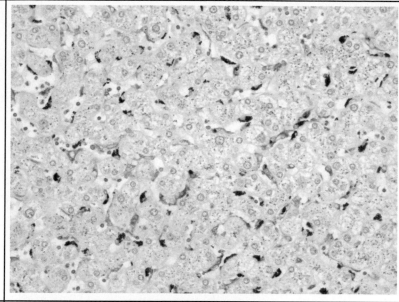

Masson Fontana

This stain is used to stain melanin and can be used in the diagnosis of malignant melanoma as well as some melanin-producing micro-organisms, e.g. *Cryptococcus*.

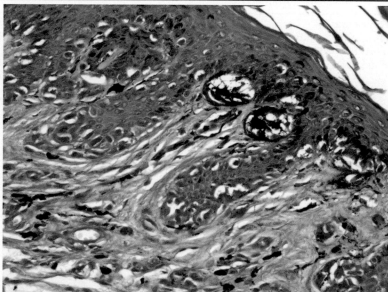

Wade-Fite

This stain is used for *Mycobacterium leprae* and atypical *Mycobacteria*.

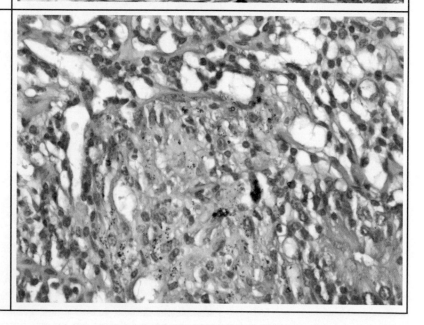

Ziehl–Neelsen

This stain can be used to demonstrate *Mycobacterium tuberculosis*. This bacterium possesses a protective capsule containing lipids that affects the rate at which dyes move into and out of the bacterium during staining. Two dyes are used: basic fuchsin mixed with phenol and methylene blue. The first dye (which is red) is forced into all the tissues in the section (including any *Mycobacteria*) by heating. The section is then exposed to acid and alcohol, which wash the red dye out of everything (except the *Mycobacteria*, which hold on to it because of the lipid capsule). All the other tissues are free to take up the contrasting blue dye, but the *Mycobacteria* remain red against a blue background.

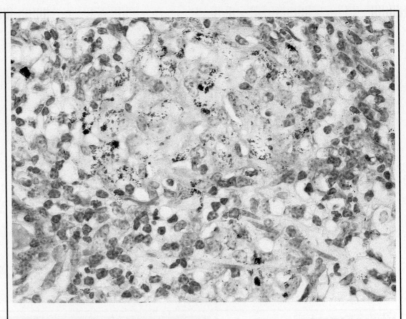

Von Kossa

This stains calcium deposits black. It can be used in the diagnosis of malakoplakia and in pseudogout.

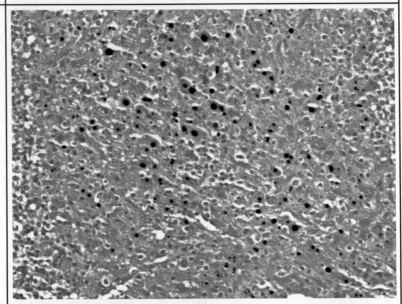

Cresyl Fast Violet

This modified stain is used to stain *Helicobacter pylori* organisms in gastric biopsies.

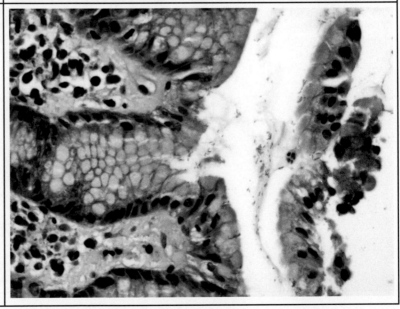

Appendix 2 – Glossary of pathological terms

Abscess – a localised collection of pus, formed from accumulation of dead and dying neutrophils and destruction of tissue

Acanthosis – an increase in the thickness of the stratum spinosum (prickle cell layer) of the epidermis

Acid- and alcohol-fast bacilli – pseudonym for mycobacteria, derived from the fact that they retain staining with carbolfuchsin after treatment with acid and alcohol

Acidophilic – staining strongly pink with the acidic dye eosin (also known as *eosinophilic*)

AIDS – acquired immune deficiency syndrome, caused by infection with the human immunodeficiency virus (HIV)

Amoeba – unicellular protozoan organism, important cause of diarrhoea worldwide

Amyloid – insoluble extracellular fibrillar protein, stains pink in routine H&E sections but best demonstrated using special stains, such as Congo red, or electron microscopy

Anaemia – deficiency of red blood cells in the blood stream

Aneurysm – abnormal dilatation of the wall of a blood vessel or the heart

Architecture – the organisation and arrangement of cells within a tissue

ARDS – adult respiratory distress syndrome, a severe form of lung disease with diffuse alveolar damage and formation of hyaline membranes in the alveoli

Asbestos – a mineral fibre used in industry and associated with development of lung fibrosis and malignant tumours, especially *mesothelioma*

Ascites – abnormal collection of fluid within the peritoneal cavity

Assmann focus – focus of granulomatous inflammation in the apex of the lung, seen in secondary tuberculosis

ATP – adenosine triphosphate

Atypical mitosis – abnormal cell division usually seen in malignant tumours, described as 'tripolar' when the chromosomes appear to divide into three groups instead of the normal two

Autolysis – self-destruction of a cell by the digestive effects of its own enzymes

β-pleated sheet – unusual form of tertiary protein structure, typically seen in *amyloid*, making the protein insoluble and resistant to digestion by normal enzymes

Basophilic – staining strongly blue-purple with the basic dye haematoxylin (also known as *haematoxyphilic*)

Bioinformatics – analysis of complex biological data using computer science, statistical analyses and mathematics

Biomedical scientist – trained scientists who usually work in a variety of laboratory environments carrying out tests and analysing samples for diagnosis and treatment of diseases

Biphasic – with two different phases, sometimes used descriptively for tumours with two different growth patterns, e.g. mesothelioma, synovial sarcoma

Birefringence – the optical property of double refraction, splitting light into two perpendicular beams, useful in identifying crystals and other substances such as *amyloid*

Breslow depth – depth of invasion of malignant melanoma, measured in millimetres from the stratum granulosum to the deepest invading tumour cell, useful in assessing likely prognosis

Bronchiectasis – abnormal permanent dilatation of the bronchi due to chronic lung infection

Bulla – on the skin, a large fluid-filled blister and, in the lung, a large cystically dilated air space

Callus – a type of granulation tissue found at the site of bone fracture and repair

Carcinoma – a malignant tumour of epithelial origin

Caseous necrosis – a form of tissue death, usually associated with tuberculosis, in which all cellular detail is lost, leaving soft, cheese-like material

Chancre – a painless ulcer that forms in the primary stage of syphilis infection

Chemokine – *cytokine* with chemotactic activity

Chemotaxis – the movement of a mediator along a chemical gradient, usually towards the site of inflammation

Cirrhosis – end stage of many types of chronic liver disease, with regenerative nodules of hepatocytes and intervening bands of fibrous scar tissue

CISH – chromogen in situ hybridisation

Clark level – depth of invasion of malignant melanoma through the normal layers of the skin, from epidermis (level 1) through to subcutaneous fat (level 5)

CMV – cytomegalovirus

Colliquative – a type of liquefactive necrosis where a solid mass becomes a viscous liquid

Consolidation – solidification of tissue, usually used to describe lung when filled with exudate fluid in pneumonia

Councilman body – a small pink globule within the liver, which is formed due to death of an individual hepatocyte, usually in acute viral hepatitis

Cribriform – sieve-like, often used to describe the architectural arrangement of cells in a tumour

Cryptogenic – term used to describe a disease of unknown origin (also called *idiopathic*)

Cytokine – small secreted molecule that controls and modulates inflammation, the immune response and haematopoiesis

Cytology – the study of cells

Dermatitis – inflammation of the skin

Desmosome – a specialised form of intercellular junction, particularly numerous in stratified squamous epithelium and giving rise to the histological appearance of 'prickles' between the cells (also known as macula adherens)

Differentiation – the process by which a cell becomes more specialised, often used in tumour pathology to describe the extent to which a tumour resembles normal tissue

Dyskeratosis – abnormal maturation of squamous epithelial cells with premature formation of keratin

Dysplasia – abnormal cell maturation, commonly used to describe pre-cancerous changes seen in epithelium

Ectopic – in the wrong place

Effusion – a collection of fluid within a body cavity

Electrophoresis – a method of separating large molecules using electrical charge, commonly used to examine serum proteins

Emphysema – abnormal and permanent dilatation of airspaces within the lungs, resulting in progressive obstruction to airflow and impaired gas exchange

Empyema – a collection of *pus* in a body cavity, typically in the pleural cavity, but also used to describe pus within the gallbladder

Endarteritis obliterans – inflammatory process affecting blood vessels, with proliferation of the intima such that it blocks the lumen of the affected vessel

Eosinophilic – staining strongly with the pink dye eosin (also known as *acidophilic*)

Epidermotropism – migrating towards the epidermis, e.g. atypical lymphocytes in mycosis fungoides

Epigenetics – external changes in gene expression that do not affect the underlying DNA sequence, such as DNA methylation

Epithelioid – cells resembling epithelial cells that are not epithelial, i.e. round to ovoid cells with plenty of cytoplasm and round to ovoid nuclei, e.g. epithelioid smooth muscle cells in epithelioid leiomyoma

Epithelioid macrophages – activated macrophages with abundant pink cytoplasm, said to resemble epithelial cells and typically seen in *granulomas*

Erosion – loss of the superficial part of an epithelial or mucosal surface (see also *ulcer*)

Extramedullary haematopoiesis – formation of blood cells outside the bone marrow, usually in the liver or spleen

Exudate – a protein-rich fluid that oozes out of damaged blood vessels, typically due to inflammation

Fascicle – a bundle, often used to describe the arrangement of smooth muscle cells in tumours

Fibrinoid – resembling fibrin, stains bright red with H&E

FISH – fluorescence in situ hybridisation

Fistula – an abnormal connection between two epithelial or endothelial surfaces

Fixation – method of preserving tissue to prevent decay, most commonly using formaldehyde, and an important first step in *tissue processing*

Frozen section – tissue samples are rapidly frozen, sectioned using a cryostat and stained, allowing very rapid production of a slide for pathological assessment

Grade – in tumour pathology, the extent to which the tumour resembles normal tissue (see also *differentiation*)

Granuloma – a collection of epithelioid macrophages and sometimes, but not always, multinucleate giant cells, with or without necrosis

Haematemesis – vomiting of blood

Haematogenous – via the bloodstream

Haematopoiesis – formation of blood cells

H&E – haematoxylin and eosin, a standard histological staining method that stains cytoplasm pink and nuclei blue-purple

Haematoxyphilic – staining intensely with the blue-purple stain haematoxylin (also known as *basophilic*)

Haemolytic anaemia – deficiency of red blood cells due to chronic red cell breakdown (lysis)

Haemoptysis – coughing up blood

Haemosiderin – a granular, brown substance containing iron, typically formed from breakdown of haemoglobin in the tissues

Hepatomegaly – enlargement of the liver

Histogenesis – differentiation of cells to form specialised tissues

HIV – human immunodeficiency virus, the cause of AIDS

HHV – human herpesvirus

HPV – human papillomavirus, the virus associated with cervical neoplasia , more recently, vulval, anal and oropharyngeal squamous cell carcinoma

Hyaline – glassy and deep pink-staining

Hyperchromasia – dark staining, usually used to describe abnormal nuclei in tumours that contain excess nuclear DNA and so stain intensely with haematoxylin

Hyperplasia – adaptation with increase in the number of cells

Hypertrophy – adaptation with increase in the size of cells

Hyperuricaemia – increased blood level of uric acid, associated with development of gout

Idiopathic – term used to describe a disease of unknown origin (see also *cryptogenic*)

Immunohistochemistry – technique using specific antibodies to identify and stain tissue components (also known as immunocytochemistry and immunoperoxidase staining)

Induration – hardening of a tissue or organ, usually due to inflammation

Infarction – tissue death due to inadequate blood supply

Interface hepatitis – inflammation disrupting the *limiting plate* of hepatocytes around the edge of the portal area

Involucrum – in osteomyelitis, a covering of new bone around the dead bony *sequestrum*

Ischaemia – insufficient blood supply

Jaundice – yellow discoloration of the tissues due to accumulation of bilirubin

Karyolysis – complete breakdown of the nuclear material of the cell, leaving an eosinophilic mass without a nucleus

Karyorrhexis – fragmentation of the pyknotic nucleus during cell necrosis

Koch's bacillus – old term for *Mycobacterium tuberculosis*

Koilocyte – an abnormal squamous cell due to infection by the human papillomavirus (HPV), may be binucleate and typically with a clear halo around an irregular, raisin-like nucleus

Langhans' giant cells – multinucleate giant cells with the nuclei arranged in a horseshoe-like pattern, typically associated with tuberculosis but not *pathognomonic*

Leukaemia – malignant disease with excess numbers of circulating white blood cells

Lichenification – leathery thickening of the skin due to chronic scratching and rubbing

Limiting plate – the layer of hepatocytes around the edge of the portal tracts in the liver

Lymphadenopathy – enlargement of lymph nodes

Lymphoma – a malignant tumour of lymphoid tissue

MALT – mucosa-associated lymphoid tissue

Microtomy – process of cutting very thin sections from tissues prior to mounting onto a glass slide

Melaena – black, altered blood in the stool, usually due to bleeding from the upper gastrointestinal tract

Melanoma – a malignant tumour of melanocytes

Mesothelioma – a malignant tumour of mesothelial cells, usually affecting the pleura, strongly associated with previous *asbestos* exposure

Metaplasia – transformation of one type of differentiated tissue to another

Monoclonal – tumour or cellular proliferation derived from a single cell

Necrosis – death of cells in a living organism

Next generation sequencing – modern sequencing technologies that allow rapid determination of the exact order of nucleotides in DNA or RNA including whole genomic analyses

NOS – not otherwise specified, a term used to denote a tumour of the most usual or common type for that particular organ (also sometimes called *NST, no special type*)

NST – no special type, a term used to denote a tumour of the most usual or common type for that particular organ, e.g. in the breast, invasive carcinoma, NST, is the most common pattern and indicates that it is not one of the special, rarer types such as tubular carcinoma

Oedema – abnormal accumulation of fluid in the tissues

Oncocyte – epithelial cell packed with mitochondria, giving the cytoplasm a pink, granular appearance

Oncogene – activated oncogenes are responsible for the development of cancers by producing abnormal proteins involved in cell growth and apoptosis (cell death)

Opsonisation – the coating of an organism marking it for *phagocytosis*. This is usually facilitated by complement proteins or antibodies

Osteoid – uncalcified bone matrix produced by osteoblasts

Osteolytic – causing breakdown of bone, typically used to describe the effect of metastatic tumour in causing apparent 'holes' in the bone on X-ray images

Osteosclerotic – causing excess deposition of bone, typically seen in cases of metastatic carcinoma from the prostate and showing areas of increased bone density on X-ray images

Palisading – lining up, usually of cells or nuclei, giving the ordered appearance of a fence

Pannus – a membrane of fibrovascular granulation tissue seen in damaged joints, typically in rheumatoid arthritis

Papillary – forming finger-like projections, typically used to describe the arrangement of tumour cells in projections around fine vascular cores

Paraneoplastic syndrome – a non-metastatic systemic effect of tumour, usually due to production of hormones, antibodies or other factors by the tumour cells

Pathognomonic – a feature so characteristic of a particular disease that it is sufficient to make the diagnosis

Pleomorphism – variation in cell shape or nuclear shape, typically associated with malignant tumours

Pneumoconiosis – a chronic lung disease caused by dust inhalation

Pneumonia – inflammation of the lung parenchyma with *consolidation* due to inflammatory exudate within the air spaces (see also *pneumonitis*)

Pneumonitis – inflammation of the lung, usually used to refer to interstitial inflammation rather than inflammation within the air spaces (see *pneumonia*)

Pneumothorax – collection of air within the pleural cavity

Polyclonal – cellular proliferation derived from multiple different cells

Polymerase chain reaction (PCR) – a method of amplifying DNA and RNA from a biological specimen

Polyp – a growth that protrudes from an epithelial surface

Pott's disease – tuberculosis affecting the spine

Pseudoepitheliomatous hyperplasia – pattern of extreme epidermal hyperplasia that may mimic carcinoma

Purulent – containing pus

Pus – green material composed of dead and dying neutrophils

Pyknosis – nuclear condensation occurring during cell necrosis

Pyogenic – pus forming

Sarcoma – a malignant tumour of mesenchymal origin

Sequestrum – a piece of dead bone, typically seen in osteomyelitis

Sinus – a blind-ended tract leading to a cavity (see also *fistula*)

Splendore-Hoeppli phenomenon – tissue reaction seen with certain infections, where organisms become encrusted with pink, proteinaceous material

Spongiosis – oedema of the epidermis, highlighting the spaces between keratinocytes with intervening 'prickles'

Stage – in tumour pathology, how far the disease has spread

Starling forces – osmotic and hydrostatic pressures that govern movement of fluid within the microcirculation

Steatosis – fatty change

Suppurative – pus forming

Tingible body macrophage – a macrophage containing many fragments of apoptotic debris in its cytoplasm, typically seen in reactive germinal centres of lymph nodes or in other sites with high rates of cell turnover

Tissue processing – preparation of tissue, including dehydration and impregnation with wax, rendering it firm enough to allow thin sections to be cut for mounting onto a glass slide

Transudate – a fluid derived from plasma that has a low protein content

Ulcer – a full-thickness defect in an epithelial or mucosal surface (see also *erosion*)

Vertical transmission – transmission of an infectious disease from a mother to her newborn baby

Vesicle – a small fluid-filled blister in the skin

Viral inclusion bodies – large collections of virus particles within infected cells that can be seen using light microscopy

Appendix 3 – Bonus E-Book Images

📷 BONUS E-BOOK IMAGES

E-Fig. 2.1 Apoptosis in normal tissues. **(A)** H&E (HP); **(B)** H&E (HP). (Reproduced from Young, B., O'Dowd, G., Woodford, P., Wheater's Functional Histology, 6th edition. 2014, Elsevier Ltd.)

E-Fig. 2.2 The mechanism of apoptosis. (Reproduced from Young, B., O'Dowd, G., Woodford, P., Wheater's Functional Histology, 6th edition. 2014, Elsevier Ltd.)

E-Fig. 3.1H Mast cells. **(A)** H&E (HP); **(B)** toluidine blue (HP); **(C)** EM ×12 000. (Reproduced from Young, B., O'Dowd, G., Woodford, P., Wheater's Functional Histology, 6th edition. Copyright 2014, Elsevier Ltd.)

E-Fig. 3.2H Endothelial cell EM ×68 000. (Reproduced from Young, B., O'Dowd, G., Woodford, P., Wheater's Functional Histology, 6th edition. Copyright 2014, Elsevier Ltd.)

E-Fig. 3.3H Neutrophils. **(A)** Giemsa (HP); **(B)** H&E (HP); **(C)** H&E (MP); **(D)** Giemsa (HP). (Reproduced from Young, B., O'Dowd, G., Woodford, P., Wheater's Functional Histology, 6th edition. Copyright 2014, Elsevier Ltd.)

E-Fig. 3.4H Neutrophil EM ×10 000. (Reproduced from Young, B., O'Dowd, G., Woodford, P., Wheater's Functional Histology, 6th edition. Copyright 2014, Elsevier Ltd.)

E-Fig. 3.5H Monocytes. **(A–C)** Giemsa (HP); **(D)** EM ×20 000. (Reproduced from Young, B., O'Dowd, G., Woodford, P., Wheater's Functional Histology, 6th edition. Copyright 2014, Elsevier Ltd.)

E-Fig. 3.6 The basics of the immune response. (Reproduced from Young, B., O'Dowd, G., Woodford, P., Wheater's Functional Histology, 6th edition. Copyright 2014, Elsevier Ltd.)

E-Fig. 4.1H Body of the stomach H&E (LP). (Reproduced from Young, B., O'Dowd, G., Woodford, P., Wheater's Functional Histology, 6th edition. Copyright 2014, Elsevier Ltd.)

E-Fig. 4.2G Chronic peptic ulcer. M/44. (Reproduced from Cooke, R., Stewart, B., Colour Atlas of Anatomical Pathology, 3rd edition. Copyright 2004, Elsevier Ltd.)

E-Fig. 4.3G Bronchiectasis. M/17. (Reproduced from Cooke, R., Stewart, B., Colour Atlas of Anatomical Pathology, 3rd edition. Copyright 2004, Elsevier Ltd.)

E-Fig. 4.4 H Tertiary (segmental) bronchus Elastic van Gieson (MP). (Reproduced from Young, B., O'Dowd, G., Woodford, P., Wheater's Functional Histology, 6th edition. Copyright 2014, Elsevier Ltd.)

E-Fig. 4.5 H Terminal portion of the respiratory tree H&E (LP). (Reproduced from Young, B., O'Dowd, G., Woodford, P., Wheater's Functional Histology, 6th edition. Copyright 2014, Elsevier Ltd.)

E-Fig. 4.6G Honeycomb lung. M/63. (Reproduced from Cooke, R., Stewart, B., Colour Atlas of Anatomical Pathology, 3rd edition. Copyright 2004, Elsevier Ltd.)

E-Fig. 4.7H Lymph node structure and vascular organisation. **(A)** H&E (LP); **(B)** schematic diagram. (Reproduced from Young, B., O'Dowd, G., Woodford, P., Wheater's Functional Histology, 6th edition. Copyright 2014, Elsevier Ltd.)

E-Fig. 4.8H Gallbladder. **(A)** H&E (LP); **(B)** H&E (MP); **(C)** H&E (LP). (Reproduced from Young, B., O'Dowd, G., Woodford, P., Wheater's Functional Histology, 6th edition. Copyright 2014, Elsevier Ltd.)

E-Fig. 4.9G Xanthogranulomatous pyelonephritis. F/60. (Reproduced from Cooke, R., Stewart, B., Colour Atlas of Anatomical Pathology, 3rd edition. Copyright 2004, Elsevier Ltd.)

E-Fig. 5.1G Pseudomembranous colitis. (Reproduced from Cooke, R., Stewart, B., Colour Atlas of Anatomical Pathology, 3rd edition. Copyright 2004, Elsevier Ltd.)

E-Fig. 5.2H Colorectal type absorptive/protective mucosa, H&E (MP). (Reproduced from Young, B., O'Dowd, G., Woodford, P., Wheater's Functional Histology, 6th edition. Copyright 2014, Elsevier Ltd.)

E-Fig. 5.3G Vertical section of the left lung and mediastinum. (Reproduced from Cooke, R., Stewart, B., Colour Atlas of Anatomical Pathology, 3rd edition. Copyright 2004, Elsevier Ltd.)

E-Fig. 5.4H Liver. **(A)** Capsule and parenchyma, H&E (MP); **(B)** architecture, H&E (LP). (Reproduced from Young, B., O'Dowd, G., Woodford, P., Wheater's Functional Histology, 6th edition. Copyright 2014, Elsevier Ltd.)

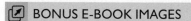

E-Fig. 5.5H Renal cortex H&E (MP). (Reproduced from Young, B., O'Dowd, G., Woodford, P., Wheater's Functional Histology, 6th edition. Copyright 2014, Elsevier Ltd.)

E-Fig. 5.6H Bone, cortical and trabecular H&E (LP). (Reproduced from Young, B., O'Dowd, G., Woodford, P., Wheater's Functional Histology, 6th edition. Copyright 2014, Elsevier Ltd.)

E-Fig. 5.7H Meninges H&E (LP). (Reproduced from Young, B., O'Dowd, G., Woodford, P., Wheater's Functional Histology, 6th edition. Copyright 2014, Elsevier Ltd.)

E-Fig. 5.8H Skin architecture H&E (LP). (Reproduced from Young, B., O'Dowd, G., Woodford, P., Wheater's Functional Histology, 6th edition. Copyright 2014, Elsevier Ltd.)

E-Fig. 5.9H Uterine cervix. (Reproduced from Young, B., O'Dowd, G., Woodford, P., Wheater's Functional Histology, 6th edition. Copyright 2014, Elsevier Ltd.)

E-Fig. 5.10H Myocardium. (A) H&E, LS (HP); (B) H&E, TS (HP). (Reproduced from Young, B., O'Dowd, G., Woodford, P., Wheater's Functional Histology, 6th edition. Copyright 2014, Elsevier Ltd.)

E-Fig. 5.11H Terminal portion of the respiratory tree. (Reproduced from Young, B., O'Dowd, G., Woodford, P., Wheater's Functional Histology, 6th edition. Copyright 2014, Elsevier Ltd.)

E-Fig. 5.12H Appendix. (A) H&E (LP); (B) H&E (MP); (C) H&E (MP). (Reproduced from Young, B., O'Dowd, G., Woodford, P., Wheater's Functional Histology, 6th edition. Copyright 2014, Elsevier Ltd.)

E-Fig. 6.1G Endometrial hyperplasia. (Reproduced from Cooke, R., Stewart, B., Colour Atlas of Anatomical Pathology, 3rd edition. Copyright 2004, Elsevier Ltd.)

E-Fig. 6.2H Myocardium. (A) H&E, LS (HP); (B) H&E, TS (HP). (Reproduced from Young, B., O'Dowd, G., Woodford, P., Wheater's Functional Histology, 6th edition. Copyright 2014, Elsevier Ltd.)

E-Fig. 6.3G Left ventricular hypertrophy. (Reproduced from Cooke, R., Stewart, B., Colour Atlas of Anatomical Pathology, 3rd edition. Copyright 2004, Elsevier Ltd.)

E-Fig. 6.4H Proliferative endometrium. (A) Early phase, H&E (LP); (B) early phase, H&E (MP); (C) early phase, H&E (HP); (D) late phase, H&E (LP); (E) late phase, H&E (HP); (F) late phase, H&E (HP). (Reproduced from Young, B., O'Dowd, G., Woodford, P., Wheater's Functional Histology, 6th edition. Copyright 2014, Elsevier Ltd.)

E-Fig. 6.5H Seminiferous tubules H&E (MP). (Reproduced from Young, B., O'Dowd, G., Woodford, P., Wheater's Functional Histology, 6th edition. Copyright 2014, Elsevier Ltd.)

E-Fig. 7.1H Uterine cervix H&E (LP). (Reproduced from Young, B., O'Dowd, G., Woodford, P., Wheater's Functional Histology, 6th edition. Copyright 2014, Elsevier Ltd.)

E-Fig. 7.2H Skin architecture. (A) Diagram; (B) H&E (LP). (Reproduced from Young, B., O'Dowd, G., Woodford, P., Wheater's Functional Histology, 6th edition. Copyright 2014, Elsevier Ltd.)

E-Fig. 7.3H Stratified squamous epithelium. (A) Diagram; (B) H&E (HP); (C) H&E (MP); (D) Papanicolaou (HP). (Reproduced from Young, B., O'Dowd, G., Woodford, P., Wheater's Functional Histology, 6th edition. Copyright 2014, Elsevier Ltd.)

E-Fig. 7.4H Transitional epithelium. (A) Diagram; (B) H&E (HP). (Reproduced from Young, B., O'Dowd, G., Woodford, P., Wheater's Functional Histology, 6th edition. Copyright 2014, Elsevier Ltd.)

E-Fig. 7.5H Simple tubular glands. (A) Diagram; (B) H&E (LP); (C) H&E (MP). (Reproduced from Young, B., O'Dowd, G., Woodford, P., Wheater's Functional Histology, 6th edition. Copyright 2014, Elsevier Ltd.)

E-Fig. 7.6H Simple branched tubular glands. (A) Diagram; (B) H&E (LP). (Reproduced from Young, B., O'Dowd, G., Woodford, P., Wheater's Functional Histology, 6th edition. Copyright 2014, Elsevier Ltd.)

E-Fig. 7.7G Secondary tumour in the liver. M/68. (Reproduced from Cooke, R., Stewart, B., Colour Atlas of Anatomical Pathology, 3rd edition. Copyright 2004, Elsevier Ltd.)

E-Fig. 7.8G Secondary carcinoma of the lung. F/59. (Reproduced from Cooke, R., Stewart, B., Colour Atlas of Anatomical Pathology, 3rd edition. Copyright 2004, Elsevier Ltd.)

E-Fig. 8.1H Muscular artery. (A) H&E (MP); (B) Elastic van Gieson (MP). (Reproduced from Young, B., O'Dowd, G., Woodford, P., Wheater's Functional Histology, 6th edition. Copyright 2014, Elsevier Ltd.)

E-Fig. 8.2G Atherosclerosis. (Reproduced from Cooke, R., Stewart, B., Colour Atlas of Anatomical Pathology, 3rd edition. Copyright 2004, Elsevier Ltd.)

E-Fig. 8.3G Atherosclerosis. (Reproduced from Cooke, R., Stewart, B., Colour Atlas of Anatomical Pathology, 3rd edition. Copyright 2004, Elsevier Ltd.)

E-Fig. 8.4G Aneurysm. (Reproduced from Cooke, R., Stewart, B., Colour Atlas of Anatomical Pathology, 3rd edition. Copyright 2004, Elsevier Ltd.)

E-Fig. 8.5G Anterior myocardial infarction. (Reproduced from Cooke, R., Stewart, B., Colour Atlas of Anatomical Pathology, 3rd edition. Copyright 2004, Elsevier Ltd.)

E-Fig. 9.1G Thrombosis of the inferior vena cava and left common iliac vein. F/70. (Reproduced from Cooke, R., Stewart, B., Colour Atlas of Anatomical Pathology, 3rd edition. Copyright 2004, Elsevier Ltd.)

E-Fig. 9.2G Thrombus in the left auricular appendage. F/85. (Reproduced from Cooke, R., Stewart, B., Colour Atlas of Anatomical Pathology, 3rd edition. Copyright 2004, Elsevier Ltd.)

E-Fig. 9.3G Pulmonary embolus. (Reproduced from Cooke, R., Stewart, B., Colour Atlas of Anatomical Pathology, 3rd edition. Copyright 2004, Elsevier Ltd.)

E-Fig. 10.1G Renal infarction. (Reproduced from Cooke, R., Stewart, B., Colour Atlas of Anatomical Pathology, 3rd edition. Copyright 2004, Elsevier Ltd.)

E-Fig. 10.2G Infarction. (Reproduced from Cooke, R., Stewart, B., Colour Atlas of Anatomical Pathology, 3rd edition. Copyright 2004, Elsevier Ltd.)

E-Fig. 10.3G Infarction. (Reproduced from Cooke, R., Stewart, B., Colour Atlas of Anatomical Pathology, 3rd edition. Copyright 2004, Elsevier Ltd.)

E-Fig. 10.4G Pulmonary infarction due to thrombo-embolism. (Reproduced from Cooke, R., Stewart, B., Colour Atlas of Anatomical Pathology, 3rd edition. Copyright 2004, Elsevier Ltd.)

E-Fig. 11.1H Elastic artery: aorta. **(A)** Elastic van Gieson (LP); **(B)** elastic van Gieson (HP). (Reproduced from Young, B., O'Dowd, G., Woodford, P., Wheater's Functional Histology, 6th edition. Copyright 2014, Elsevier Ltd.)

E-Fig. 11.2G Cutaneous haemangioma. (Reproduced from Cooke, R., Stewart, B., Colour Atlas of Anatomical Pathology, 3rd edition. Copyright 2004, Elsevier Ltd.)

E-Fig. 11.3G The left ventricular outflow tract demonstrating features of hypertrophic cardiomyopathy. (Reproduced from Cooke, R., Stewart, B., Colour Atlas of Anatomical Pathology, 3rd edition. Copyright 2004, Elsevier Ltd.)

E-Fig. 11.4H Cardiac muscle. **(A)** H&E, LS (MP); **(B)** H&E, TS (HP); **(C)** H&E, polarised light, LS (HP); **(D)** H&E, LS (HP). (Reproduced from Young, B., O'Dowd, G., Woodford, P., Wheater's Functional Histology, 6th edition. Copyright 2014, Elsevier Ltd.)

E-Fig. 11.5H Heart: left ventricular wall H&E (LP). (Reproduced from Young, B., O'Dowd, G., Woodford, P., Wheater's Functional Histology, 6th edition. Copyright 2014, Elsevier Ltd.)

E-Fig. 11.6H Heart valve H&E (LP). (Reproduced from Young, B., O'Dowd, G., Woodford, P., Wheater's Functional Histology, 6th edition. Copyright 2014, Elsevier Ltd.)

E-Fig. 11.7G Rheumatic valve disease affecting the aortic valve. (Reproduced from Cooke, R., Stewart, B., Colour Atlas of Anatomical Pathology, 3rd edition. Copyright 2004, Elsevier Ltd.)

E-Fig. 11.8G Acute bacterial endocarditis affecting the mitral valve. (Reproduced from Cooke, R., Stewart, B., Colour Atlas of Anatomical Pathology, 3rd edition. Copyright 2004, Elsevier Ltd.)

E-Fig. 12.1H Nasal mucosa H&E (HP). (Reproduced from Young, B., O'Dowd, G., Woodford, P., Wheater's Functional Histology, 6th edition. Copyright 2014, Elsevier Ltd.)

E-Fig. 12.2H Nasopharynx H&E (HP). (Reproduced from Young, B., O'Dowd, G., Woodford, P., Wheater's Functional Histology, 6th edition. Copyright 2014, Elsevier Ltd.)

E-Fig. 12.3H Larynx H&E (LP). (Reproduced from Young, B., O'Dowd, G., Woodford, P., Wheater's Functional Histology, 6th edition. Copyright 2014, Elsevier Ltd.)

E-Fig. 12.4H Trachea H&E (MP). (Reproduced from Young, B., O'Dowd, G., Woodford, P., Wheater's Functional Histology, 6th edition. Copyright 2014, Elsevier Ltd.)

E-Fig. 12.5H Terminal portion of the respiratory tree H&E (LP). (Reproduced from Young, B., O'Dowd, G., Woodford, P., Wheater's Functional Histology, 6th edition. Copyright 2014, Elsevier Ltd.)

E-Fig. 12.6G Lobar pneumonia. (Reproduced from Cooke, R., Stewart, B., Colour Atlas of Anatomical Pathology, 3rd edition. Copyright 2004, Elsevier Ltd.)

E-Fig. 12.7G Bronchogenic carcinoma. (Reproduced from Cooke, R., Stewart, B., Colour Atlas of Anatomical Pathology, 3rd edition. Copyright 2004, Elsevier Ltd.)

E-Fig. 12.8G Mesothelioma. (Reproduced from Cooke, R., Stewart, B., Colour Atlas of Anatomical Pathology, 3rd edition. Copyright 2004, Elsevier Ltd.)

E-Fig. 13.1H Tongue, anterior two-thirds H&E (LP). (Reproduced from Young, B., O'Dowd, G., Woodford, P., Wheater's Functional Histology, 6th edition. Copyright 2014, Elsevier Ltd.)

E-Fig. 13.2H Parotid gland H&E (LP). (Reproduced from Young, B., O'Dowd, G., Woodford, P., Wheater's Functional Histology, 6th edition. Copyright 2014, Elsevier Ltd.)

E-Fig. 13.3H Components of the wall of the gastrointestinal tract. **(A)** Colon, H&E (HP); **(B)** oesophagus, H&E (LP); **(C)** colon H&E (HP). (Reproduced from Young, B., O'Dowd, G., Woodford, P., Wheater's Functional Histology, 6th edition. Copyright 2014, Elsevier Ltd.)

E-Fig. 13.4H Oesophago-gastric junction H&E (LP). (Reproduced from Young, B., O'Dowd, G., Woodford, P., Wheater's Functional Histology, 6th edition. Copyright 2014, Elsevier Ltd.)

E-Fig. 13.5G Chronic peptic ulcer. M/44. (Reproduced from Cooke, R., Stewart, B., Colour Atlas of Anatomical Pathology, 3rd edition. Copyright 2004, Elsevier Ltd.)

E-Fig. 13.6H Gastric body mucosa. (Reproduced from Young, B., O'Dowd, G., Woodford, P., Wheater's Functional Histology, 6th edition. Copyright 2014, Elsevier Ltd.)

E-Fig. 13.7G Linitis plastica. F/68. (Reproduced from Cooke, R., Stewart, B., Colour Atlas of Anatomical Pathology, 3rd edition. Copyright 2004, Elsevier Ltd.)

E-Fig. 13.8H Small intestine, monkey. **(A)** Duodenum, H&E (LP); **(B)** Ileum, H&E (MP). (Reproduced from Young, B., O'Dowd, G., Woodford, P., Wheater's Functional Histology, 6th edition. Copyright 2014, Elsevier Ltd.)

E-Fig. 13.9G Crohn's disease of the terminal ileum. M/21. (Reproduced from Cooke, R., Stewart, B., Colour Atlas of Anatomical Pathology, 3rd edition. Copyright 2004, Elsevier Ltd.)

E-Fig. 13.10H Appendix. **(A)** H&E (LP); **(B)** H&E (MP); **(C)** H&E (MP). (Reproduced from Young, B., O'Dowd, G., Woodford, P., Wheater's Functional Histology, 6th edition. Copyright 2014, Elsevier Ltd.)

E-Fig. 13.11H Colon. **(A)** H&E (LP); **(B)** H&E (MP); **(C)** Alcian blue/van Gieson (MP); **(D)** Alcian blue/van Gieson (HP); **(E)** H&E (HP). (Reproduced from Young, B., O'Dowd, G., Woodford, P., Wheater's Functional Histology, 6th edition. Copyright 2014, Elsevier Ltd.)

E-Fig. 13.12G Acute ulcerative colitis. F/16. (Reproduced from Cooke, R., Stewart, B., Colour Atlas of Anatomical Pathology, 3rd edition. Copyright 2004, Elsevier Ltd.)

E-Fig. 13.13G Benign tubular adenomatous polyps of the colon. M/46. These were asymptomatic. (Reproduced from Cooke, R., Stewart, B., Colour Atlas of Anatomical Pathology, 3rd edition. Copyright 2004, Elsevier Ltd.)

E-Fig. 13.14G Villous adenoma of the rectum. F/48. (Reproduced from Cooke, R., Stewart, B., Colour Atlas of Anatomical Pathology, 3rd edition. Copyright 2004, Elsevier Ltd.)

E-Fig. 13.15H Immunohistochemical staining for mismatch repair proteins. **(A)** MLH1 (MP); **(B)** PMS2 (MP); **(C)** MSH2 (MP); **(D)** MSH6 (MP).

E-Fig. 13.16G Adenocarcinoma of the rectum. M/70. (Reproduced from Cooke, R., Stewart, B., Colour Atlas of Anatomical Pathology, 3rd edition. Copyright 2004, Elsevier Ltd.)

E-Fig. 13.17G Diverticulosis of the colon. (Reproduced from Cooke, R., Stewart, B., Colour Atlas of Anatomical Pathology, 3rd edition. Copyright 2004, Elsevier Ltd.)

E-Fig. 14.1H Hepatocytes. **(A)** H&E (HP); **(B)** PAS/haematoxylin (HP). (Reproduced from Young, B., O'Dowd, G., Woodford, P., Wheater's Functional Histology, 6th edition. Copyright 2014, Elsevier Ltd.)

E-Fig. 14.2H Portal tract H&E (MP). (Reproduced from Young, B., O'Dowd, G., Woodford, P., Wheater's Functional Histology, 6th edition. Copyright 2014, Elsevier Ltd.)

E-Fig. 14.3H Hepatic vasculature and biliary system. (Reproduced from Young, B., O'Dowd, G., Woodford, P., Wheater's Functional Histology, 6th edition. Copyright 2014, Elsevier Ltd.)

E-Fig. 14.4H Liver architecture. **(A)** Diagram of the liver lobule; **(B)** Pig, H&E (LP); **(C)** Human, H&E (LP); **(D)** Diagram of the simple acinus; **(E)** Diagram of acinar agglomerate. (Reproduced from Young, B., O'Dowd, G., Woodford, P., Wheater's Functional Histology, 6th edition. Copyright 2014, Elsevier Ltd.)

E-Fig. 14.5G Cirrhosis. (Reproduced from Cooke, R., Stewart, B., Colour Atlas of Anatomical Pathology, 3rd edition. Copyright 2004, Elsevier Ltd.)

E-Fig. 14.6G Hepatocellular carcinoma. (Reproduced from Cooke, R., Stewart, B., Colour Atlas of Anatomical Pathology, 3rd edition. Copyright 2004, Elsevier Ltd.)

E-Fig. 14.7H Bile canaliculi. **(A)** Enzyme histochemical staining for ATPase (HP); **(B)** Iron haematoxylin (HP). (Reproduced from Young, B., O'Dowd, G., Woodford, P., Wheater's Functional Histology, 6th edition. Copyright 2014, Elsevier Ltd.)

E-Fig. 14.8H Gallbladder. **(A)** H&E (LP); **(B)** H&E (MP); **(C)** H&E (LP). (Reproduced from Young, B., O'Dowd, G., Woodford, P., Wheater's Functional Histology, 6th edition. Copyright 2014, Elsevier Ltd.)

E-Fig. 14.9H Exocrine pancreas. **(A)** H&E (MP); **(B)** H&E (HP); **(C)** EM ×8500. (Reproduced from Young, B., O'Dowd, G., Woodford, P., Wheater's Functional Histology, 6th edition. Copyright 2014, Elsevier Ltd.)

E-Fig. 14.10G Acute pancreatitis. (Reproduced from Cooke, R., Stewart, B., Colour Atlas of Anatomical Pathology, 3rd edition. Copyright 2004, Elsevier Ltd.)

E-Fig. 14.11G Chronic pancreatitis. The pancreas is shrunken due to atrophy and fibrosis of the exocrine component, giving it a white appearance. Multiple calculi are seen throughout the head, which obstruct the ductal system. (Reproduced from Cooke, R., Stewart, B., Colour Atlas of Anatomical Pathology, 3rd edition. Copyright 2004, Elsevier Ltd.)

E-Fig. 15.1H Kidney H&E (LP). (Reproduced from Young, B., O'Dowd, G., Woodford, P., Wheater's Functional Histology, 6th edition. Copyright 2014, Elsevier Ltd.)

E-Fig. 15.2H Renal corpuscle. **(A)** Schematic diagram; **(B)** PAS (HP). (Reproduced from Young, B., O'Dowd, G., Woodford, P., Wheater's Functional Histology, 6th edition. Copyright 2014, Elsevier Ltd.)

E-Fig. 15.3H (A) Renal cortex H&E (MP), proximal and distal convoluted tubules. (B) PCT, Azan (HP); (C) PCT, PAS (HP); (D) DCT, H&E (HP); (E) DCT, PAS (HP). (Reproduced from Young, B., O'Dowd, G., Woodford, P., Wheater's Functional Histology, 6th edition. Copyright 2014, Elsevier Ltd.)

E-Fig. 15.4H Glomerulus. (A) SEM ×1500; (B) SEM ×6000. (Reproduced from Young, B., O'Dowd, G., Woodford, P., Wheater's Functional Histology, 6th edition. Copyright 2014, Elsevier Ltd.)

E-Fig. 15.5H Glomerulus. (A) EM ×4800; (B) EM ×14 000; (C) EM ×30 000. (Reproduced from Young, B., O'Dowd, G., Woodford, P., Wheater's Functional Histology, 6th edition. Copyright 2014, Elsevier Ltd.)

E-Fig. 15.6 Amyloidosis.

E-Fig. 15.7G Diabetic kidneys with pyelonephritis and papillary necrosis. M/47. (Reproduced from Cooke, R., Stewart, B., Colour Atlas of Anatomical Pathology, 3rd edition. Copyright 2004, Elsevier Ltd.)

E-Fig. 15.8G Oncocytoma. M/65. (Reproduced from Cooke, R., Stewart, B., Colour Atlas of Anatomical Pathology, 3rd edition. Copyright 2004, Elsevier Ltd.)

E-Fig. 15.9G Renal cell carcinoma. (Reproduced from Cooke, R., Stewart, B., Colour Atlas of Anatomical Pathology, 3rd edition. Copyright 2004, Elsevier Ltd.)

E-Fig. 15.10G Wilms' tumour. F/5. (Reproduced from Cooke, R., Stewart, B., Colour Atlas of Anatomical Pathology, 3rd edition. Copyright 2004, Elsevier Ltd.)

E-Fig. 15.11H Transitional epithelium H&E (HP). (Reproduced from Cooke, R., Stewart, B., Colour Atlas of Anatomical Pathology, 3rd edition. Copyright 2004, Elsevier Ltd.)

E-Fig. 15.12G Carcinoma of the bladder. M/88. (Reproduced from Cooke, R., Stewart, B., Colour Atlas of Anatomical Pathology, 3rd edition. Copyright 2004, Elsevier Ltd.)

E-Fig. 16.1H Thymus. (A) Infant, H&E (LP); (B) adult, H&E (LP). (Reproduced from Young, B., O'Dowd, G., Woodford, P., Wheater's Functional Histology, 6th edition. Copyright 2014, Elsevier Ltd.)

E-Fig. 16.2H Spleen H&E (LP). (Reproduced from Young, B., O'Dowd, G., Woodford, P., Wheater's Functional Histology, 6th edition. Copyright 2014, Elsevier Ltd.)

E-Fig. 16.3H Palatine tonsil H&E (LP). (Reproduced from Young, B., O'Dowd, G., Woodford, P., Wheater's Functional Histology, 6th edition. Copyright 2014, Elsevier Ltd.)

E-Fig. 16.4H Gut-associated lymphoid tissue. (A) Peyer's patch, H&E (MP); (B) the appendix, immunohistochemical stain for CD20 (LP). (Reproduced from Young, B., O'Dowd, G., Woodford, P., Wheater's Functional Histology, 6th edition. Copyright 2014, Elsevier Ltd.)

E-Fig. 16.5H Lymph node structure and vascular organisation. (A) H&E (LP); (B) schematic diagram. (Reproduced from Young, B., O'Dowd, G., Woodford, P., Wheater's Functional Histology, 6th edition. Copyright 2014, Elsevier Ltd.)

E-Fig. 16.6G Secondary tumour in a lymph node. F/43. (Reproduced from Cooke, R., Stewart, B., Colour Atlas of Anatomical Pathology, 3rd edition. Copyright 2004, Elsevier Ltd.)

E-Fig. 16.7G Malignant lymphoma of the small intestine. (Reproduced from Cooke, R., Stewart, B., Colour Atlas of Anatomical Pathology, 3rd edition. Copyright 2004, Elsevier Ltd.)

E-Fig. 16.8H Normal bone marrow H&E (LP). (Reproduced from Young, B., O'Dowd, G., Woodford, P., Wheater's Functional Histology, 6th edition. Copyright 2014, Elsevier Ltd.)

E-Fig. 16.9G Multiple myeloma. (Reproduced from Cooke, R., Stewart, B., Colour Atlas of Anatomical Pathology, 3rd edition. Copyright 2004, Elsevier Ltd.)

E-Fig. 16.10 Amyloidosis.

E-Fig. 17.1H Apocrine secretion. (A) H&E (MP); (B) H&E (HP). (Reproduced from Young, B., O'Dowd, G., Woodford, P., Wheater's Functional Histology, 6th edition. Copyright 2014, Elsevier Ltd.)

E-Fig. 17.2H Endocervix. (A) H&E (LP); (B) H&E (MP). (Reproduced from Young, B., O'Dowd, G., Woodford, P., Wheater's Functional Histology, 6th edition. Copyright 2014, Elsevier Ltd.)

E-Fig. 17.3H Cervical cytology Papanicolou (HP). (Reproduced from Young, B., O'Dowd, G., Woodford, P., Wheater's Functional Histology, 6th edition. Copyright 2014, Elsevier Ltd.)

E-Fig. 17.4H Uterine cervix H&E (LP). (Reproduced from Young, B., O'Dowd, G., Woodford, P., Wheater's Functional Histology, 6th edition. Copyright 2014, Elsevier Ltd.)

E-Fig. 17.5H Myometrium. (A) H&E (MP); (B) H&E (HP). (Reproduced from Young, B., O'Dowd, G., Woodford, P., Wheater's Functional Histology, 6th edition. Copyright 2014, Elsevier Ltd.)

E-Fig. 17.6G Leiomyoma. (Reproduced from Cooke, R., Stewart, B., Colour Atlas of Anatomical Pathology, 3rd edition. Copyright 2004, Elsevier Ltd.)

E-Fig. 17.7G Endometriotic cyst of ovary (endometrioma). (Reproduced from Cooke, R., Stewart, B., Colour Atlas of Anatomical Pathology, 3rd edition. Copyright 2004, Elsevier Ltd.)

E-Fig. 17.8G Endometrial carcinoma. (Reproduced from Cooke, R., Stewart, B., Colour Atlas of Anatomical Pathology, 3rd edition. Copyright 2004, Elsevier Ltd.)

E-Fig. 17.9H Early placenta. (A) H&E (LP); (B) H&E (MP); (C) H&E (HP). (Reproduced from Young, B., O'Dowd, G., Woodford, P., Wheater's Functional Histology, 6th edition. Copyright 2014, Elsevier Ltd.)

E-Fig. 17.10H Fallopian tube. (A) H&E (LP); (B) H&E (MP); (C) H&E (HP); (D) Azan (HP). (Reproduced from Young, B., O'Dowd, G., Woodford, P., Wheater's Functional Histology, 6th edition. Copyright 2014, Elsevier Ltd.)

E-Fig. 17.11G Mucinous cystadenoma. (Reproduced from Cooke, R., Stewart, B., Colour Atlas of Anatomical Pathology, 3rd edition. Copyright 2004, Elsevier Ltd.)

E-Fig. 17.12G Mature cystic teratoma (dermoid cyst). (Reproduced from Cooke, R., Stewart, B., Colour Atlas of Anatomical Pathology, 3rd edition. Copyright 2004, Elsevier Ltd.)

E-Fig. 18.1H Breast. **(A)** H&E (LP); **(B)** H&E (MP); **(C)** H&E (HP); **(D)** H&E (HP); **(E)** immunohistochemical stain for smooth muscle actin (MP). (Reproduced from Young, B., O'Dowd, G., Woodford, P., Wheater's Functional Histology, 6th edition. Copyright 2014, Elsevier Ltd.)

E-Fig. 18.2H Breast during pregnancy. **(A)** H&E (LP); **(B)** H&E (MP). (Reproduced from Young, B., O'Dowd, G., Woodford, P., Wheater's Functional Histology, 6th edition. Copyright 2014, Elsevier Ltd.)

E-Fig. 18.3G Fat necrosis. F/42. (Reproduced from Cooke, R., Stewart, B., Colour Atlas of Anatomical Pathology, 3rd edition. Copyright 2004, Elsevier Ltd.)

E-Fig. 18.4G Fibrocystic disease of the breast. F/35. (Reproduced from Cooke, R., Stewart, B., Colour Atlas of Anatomical Pathology, 3rd edition. Copyright 2004, Elsevier Ltd.)

E-Fig. 18.5G Fibroadenoma. F/18. (Reproduced from Cooke, R., Stewart, B., Colour Atlas of Anatomical Pathology, 3rd edition. Copyright 2004, Elsevier Ltd.)

E-Fig. 18.6G Carcinoma of the breast. F/70. (Reproduced from Cooke, R., Stewart, B., Colour Atlas of Anatomical Pathology, 3rd edition. Copyright 2004, Elsevier Ltd.)

E-Fig. 18.7G Mucinous carcinoma of the breast. F/70. (Reproduced from Cooke, R., Stewart, B., Colour Atlas of Anatomical Pathology, 3rd edition. Copyright 2004, Elsevier Ltd.)

E-Fig. 18.8H The nipple H&E (LP). (Reproduced from Young, B., O'Dowd, G., Woodford, P., Wheater's Functional Histology, 6th edition. Copyright 2014, Elsevier Ltd.)

E-Fig. 18.9G Paget's disease of the nipple. F/39. (Reproduced from Cooke, R., Stewart, B., Colour Atlas of Anatomical Pathology, 3rd edition. Copyright 2004, Elsevier Ltd.)

E-Fig. 19.1H Testis, monkey H&E (LP). (Reproduced from Young, B., O'Dowd, G., Woodford, P., Wheater's Functional Histology, 6th edition. Copyright 2014, Elsevier Ltd.)

E-Fig. 19.2H Seminiferous tubule. **(A)** H&E (HP); **(B)** diagram. (Reproduced from Young, B., O'Dowd, G., Woodford, P., Wheater's Functional Histology, 6th edition. Copyright 2014, Elsevier Ltd.)

E-Fig. 19.3G Seminoma of the testis. M/40. (Reproduced from Cooke, R., Stewart, B., Colour Atlas of Anatomical Pathology, 3rd edition. Copyright 2004, Elsevier Ltd.)

E-Fig. 19.4G Combined teratoma and seminoma of the testis. M/20. (Reproduced from Cooke, R., Stewart, B., Colour Atlas of Anatomical Pathology, 3rd edition. Copyright 2004, Elsevier Ltd.)

E-Fig. 19.5H Prostate gland, dog H&E (LP). (Reproduced from Young, B., O'Dowd, G., Woodford, P., Wheater's Functional Histology, 6th edition. Copyright 2014, Elsevier Ltd.)

E-Fig. 19.6G Benign prostatic hypertrophy. M/84. (Reproduced from Cooke, R., Stewart, B., Colour Atlas of Anatomical Pathology, 3rd edition. Copyright 2004, Elsevier Ltd.)

E-Fig. 20.1G Acromegaly typical clinical manifestations. (Reproduced from Cooke, R., Stewart, B., Colour Atlas of Anatomical Pathology, 3rd edition. Copyright 2004, Elsevier Ltd.)

E-Fig. 20.2G Hashimoto's thyroiditis. (Reproduced from Cooke, R., Stewart, B., Colour Atlas of Anatomical Pathology, 3rd edition. Copyright 2004, Elsevier Ltd.)

E-Fig. 20.3G Follicular adenoma. (Reproduced from Cooke, R., Stewart, B., Colour Atlas of Anatomical Pathology, 3rd edition. Copyright 2004, Elsevier Ltd.)

E-Fig. 20.4G Multinodular goitre. (Reproduced from Cooke, R., Stewart, B., Colour Atlas of Anatomical Pathology, 3rd edition. Copyright 2004, Elsevier Ltd.)

E-Fig. 20.5G Phaeochromocytoma. (Reproduced from Cooke, R., Stewart, B., Colour Atlas of Anatomical Pathology, 3rd edition. Copyright 2004, Elsevier Ltd.)

E-Fig. 20.6G Neuroblastoma. (Reproduced from Cooke, R., Stewart, B., Colour Atlas of Anatomical Pathology, 3rd edition. Copyright 2004, Elsevier Ltd.)

E-Fig. 20.7H Anterior pituitary. **(A)** H&E (HP); **(B)** Azan (HP); **(C)** immunohistochemical method for growth hormone (HP); **(D)** EM ×4270. (Reproduced from Young, B., O'Dowd, G., Woodford, P., Wheater's Functional Histology, 6th edition. Copyright 2014, Elsevier Ltd.)

E-Fig. 20.8H Thyroid gland. **(A)** H&E (LP); **(B)** immunohistochemical method for CD34. (Reproduced from Young, B., O'Dowd, G., Woodford, P., Wheater's Functional Histology, 6th edition. Copyright 2014, Elsevier Ltd.)

E-Fig. 21.1H Epidermis H&E (HP). (Reproduced from Young, B., O'Dowd, G., Woodford, P., Wheater's Functional Histology, 6th edition. Copyright 2014, Elsevier Ltd.)

E-Fig. 21.2H Epidermis. Epoxy resin section, toluidine blue (HP). (Reproduced from Young, B., O'Dowd, G., Woodford, P., Wheater's Functional Histology, 6th edition. Copyright 2014, Elsevier Ltd.)

E-Fig. 21.3G Atopic dermatitis. (Courtesy of Dr Girish Gupta, Mr John Biagi, and the staff of the Department of Medical Illustration, NHS Lanarkshire)

E-Fig. 21.4G Chronic dermatitis. (Courtesy of Dr Girish Gupta, Mr John Biagi, and the staff of the Department of Medical Illustration, NHS Lanarkshire)

E-Fig. 21.5G Psoriasis. (Courtesy of Dr Girish Gupta, Mr John Biagi, and the staff of the Department of Medical Illustration, NHS Lanarkshire)

E-Fig. 21.6G Seborrhoeic keratosis. (Courtesy of Dr Girish Gupta, Mr John Biagi, and the staff of the Department of Medical Illustration, NHS Lanarkshire)

E-Fig. 21.7G Nodular basal cell carcinoma. (Courtesy of Dr Girish Gupta, Mr John Biagi, and the staff of the Department of Medical Illustration, NHS Lanarkshire)

E-Fig. 21.8G Superficial basal cell carcinoma. (Courtesy of Dr Girish Gupta, Mr John Biagi, and the staff of the Department of Medical Illustration, NHS Lanarkshire)

E-Fig. 21.9G Squamous cell carcinoma. (Courtesy of Dr Girish Gupta, Mr John Biagi, and the staff of the Department of Medical Illustration, NHS Lanarkshire)

E-Fig. 21.10H Melanocytes. **(A)** H&E (HP); **(B)** H&E, pigmented skin (MP); **(C)** immunohistochemistry for melanA (MP); **(D)** dual immunohistochemistry for melanA (*red*) and langerin (*brown*) (MP). (Reproduced from Young, B., O'Dowd, G., Woodford, P., Wheater's Functional Histology, 6th edition. Copyright 2014, Elsevier Ltd.)

E-Fig. 21.11G Benign naevus. (Courtesy of Dr Girish Gupta, Mr John Biagi, and the staff of the Department of Medical Illustration, NHS Lanarkshire)

E-Fig. 21.12G Malignant melanoma. (Courtesy of Dr Girish Gupta, Mr John Biagi, and the staff of the Department of Medical Illustration, NHS Lanarkshire)

E-Fig. 21.13G Dermatofibroma. (Courtesy of Dr Girish Gupta, Mr John Biagi, and the staff of the Department of Medical Illustration, NHS Lanarkshire)

E-Fig. 22.1H Bone, cortical and trabecular H&E (LP). (Reproduced from Young, B., O'Dowd, G., Woodford, P., Wheater's Functional Histology, 6th edition. Copyright 2014, Elsevier Ltd.)

E-Fig. 22.2H Active osteoblasts and osteoid. **(A)** H&E (HP); **(B)** undecalcified resin section, Goldner trichrome stain (HP). (Reproduced from Young, B., O'Dowd, G., Woodford, P., Wheater's Functional Histology, 6th edition. Copyright 2014, Elsevier Ltd.)

E-Fig. 22.3H Osteoclasts. **(A)** H&E (HP); **(B)** undecalcified resin section, Goldner trichrome (HP). (Reproduced from Young, B., O'Dowd, G., Woodford, P., Wheater's Functional Histology, 6th edition. Copyright 2014, Elsevier Ltd.)

E-Fig. 22.4G Acute osteomyelitis. (Reproduced from Cooke, R., Stewart, B. Colour Atlas of Anatomical Pathology, 3rd edition. Copyright 2004, Elsevier Ltd.)

E-Fig. 22.5G Chronic osteomyelitis. (Reproduced from Cooke, R., Stewart, B. Colour Atlas of Anatomical Pathology, 3rd edition. Copyright 2004, Elsevier Ltd.)

E-Fig. 22.6G Osteoporosis. (Reproduced from Cooke, R., Stewart, B., Colour Atlas of Anatomical Pathology, 3rd edition. Copyright 2004, Elsevier Ltd.)

E-Fig. 22.7G Paget's disease. (Reproduced from Cooke, R., Stewart, B., Colour Atlas of Anatomical Pathology, 3rd edition. Copyright 2004, Elsevier Ltd.)

E-Fig. 22.8G Osteoid osteoma in the proximal phalanx of a finger. (Reproduced from Cooke, R., Stewart, B., Colour Atlas of Anatomical Pathology, 3rd edition. Copyright 2004, Elsevier Ltd.)

E-Fig. 22.9G Osteogenic sarcoma. (Reproduced from Cooke, R., Stewart, B., Colour Atlas of Anatomical Pathology, 3rd edition. Copyright 2004, Elsevier Ltd.)

E-Fig. 22.10H Hyaline cartilage. **(A)** H&E (MP); **(B)** thin epoxy resin section, toluidine blue (HP). (Reproduced from Young, B., O'Dowd, G., Woodford, P., Wheater's Functional Histology, 6th edition. Copyright 2014, Elsevier Ltd.)

E-Fig. 22.11G Benign chondroma. (Reproduced from Cooke, R., Stewart, B., Colour Atlas of Anatomical Pathology, 3rd edition. Copyright 2004, Elsevier Ltd.)

E-Fig. 22.12G Chondrosarcoma arising in the scapula. (Reproduced from Cooke, R., Stewart, B., Colour Atlas of Anatomical Pathology, 3rd edition. Copyright 2004, Elsevier Ltd.)

E-Fig. 22.13G Osteochondroma on a rib. (Reproduced from Cooke, R., Stewart, B., Colour Atlas of Anatomical Pathology, 3rd edition. Copyright 2004, Elsevier Ltd.)

E-Fig. 22.14G Synovial cyst or ganglion removed from near a joint. (Reproduced from Cooke, R., Stewart, B., Colour Atlas of Anatomical Pathology, 3rd edition. Copyright 2004, Elsevier Ltd.)

E-Fig. 22.15G Giant cell tumour of tendon sheath (nodular tenosynovitis). (Reproduced from Cooke, R., Stewart, B., Colour Atlas of Anatomical Pathology, 3rd edition. Copyright 2004, Elsevier Ltd.)

E-Fig. 22.16H White adipose tissue. **(A)** H&E (HP); **(B)** EM ×6000. (Reproduced from Young, B., O'Dowd, G., Woodford, P., Wheater's Functional Histology, 6th edition. Copyright 2014, Elsevier Ltd.)

E-Fig. 22.17G Benign subcutaneous lipoma. (Reproduced from Cooke, R., Stewart, B., Colour Atlas of Anatomical Pathology, 3rd edition. Copyright 2004, Elsevier Ltd.)

E-Fig. 23.1H Grey matter H&E (HP). (Reproduced from Young, B., O'Dowd, G., Woodford, P., Wheater's Functional Histology, 6th edition. Copyright 2014, Elsevier Ltd.)

E-Fig. 23.2H Astrocytes. (A) Diagram; (B) immunohistochemical method for glial fibrillary acidic protein (HP); (C) EM ×12 000; (D) EM ×57 500. (Reproduced from Young, B., O'Dowd, G., Woodford, P., Wheater's Functional Histology, 6th edition. Copyright 2014, Elsevier Ltd.)

E-Fig. 23.3H White matter CNS myelin and oligodendrocytes. (A) H&E (MP); (B) H&E (HP); (C) TS, solochrome cyanin (HP); (D) LS, solochrome cyanin (HP); (E) EM ×13 000; (F) schematic diagram. (Reproduced from Young, B., O'Dowd, G., Woodford, P., Wheater's Functional Histology, 6th edition. Copyright 2014, Elsevier Ltd.)

E-Fig. 23.4H (A) diagram; (B) ricinus communis agglutinin (HP); (C) immunohistochemical method for CD68 (MP). (Reproduced from Young, B., O'Dowd, G., Woodford, P., Wheater's Functional Histology, 6th edition. Copyright 2014, Elsevier Ltd.)

E-Fig. 23.5H Ependyma H&E (HP). (Reproduced from Young, B., O'Dowd, G., Woodford, P., Wheater's Functional Histology, 6th edition. Copyright 2014, Elsevier Ltd.)

E-Fig. 23.6H Meninges. (A) Diagram; (B) dura mater, H&E (MP); (C) H&E (LP). (Reproduced from Young, B., O'Dowd, G., Woodford, P., Wheater's Functional Histology, 6th edition. Copyright 2014, Elsevier Ltd.)

E-Fig. 23.7G Acute bacterial meningitis. (Reproduced from Cooke, R., Stewart, B., Colour Atlas of Anatomical Pathology, 3rd edition. Copyright 2004, Elsevier Ltd.)

E-Fig. 23.8G Massive intracerebral haemorrhage. (Reproduced from Cooke, R., Stewart, B., Colour Atlas of Anatomical Pathology, 3rd edition. Copyright 2004, Elsevier Ltd.)

E-Fig. 23.9G Extradural haemorrhage. (Reproduced from Cooke, R., Stewart, B., Colour Atlas of Anatomical Pathology, 3rd edition. Copyright 2004, Elsevier Ltd.)

E-Fig. 23.10G Middle cerebral artery territory infarct. (Reproduced from Cooke, R., Stewart, B., Colour Atlas of Anatomical Pathology, 3rd edition. Copyright 2004, Elsevier Ltd.)

E-Fig. 23.11G Meningioma. (Reproduced from Cooke, R., Stewart, B., Colour Atlas of Anatomical Pathology, 3rd edition. Copyright 2004, Elsevier Ltd.)

INDEX

Page numbers followed by "f" indicate figures, "t" indicate tables, and "b" indicate boxes